CLINICAL
PEDIATRIC
UROLOGY

SECOND EDITION

Edited by

PANAYOTIS P. KELALIS, M.D., M.S., F.A.A.P., F.A.C.S.

Professor of Urology and Chairman, Department of Urology
Head, Section of Pediatric Urology
Mayo Clinic and Mayo Foundation
Rochester, Minnesota

LOWELL R. KING, M.D., F.A.A.P., F.A.C.S.

Professor of Urology and Associate Professor of Pediatrics
Head, Section of Pediatric Urology
Division of Urology
Duke University Medical Center
Durham, North Carolina

and

A. BARRY BELMAN, M.D., M.S., F.A.A.P., F.A.C.S.

Professor of Urology and Child Health and Development
George Washington University
School for Health Sciences
Chairman, Department of Pediatric Urology
Children's Hospital National Medical Center
Washington, D.C.

1985
W. B. Saunders Company
PHILADELPHIA □ LONDON □ TORONTO □ MEXICO CITY □ RIO DE JANEIRO □ SYDNEY □ TOKYO

W. B. Saunders Company: West Washington Square
Philadelphia, PA 19105

1 St. Anne's Road
Eastbourne, East Sussex BN21 3UN, England

1 Goldthorne Avenue
Toronto, Ontario M8Z 5T9, Canada

Apartado 26370 — Cedro 512
Mexico 4, D.F., Mexico

Rua Coronel Cabrita, 8
Sao Cristovao Caixa Postal 21176
Rio de Janeiro, Brazil

9 Waltham Street
Artarmon, N.S.W. 2064, Australia

Ichibancho, Central Bldg., 22-1 Ichibancho
Chiyoda-Ku, Tokyo 102, Japan

Library of Congress Cataloging in Publication Data
Main entry under title:

Clinical pediatric urology.

Includes index.
1. Pediatric urology.   I. Kelalis, Panayotis P.,
1932–   . II. King, Lowell R. III. Belman, A. Barry,
1938–   . [DNLM: 1. Urologic diseases — In infancy and
childhood. WS 320 C643]
RJ466.C53 1985   618.92'6   83-20294
ISBN 0-7216-5349-9 (set)
ISBN 0-7216-5347-2 (v. 1)
ISBN 0-7216-5348-0 (v. 2)

Volume I ISBN   0–7216–5347–2
Volume II ISBN 0–7216–5348–0
SET ISBN   0–7216–5349–9

Clinical Pediatric Urology

Last digit is the print number: 9   8   7   6   5   4   3   2   1

Contributors

TERRY D. ALLEN, M.D.
Professor of Urology, University of Texas Health Science Center at Dallas, Southwestern Medical School; Attending Urologist, Children's Medical Center, Parkland Memorial Hospital, Dallas Veterans' Administration Medical Center, Baylor University Medical Center, and Presbyterian Hospital of Dallas, Dallas, Texas

DAVID M. BARRETT, M.D.
Associate Professor of Urology, Mayo Medical School; Consultant, Department of Urology and Section of Pediatric Urology, Mayo Clinic and Mayo Foundation, Rochester, Minnesota

STUART B. BAUER, M.D.
Assistant Professor of Urology (Surgery), Harvard Medical School; Director, Neurology Section, and Associate in Surgery (Urology), Children's Hospital Medical Center, Boston, Massachusetts

JEAN B. BELASCO, M.D.
Assistant Professor of Pediatrics, University of Pennsylvania School of Medicine; Assistant Physician, Division of Oncology, Children's Hospital of Philadelphia, Philadelphia, Pennsylvania

A. BARRY BELMAN, M.D., M.S., F.A.A.P., F.A.C.S.
Professor of Urology and Child Health and Development, George Washington University School for Health Sciences; Chairman, Department of Pediatric Urology, Children's Hospital National Medical Center, Washington, D.C.

RALPH C. BENSON, JR., M.D.
Associate Professor of Urology, Mayo Medical School; Consultant, Department of Urology, Mayo Clinic, Rochester, Minnesota

WILLIAM A. BROCK, M.D., F.A.C.S., F.A.A.P.
Associate Clinical Professor of Surgery/Urology, Associate Clinical Professor of Pediatrics, University of California, San Diego, School of Medicine; Chief of Urology, Children's Hospital and Health Center, San Diego; Attending Urologist, University of California, San Diego, Medical Center, San Diego, California

STANLEY A. BROSMAN, M.D.
Clinical Professor of Urology, University of California, Los Angeles, Medical School; Attending Urologist, UCLA Center for the Health Sciences; Clinical Attending Urologist, Harbor General-UCLA Medical Center; Consultant, Wadsworth Veterans' Administration Hospital, Los Angeles, California; Attending Urologist, St. John's Hospital, Oxnard, California, and Santa Monica Hospital, Santa Monica, California

JAY D. BURSTEIN, M.D.
Senior Resident, Mt. Sinai Hospital, Chicago, Illinois

ANTHONY A. CALDAMONE, M.D.
Assistant Professor of Urology, Case Western Reserve University School of Medicine; Head, Pediatric Urology, Rainbow Babies' and Children's Hospital, Cleveland, Ohio

ARNOLD H. COLODNY, M.D.
Associate Professor of Surgery, Harvard Medical School; Senior Surgeon and Associate Director, Division of Urology, Children's Hospital, Boston, Massachusetts

MATTHEW CRAWFORD, M.B., B.S., F.F.A.R.A.C.S.
Instructor, Mayo Medical School; Special Clinical Fellow in Anesthesia, St. Mary's Hospital, Rochester, Minnesota

GIULIO J. D'ANGIO, M.D.
Professor of Radiation Therapy, Professor of Pediatric Oncology, Professor of Radiology, University of Pennsylvania School of Medicine; Director, Children's Cancer Research Center, Children's Hospital of Philadelphia; Radiation Therapist, Hospital of the University of Pennsylvania, Philadelphia, Pennsylvania

BRIAN DAWSON, M.B., B.S., F.F.A.R.C.S.
Associate Professor, Mayo Medical School; Consultant Anesthesiologist, Mayo Clinic and St. Mary's Hospital, Rochester, Minnesota

JOHN W. DUCKETT, M.D.
Professor of Urology, University of Pennsylvania School of Medicine; Director, Division of Urology, Children's Hospital of Philadelphia, Philadelphia, Pennsylvania

RICHARD M. EHRLICH, M.D.
Professor of Surgery/Urology, University of California, Los Angeles, Medical Center, Los Angeles, California

R. BRUCE FILMER, M.B., B.S., F.R.C.S., F.R.A.C.S., F.A.C.S.
Clinical Lecturer in Paediatric Urology, University of Sydney, Sydney, New South Wales; Consulting Paediatric Urologist, Royal Alexandra Hospital for Children, Camper Down, New South Wales; Paediatric Urologist, Westmead Medical Centre, Westmead, New South Wales, Australia

RICHARD N. FINE, M.D.
Professor of Pediatrics, University of California, Los Angeles, Center for the Health Sciences; Head, Division of Pediatric Nephrology, UCLA Clinics and Hospital; Consultant, Cedars-Sinai Medical Center, Los Angeles, California; Consultant, Olive View Medical Center, Van Nuys, California; Consultant, Kern County Medical Center, Bakersfield, California

CASIMIR F. FIRLIT, M.D., Ph.D.
Professor of Urology, Northwestern University Medical School; Chairman, Division of Urology, and Head of Renal Transplantation, Children's Memorial Hospital, Chicago, Illinois

WILLIAM L. FURLOW, M.D.
Professor of Urology, Mayo Medical School; Consultant, Department of Urology, Mayo Clinic and Mayo Foundation, Rochester, Minnesota

GERALD S. GILCHRIST, M.D.
Professor and Vice-Chairman, Department of Pediatrics, Mayo Medical School; Consultant in Pediatric Hematology and Oncology, Mayo Clinic and Mayo Foundation, Rochester, Minnesota

KENNETH I. GLASSBERG, M.D.
Associate Professor of Urology, State University of New York, Downstate Medical Center, College of Medicine; Director, Division of Pediatric Urology, State University Hospital, Downstate Medical Center and Kings County Hospital Center; Director of Pediatric Urology, Long Island College Hospital, Brooklyn, New York

EDMOND T. GONZALES, JR., M.D.
Professor of Urology, Baylor College of Medicine; Director of Pediatric Urology, Texas Children's Hospital, Houston, Texas

W. GRAHAM GUERRIERO, M.D.
Associate Professor of Urology, Baylor College of Medicine; Deputy Chief of Urology, Ben Taub Hospital, Houston, Texas

W. HARDY HENDREN, M.D.
Professor of Surgery, Harvard Medical School; Chief of Surgery, Children's Hospital of Boston; Visiting Surgeon, Massachusetts General Hospital, Boston, Massachusetts

TERRY W. HENSLE, M.D.
Associate Professor of Urology, College of Physicians and Surgeons, Columbia University; Director of Pediatric Urology, Babies' Hospital, Columbia-Presbyterian Medical Center, New York, New York

ALAN D. HOFFMAN, M.D.
Assistant Professor of Diagnostic Radiology, Mayo Medical School; Consultant in Radiology, Mayo Clinic and Mayo Foundation, Rochester, Minnesota

GEORGE W. KAPLAN, M.D., M.S., F.A.A.P., F.A.C.S.
Clinical Professor of Surgery and Pediatrics and Chief of Pediatric Urology, University of California, San Diego, School of Medicine; Senior Staff, Children's Hospital of San Diego; Attending Staff, University Hospital, San Diego; Consultant, U.S. Naval Hospital and Kaiser Foundation Hospital, San Diego, California

EVAN J. KASS, M.D., F.A.A.P., F.A.C.S.
Associate Professor of Urology and Child Health and Development, George Washington University Medical Center; Vice Chairman, Department of Urology, Children's Hospital National Medical Center, Washington, D.C.

PANAYOTIS P. KELALIS, M.D., M.S., F.A.A.P., F.A.C.S.
Professor of Urology and Chairman, Department of Urology; Head, Section of Pediatric Urology, Mayo Clinic and Mayo Foundation, Rochester, Minnesota

LOWELL R. KING, M.D., F.A.A.P., F.A.C.S.
Professor of Urology and Associate Professor of Pediatrics; Head, Section of Pediatric Urology, Division of Urology, Duke University Medical Center, Durham, North Carolina

GEORGE T. KLAUBER, M.D.
Professor of Urology and Pediatrics, Tufts University School of Medicine; Attending Urologist and Chief of Pediatric Urology, Boston Floating Hospital for Infants and Children and New England Medical Center, Boston, Massachusetts

STANLEY J. KOGAN, M.D.
Adjunct Professor of Urology, New York Medical College; Co-Director, Section of Pediatric Urology, Westchester County Medical Center, Valhalla, New York; Attending Pediatric Urologist, Albert Einstein College Hospital, Montefiore Medical Center, Jacobi City Hospital, and North Central Bronx City Hospital; Co-Director of Pediatric Urology, Misericordia Hospital, New York, New York

STEPHEN A. KRAMER, M.D.
Assistant Professor of Urology, Mayo Medical School; Consultant, Department of Urology, Section of Pediatric Urology, Mayo Clinic and Mayo Foundation; Consultant, St. Mary's Hospital, Rochester, Minnesota

R. LAWRENCE KROOVAND, M.D., F.A.A.P., F.A.C.S.
Associate Professor of Urology, Wayne State University School of Medicine; Associate Chief, Pediatric Urology, Children's Hospital of Michigan, Detroit, Michigan

JACQUES M. LEMIRE, M.D., F.R.C.P.(C)
Research Fellow, Division of Pediatric Nephrology, University of California, Los Angeles, Medical Center, Los Angeles, California

SELWYN B. LEVITT, M.D.
Adjunct Clinical Professor of Urology, New York Medical College; Co-Director, Section of Pediatric Urology, Westchester County Medical Center, Valhalla, New York; Attending Pediatric Urologist, Albert Einstein College Hospital, Montefiore Hospital and Medical Center, and Bronx Municipal Hospital Center, New York, New York

MASSOUD MAJD, M.D.
Professor of Radiology and Child Health and Development, George Washington University School of Medicine; Director, Section of Nuclear Medicine, Department of Radiology, Children's Hospital National Medical Center, Washington, D.C.

REZA S. MALEK, M.D., M.S., F.R.C.S.(C), F.A.C.S., F.A.A.P.
Associate Professor of Urology, Mayo Medical School; Consultant, Section of Pediatric Urology, Department of Urology, Mayo Clinic; Consultant in Urology and Pediatric Urology, Rochester Methodist Hospital and St. Mary's Hospital, Rochester, Minnesota

DAWN S. MILLINER, M.D.
Assistant Professor of Medicine, Mayo Medical School; Consultant in Pediatric Nephrology and in Nephrology and Internal Medicine, Mayo Clinic and Mayo Foundation, Rochester, Minnesota

DONALD I. MOEL, M.D.
Assistant Professor of Pediatrics, Northwestern University Medical School; Division Head, Pediatric Nephrology, Children's Memorial Hospital, Chicago, Illinois

ANDREW C. NOVICK, M.D.
Head, Section of Renal Transplantation, Department of Urology, Cleveland Clinic, Cleveland, Ohio

ALAN D. PERLMUTTER, M.D.
Professor of Urology, Wayne State University School of Medicine; Chief, Department of Pediatric Urology, Children's Hospital of Michigan, Detroit, Michigan

RONALD RABINOWITZ, M.D., F.A.A.P., F.A.C.S.
Associate Professor of Urology, Associate Professor of Pediatrics, University of Rochester School of Medicine and Dentistry; Attending Pediatric Urologist, Strong Memorial Hospital; Chief of Urology, Rochester General Hospital; Pediatric Urologist, University of Rochester Birth Defects Center, Rochester, New York

ALAN B. RETIK, M.D.
Professor of Surgery (Urology), Harvard Medical School; Chief, Division of Urology, Children's Hospital Medical Center, Boston, Massachusetts

KENNETH N. ROSENBAUM, M.D.
Associate Professor of Child Health and Development, George Washington University School for

Health Sciences; Director, Clinical Genetics and Genetics Laboratory, Children's Hospital National Medical Center, Washington, D.C.

GRANNUM R. SANT, M.D.

Assistant Professor of Urology, Tufts University School of Medicine; Assistant Surgeon, Department of Urology, Tufts–New England Medical Center Hospital, Boston, Massachusetts

ARNOLD SHKOLNIK, M.D.

Associate Professor of Clinical Radiology, Northwestern University Medical School; Attending Radiologist and Chief, Section of Ultrasound, Children's Memorial Hospital, Chicago, Illinois

WILLIAM A. SMITHSON, M.D.

Assistant Professor of Pediatrics, Mayo Medical School; Consultant in Pediatrics and Pediatric Hematology-Oncology, Mayo Clinic, Rochester, Minnesota

GUNNAR B. STICKLER, M.D., Ph.D.

Professor of Pediatrics, Mayo Medical School and Mayo Clinic, Rochester, Minnesota

ROBERT L. TELANDER, M.D.

Associate Professor and Head, Section of Pediatric Surgery, Mayo Medical School; Consultant in Pediatric Surgery, Mayo Clinic and Mayo Foundation and St. Mary's Hospital, Rochester, Minnesota

R. DIXON WALKER, III, M.D.

Director, Pediatric Urology, and Professor of Surgery and Pediatrics, University of Florida College of Medicine; Pediatric Urologist, Shands Teaching Hospital, Gainesville, Florida

ROBERT A. WEISS, M.D.

Assistant Professor of Pediatrics, Albert Einstein College of Medicine; Attending Pediatrician and Co-Director, Children's Kidney Center at Hospital of the Albert Einstein College of Medicine; Attending Pediatrician, Bronx Municipal Hospital Center and Montefiore Hospital and Medical Center, New York, New York

ROBERT M. WEISS, M.D.

Professor of Surgery/Urology, Yale University School of Medicine; Attending Physician, Yale–New Haven Hospital, New Haven, Connecticut

JOHN R. WOODARD, M.D.

Professor of Surgery (Urology) and Director of Pediatric Urology, Emory University School of Medicine; Chief of Urology, Henrietta Egleston Hospital for Children; Active Staff, Emory University Hospital and Grady Memorial Hospital; Courtesy Staff, Scottish Rite Children's Hospital, Atlanta, Georgia

DONALD ZIMMERMAN, M.D.

Assistant Professor of Pediatrics, Mayo Medical School; Consultant in Pediatric Endocrinology and Metabolism, Mayo Clinic; Attending Pediatrician, St. Mary's Hospital, Rochester, Minnesota

Preface to The Second Edition

In the eight years since the publication of the First Edition of Clinical Pediatric Urology, a number of significant changes have occurred. Although not duly recognized by certification, pediatric urology has become accepted as a bona fide subspecialty of urology by most of our peers. At this time, pediatric urologists can be found at almost all major medical centers, most of whom devote virtually all their time to the urologic problems of infants and children. The contributors to this Second Edition reflect this change.

The professional organizations related to the pediatric concept of the specialty also have demonstrated significant growth. The Section on Urology of the American Academy of Pediatrics has blossomed into a dynamic organization with thought-provoking scientific meetings attended faithfully by those who devote all or most of their time to pediatric urology. Meanwhile, the Society for Pediatric Urology has matured and plays a respected and influential role at the annual meeting of the American Urological Association. These two societies have done much both to foster and to further the information contained in these volumes.

Almost all chapters in this Second Edition have been completely rewritten and many new chapters have been added, reflecting changes in the field. Although it is difficult to have a work of this magnitude entirely up-to-date at the time of publication, every effort has been made to include the state-of-the-art practice without including areas that we considered to be "fads."

This edition, like the first, is meant to be a complete work covering all aspects of pediatric urology. Unfortunately, omissions must certainly exist, and the editors would be grateful if these could be called to their attention so that they can be rectified in future editions. As in the First Edition, editing was kept to a minimum to reflect both the style and the philosophy of the individual authors.

We are deeply indebted to the contributors, both present and past, for their efforts and cooperation despite heavy commitments and other responsibilities. Those authors who have written chapters in this edition for the first time relied heavily on the efforts of previous authors for ideas, information, and illustrations. We are all grateful.

It is again with gratitude that we mention the help of our secretaries, Ms. Dixie Schmidt, Janet Abernathy, Karla Chaucer, Hilary Kavanagh, Debra Souders, Catherine Evans, and especially Mrs. Betty Calkins of the Section of Publications at the Mayo Clinic. Their efficiency and hard work are greatly appreciated.

PANAYOTIS P. KELALIS
LOWELL R. KING
A. BARRY BELMAN

Contents

PRESENTATION OF UROGENITAL DISORDERS IN CHILDREN

R. DIXON WALKER, III

The child with urologic disease presents with special problems quite different from those of the adult. In some instances, the urologist will need his sharpest diagnostic acumen to establish a diagnosis. The child is often unable to convey his symptoms in any meaningful way, and is incapable of comprehending the seriousness of his disease. Symptomatology is frequently vague, and the inadequate vocabulary of the child may impede its meaningful expression. Indeed, the description of symptoms may have to be secured at second hand from the parents, whose impressions may be distorted by their own intellectual capacity and emotional responses. The urologist must be aware of congenital and acquired diseases in other organ systems, because they can seriously affect genitourinary pathology. Examination of the pediatric patient must be especially meticulous and thorough so that all pathologic conditions can be discovered. Moreover, in managing genitourinary problems, one must deal with the anxiety of the child and of the family as well as the disease itself.

SYMPTOMS OF GENITOURINARY DISORDER

Generalized Symptoms

Symptoms elicited from the child or the parent may be systemic, or they may be confined to a specific anatomic area of the urinary tract. Many urologic diseases are first seen with symptomatology that one usually associates with other organ systems. Nausea and vomiting occur with uremia, acidosis, and acute pyelonephritis, or in association with ureteropelvic or ureteral obstruction. Metabolic acidosis is associated with weakness, and bone pain may be secondary to disturbances of calcium and potassium metabolism.

Uremia results in multisystemic symptoms. In addition to nausea and vomiting, these include apathy, lethargy, coma, muscle twitching, headache, vertigo, anorexia, poor growth, melena, dyspnea, or other signs of congestive heart failure. Headache is a frequent accompaniment of hypertension, and if hypertensive encephalopathy occurs, many of the neurologic findings can mimic those seen in uremia.

Abdominal Pain

Abdominal pain can be related to acute infection or to distention of a hollow viscus. Patients with acute pyelonephritis may present either with vague abdominal symptoms or with acute flank pain. Nausea and vomiting frequently precede the pain and sometimes are the only symptoms immediately apparent. Pain caused by distention of the renal pelvis or ureter can usually be distinguished by studying the history. Renal pelvic pain is most often localized in the flank, with little radiation. Acute ureteral distention is characterized by sharp pain which may radiate into the groin. Flank pain that is brought on by overhydration should always alert one to the possibility of an underlying obstruction of the ureteropelvic junction. It is surprising that patients suffering from severe hydronephrosis may report no pain associated with it or may report only vague, non-specific pain, not infrequently accompanied by nausea and vomiting.

Abdominal Mass

It is not unusual for a child to present with an abdominal mass, usually discovered accidentally by the parents or the physician. The first manifestation of a wide variety of pathologic and nonpathologic conditions, including distended bladder, polycystic kidneys, multi-cystic kidney, Wilms' tumor, neuroblastoma, hydronephrosis, and renal vein thrombosis, may be an abdominal mass. The differential diagnosis of abdominal masses is discussed more extensively in Chapter 5.

Abnormal Voiding

The infant or child who exhibits symptoms of urinary retention or who has difficulty in initiating voiding may be suffering from serious underlying disease. Urologic evaluation is always indicated in such children. Although urine output is normally low in the first two days of life, about 90 per cent of all newborn infants void at least once during their first 24 hours of life, and virtually all have voided by the time they are 48 hours old. Table 1–1 shows normal 24-hour urine output in infants and children.

In the male neonate, anuria or urinary retention should alert one to the possibility of posterior urethral valves. Retention in the older child is likewise usually associated with urethral obstruction, but it can also occur with neurogenic bladder. Urethral obstruction may also be due to extreme meatal stenosis or

Table 1–1. Average 24-Hour Urine Output in Infants and Children

Age	Output in ml
Birth to 48 hours	15 to 60
3 to 10 days	100 to 300
10 days to 2 months	250 to 450
2 months to 1 year	400 to 500
1 to 3 years	500 to 600
3 to 5 years	600 to 700
5 to 8 years	650 to 1000
8 to 14 years	800 to 1400

From Campbell MF, Harrison JH: Urology. Vol 2. Third ed. Philadelphia, WB Saunders Co., 1970.

urethral stricture. Difficulty with voiding can also occur with acute urethritis or cystitis, although the presence of frequency, urgency, or dysuria more commonly suggests these diagnoses. Retention may also rarely be a manifestation of a severe psychiatric disorder.

Hematuria, be it microscopic, gross, total, initial, or terminal, may be secondary to pathologic conditions at any anatomic level. This is discussed in detail in Chapter 6.

Polyuria is not a common presenting symptom; however, it does occur more often than has been appreciated. Parents usually relate a history of frequent voiding, and it is important to ascertain whether this is of small or of large amount. If the amount voided cannot be definitely established, it is worthwhile to measure a total 24-hour urine volume. Polyuria is frequently associated with polydipsia, and can be seen in a variety of pathologic conditions. Diabetes mellitus and diabetes insipidus are the conditions most commonly associated with polyuria. However, any disorder that results in a severe concentration defect can be responsible for polyuria. Such disorders include chronic pyelonephritis, hydronephrosis, renal cystic disease, and severe renal dysplasia.

Incontinence and Enuresis

Incontinence and enuresis, which are common problems in children, can be frustrating to both parents and physician. One must remember that both these problems are symptoms, not diagnoses, and that a cause should be sought. In many instances, no etiologic factor can be isolated. Enuresis rarely is secondary to urinary tract disease and is usually self-limiting. The presence of daytime urinary incontinence in an otherwise normal child more than 3½ years of age indicates the need for a thorough, unbiased workup, often including complete neurologic and physical examinations, intravenous pyelogram, cystourethrogram, and possibly urodynamic evaluation.

Continual dampness associated with normal voiding strongly suggests ureteral ectopia. Urge incontinence may be secondary to acute or chronic cystitis, occult neuropathic bladder, or uninhibited bladder contractions. Overflow incontinence is most often seen in the patient with myelodysplasia. Incontinence can be anticipated when there is dysfunction of the sphincters. This may be functional (dyssynergia), iatrogenic, or secondary to abnormalities such as exstrophy of the bladder after closure, urogenital sinus, or absence of the urethra in females. Continued leakage after voiding can be seen in the patient with a patulous urethra or a urethral diverticulum. A very patulous urethra can be related to congenital absence of the corpus spongiosum; it can also occur after hypospadias or epispadias repair. Urethral diverticula in the male may be associated with anterior urethral values and distal obstruction.

ASSOCIATION OF GENITOURINARY WITH OTHER ORGANIC ANOMALIES

The association of genitourinary anomalies with anomalies in other organ systems has been well established. Within the urinary tract, two or more anomalies are frequently combined. Multiple defects may be coincidental or related. Genetic mutations, as well as abnormal genetic patterns, at times manifest themselves in more than one organ system. Teratogenic agents may affect two different organ systems during development. Lastly, the maldevelopment of one organ system may so affect the fetal environment that abnormalities of other organ systems appear. An understanding of these relationships is important in planning reparative procedures in children and in giving genetic counseling to parents.

Syndromes involving the genitourinary tract to a major or minor extent are legion, and no attempt is made to include them all here. Rather, selected syndromes will be employed as examples of problems involving an interrelationship between two organ systems. Cryptorchidism, hypospadias, and Wilms' tumor are discussed in other chapters and will only briefly be discussed here.

Upper Urinary Tract Anomalies

ASSOCIATION WITH CRYPTORCHIDISM AND HYPOSPADIAS. Cryptorchidism is one of the more common abnormalities of the genitourinary tract. A frequently encountered question regarding management concerns the need for excretory urography. Campbell and Harrison found at autopsy that 33 per cent of patients with undescended testes had associated genitourinary abnormalities. Felton, as well as Farrington and Kerr, demonstrated that cryptorchidism is associated with significant pathologic lesions of the urinary tract. However, Watson et al found only 3 per cent displaying significant abnormalities on the excretory urogram; although they agreed with previous investigators that excretory urography should probably be done, they suggested cautioning parents that the chance of finding a significant lesion is small. Donohue et al found only 2 major radiologic abnormalities in 100 cryptorchid patients.

The problem has been with the interpretation of the aforementioned data. For those who see large numbers of cryptorchid patients, these data indicate a low yield and, in Noble and Wacksman's study, 70 per cent of pediatric urologists did not routinely obtain an excretory urogram in patients with undescended testicle. One can conclude that the yield is quite low, probably not significantly different from what would be found in the normal population, and that excretory urography therefore is not routinely indicated. An exception to this is that an excretory urogram or sonogram is desirable if, on exploration, no vas deferens or epididymis is identified.

In children with hypospadias, a higher number of significant lesions is found. Bauer et al investigated only those boys who had associated urinary tract infection and found that 10 of 39 had abnormalities, 2 of which required surgery. Shima et al found 6 cases of ureteropelvic junction obstruction in 272 patients. All of the patients had proximal hypospadias and none of 29 patients with glandular hypospadias had an upper tract anomaly. Vesicoureteral reflux was found in 4 of 272 patients, an incidence probably similar to that in the normal population. Noble and Wacksman's survey indicated that about 50 per cent of pediatric urologists currently obtain an excretory urogram on boys with hypospadias. A reasonable compromise might be to do abdominal ultrasound rather than a urogram as a screening study, since this is less invasive and expensive and will probably screen adequately for significant anomalies. Urography can then be performed in patients with positive or equivocal findings on abdominal ultrasound.

Wilms' Tumor

ASSOCIATION WITH HEMIHYPERTROPHY AND ANIRIDIA. The incidence of hemihypertrophy is not known but is thought to be very low. It appears to be less common than aniridia, which has an incidence of 1 in 50,000 (Fontana et al). In patients with hemihypertrophy, there is an increased incidence of Wilms' tumor, adrenocortical tumors, hepatoblastoma, mental deficiency, clubbed feet, syndactyly, congenital heart disease, cryptorchidism, and hypospadias (Bjorklund). Wilms' tumor and hemihypertrophy may occur on opposite sides. Newer knowledge suggests that the anomalies associated with Wilms' tumor may be divided into four types: hemihypertrophy, hamartoma, visceral cytomegaly (Beckwith-Wiedemann syndrome), and malignant tumors of the adrenal and liver (Miller, 1981).

The incidence of congenital aniridia (1 in 50,000) is almost the same as that of exstrophy of the bladder. Aniridia is associated with congenital glaucoma and cataracts (Miller et al); there is usually a strong family history, with 65 per cent of affected children having an affected parent. In children with both aniridia and Wilms' tumor, however, there is usually no family history of aniridia (Mackintosh et al). It has been suggested that aniridia in these instances is due to a genetic mutation, and the absence of family history has led to the use of the term "congenital sporadic aniridia."

Genitourinary Tract Anomalies

ASSOCIATION WITH CARDIOVASCULAR AND PULMONARY ANOMALIES. The incidence of anomalies of the urinary tract is sufficiently high in patients with congenital cardiac defects to warrant evaluation (Table 1–2). This is usually done as part of cardiac angiography. Fluoroscopy and excretory urography are easily performed while the contrast medium is being concentrated and excreted from the kidneys. Humphry and Munn were usually able to visualize the urinary tract after cardiac catheterization. Newman and associates found that 3.9 per cent of patients undergoing cardiac catheterization had abnormal urograms. This figure may be erroneously low. An incidence of 12 per cent was found in the joint Canadian study and by King. Five per cent of these patients required urologic surgery. Carlton and Scott found that 35 per cent of patients with anomalies of two organ systems had involvement of the cardiovascular system and the genitourinary tract. The incidence of cardiovascular anomalies in association with horseshoe kidney is 11 per cent (Boatman et al). Thirty per cent of children with crossed or pelvic renal ectopia have been found to have cardiovascular anomalies

Table 1–2. Renal Anomalies Found on Intravenous Pyelogram after Cardiac Catheterization*

Type of Urinary Tract Abnormality	Number Found	Cardiac Patients Exhibiting Lesion (Per Cent)
Hydroureteronephrosis	18	4.06
Unilateral renal agenesis	4	0.90
Significant renal dysplasia	3	0.68
Fused kidney	2	0.45
Accessory renal mass	2	0.45
Ectopic kidney (in pelvis)	1	0.22
Large extrarenal pelvis without caliectasis	1	0.22
Duplication of collecting system	17	3.80
TOTAL	48	10.78

From King LR: Other congenital abnormalities. *In* Pediatric Surgery. Vol 2. Third ed. Edited by O Swenson. New York, Appleton-Century-Crofts, Inc., 1969.

* One film exposed after cardiac catheterization study performed because of congenital heart disease, 443 consecutive patients.

(Kelalis et al, 1973b). In a recent study by Engle, anomalies of the urinary tract were found in 7.7 per cent of children who had post-angiocardiographic screening. In children with severe cardiac anomalies, the incidence is 28.5 per cent urologic abnormalities. On review of the 26 urologic abnormalities discussed by Engle, only 5 obstructed kidneys would have required surgical intervention, so that the incidence of "surgically significant abnormalities" may be as low as 1.8 per cent.

Urinary tract anomalies also occur associated with pneumothorax and pneumomediastinum in the newborn. Bashour and Balfe found that 19 per cent of neonates with spontaneous pneumothorax or mediastinum had renal anomalies. All of the renal anomalies were significant and included posterior urethral valves, infantile polycystic kidneys, renal agenesis, and multicystic renal dysplasia.

ASSOCIATION WITH NEUROLOGIC AND MUSCULOSKELETAL ANOMALIES. The obvious association of myelomeningocele with abnormalities of the genitourinary tract manifests itself principally in the form of the accompanying neurogenic bladder, with all its sequelae. This relationship is based upon cause and effect and not upon a common genetic or teratogenic source. Absence of the sacral segments predisposes the child to a neurogenic bladder. If as many as three sacral segments are absent, the possibility of neurogenic bladder is greatly enhanced (Williams and Nixon).

Vitko et al found that approximately one third of children with kyphosis or scoliosis also had some type of genitourinary anomaly. Avascular necrosis of the head of the femur has been found associated with genitourinary abnormalities in 4.3 per cent of patients (Catterall et al). It has also been reported that children with oligodactyly, ectrodactyly, brachydactyly, and polydactyly have an increased incidence of renal agenesis and ureteral duplication (Curran and Curran).

ASSOCIATION WITH GASTROINTESTINAL ANOMALIES. Williams and Grant have stated that urologic problems seen with imperforate anus either are coexistent congenital disorders of the genitourinary tract or are the result of associated anomalies of the spinal cord; other problems include complications of the accompanying fistula, or they arise as complications from the definitive surgery. Seventeen to 38 per cent of patients with imperforate anus have associated genitourinary anomalies. The level of rectal atresia correlates with the number of anomalies seen, with a greater number of anomalies existing in patients with high rectal atresia (see Chapter 19).

The incidence of renal anomalies is increased in infants with tracheoesophageal fistula. Both these disorders are associated with anomalies in other organ systems (Temtamy and Miller).

ASSOCIATION WITH ANOMALIES OF FACIAL DEVELOPMENT. In the mid-1940's, Potter described a case of abnormal facial development combined with renal agenesis and oligohydramnios. Numerous similar cases have since been added to the literature, and the abnormality has come to be known as Potter's syndrome. Potter has suggested that the term "renal nonfunction syndrome" be substituted. Controversy still exists about the reason for the apparent association of abnormalities Potter described. Thomas and Smith felt that all the nonrenal features of the syndrome could be caused by prolonged fetal compression secondary to oligohydramnios. Potter has disagreed, however, and states that the prominent facial semicircular folds and the malposition of the ears cannot be explained on the basis of fetal compression.

Many patients have malformed ears but no other facial abnormalities. Hilson reviewed a series of patients with malformed ears and found a wide range of genitourinary disorders besides renal agenesis, including duplication, cystic disease, hydronephrosis, and hypospadias. Taylor thought that renal abnormalities were much more likely to be found in children with underdeveloped facial bones and abnormal ears.

ASSOCIATION OF RENAL-GENITAL WITH MULTISYSTEMIC ANOMALIES. Because of the large number of renal-genital anomalies found to be associated with multisystemic defects, and because of the lack of continuity between them, these entities are not discussed in detail here. Table 1–3 contains a list of some of the more common syndromes and their relationships.

EXAMINATION

Examination of the pediatric patient with suspected genitourinary disease will yield a quantity of useful data directly proportional to the diligence of the examiner and the thoroughness of the examination. In pediatric urology, perhaps even more than in adult urology, it is imperative that the scope of the examination encompass more than the abdomen and genitalia.

Neonatal Examination

Approximately 27 per cent of infants with a single umbilical artery have been found to have associated urogenital defects (Bourne and Bernirschke). This figure has been challenged, however. It has been stated that the incidence of genitourinary abnormalities is not increased in infants with a single umbilical artery (Froehlich and Fujikura). Nevertheless, initial examination of the neonate should include examination of the placenta. The urologist is not part of the delivery team and, therefore, will have to rely on examination of the placenta by the obstetrician or the pediatrician.

Impaired respiration may signify that a large intra-abdominal mass is compromising the pulmonary tree. The general physical examination may reveal abnormalities that have a high rate of association with genitourinary disease. Abnormalities of the ears, particularly in association with abnormal facial bones, should alert the physician to the possibility of associated renal abnormalities (Taylor). Imperforate anus is closely associated with abnormalities of the kidney and the

Table 1–3. Multisystemic Anomalies with Genitourinary Pathology

Syndrome	Cardiovascular	Gastrointestinal	Neurologic	Integument	Musculoskeletal	Facial	Genital	Urinary
Prune Belly (Waldbaum and Marshall)		Occasional			Abdominal muscles absent		Undescended testicles	Hydronephrosis
Russell-Silver (Haslam et al)					Short stature Hemihypertrophy Short arms	Craniofacial dysostosis		Nonspecific renal anomalies
Curran					Acral anomalies			Renal agenesis Duplication
Turner Winter			Middle ear abnormalities				Vaginal atresia	Renal anomalies
Rüdiger			Motor instability		Short extremities Thick palms	Coarse facial features		Hydronephrosis
Goyer			Hearing loss	Ichthyosis				Renal disease
Von Hippel-Lindau (Malek and Green; Richards et al)		Pancreatic cysts	Cerebral medullary angioblastic tumor					Hypernephroid benign tumor
Holt-Oram (Silver et al)	Atrial septal defect				Defects of upper limb			Renal anomalies
Neonatal Ascites (Garrett et al; Lord)		Portohepatic obstruction Bowel perforation						Hydronephrosis
Turner's Female (XO) (Persky and Owens)					Wide chest Cubitus valgus	Webbed neck		Renal anomalies (70%)
Turner's Male (Noonan's) (Redman)					Wide chest Cubitus valgus	Webbed neck	Small testicles	Renal anomalies (50%)

Caudal Regression (Miller)		Imperforate anus		Inversion feet LS spine anomalies			Uterine and vaginal agenesis	Renal agenesis
Vater (Temtamy and Miller)	Ventricular septal defect	Imperforate anus Tracheo-esophageal fistula		Vertebral defects Radial dysplasia Polydactyly Syndactyly				Renal dysplasia
Robinow's (Wadlington et al)				Hemihypertrophy			Small genitalia	
"G" (Opitz et al)		Neuromuscular defect of esophagus				Abnormal fascies Low-set ears	Hypospadias	
Smith-Lemli-Opitz (Ferrier)			Retardation	Syndactyly		Short upturned nose Microcephaly Epicanthal folds	Hypospadias Cryptorchidism	
Donohue's "Leprechaunism" (Gorlin and Sedano)					Hirsutism	Elfin face Prominent eyes Thick lips Low-set ears	Enlarged penis or clitoris	
Trisomy 13 (Hecht)	Ventricular and atrial septal defects	Omphalocele	Deafness Retardation	Polydactyly		Low-set ears	Cryptorchidism	Duplication Hydronephrosis
Trisomy 18 (Hecht)	Ventricular septal defect Patent ductus	Neonatal hepatitis TE fistula Malrotation	Retardation Hydrocephalus			Low-set ears Choanal atresia Cleft palate	Prominent clitoris Cryptorchidism	Horseshoe kidney Duplication Hydronephrosis
Trisomy 21 (Hecht)	Increased cardiac anomalies	Duodenal obstruction	Retardation	Muscle hypotonia		High arched palate	Small penis Cryptorchidism	Renal dysplasia

lower urinary tract. The presence of a meningomyelocele is usually predictive of future urologic problems. The abdomen should be examined thoroughly. Not infrequently, multicystic kidney and hydronephrosis secondary to ureteropelvic junction obstruction have an abdominal mass as their only presenting finding.

Indeed, the correlation between congenital anomalies is sufficient that the finding of any defect on physical examination should alert one to the possibility of accompanying genitourinary disease, and appropriate screening tests should be considered to ascertain whether it is present.

General Evaluation

Examination of an infant or child should include both a general physical examination and a more extensive and sophisticated examination of the genitourinary tract.

Increased blood pressure is frequently associated with genitourinary pathology, and techniques of obtaining correct readings in the child are different from those used in the adult. Blood pressure cuffs should be of such size as to cover two thirds of the arm. If the blood pressure is difficult to auscultate, the Doppler ultrasound instrument may be used to considerable advantage (Dweck et al).

Assessment of growth is very important in children with renal disease. Growth may be severely retarded in children with renal failure, and a pattern of retarded growth may be the only clinical manifestation of renal tubular acidosis (RTA). Abnormalities of bone development may also be due to secondary hyperparathyroidism, a complication of renal failure.

A number of congenital and acquired conditions that are often seen on physical examination may be related to genitourinary disease. These abnormalities are described in the preceding section discussing the relationships of urinary disorders to genitourinary and other anomalies.

Abdomen

Examination of a structure has traditionally included inspection, palpation, percussion, and auscultation.

Inspection of the abdomen should include not only an evaluation of abdominal size, but also inspection for abdominal masses. The presence of umbilical drainage should be noted, as should the condition of the skin.

Anomalies such as gastroschisis, omphalocele, exstrophy of the bladder or cloaca, and prune-belly syndrome will be readily apparent if present.

Palpation should be directed to the deep abdominal structures, as well as to the superficial musculature and flank. If present, superficial urachal cysts are situated in the midline. One should try to distinguish between ascitic fluid, bladder distention, the presence of intra-abdominal or retroperitoneal masses, and hepatic or splenic enlargement. Ascites can be distinguished by its fluid wave. The presence of an abdominal mass should strongly alert one to the possibility of genitourinary disease, because approximately 50 per cent of these masses will be related to the urinary tract (Melicow and Uson). The differential diagnosis of abdominal masses is discussed more fully in Chapter 5.

Percussion and auscultation are perhaps of less importance in diagnosing genitourinary disease than are palpation and inspection, although percussion can give evidence of ascitic fluid or even of hydronephrotic fluid if the kidney is large.

Female Genitalia

Abnormalities related to the clitoris include complete absence, as well as hypertrophy. Clitoral hypertrophy may be a manifestation—and perhaps the only physical sign—of adrenogenital syndrome, and should be evaluated with appropriate hormonal and genetic studies (see Chapters 18, 25, and 26).

The labia in the female child should be well developed, with an adequate introitus. Imperforate hymen may be associated with hydrocolpos or hematocolpos. The vagina should be inspected for the presence of foreign bodies. The urethral meatus should be just ventral to the vaginal introitus. Its absence from this location may signify that the patient has hypospadias or a urogenital sinus. In black pubescent or prepubescent girls, a circumferential prolapse of urethral mucosa may present as a bleeding necrotic urethral mass. A prolapsed ureterocele will also appear as a perineal mass and may be difficult to distinguish from hydrocolpos.

Male Genitalia

Examination of the male genitalia should include the urethral meatus, the penis, and the scrotal contents.

The male urethral meatus should be a cleft

Table 1–4. Meatal Calibration of Male Neonates

Calibration in French Units	Number of Cases
4	9
5	0
6	10
7	32
8	40
9	3
10	5
11	0
12	1

From Allen JS, Summers JL, Wilkerson JE: Meatal calibration of newborn boys. J Urol 107:498, 1972.

or slit at the tip or on the ventral surface of the glans penis. Meatal stenosis is characterized by a rounded, nonelastic meatus; it may be associated with minimal urethral obstruction. The diagnosis should be confirmed with calibration of the meatus by bougie or, preferably, by observation of the urinary stream or a urine flow rate.

Table 1–4 indicates average meatal size in the newborn. By 18 months of age, 90 per cent of boys will have a urethral meatus larger than 12 French units in size (Berry and Cross). The significance of the rounded, small meatus has not been definitely established, and its relationship to renal disease, urinary tract infection, and enuresis is incompletely understood. In asymptomatic patients, meatotomy should be reserved for those with objective evidence of a voiding disturbance. Hypospadias is easily recognized by the triad of ventral urethral meatus, ventral chordee, and incomplete formation of the foreskin. The meatus is usually small.

Other abnormalities of the penis include chordee without hypospadias, penile torsion, webbed penis, and translocation of the penis into the scrotum or the perineum. Microphallus, as a category of abnormality, should be restricted to boys who truly have very small penises. Hinman's data indicate that the median length of the penis, stretched, or on erection, at birth is 3.75 cm. At age 1, it is 4.59 cm. In most cases of microphallus, the length at birth is less than 1 cm. In an obese youngster, a large mound of superficial fat may partially conceal the penis. This mound should be retracted and the penile length and

circumference measured. In most instances, an obese boy will be found to have a penis of normal size. A prepubertal boy with a large phallus should be suspected of having male adrenogenital syndrome or congenital absence of erectile tissue. A large flaccid penis is characteristic of congenital absence of the corpora cavernosa. There appears to be a spectrum of severity: In some boys, erectile tissue is totally absent, whereas in others, only the corpus spongiosum is missing. Absence of the corpus spongiosum is often associated with megalourethra, some types of which are correctable and ultimately compatible with normal male function.

The scrotum and its contents should be evaluated thoroughly. It must be established not only that testes are present bilaterally, but also that the vas deferens and epididymis are present. These structures may be difficult to palpate in children, but their absence may signal failure of the metanephric kidney to develop on the ipsilateral side.

Testes retract easily because of the activity of the cremasteric muscle. An overactive cremasteric muscle can be circumvented by trapping the testicle at the external ring or by examining the patient while he is in a squatting position. Acute scrotal swelling may be related to hydrocele, or to torsion of the testicle or its appendages. Transillumination and herniography are helpful in differentiating these abnormalities. The thickened spermatic cord can often be palpated in torsion. If there is associated pain, it may be an indication of torsion of the testicle; however, torsion in children is not infrequently free of pain. The "blue dot sign" may indicate torsion of the appendix testis or appendix epididymis (Dresner). The Doppler ultrasound instrument with pencil attachment should be used in evaluating blood flow in the acute scrotum. Epididymitis is almost unknown in boys and should be diagnosed only when there is associated pyuria and fever and good blood flow in Doppler examination. Acute solid scrotal swelling should usually be assumed to be caused by torsion unless proved otherwise by surgery.

Voiding

Observations of voiding are of particular value in boys, because most obstructive lesions of the urethra lead to abnormal voiding patterns. These deviations from the normal voiding pattern are subject to varying interpretations, but if they are correlated with positive anatomic findings, a pathologic condition is indicated. Children with posterior urethral valves will often strain to urinate and exhibit dribbling and an insufficient stream. Attempts to urinate may be associated with contortions of the face and a considerable increase in intra-abdominal pressure. Urethral strictures, which are usually a complication of hypospadias repair or urethral instrumentation, may also be associated with straining to urinate. Boys with hesitancy and intermittent flow probably have inability to relax the external or internal sphincter and require urodynamic evaluation. A child with apparent meatal stenosis usually does not strain while voiding and has no difficulty in starting his stream. A child with severe meatal stenosis, on the other hand, may have a very thin, high-velocity, and angulated stream. Urethral diverticula, often secondary to the presence of anterior urethral valves, and megalourethra with inadequate corpora spongiosa may be demonstrated on voiding as the urethra dilates and fills under increased pressure. The uncircumcised boy with severe phimosis may balloon his foreskin as he voids, but the urethra itself should not distend.

Rectal Examination

Examination of the rectum can be invaluable in providing information about both the male and the female patient. Suspected foreign bodies in the vagina can often be confirmed by rectal examination. Abnormalities of the wolffian or müllerian duct structures, such as müllerian duct cysts and seminal vesicle cysts, can be palpated by rectal examination. The extent of pelvic tumors can also be estimated by rectal examination. In a myelodysplastic child or a child in whom neurogenic bladder is suspected, rectal examination can yield information regarding sphincter tone. Examination of the rectal sphincter should also be performed prior to urinary diversion by ureterosigmoidostomy or other procedures after which the anal sphincter will provide urinary continence.

Neurologic Evaluation

A large percentage of the urologist's patients will be children in whom it is imperative to determine whether there is a neurologic deficit, including children with enuresis, incontinence, traumatic lesions, and myelodysplasia. Neurologic examination of the very young child is difficult because it requires accurate evaluation of subjective responses. The bulbocavernosus reflex is elicited by squeezing the glans or clitoris and noting a rectal sphincter contraction by digital examination or observation. The presence of this reflex is objective evidence that the reflex arc to the sphincter is intact. Intact sensation can be determined by examining responses to pinprick or soft touch in the perineum, the perianal area, and the genital areas. Proprioception can be elicited as the bladder is filled through an indwelling catheter. Distinguishing between hot and cold water in the bladder requires definite responses, and consequently such a test is usually not reliable in the younger child.

DIAGNOSIS AND MANAGEMENT OF FETAL ABNORMALITIES

Since the advent of fetal ultrasound and amniocentesis with analysis of specific fetal proteins, the urologist is occasionally called upon to evaluate and monitor a fetus with a genitourinary abnormality.

The diagnosis of fetal abnormalities by ultrasound is discussed in the chapter on abdominal ultrasound. This technique analyzes sound waves as they are transmitted through a substance, reflected, and measured by an ultrasonic detector. Static studies such as the B-mode scan provide a cross section of the structure from which one can measure size and consistency. Real time ultrasound allows one to observe the urinary tract "in motion"; thus, motility can be assessed. Although the resolution is not as clear as in other radiologic studies, the noninvasiveness of the examination makes it quite popular in intrauterine evaluation. The fetus can be evaluated as early as the sixth gestational week, although the precise diagnosis of genitourinary abnormalities usually cannot be accomplished until the second or third trimester. A number of genitourinary conditions suspected on fetal ultrasound have been confirmed at birth. These include multicystic kidney, ureteropelvic junction obstruction, posterior urethral valves, hydrocele, renal dysplasia, sacrococcygeal teratoma, and megaureter.

Immunoelectrophoresis of amniotic fluid allows the perinatologist to analyze specific fetal proteins. Abnormal levels may be suggestive of fetal disease processes. Alpha-fetoprotein is elevated in the amniotic fluid of fetuses who have large myelomeningoceles, congenital nephrosis, sacrococcygeal teratoma, and polycystic kidneys. Brock has identified a new fetal protein whose chemical structure has not been clearly delineated that may also be linked to neural tube defects. Milunsky and Tulchinsky recently reported the prenatal diagnosis of adrenal hyperplasia by measuring amniotic fluid levels of adrenal hormones and their precursors.

The management of genitourinary abnormalities in the fetus is a more complex issue. Harrison et al have outlined a thoughtful, thorough and aggressive approach to the management of fetal lesions. Treatment involving early delivery or interventional surgery has to be put into the perspective that hydronephrosis is often markedly improved when diagnosed and repaired in the neonatal period. Whether it is beneficial to operate upon severely obstructed kidneys in utero or after induced early delivery is not known yet, and will require comparison with patients allowed to go to full gestation. This issue was recently explored by a panel of experts who debated the ethical and medical issues surrounding fetal intervention (Duckett et al). Although members of this panel were not in total agreement, one can draw some conclusions from their discussions. The emphasis on fetal intervention focuses on an important issue, that modern fetal ultrasound techniques allow early diagnosis of intrauterine anomalies and expedite correction of these after normal delivery. It is not known at present whether fetal intervention is indicated for relief of hydronephrosis. Such intervention is not standard treatment, and should be limited to a few centers that are studying the possibilities in both clinical and research facilities. The burden of proof is on these centers to show that such infants do better than they would if they had been allowed to proceed to term. Renal dysplasia is the process that is most frequently linked to early postnatal renal deaths, and there is currently no evidence to suggest that early fetal intervention will prevent this.

SPECIAL PROBLEMS OF CHILDREN WITH UROGENITAL DISEASE

Psychologic Considerations

ATTITUDINAL FACTORS. Awareness of psychologic considerations specific to children is vitally important to successful medical management because all manifestations of disease in children must be taken into account in planning the treatment of the child's illness. Neither child nor parent is in a position to alter the course of management, and the urologist, in cooperative communication with the pediatrician, must assume that responsibility.

The attitude of the child toward his disease will affect his recovery and must, therefore, be carefully evaluated by the urologist. All sick children display anxiety, and the anxiety of the sick child is likely to differ both in origin and in effect from that of the sick adult. The child views his misfortune in terms of his immediate discomfort and lacks the psychologic maturity and emotional control to cope with what is happening to him.

SEPARATION ANXIETY. The sick child is anxious because of his illness and pain, because he senses anxiety in his parents, and because the surroundings in the physician's office or the hospital are strange. The younger the child, the more he has relied upon his parents for control over his environment. Now, hospitalization has placed him in an environment where he can make few decisions for himself, and where he is manipulated by a variety of people, many of them total strangers to him, and all of them outside his immediate family. He has no choice of bed, room, clothing, or food. Often he is placed in a bleak room, and his body is routinely assaulted by repeated examinations, painful venipuncture, and frightening machinery. He may be asked to inhale gases that have a peculiar smell and that induce a sleep from which he awakens, not rested and invigorated, but suffering from sore throat and incisional pain, and unable to eat, void, defecate, or even talk. Moreover, he may find himself in yet more unusual and threatening surroundings, i.e., an intensive care unit.

The attitude and emotional responses of the child to his illness and hospitalization do not remain static, but will change as he progresses from the neonatal state to infancy, then through early childhood onward to adolescence. The neonate or infant has no comprehension of the disease process and is totally dependent on external forces. As the child grows, he begins to identify with his surroundings and particularly with his mother. Thus, hospitalization during this early childhood period results primarily in separation anxiety (Edleston). The child is often able to comprehend the nature of this anxiety, even though he may not understand its origin. Separation anxiety can be relieved, at least in part, by allowing the parent to stay with the hospitalized child.

EMASCULATION ANXIETY. Other anxieties have to do with the illness itself and vary with age. A child is not able to appreciate the nuances of his disease. He may be told that he will have an operation on his penis, but he does not have sufficient knowledge to interpret this information properly. Will he regard the procedure positively as one of reconstruction, or fear it as a process of emasculation? If his response is one of fear, will this fear be reinforced with each successive operation?

A 1973 study indicates that separation from the mother is most responsible for anxiety in the hypospadias patient aged 1½ to 3 (Kelalis et al, 1973a). After age 3, the patient tends to develop anxiety about his genitalia; the anxiety progresses with increasing age and reaches a maximum at puberty. Robertson and Walker confirmed the existence of anxiety about genital abnormalities in older boys with hypospadias and demonstrated that this type of anxiety is quite different from that suffered by children with more obvious congenital abnormalities like cleft lip or palate.

TIMING OF ELECTIVE GENITAL SURGERY. The best time to do elective genital surgery remains controversial. The aforementioned data suggest that the problem with separation anxiety can largely be surmounted by having the mother stay with the child. Manley and Epstein have performed hypospadias repair successfully in 17 boys less than 18 months of age. Belman and Kass reported similar results in 37 children under 1 year of age. In the hands of experienced pediatric anesthesiologists, the anesthetic risk in healthy infants is no different from that in older children. Penile size does not change significantly between 1 and 3 years of age. Boys with undescended testicles at age 1 are extremely unlikely to have these testes descend spontaneously, at least until puberty. Histologic damage has been observed in the undescended testicle by 12 months of age. These data suggest that orchiopexy and hypospadias repair should be done at 1 year of age or early in the second year of life.

PROBLEMS OF ADOLESCENCE. Although the beginning and end of adolescence are not well defined, it is known that there are specific problems related to this period of intense physical and emotional growth. These are related to emancipation from dependency on parents, establishment of personal and sexual identity, development of personal moral and ethical codes, and the choosing of a career and lifestyle. Particular medical problems of adolescence are high suicide and accident rates, drug abuse, and increased incidence of venereal disease. The urologist must be aware that body image is extremely important to the adolescent, and that such treatments as steroids, tumoricidal drugs, and urinary diversion procedures are likely to meet with great resistance.

TERMINAL ILLNESS. Terminal disease and approaching death in the child present even more complex psychologic problems. It is probable that children with terminal disease have some foreknowledge of death. Experience indicates that children can be very perceptive of a terminal illness; such apprehension probably produces the ultimate separation anxiety.

Medical Evaluation

From the urologic standpoint, the child should be medically evaluated in a context quite different from the approach used in adults. The urologist must, on occasion, reorient his thinking because symptoms in a child may have causes vastly different from those in adults.

On the basis of initial history and physical examination, one can exclude unlikely diagnoses, leaving a list of diseases that require further investigation including laboratory tests, radiologic evaluation, and pathologic examination of tissue. Investigational tests should be considered in the context of their risk to the patient and their relative cost. Tests that carry little or no risk and are inexpensive are usually preferred as preliminary screening devices. Such tests can usually be done on an outpatient basis. Tests of higher risk and greater costs should be reserved for specific indications.

Many diagnoses can be excluded by history and physical examination. Preliminary screening tests may include laboratory investigation with blood studies, urinalysis, and urine culture. These involve virtually no risk and little cost. Renal ultrasound is noninvasive and an excellent screening method for diagnosing obstructive uropathy. Studies with a minimal risk in relation to the diagnostic benefit achieved may include intravenous pyelography, cystourethrography, renal scan, urine concentration tests, and renal clearances. With modern anesthetic techniques, cystoscopy also carries a low risk, but does not have a yield high enough to justify its use in many patients. Higher-risk studies that require specific indications include aortography of any type and renal biopsy. Using this sort of progressive logical approach to the child with urologic disease, one may most expeditiously proceed with the evaluation at the lowest possible cost, avoiding the temptation of making a superficial and rapid diagnosis early in the course of evaluation which might prevent or delay discovery of a more serious underlying disease.

BIBLIOGRAPHY

TEXTBOOK REFERENCES

Campbell MF, Harrison JH: Urology. Vol 2. Third ed. Philadelphia, WB Saunders Co., 1970, pp 1629, 1730.

Engle MA: Associated urologic anomalies in infants and children with congenital heart disease. In Associated Congenital Anomalies. Edited by M El-Shafie and CH Klippel. Baltimore, Williams & Wilkins, 1981, pp 137–142.

Ferrier PE: Disorders of sexual differentiation. In Metabolic, Endocrine, and Genetic Disorders of Children. Vol 2. Edited by VC Kelley. Hagerstown, Md., Harper & Row, Publishers, 1974, pp 573–583.

Hecht F: Autosomal chromosome abnormalities. In Metabolic, Endocrine, and Genetic Disorders of Children. Vol 1. Edited by VC Kelley. Hagerstown, Md., Harper & Row, 1974, pp 101–142.

King LR: Other congenital abnormalities. In Pediatric Surgery. Vol 2. Third ed. Edited by O Swenson. New York, Appleton-Century-Crofts, Inc., 1969, pp 1116–1127.

Miller RW: Relation between cancer and congenital malformations. In Associated Congenital Anomalies. Edited by M El-Shafie and CH Klippel. Baltimore, Williams & Wilkins, 1981, pp 67–70.

REVIEW ARTICLES

Allen JS, Summers JL, Wilkerson JE: Meatal calibration of newborn boys, J Urol 107:498, 1972.

Bashour BN, Balfe JW: Urinary tract anomalies in neonates with spontaneous pneumothorax and/or pneumomediastinum. Pediatrics 59(Suppl 6, pt 2):1048, 1977.

Bauer SB, Bull MJ, Retik AB: Hypospadias: a familial study. J Urol 121:474, 1979.

Belman AB, Kass EJ: Hypospadias repair in children less than one year of age. J Urol 128:1273, 1982.

Berry CD Jr, Cross RR Jr: Urethral meatal caliber in circumcised and uncircumcised males. Am J Dis Child 92:152, 1956.

Bjorklund S-I: Hemihypertrophy and Wilms's tumour. Acta Paediatr Scand 44:287, 1955.

Boatman DL, Kolln CP, Flocks RH: Congenital anomalies associated with horseshoe kidney. J Urol 107:205, 1972.

Bourne GL, Bernirschke K: Absent umbilical artery: a review of 113 cases. Arch Dis Child 35:534, 1960.

Brock DJH: Foeto-specific proteins in prenatal diagnosis. Biochem Soc Trans 7:1179, 1979.

Carlton CE Jr, Scott R Jr: Incidence of urological anomalies in association with major nonurological anomalies. J Urol 84:43, 1960.

Catterall A, Roberts GC, Wynne-Davies R: Association of Perthes' disease with congenital anomalies of genitourinary tract and inguinal region. Lancet 1:996, 1971.

Curran AS, Curran JP: Associated sacral and renal malformations: a new syndrome? Pediatrics 49:716, 1972.

Donohue RE, Utley WLF, Maling TM: Excretory urography in asymptomatic boys with cryptorchidism. J Urol 109:912, 1973.

Dresner ML: Torsed appendage: diagnosis and management; blue dot sign. Urology 1:63, 1973.

Duckett JW, Harrison MR, deLorimier AA, Arant BS, Bellinger MF, Kroovand RL, Bernstein J: Fetal intervention for obstructive uropathy. Dialog Ped Urol 5:1, 1982.

Dweck HS, Reynolds DW, Cassady G: Indirect blood pressure measurement in newborns. Am J Dis Child 127:492, 1974.

Edelston J: Separation anxiety in young children: a study of hospital cases. Genet Psychol Monogr 28:3, 1943.

Farrington GH, Kerr IH: Abnormalities of the upper urinary tract in cryptorchidism. Br J Urol 41:77, 1969.

Felton LM: Should intravenous pyelography be a routine procedure for children with cryptorchidism or hypospadias? J Urol 81:335, 1959.

Filly RA: Detection of fetal malformations with ultrasonic B-scans. Birth Defects 15:45, 1979.

Fontana VJ, Ferrara A, Perciaccante R: Wilms's tumor and associated anomalies. Am J Dis Child 109:459, 1965.

Froehlich LA, Fujikura T: Follow-up of infants with single umbilical artery. Pediatrics 52:6, 1973.

Garrett RA, Franken EA Jr: Neonatal ascites: perirenal urinary extravasation with bladder outlet obstruction. J Urol 102:627, 1969.

Gorlin RJ, Sedana H: Leprechaunism—Donohue's syndrome. Mod Med 40:86 (Dec 11), 1972.

Goyer RA, Reynolds J Jr, Burke J, et al: Hereditary renal disease with neurosensory hearing loss, proteinuria and ichthyosis. Am J Med Sci 256:166, 1968.

Harrison MR, Golbus MS, Filly RA: Management of the fetus with a correctable congenital defect. JAMA 246:774, 1981.

Haslam RHA, Berman W, Heller RM: Renal abnormalities in the Russell-Silver syndrome. Pediatrics 51:216, 1973.

Hilson D: Malformation of ears as sign of malformation of genitourinary tract. Br Med J 2:785, 1957.

Hinman F Jr: Microphallus: characteristics and choice of treatment from a study of 20 cases. J Urol 107:499, 1972.

Humphry A, Munn HD: Abnormalities of the urinary tract in association with congenital cardiovascular disease. Can Med Assoc J 95:143, 1966.

Kelalis PP, Bunge R, Barkin M: The timing of elective surgery on the genitalia of male children with particular reference to undescended testes and hypospadias. (Report by the Action Committee on surgery on the genitalia of male children.) American Academy of Pediatrics, Section on Urology, Chicago, October, 1973a.

Kelalis PP, Malek RS, Segura JW: Observations on renal ectopia and fusion in children. J Urol 110:588, 1973b.

Lord JM: Foetal ascites. Arch Dis Child 28:298, 1953.

Mackintosh TF, Girdwood TG, Parker DJ, et al: Aniridia

and Wilms's tumour (nephroblastoma). Br J Ophthalmol 52:846, 1968.

Malek RS, Greene LF: Urologic aspects of Hippel-Lindau syndrome. J Urol 106:800, 1971.

Manley CB, Epstein ES: Early hypospadias repair. J Urol 125:698, 1981.

Melicow MM, Uson AC: Palpable abdominal masses in infants and children: a report based on a review of 653 cases. J Urol 81:705, 1959.

Miller RW, Fraumeni JF Jr, Manning MD: Association of Wilms's tumor with aniridia, hemihypertrophy and other congenital malformations. N Engl J Med 270:922, 1964.

Miller SF: Transposition of the external genitalia associated with the syndrome of caudal regression. J Urol 108:818, 1972.

Milunsky A, Tulchinsky D: Prenatal diagnosis of congenital adrenal hyperplasia due to 21-hydroxylase deficiency. Pediatrics 59:768, 1977.

Newman H, Molthan ME, Osborn WF: Urinary tract anomalies in children with congenital heart disease. Am J Roentgenol Radium Ther Nucl Med 106:52, 1969.

Noble MJ, Wacksman J: Screening excretory urography in patients with cryptorchidism or hypospadias: a survey and review of the literature. J Urol 124:98, 1980.

Opitz JM, Frias JL, Gutenberger JE, et al: The G syndrome of multiple congenital anomalies. Birth Defects 5(pt II):95, 1969.

Persky L, Owens R: Genitourinary tract abnormalities in Turner's syndrome (gonadal dysgenesis). J Urol 105:309, 1971.

Potter EL: Facial characteristics of infants with bilateral renal agenesis. Am J Obstet Gynecol 51:885, 1946.

Potter EL: Oligohydramnios: further comment. J Pediatr 84:931, 1971.

Redman JF: Noonan's syndrome and cryptorchidism. J Urol 109:909, 1973.

Richards RD, Mebust WK, Schimke RN: A prospective study on Von Hippel-Lindau disease. J Urol 110:27, 1973.

Robertson M, Walker D: Psychological factors in hypospadias repair. J Urol 113:698, 1975.

Rudiger RA, Schmidt W, Loose DA, et al: Severe developmental failure with coarse facial features, distal limb hypoplasia, thickened palmar creases, bifid uvula, and ureteral stenosis: a previously unidentified familial disorder with lethal outcome. J Pediatr 79:977, 1971.

Shima H, Ikoma F, Terakawa T, Satuh Y, Nagata H, Shimada K, Nagano S: Developmental anomalies associated with hypospadias. J Urol 122:619, 1979.

Silver W, Steier M, Schwartz O, et al: The Holt-Oram syndrome with previously undescribed associated anomalies. Am J Dis Child 124:911, 1972.

Taylor WC: Deformity of ears and kidneys. Can Med Assoc J 93:107, 1965.

Temtamy SA, Miller JD: Extending the scope of the VATER association: definition of the VATER syndrome. J Pediatr 85:345, 1974.

Thomas IT, Smith DW: Oligohydramnios, cause of the nonrenal features of Potter's syndrome, including pulmonary hypoplasia. J Pediatr 84:811, 1974.

Turner G: A second family with renal, vaginal, and middle ear anomalies (letter). J Pediatr 76:641, 1970.

Virnig NL, Reynolds JW: Reliability of flush blood pressure measurements in the sick newborn infant. J Pediatr 84:594, 1974.

Vitko RJ, Cass AS, Winter RB: Anomalies of the genitourinary tract associated with congenital scoliosis and congenital kyphosis. J Urol 108:655, 1972.

Wadlington WB, Tucker VL, Schimke RN: Mesomelic dwarfism with hemivertebrae and small genitalia (the Robinow syndrome). Am J Dis Child 126:202, 1973.

Waldbaum RS, Marshall VF: The prune belly syndrome: a diagnostic therapeutic plan. J Urol 103:668, 1970.

Watson RA, Lennox KW, Gangai MP: Simple cryptorchidism: the value of the excretory urogram as a screening method. J Urol 111:789, 1974.

Williams DI, Grant J: Urological complications of imperforate anus. Br J Urol 41:660, 1969.

Williams DI, Nixon HH: Agenesis of the sacrum. Surg Gynecol Obstet 105:84, 1957.

Winter JSD, John G, Mellman WJ, et al: A familial syndrome of renal, genital, and middle ear anomalies. J. Pediatr 72:88, 1968.

2

ANESTHETIC MANAGEMENT

Brian Dawson and Matthew Crawford

Anesthetic management and supportive care of children undergoing urologic procedures is essentially similar to that for other pediatric surgical operations. The goals are:

1. Adequate preoperative evaluation and preparation.
2. A surgical procedure free of pain and patient awareness.
3. Minimal disturbance of body functions.
4. A comfortable and uneventful postoperative course.

However, children undergoing urologic procedures do present special considerations:

1. Anomalies of the genitourinary tract are associated with a high incidence of other congenital anomalies.
2. A high incidence of multiple surgical procedures requiring repeated anesthetic administrations.
3. An altered drug pharmacology in patients with impaired renal function. However, the majority of children undergoing urologic surgery have normal renal function.
4. Over 50 per cent of all urologic pediatric patients can be safely managed on an outpatient basis.
5. Most procedures are elective—at the Mayo Clinic only 1 per cent are considered urgent.
6. Unusual positions on the operating table have the potential for impairment of respiratory and circulatory function.
7. The intimate relationship of the kidney to the diaphragm carries the attendant risk of pneumothorax.

PREOPERATIVE PREPARATION

Examination

Before surgery, the child undergoes a history and physical examination, comple-

mented by laboratory studies, to determine the safety of administration of anesthesia.

Important aspects of the history include:

1. Personal anesthetic history.
   a. Drugs used and any resulting complications.
2. Family anesthetic history. Certain anesthetic complications may be familial.
   a. Malignant hyperpyrexia.
   b. Abnormally prolonged response to succinylcholine.
3. Allergies.
   a. Specific drug allergies.
   b. Allergic rhinitis.
   c. Asthma.
4. Recent exposure to infectious diseases.
5. History of hepatitis.
6. Personal and family history of bleeding.
7. Duration and type of current medications.

During the physical examination, the anesthesiologist is particularly interested in abnormalities of the mouth or neck that may impair respiration, the presence of loose teeth, and the existence of any cardiac pulmonary, renal, or neuromuscular disease that may modify anesthetic management.

Basic laboratory studies *traditionally* include chest roentgenogram, concentrations of hemoglobin, and urinalysis supplemented by additional tests as dictated by the underlying disease. In children with urologic problems, these may include determination of serum electrolytes, serum creatinine, and blood urea nitrogen, assessment of acid-base balance, and specific urologic roentgenograms. Blood is cross-matched as required.

For conservation of manpower and the family's financial resources, it is suggested that if no essential change in health has occurred after an extensive workup in the 6 months prior to surgery, no further detailed physical examination or laboratory studies are required. Furthermore, it has been suggested that elective pediatric surgery is not an indication for routine preoperative chest roentgenography. Rather, chest roentgenograms should be obtained preoperatively in children only when clinically indicated (Farnsworth et al).

The most common problem in preoperative evaluation is the possible coexistence of the common cold. Allergic rhinitis, teething, and chronic ear infections may result in runny noses. Many children with urologic problems have urinary tract infections causing preoperative temperature elevations. Preoperative temperature elevation also may result from dehydration due to unnecessarily prolonged withholding of fluids. The authors of this chapter will proceed with anesthesia unless the runny nose is obviously purulent or there is clear evidence of significant pharyngeal, laryngeal, or pulmonary infection. In sum, it is quite rare for elective surgery to be postponed for anesthetic reasons.

Psychologic Preparation

Certain factors may influence the behavior of a child in hospital. These include:

1. Separation from home and family.
2. Placement in an unfamiliar environment with unfamiliar people.
3. The need to undergo strange and painful procedures, particularly surgery and anesthesia.
4. Exposure to many people, including other children, with the risk of cross-infection.

No matter how busy the schedule, there should always be time for a reasonable explanation to the child (if old enough to comprehend) and to his parents concerning what will or will not happen to him. At the same time, the anesthesiologist can discharge his professional duties of disclosing to the parents the procedures, risks, and likely outcome of the anesthetic management, and its alternatives. The positive aspects should be stressed as well as the risks of complications (Orwoll). The parents can be told that the risks of anesthesia during elective surgery on otherwise healthy children is somewhat less than the risk of driving to and from the hospital.

Many of the psychologic problems of hospital admission can be avoided by performing surgery as an outpatient procedure with the patient under general anesthesia. This popular innovation facilitates the delivery of quality health care to children at reduced cost (Reed et al).

Physical Preparation

Should the magnitude of surgery require hospital admission, baseline values of vital signs are obtained in the pediatric ward and the child is familiarized with postoperative equipment. It should be noted that the normal blood pressure ranges from 70 mm Hg systolic at birth to 80 mm Hg at 1 year and 100 mm Hg at 10 years of age.

In order to reduce the risk of aspiration of vomitus, children are denied solid food after the evening meal. However, thirst may be satisfied by permitting plain water to drink up to 4 hours before surgery. Infants may be permitted bottle feeding up to 4 hours before surgery, the last bottle consisting of sweetened water. It is important to give fluid and calories to infants prior to surgery to prevent restlessness, elevated temperature, acidosis, dehydration, and hypoglycemia. Intravenous fluids with 5 or 10 per cent dextrose may be started preoperatively as required.

PREMEDICATION. Premedication for the hospitalized child may be administered as shown in Table 2–1 (Dawson and Lynn). A wide variety of drugs are available, but this

Table 2–1. Guide for Premedication in Children*

Weight (kg)	Pentobarbital (2 h before operation)†	Meperidine (45 min before operation, intramuscularly)	Atropine
0 to 10	0	0	0.1 mg
10 to 20	30 mg (by rectum)	1 mg/kg	0.2 mg
20 to 30	45 mg (by rectum)	1 mg/kg	0.3 mg
30 to 40	60 mg (by mouth)	1 mg/kg	0.4 mg
>40	90 mg (by mouth)	1 mg/kg	0.4 mg

Modified from Dawson B, Lynn HB: The pediatric patient in the operating room. Surg Clin North Am 45:949, 1965.
* This guide may be varied according to physical and emotional status of the patient.
† Pentobarbital is omitted for emergency surgery.

regimen has proved reliable for us. Dosages may be modified according to the physical and emotional status of the child. Correct timing of drug administration is perhaps the most important factor in premedication so that the child arrives in the operating room drowsy, yet cooperative. Atropine sulfate is used to reduce salivation and secretions of the respiratory tract and to decrease endogenous vagal activity and the exogenous vagal effects of certain drugs (e.g., succinylcholine) that tend to cause a reduction in the heart rate. Glycopyrrolate is an excellent long-acting substitute for atropine that probably does not cross the blood-brain barrier. The dosage is about half that for atropine (Lavis et al). Both atropine and glycopyrrolate should be omitted preoperatively in patients with a significant pyrexia, to avoid further elevations of temperature and heart rate. Oral diazepam 0.4 mg/kg may be used preoperatively, but its effect may be unpredictable.

Transportation to and from the Operating Room

Small infants and neonates are exposed to risks during transportation to and from the operating room. To maintain normal temperature a heated incubator or console should be used; alternatively, the baby should be wrapped and the head covered. An electrocardiogram and a precordial stethoscope should be used for monitoring. Adequate O_2 and air with ventilatory and intubation equipment should be available together with personnel who know how to use them.

ANESTHETIC MANAGEMENT AND SUPPORTIVE CARE

Anesthetic Management

The anesthetic management of the pediatric urologic patient in the operating room is based on maintaining:

1. Insensitivity to pain and nonawareness of surroundings.
2. A patent airway at all times.
3. Adequate ventilation and oxygenation.
4. Smooth induction of and recovery from anesthesia.
5. Adequate muscular relaxation.
6. Minimal interference with circulation.
7. Minimal disturbance of renal function.
8. Normal body temperature.
9. Adequate monitoring.
10. Adequate and appropriate intravenous therapy.

Although children are usually given a general anesthetic to produce insensitivity to pain, there has been a rapidly growing interest in the supplemental use of regional and local nerve block to produce better postoperative analgesia (vide infra).

Equipment

Any of the wide range of anesthetic delivery systems, intelligently used, may be applied safely in children provided there is:

1. Minimal total dead space.
2. Minimal air-flow resistance.
3. Minimal valve-opening pressure.
4. Adequate inspired gas flow.
5. Satisfactory gas flow mixtures.

These limitations will serve to ensure adequate oxygen flow to the lungs and carbon dioxide removal from the lungs.

In children weighing less than 20 kg, a Rees modification of the Ayre T-piece is often preferred; this is simple and lightweight, has no valves, and is easily sterilized. Inspired gases delivered by the system are completely dry; this may result in heat and water loss and alterations in the respiratory tract. Consequently, a humidifier should be connected to the inspired gas line to provide heated humidification of inspired gases. Children weighing more than 20 kg are usually anesthetized using an adult circle absorber system. Such apparatus has been used with safety in neonates (Graff et al).

There has been growing concern over the effect of prolonged exposure of operating room personnel to minute concentrations of waste anesthetic gases contaminating the operating room atmosphere (Cohen). Regardless of the anesthetic apparatus used, the attachment of a relatively cheap scavenger device to prevent this contamination is mandatory today.

Induction

In infants and young children with an established intravenous route and all older children, anesthesia may be induced with sodium thiopental 5 mg/kg. Otherwise anesthesia may be induced with an inhalational anesthetic mixture, usually oxygen, nitrous oxide, and halothane. During induction, the operat-

Table 2 – 2. Endotracheal Tube Size

For Infants under 1 Year of Age:

<3 months: 3.0 mm internal diameter

3 to 6 months: 3.5 mm internal diameter

6 to 12 months: 4.0 mm internal diameter

For Children over 1 Year of Age:

$$\frac{\text{Age in years}}{4} + 4.5 \text{ mm internal diameter}$$

ing room should be completely quiet, for all sounds seem acutely amplified to the patient at this time. The child should not be examined or tampered with until he has been completely anesthetized; any unwarranted intrusions can easily trigger laryngospasm.

Neonates may be intubated while awake; in older infants and children intubation is accomplished after induction, with or without succinylcholine. Many children undergoing urologic operations can be safely anesthetized without endotracheal intubation — for example, cystoscopy and surgery on the external genitalia. In these cases a depth of anesthesia appropriate for the surgical stimulus must be maintained; an appropriately sized endotracheal tube, a laryngoscope, and a syringe containing succinylcholine are always kept ready. A formula for probable endotracheal tube size has served us well (Table 2 – 2) (Dawson and Lynn).

Drugs

ANESTHETIC AGENTS. Halothane (Fluothane) has been established as a most satisfactory and safe anesthetic agent in children. In an extensive review, Carney and Van Dyke noted only 11 reports of possible halothane hepatitis in children, who constituted 12 per cent of the surgical cases and received halothane for 91 per cent of their operations. The striking lack of hepatic complications from repeat exposure to halothane is important in the management of multiple urologic procedures. Halothane has not been associated with renal complications. Methoxyflurane (Pentrane), on the other hand, has been associated with renal tubular necrosis and renal failure, apparently owing to serum inorganic fluoride, an end product of methoxyflurane metabolism. Methoxyflurane is little used today and is mainly of historical interest. Enflurane (Ethrane), more recently introduced and widely used, has a more limited metabolism that results in low levels of serum

inorganic fluoride. Its use in patients with impaired renal function has not been clearly established. Isoflurane (Forane), a structural isomer of enflurane, has the least metabolism of any halogenated volatile anesthetic agent, less than 0.2 per cent. Serum fluoride levels are significantly less than with enflurane, and isoflurane would seem to be a valuable anesthetic agent in patients with impaired renal function. Another advantage is that isoflurane does not sensitize the heart to the effects of exogenous and endogenous epinephrine as does halothane. This results in significantly fewer arrhythmias. Unfortunately, induction of anesthesia in children is more stormy with isoflurane than with halothane owing to the more irritant effects of isoflurane on the respiratory tract. Prior induction with thiopental or halothane can be employed.

Parenteral agents are used with nitrous oxide to produce balanced anesthesia (Lundy) — for example, sodium thiopental as a hypnotic; analgesia with nitrous oxide often complemented with narcotic; and muscle relaxants. Although these techniques can be applied to small infants, they are more commonly used in older children. Patient awareness during surgery is a serious complication when balanced anesthesia becomes unbalanced, usually as a result of too much analgesia and muscular relaxation and too little hypnosis. Alertness to the signs of lightening anesthesia, which are similar to the signs of fright, will prevent this complication. Ketamine is little used in pediatric urology owing to postoperative side effects including hallucinations. However, it is still a useful agent to have for the intramuscular induction of anesthesia in a completely refractory child.

Much has been written on individual drug dosages in children. This commits an impossible task to the memory. A safe approximation to the dose of any drug in a child is

$$\frac{\text{weight in kilograms}}{70} \times \text{adult dose,}$$

70 being the weight in kg of the average adult.

MUSCLE RELAXANTS. Adequate muscular relaxation is necessary for intra- and extraperitoneal procedures on the kidney, ureter, and bladder. However, disagreement about the definition of adequacy can attenuate the rapport between anesthesiologist and surgeon. This may be avoided by a clear understanding of each other's problems, by the knowledge that the action of any muscle relaxant may be prolonged by the presence of impaired renal function, and by the intelligent use of a peripheral nerve stimulator to monitor muscle relaxant activity.

Continued muscle relaxation may be an important cause of hypoventilation and hypoxia at the conclusion of surgery. It must be recognized and treated promptly. This may be done with continuous positive-pressure ventilation or, more appropriately, by pharmacologic reversal of the muscle relaxant effect by an anticholinesterase (Neostigmine). This may result in bradycardia and requires prior treatment with atropine. Muscle relaxants are of two types:

1. The short-acting depolarizing drugs, which include succinylcholine. Use of succinylcholine in small children can be associated with bradycardia and arrhythmias (Leigh et al).
2. The long-acting nondepolarizing drugs such as pancuronium (Pavulon), D-tubocurarine (curare), and metocurine (Metubine). Two new shorter-acting nondepolarizing drugs, actracurium and vecuronium, are being tested and may be of great value in pediatric urology.

VENTILATION IMPAIRMENT. Many factors may contribute to impairment of ventilation during anesthesia and surgery; these include the premedication, anesthetic drugs, and muscle relaxants, as well as the operative position of the patient, retraction for surgical exposure, and the presence of large surgical masses. Consequently the anesthesiologist should ensure adequacy of ventilation and the airway at all times.

Supportive Care

Intravenous Infusion

An intravenous infusion is started on all children who undergo urologic surgery except those undergoing minor surgical procedures. (Many anesthesiologists believe, with justification, that one should be started on *every* child who is a urologic surgical patient.) This is usually accomplished with a percutaneous needle and occasionally by a cutdown. In patients requiring preoperative intravenous fluid therapy, this procedure is obviously done on the ward; otherwise, it is best done in the operating room after the child has been anesthetized. Venous dilatation from the peripheral action of anesthetic agents facilitates intravenous cannulation. The modest prolongation of anesthesia time needed for the occa-

sional cutdown in small infants is not considered to be detrimental.

The arm is the best site for intravenous administration in children undergoing urologic surgery. Venous return from the leg may be impaired by pressure on the inferior vena cava from retraction or from an intra-abdominal mass, and it is not unknown for the inferior vena cava to be unintentionally opened during removal of large tumors; either circumstance will render an intravenous site in the leg ineffective, usually at a time when it is most needed. In infants, the external jugular and preauricular veins are very useful sites for intravenous administration. A graduated volume-control device is used on all intravenous lines to prevent fluid overloading. We have found the Buretrol device to be most satisfactory.

Intravenous fluid therapy in the operating room is based on providing maintenance fluid requirements and any necessary replacement fluids. Preoperative fluid deficits are corrected before the child is committed to elective surgery and in all but the most urgent emergency procedures. Maintenance fluid is given as 5 per cent dextrose in 0.2 per cent sodium chloride at the rate of 4 ml/kg per hour in small infants, whereas Ringer's lactate with 5 per cent dextrose is used in older children. The intravenous volume control device is filled with 1 hour's supply at a time.

All intravenous fluids in children should contain 5 per cent dextrose to provide a caloric intake and prevent hypoglycemia. Ten per cent dextrose is employed in neonates. Replacement fluids are 5 per cent dextrose in Ringer's lactate solution and whole blood. Five per cent dextrose in Ringer's lactate solution is used to replace fluid lost as transudate into the bowel and peritoneal cavity during surgical procedures on the kidney, ureter, and bladder. Seven to 10 ml/kg per hour are usually required, but the exact volume given is determined by the patient's physical signs. Most children undergoing major urologic surgery have a urethral catheter in place; urine output can be a useful guide to adequacy of fluid replacement after completion of the surgical repair.

REPLACEMENT OF BLOOD. Warmed whole blood remains the best replacement fluid for blood lost in the operating room. The blood volume of small children is estimated at 85 ml/kg. Serious alterations in hemodynamics will occur if this volume is not maintained. Estimates of blood loss and adequacy of replacement are based on fluctuations of pulse rate and arterial blood pressure, supplemented by intelligent interpretation of alterations in central venous pressure.

Other factors that affect not only central venous pressure but also pulse rate and arterial blood pressure are (1) the myocardial depressant and peripheral circulatory actions of anesthetic drugs, (2) positive-pressure ventilation, (3) patient position, and (4) surgical interference with venous return. It must be noted further that with the elimination of these factors in the postoperative period, the clinical picture will change. Gravimetric and colorimetric methods for the quantitative determination of blood loss have their advocates and are of value; however, neither method can take into consideration the blood lost on and under the surgical drapes. Also, these methods are of least value when they are most needed, namely, in the presence of a brisk hemorrhage. The suspicious and discerning eye of the anesthesiologist remains the most valuable adjunct to monitoring the patient's physical signs in determining the need for replacing blood loss.

Miscellaneous Hazards

PATIENT POSITIONING. Patients undergoing urologic operations are often placed in unusual positions on the operating table. This results in some impairment of respiration (which should be corrected by controlled ventilation) and of circulation because of venous pooling in dependent parts and of impairment of flow in the inferior vena cava. The senior author (B.D.) has also seen two cases of nonfatal air emboli in patients undergoing removal of a large renal mass while they were in a combined kidney–head down position. The inferior vena cava was accidentally opened in both instances.

Whatever position is used, it is necessary to be certain that peripheral nerves are free from pressure and that the patient is not in contact with metal. Cystoscopic procedures are often carried out in darkened rooms; a sufficient light source must be present at the head of the table to permit continuous monitoring of the patient's physical signs and observation of the anesthesia apparatus to ensure correct function. Anything less than these precautions jeopardizes patient safety.

PNEUMOTHORAX. The intimate relationship of the diaphragm to the posterior aspect of the kidney occasionally results in the accidental opening of the pleural cavity. This is more likely to occur with anatomic distortion, as in re-exploration or in the presence of

a large mass; it is unlikely to be a problem when controlled positive-pressure ventilation is used. The diaphragmatic hole is closed surgically; a catheter may be placed in the pleural space, to be withdrawn during positive-pressure inspiration at subcutaneous tissue closure. After kidney surgery, the child's chest should always be checked with a stethoscope, and if necessary a chest roentgenogram should be done. The remote possibility of tension pneumothorax arising from perforation of a lung should always be considered.

REDUCED RENAL FUNCTION. The combination of anesthesia and surgery usually results in reduced renal function. Factors contributing to this include diminished renal blood flow caused by myocardial depression; increased sympathetic activity; hypotension; renal vasoconstriction; and increased release of antidiuretic hormone. Anesthetic drugs and surgical manipulation and retraction share the responsibility for these changes. The neuroleptic agents droperidol and fentanyl, used to supplement nitrous oxide in balanced anesthesia, produce little change in renal function (Gorman and Craythorne) and thus may have an important place in renal surgery. After completion of surgical repair on the kidney, ureter, or bladder, the urologist is anxious to improve renal function and urine output with diuretics. We have used mannitol very successfully in children, administering a dosage of 0.5 g/kg, occasionally supplemented by furosemide (Lasix).

Temperature Control

Maintenance of normal body temperature during operation is essential in the pediatric patient. Unintentional hypothermia and, in particular, malignant hyperpyrexia have been associated with mortality.

The child who is under anesthesia with muscle relaxation loses his major source of heat production, muscle activity. He will tend to come into equilibrium with his thermal environment. Unintentional hypothermia can ensue, resulting in hypoventilation, hypotension, delayed drug metabolism from impaired enzyme activity, and delayed return of consciousness. Severe cooling may result in death.

In addition, with the return of consciousness and muscular activity, the child will shiver; this causes a significant increase in oxygen consumption—an additional postoperative hazard in the child exposed to the risk of hypoxia from multiple causes.

Unintentional hypothermia is prevented by maintaining the operating room temperature at 22° C at a minimum; this should be satisfactory for all occupants. Those who insist on arctic conditions for the practice of their operative skills may be reminded that a minimum operating room temperature of 20° C (68° F) is required (Joint Commission on Accreditation of Hospitals Manual and NFPA Code 56A, revised in 1971). But even 20° C is too cold for the anesthetized child. A water mattress warmed to 37.5° C; warmed, humidified inspired gas; and heating lamps will assist in maintaining normothermia.

Elevation of temperature can also occur. Causes include hypermetabolic states, infection, dehydration, and excessive medication with atropine. The most sinister cause, however, is malignant hyperpyrexia (Britt and Kalow; Ryan and Kerr). This can occur in young and otherwise healthy individuals; often there is some history of skeletal muscle abnormality, and the disorder may occur in families as an autosomal dominant trait — hence the need for a good family anesthetic history. Characteristically, induction of anesthesia is followed by tachycardia, tachypnea, and a rapid increase in body temperature because of intense metabolic derangements from abnormal skeletal muscle activity. In many cases, but not all, there has been an abnormal response to succinylcholine, manifested in the form of muscle rigidity. Arterial blood gas analysis reveals severe metabolic and respiratory acidosis, hypoxemia, hyperkalemia, myoglobinemia, and myoglobinuria.

Treatment of this very serious complication begins with early recognition by clinical signs and body temperature elevation. This implies that temperature should be monitored in all patients who are under anesthesia. Anesthesia is discontinued, and 100 per cent oxygen is used to ventilate the patient's lungs. The patient is cooled by every available means; these include intravenous ice-cold fluids, immersion in ice-cold water, circulation of ice-cold water through the mattress, and cooling of body cavities. The severe acidosis is treated with liberal quantities of sodium bicarbonate. Urinary output is maintained with furosemide and mannitol to prevent renal failure. Dantrolene has been demonstrated to prevent and reverse all the symptoms of malignant hyperthermia in an average dose of up to 2.5 mg/kg (Gronert). Dantrolene should be available in all institutions where general anesthesia is used.

Early arterial blood gas analysis differen-tiates malignant hyperpyrexia from other hyperthermic states. In many children undergoing surgery on the ureter and bladder, moderately elevated body temperatures occur during or immediately after surgery, probably from bacteremia.

Cardiac Resuscitation

The ultimate emergency — the need for cardiac resuscitation — may happen while the child is in the operating room. External cardiac compression can be easily and effectively performed on the pediatric patient (Mathews et al; Thaler and Stobie). Every urologist doing pediatric practice should understand how to perform this procedure. In the infant, the midsternum is compressed at a rate of 60 per minute; not unless the child is at least 6 years old may the heel of the hand be applied to the lower sternum immediately above the xiphisternum.

There should be a brief pause after each third compression to permit the anesthesiologist to ventilate the lungs adequately with 100 per cent oxygen. (It is assumed that an airway and an intravenous route have been established.) The child should be kept warm. Drug therapy includes sodium bicarbonate for control of metabolic acidosis; epinephrine, isoproterenol, and calcium for myocardial inotropic effect; and lidocaine (Xylocaine) for treatment of myocardial irritability. Concentration and starting dosage of these drugs for infants are listed in Table 2–3.

In infants and children, it is important that these drugs be given by syringe and not in continuous intravenous drip. One of the worst hazards facing the resuscitated child is accidental fluid overload, which severely taxes an already heavily stressed heart. The volumes of all fluids administered should be accurately recorded. Arterial blood gas analysis should be available, and defibrillation

Table 2–3. Drugs Used in Cardiac Resuscitation

Drug (concentration)	Dosage ml/kg
Epinephrine, 1:10,000	0.2
Calcium chloride, 100 mg/ml	0.1
Sodium bicarbonate, 44.6 mEq/50 ml	2.0
Lidocaine, 10 mg/ml	0.15
Isoproterenol, 1:5000	0.02

should be performed as necessary with direct-current discharge.

If external cardiac compression is unsuccessful, open-chest compression should be performed; conditions necessitating the use of this approach include pericardial tamponade, pneumothorax and pneumomediastinum, severe hemorrhage and hypovolemia, air embolus, and flail chest. One continues as long as there is hope of survival with the cerebrum intact. Monitoring includes electrocardiography and measurement of body temperature, blood gases, and urinary output. The child is cooled if hyperthermia occurs.

If signs of cerebral irritability appear, dehydration therapy is instituted with mannitol in a dosage of 0.5 g/kg. Dexamethasone (Decadron) may also be given intravenously in a dose of up to 8 mg. Encouraging signs in resuscitation include rapid return of consciousness, rapid return of spontaneous respiration with arterial carbon dioxide tension in the normal range, and pupillary reaction to light. Discouraging signs include persistent apnea with arterial carbon dioxide tension at or above normal range, convulsions, hyperpyrexia, and decerebrate activity. An electroencephalogram is helpful at this stage.

Monitoring

From the previous paragraphs it is possible to summarize monitoring requirements for the pediatric urologic patient in the operating room:

1. Mandatory.
   a. Heart action by precordial or esophageal stethoscope complemented by electrocardiography.
   b. Breath sounds by precordial or esophageal stethoscope.
   c. Arterial blood pressure by sphygmomanometer or ultrasound apparatus, or directly by intra-arterial needle.
   d. Body temperature.
   e. Degree of muscle relaxation determined by a peripheral nerve stimulator.
   f. Concentration of oxygen in the inspired gas mixture, using an oxygen analyzer.
2. Optional.
   a. Urinary output—this should be considered mandatory in major procedures.
   b. Central venous pressure.
   c. Blood gas analysis.
   d. Blood glucose—this should be considered mandatory in neonates.

REGIONAL ANESTHESIA

Regional Anesthesia in Pediatric Urology

Local anesthesia as a supplement to light general anesthesia is becoming a more commonly utilized technique in pediatric surgery. By employing a regional technique, the depth of general anesthesia to which the patient is subjected can be greatly reduced. Many operations can be performed without endotracheal intubation, as the risk of laryngeal spasm from surgical stimulation is greatly reduced.

With the use of long-acting local anesthetic solutions such as bupivacaine, analgesia for 4 to 6 hours is common, greatly reducing or eliminating the need for other postoperative analgesics. The patient's early postoperative period is much smoother than the stormy scene that may follow general anesthesia alone.

Caudal Anesthesia

Caudal anesthesia is particularly suited to surgery below the umbilicus, as the sacral, lumbar, and lower thoracic dermatomes can be safely and easily blocked by this route (Campbell; Lourey and McDonald; Fortuna).

Agents commonly used include 1 or 2 per cent solutions of lidocaine or mepivacaine or 0.25 to 0.5 per cent bupivacaine. These agents may be used with or without epinephrine.

In practice a dosage regimen of 0.5 ml/kg of these solutions injected via the sacral hiatus consistently spreads to block the upper lumbar dermatomes and occasionally the lower thoracic segments (Schulte-Steinberg). Higher levels of blockade may be obtained with increasing volume; however, epinephrine is required with these higher dosages. The total dosage per kg should always be checked to ensure that it is below the recommended dose level, e.g., bupivacaine 2 to 3 mg/kg (Schulte-Steinberg).

Technique

Following induction of general anesthesia, the patient is placed in a lateral decubitus position and the sacral area is prepared with povidone-iodine (Betadine). The sacral hiatus is palpated as a depression in the midline between the sacral cornua proximal to the sacrococcygeal joint. A 21-gauge short bevel scalp vein needle is inserted at the level of the sacral hiatus and directed cephalad at an angle of 65 to 70 degrees to the skin. The bevel of the needle is directed toward the feet to reduce the incidence of interosseous injection.

A characteristic "give" is usually felt as the needle pierces the sacrococcygeal ligament. Care is taken not to advance the needle more than 5 mm up through the sacral canal so as to avoid a spinal tap. The syringe should be aspirated prior to injection of any solution; should blood or CSF be obtained, the procedure should be abandoned.

A test dose of 1 ml of local anesthetic solution is injected and should meet minimal resistance. If the needle is posterior to the caudal canal a subcutaneous swelling will rapidly develop. Intravascular or subarachnoid injection may result in a rapid onset of hypotension. After correct placement of the needle has been determined, the remainder of the dosage should be administered at about 1 ml per second, with repeated attempts at aspiration.

Following the injection, the patient is returned to the supine position and skin preparation for surgery is commenced. If there is no response to surgical stimulation, indicating a successful block, the initial concentration of volatile anesthetic agent can be markedly reduced.

Complications of the technique are the same as those in adults and have been previously recorded (Schulte-Steinberg). The major possible complications of the technique include:

1. Dural puncture with subsequent high spinal blockade.
2. Intravascular or intraosseous injection with resultant high blood levels of local anesthetic solution causing convulsions or cardiovascular depression.
3. Intrapelvic injection resulting from failure to identify the sacral canal.

Contraindications, of course, include infections of the sacrococcygeal regions, disease of the central nervous system, gross spinal deformities, and coagulation defects.

If care is taken in patient selection, needle placement, and aspiration technique, the complications will be minimized.

Penile Block

Circumcision may cause much postoperative pain despite narcotic analgesia. Intraoperatively it is well known to cause marked laryngospasm even with deep anesthesia. Block of the dorsal nerves of the penis is a safe and effective way to overcome these problems (Bacon).

Sensation of most of the shaft and glans of the penis is transmitted by the dorsal penile nerves. These nerves and their accompanying end artery emerge under the symphysis pubis close to the midline and transverse the dorsum of the penis. Here they can be easily blocked by small volumes of local anesthetic solution. However, use of a non-epinephrine-containing solution is mandatory owing to the anatomy of the blood supply of the penis.

Technique

Following induction of general anesthesia, the skin overlying the symphysis pubis is prepared with betadine. The index and middle fingers of the left hand are slightly abducted and placed to palpate the symphysis pubis. A syringe with a 23-gauge needle and filled with 0.5 per cent plain bupivacaine is held in the right hand. The needle is inserted between the two abducted fingers of the left hand at right angles to the skin and advanced until contact is made with the symphysis pubis. It is then redirected to pass just inferior to the lower border of the arch of the symphysis. The syringe is aspirated to exclude blood vessel perforation and the solution is injected. A dosage regimen commencing at 0.2 ml/kg at birth and tapering to 0.1 ml/kg at age 10 years has been found satisfactory.

Postoperative analgesia can be assured for at least 6 hours following a successful block.

Regional Nerve Block

Supplemental regional nerve block with bupivacaine has been successfully used to supplement general anesthesia in children (Shandling and Steward). This reduces the general anesthetic requirements and the need for postoperative analgesics. The technique is applicable to all operations on the external genitalia, including hydrocelectomy and orchiopexy, and is particularly appropriate in outpatient surgery. While bupivacaine 0.5 per cent is recommended, motor blockade may be avoided by the use of 0.25 per cent bupivacaine.

IMPAIRED RENAL FUNCTION

The child with impaired renal function poses numerous problems and challenges to the anesthesiologist:

1. Acid-base imbalance. There is increasing metabolic acidosis, producing an adverse effect on most of the body's systems.
2. Electrolyte imbalance.
   a. Hyperkalemia secondary to the metabolic acidosis.
   b. Hypernatremia is usual but hyponatremia is occasionally seen.
   c. Other electrolyte abnormalities.
3. Hypertension.
4. Severe anemia. This results in an increased cardiac output, which may result in high-output cardiac failure.
5. The child may be on numerous medications, all of which should be continued up to the time of surgery.
6. There is a high risk of infection.

Anesthetic management of these patients is dictated by the above limitations and includes very careful monitoring, blood transfusions to maintain a hemoglobin level of 9 g/100 ml, sterile techniques if possible, and avoidance of myocardial depression. Shock may result from anesthesia administered soon after dialysis because of the possible presence of hypovolemia. Light halothane or isoflurane anesthesia is most appropriate. Muscle relaxants are usually required in reduced dosage and must be carefully monitored with a blockade monitor. An advantage of isoflurane is the degree of muscle relaxation obtained, which may obviate the need for muscle relaxants. Succinylcholine, with prior treatment with a small dose of nondepolarizing muscle relaxant to prevent muscle fasciculations, may be used carefully in the absence of significant reduction or elevation in serum potassium levels. Intravenous fluids should be used with care to avoid overloading and central venous pressure should be monitored. Five per cent dextrose with 0.2 per cent NaCl is most appropriate. Perioperative arterial blood gases and electrolyte levels should be checked at regular intervals and adjustments made.

RENAL TRANSPLANTATION

Anesthetic management in renal transplantation follows the same principles as those for the patient with impaired renal function. Usually the child has had recent dialysis and is in chemical and electrolyte balance. The child may be anesthetized with isoflurane, which offers a considerable degree of muscle relaxation; it is virtually nonmetabolized and therefore is excreted through the lungs, but it does produce some myocardial depression. Alternatively droperidol, fentanyl citrate (Sublimaze), and diazepam (Valium) may be used; these produce little myocardial depression and do not rely on the kidneys for elimination, but do require supplemental muscle relaxants. Either technique appears to work well, providing modest doses for every drug. Hypotension should be corrected with dopamine. Intravenous fluids should be carefully managed and central venous pressure continuously monitored.

POSTOPERATIVE CARE

Emergence from Anesthesia

The conclusion of surgery and the emergence from anesthesia are potentially dangerous periods. The child should be awakening and responding to stimuli. Endotracheal extubation should receive all the attention to detail given to intubation. At this critical time, the potential for hypoxia is great; the possible causes include residual relaxation, hypothermia, continuing effect of central nervous system depressant drugs, and splinting of the muscles of respiration by pain, surgical dressings, or gastric dilatation. The possibility of pneumothorax following renal surgery should always be considered, and the chest should be examined. The risky journey from the operating room to the recovery room should be made with the child breathing oxygen and with the attendance of a member of the anesthesia group and one of the surgical team.

The Recovery Room

The child continues to receive intensive care in the recovery room under the attention of trained personnel. Here, vital signs are continually monitored; the airway is checked, and ventilation is measured with a Wright spirometer. The dressings are inspected for possible bleeding. The child breathes humidified oxygen and receives necessary pain medication. Excessive nausea and vomiting are treated with promethazine (Phenergan) or trimethobenzamide (Tigan) suppositories. Urinary output is carefully measured. When the child is fully awake and in satisfactory condition and has been checked by both anesthesiologist and urologist, he is sent to the postoperative ward or, in rare instances, to the intensive care unit.

Postoperative Intravenous Fluid Therapy

During the postoperative period, the child who does not have impaired renal function receives intravenous fluid therapy to supply maintenance and replacement fluids only until he can adequately ingest, retain, and absorb oral fluids. The management of the child with azotemia is reviewed in Chapter 28.

Guidelines for maintenance intravenous fluid vary widely both for composition and for volume (Bennett et al; Herbert et al; Wylie and Churchill-Davidson). We use, as a starting point, 5 per cent dextrose in 0.2 per cent sodium chloride, 100 ml/kg per 24 hours, except that infants less than 7 days old receive 50 ml/kg per 24 hours. These dosages must be constantly adjusted according to the clinical response.

Fluid overload in the child is an ever-present danger that can be avoided only by the following measures:

1. Writing down explicit instructions.
2. Carefully monitoring the patient's pulse, arterial blood pressure, central venous pressure (optional), and urine volume (normal is 15 to 30 ml per hour); chest auscultation; and regularly weighing infants.
3. Using controlled-volume administration, for example with one of the following:
   a. Controlled-volume container (such as Buretrol).
   b. Volume-control minidrop intravenous regulator.
   c. Holter intravenous pump.

Requirements for maintenance fluids will be increased by fever and excessive sweating and decreased by an atmosphere with high humidity. Because of the infant's propensity to hypoglycemia in the postoperative period, all intravenous fluids should contain 5 per cent dextrose.

Replacement fluids are given as 5 per cent dextrose in Ringer's lactate or as whole blood, as required. The volume required is determined by the response of the pulse and by arterial blood pressure, central venous pressure, and urine output. Additional electrolytes, especially potassium, are given in quantities determined by serum electrolyte levels. When large volumes of replacement fluid are required, arterial blood gas determinations will reveal metabolic derangements that may require correction. Very rarely, in major urologic surgery, a period of parenteral alimentation may be required to supply nutritional requirements and to rest the gastrointestinal tract (Buntain et al).

The Intensive Care Unit

The intensive care unit has evolved in recent years to continue on a longer-term basis the intensive care given to the child in the operating room and recovery room. Consequently, the most important component of the intensive care facility is a specially trained, dedicated staff whose skilled use and intelligent interpretation of the elaborate monitoring and therapeutic equipment ensure the best in continuing care for the acutely ill child. Physicians of various specialties share in and contribute to this care; however, one physician must have the ultimate responsibility and authority. In the case of the pediatric urologic patient, that physician clearly is the pediatric urologist. Intensive care is expensive care, however; consequently, it should be used only when necessary, and the child should be transferred to the pediatric ward as soon as his condition safely permits.

OUTPATIENT SURGERY FOR PEDIATRIC UROLOGY

Numerous pediatric urologic procedures can be safely performed on an outpatient basis, especially cystoscopy, minor surgery on the external genitalia, hydrocelectomy, and orchiopexy. These procedures comprise over 50 per cent of a busy pediatric urologic practice.

The advantages for the child and his family are considerable. These include minimal separation from parents with reduction in psychological disturbance, less disruption of the family routine, considerable reduction in cost, and reduced risk of nosocomial infections from cross-contamination (Othersen and Clatworthy).

Preoperative evaluation and preparation are no different from that for inpatient surgery, with the exception that premedication is frequently omitted. However, premedication is desirable for children returning for multiple surgeries. Anesthetic management is also similar to that for inpatient surgery. Experience has shown that fears of postoperative problems from endotracheal intubation in the outpatient are unfounded if intubation is skillfully done (Levy and Coakley; Trump). From 1970 to 1980, 7466 children were intubated at the Surgicenter in Phoenix. Only one patient was admitted to the hospital; this child had moderately severe croup which was treated overnight with humidification and racemic epinephrine, and the child was dismissed the following day (Reed WA, personal communication, 1981).

Following surgery, the child should be transferred to the outpatient recovery room in the care of an anesthesiologist and a member of the surgical team. There the patient is carefully monitored. When all is in order, the child may be released in the custody of his parents after an average stay in the recovery room of about 2 hours. Before release, the child should be pain-free, the operative site completely dry, and nausea or vomiting under control. The child should be able to retain oral fluid intake and preferably have voided, although this is not always possible. On release, the parents should receive written instructions and telephone numbers of those whom they should call if problems arise. The most common cause of postoperative admission to the hospital is bleeding, and it cannot be emphasized enough that the operative site must be absolutely dry on dismissal from the institution. The efficacy and safety of outpatient surgery in children has been clearly established, and further growth can be expected in the years ahead.

BIBLIOGRAPHY

Bacon AK: An alternative block for post-circumcision analgesia. Anaesth Inten Care 5:63, 1977.

Bennett EJ, Daughety MJ, Jenkins MT: Some controversial aspects of fluids for the anesthetized neonate. Anesth Analg (Cleve) 49:478, 1970.

Britt BA, Kalow W: Malignant hyperthermia: a statistical review. Can Anaesth Soc J 17:293, 1970.

Buntain WL, Lynn HB, Cloutier MD, et al: Management of the pediatric surgical patient. Mayo Clin Proc 47:654, 1972.

Campbell MF: Caudal anesthesia in children. J Urol 30:245, 1933.

Carney FMT, Van Dyke RA: Halothane hepatitis: a critical review. Anesth Analg (Cleve) 51:135, 1972.

Cohen DD, Dillon JB: Anesthesia for outpatient surgery. JAMA 196:1114, 1966.

Cohen EN (Chairman): Occupational disease among operating room personnel: a national study. (Report of an Ad Hoc Committee on the Effect of Trace Anesthetics on the Health of Operating Room Personnel, American Society of Anesthesiologists). Anesthesiology 41:321, 1974.

Dawson B, Lynn HB: The pediatric patient in the operating room. Surg Clin North Am 45:949, 1965.

Farnsworth PB, Steiner E, Klein RM, et al: The value of routine preoperative chest roentgenograms in infants and children. JAMA 244:582, 1980.

Ford JL, Reed WA: The Surgicenter: an innovation in the delivery and cost of medical care. Ariz Med 26:801, 1969.

Fortuna A: Caudal analgesia: a simple and safe technique in paediatric surgery. Br J Anaesth 39:165, 1967.

Gorman HM, Craythorne NWB: The effects of a new neuroleptanalgesia agent (Innovar) on renal function in man. Acta Anaesthesiol Scand (Suppl) 24:111, 1966.

Graff TD, Holzman RS, Benson DWL: Acid-base balance in infants during halothane anesthesia with the use of an adult circle-absorption system. Anesth Analg (Cleve) 43:583, 1964.

Gronert GA: Malignant hyperthermia. Anesthesiology 53:395, 1980.

Herbert WI, Scott EB, Lewis GB Jr: Fluid management of the pediatric surgical patient. Anesth Analg (Cleve) 50:376, 1971.

Lavis DM, Lunn JN, Rosen M: Glycopyrrolate in children. J Pediatr Surg 15:477, 1980.

Leigh MD, McCoy DD, Belton MK, et al: Bradycardia following intravenous administration of succinylcholine chloride to infants and children. Anesthesiology 18:698, 1957.

Levy M-L, Coakley CS: Survey of "in and out surgery"—first year. South Med J 61:995, 1968.

Lourey CJ, McDonald JH: Caudal anaesthesia in infants and children. Anaesth Intens Care 1:547, 1973.

Lundy JS: Balanced anesthesia. Minn Med 9:399, 1926.

Mathews DH, Avery ME, Jude JR: Closed-chest cardiac massage in the newborn infant. JAMA 183:964, 1963.

Mazze RI, Trudell JR, Cousins MJ: Methoxyflurane metabolism and renal dysfunction: clinical correlation in man. Anesthesiology 35:247, 1971.

Orwoll G: The doctor's duty of disclosure. Anesth Analg (Cleve) 53:759, 1974.

Othersen HB Jr, Clatworthy HW Jr: Outpatient herniorrhaphy for infants. Am J Dis Child 116:78, 1968.

Reed WA, Crouch BL, Ford JL: Anesthesia and operations on outpatients. Clin Anesth 10:335, 1974.

Ryan JF, Kerr WS Jr: Malignant hyperthermia: a catastrophic complication. J Urol 109:879, 1973.

Schulte-Steinberg O: Neural blockade for pediatric surgery. In Neural Blockade in Clinical Anesthesia and Management of Pain. Edited by Cousins MJ, Bridenbaugh PO. Philadelphia, JB Lippincott Co., 1980, pp 503–523.

Shandling B, Steward DJ: Regional analgesia for postoperative pain in pediatric outpatient surgery. J Pediatr Surg 15:477, 1980.

Shirkey HC: Drug dosage for infants and children. JAMA 193:443, 1965.

Thaler MM, Stobie GHC: An improved technic of external cardiac compression in infants and young children. N Engl J Med 269:606, 1963.

Trump D: Discussion of Dr. Thomas S. Morse's paper on outpatient surgical procedures. Meeting of the American Association of Pediatric Surgeons, Hamilton, Bermuda, April 23, 1971.

Wylie WD, Churchill-Davidson HC: A Practice of Anaesthesia. Third ed. London, Lloyd-Luke (Medical Books), 1972, p 731.

3

OFFICE AND OUTPATIENT PEDIATRIC UROLOGY

RONALD RABINOWITZ AND ANTHONY A. CALDAMONE

Over the past century, the pediatric aspect of urology has advanced from a small percentage of urologic practice to a subspecialty of urology whose practitioners treat children predominantly or exclusively (Bicknell). While pediatric urologists see a wide range of unusual, complex, challenging, and interesting prenatal, congenital, and acquired conditions, the basic practice of pediatric urology begins with the office and outpatient evaluation, and often includes office or outpatient surgical procedures. Indeed, except for major reconstructive procedures, a progressively larger percentage of pediatric urologic practice is completed without necessity for overnight hospitalization.

OFFICE PEDIATRIC UROLOGY

The office of the pediatric urologist usually serves as the place of initial contact with the patient and the patient's family. It is the setting for the history, physical examination, discussion of diagnosis, proposed evaluation, and review of evaluation, as well as the location for minor surgical procedures. While it must be a comfortable area for adult discussion, the object of everyone's concern, the child, must also be made to feel at ease. The physician should direct a significant part of his attention to the patient. It is often helpful to greet the child first, thereby demonstrating who is the focus of attention. Every effort should be made to make the child feel that the physician is a friend, not a foe. Appropriate toys, puzzles, children's books, and cartoon wallpaper may be very helpful. As in the pediatrician's office and the operating room, the ambient temperature should be comfortably warm for the child.

History

Examination of the child for urologic complaints was thoroughly outlined over 30 years ago by Campbell (1951). Although the indications for various diagnostic studies have changed and the techniques and studies have been altered, improved, and advanced, the basic aspects of the physical examination and urinalysis were concisely outlined and appropriately emphasized. Procedures were given for examination of the child's abdomen, genitalia, and rectum.

A 10-year review of the pediatric aspect of a urologic practice was published in 1962 by Tudor et al. There were 1622 girls (67 per cent) and 781 boys. Of the total, 59 per cent (1417) were seen because of urinary infections, the vast majority in females. There were 578 anomalies seen. Thirty-seven of the 71 renal anomalies were ureteropelvic junction obstructions. Of the genital anomalies, there were 80 cases of cryptorchidism, hernia, or hydrocele and 15 testicular torsions. Penile problems included 69 cases of hypospadias, 166 meatal stenoses, and 31 urethral strictures. Of the 1196 upper tract studies in girls with "bladder neck syndrome," 7.5 per cent were abnormal. Of the 291 of these girls who had cystograms, 30 (10 per cent) demonstrated reflux.

Office Population

In a busy two-physician pediatric urology practice in 1981, 2395 children were seen

(Kroovand). This number is comparable to the entire 10-year experience reported two decades earlier (Tudor et al). In Kroovand's review, unlike that of Tudor, 64 per cent of patients were boys. Of the 682 new patients, 43.5 per cent were seen because of voiding dysfunction with or without infection (69 per cent of these 297 children were girls). There were 102 hypospadiacs, 109 with cryptorchidism, hernia, or hydrocele, and 34 with meatal stenosis. One hundred eighty-three children with urinary tract infections were evaluated with excretory urograms and voiding cystourethrograms. Forty-four per cent (81) had reflux. Including follow-up studies, 562 excretory urograms and 350 voiding cystourethrograms were performed, along with 3 renal scans and 131 ultrasound examinations. Seven hundred two children (79 per cent boys) underwent a surgical procedure during that year (29 per cent of the total number of children seen). Of the new patients seen, 77 per cent were referred by pediatricians or family practitioners, 8 per cent by other urologists, 3 per cent by pediatric surgeons, and 12 per cent from patient families. Forty-four per cent of the 682 new patients underwent a surgical procedure.

This review of the practice of Kroovand and Perlmutter was quite similar to the single physician practice of one of the authors of this chapter (R.R.), who saw 1574 children in 1982 (56 per cent boys). Many of the diagnostic categories and percentages were similar. Of the 533 new patients, 48 per cent had urinary infections, voiding dysfunction, or both (81 per cent of these 256 children were girls). There were also 71 hypospadiacs, 82 with cryptorchidism, hernia, or hydrocele, and 32 with meatal stenosis. Of the new patients, 163 had excretory urograms and 179 had voiding cystourethrograms. Forty-one per cent of the new patients with urinary tract infections had vesicoureteral reflux. Including follow-up studies, there were 267 excretory urograms, 387 voiding cystourethrograms, 86 renal scans, 55 nuclear cystograms, and 84 ultrasound examinations. These numbers reflect the increasing use of radioisotopes in pediatric urology (Bueschen and Witten; Majd and Belman). During the year, 338 children (72 per cent boys) underwent a surgical procedure (21 per cent of the total number of children seen). Eighty per cent of the new patients seen were referred by pediatricians, 6 per cent by family practitioners, 5 per cent by other urologists, and 5 per cent by pediatric surgeons, and 4

per cent were brought in directly by the childrens' families.

Office Management of Commonly Referred Conditions

URINARY TRACT INFECTIONS AND VESICOURETERAL REFLUX. One of the most common conditions referred to the pediatric urologist is a urinary tract infection. Many children will have had culture documentation, while others may have had only an abnormal urinalysis. Culture documentation is imperative, and once infection is documented, treatment is instituted and uroradiographic evaluation (excretory urogram and voiding cystourethrogram) is indicated (Hollerman). In the past, it was thought that evaluation of girls could be delayed until the second or third infection, but follow-up studies indicate that the vast majority (80 per cent in white female children) will get a recurrence and about one third will have reflux (Smellie et al; Fair et al; Kunin; Savage et al; Parkkulainen and Kosunen). If there is a question about the validity of a culture obtained from a urine collection bag or voided urine specimen, the bladder is catheterized with a small (5 French) feeding tube, or suprapubic aspiration is performed. Both of these methods are easily carried out in the office. Treatment of the infection is initiated once the diagnosis is presumed or confirmed. The child with severe clinical upper-tract infection, systemic symptoms, and possible sepsis is hospitalized for parenteral antibiotics and fluid balance. With a less serious infection that appears to involve the upper urinary tract, outpatient treatment with oral broad-spectrum antibiotics is usually sufficient. Clinical lower-tract infections and those with asymptomatic bacteriuria are also treated with oral agents.

It is the contention of some that those children without signs of upper-tract infection need not be evaluated radiographically. This view is difficult to defend in the light of the very high rate of recurrence of infection and the fact that unrecognized previous urinary tract infections are quite common in children (Kunin; Savage et al; Smellie et al). The timing of the uroradiographic investigation may be important. If the child is quite ill or does not respond reasonably quickly, obstruction must be promptly ruled out. This is accomplished in girls with an excretory urogram or sonogram to evaluate the upper urinary tract. In boys, a cystourethrogram must be performed to rule out a posterior urethral valve. The voiding cystourethrogram to evaluate for bladder abnormalities and reflux is less urgent in girls. If the child responds promptly to treatment, waiting 4 to 6 weeks for the radiographic studies allows for resolution of the associated edema and inflammation that accompany the infection and might distort interpretation of the films (van Gool and Tanagho; Pais and Retik; Grana et al). Since the risk of reflux and recurrence is high, the febrile child with a urinary tract infection should be maintained on a prophylactic dosage of an antibiotic in the interim until the radiographic results are known (Belman). Performing an expression cystogram with the patient under anesthesia should be discouraged. The discomfort incurred by an awake child treated by trained sympathetic personnel is minimal, and there is some risk incurred with anesthesia, however slight. In addition, the sensitivity of the cystogram in demonstrating reflux is reduced in the asleep state (Vlahakis et al).

The most common major structural anomaly found in children with urinary infection is vesicoureteral reflux. The combination of reflux and infection markedly increases the risk for renal parenchymal loss and scarring (Ransley and Risdon; Lenaghan et al). Therefore, once reflux is documented, long-term prophylaxis with a safe antibacterial is begun. Resolution of the reflux will occur in a large percentage of these children (Normand and Smellie; Edwards et al).

Cystoscopy to evaluate the ureterovesical junctions is rarely indicated as routine, as it does not alter the treatment plan (Johnson et al). Those children who have more severe grades of reflux (IV and V) and/or breakthrough pyelonephritis will probably require surgical correction. Cystoscopy may be carried out at that time (Scott and Stansfeld; Rolleston et al; Willscher et al). The remainder may be managed with interval evaluations that initially include an excretory urogram or renal scan every 2 years and an annual voiding cystourethrogram. The time interval for these studies is somewhat arbitrary and may be increased after 2 years to a voiding cystourethrogram every 18 months and an IVP every 3 years. Direct (catheter) nuclear cystograms may be interspersed with voiding cystourethrograms, and radioisotope differential renal scans are especially helpful in evaluating the function of chronically scarred kidneys.

ENURESIS. Many children are seen in the pediatric urologic office with the complaint of wetting. In the absence of a history of urinary tract infection, if the only symptom is nocturnal enuresis and the physical examination is normal, radiographic and cystoscopic investigation is not indicated in this group (Perlmutter). Treatment, if indicated, can be conditioning with an enuresis alarm or use of a pharmacologic agent. It is important to recall the self-limited nature of this process. The primary role of the pediatric urologist who is referred a child with bedwetting is to provide information and reassurance, and secondarily to select out those children in whom further evaluation or treatment is indicated. It is often helpful to describe this condition as a specific defect that will improve with time, in order to relieve any blame that has been placed on the child as a result of attributing this to laziness or retaliation. If the wetting is associated with urinary infection or other signs or symptoms such as gastrointestinal problems, gait abnormalities, or wetting with a normal voiding pattern, all of which are suggestive of structural pathology (e.g., urinary obstruction, ectopic ureter, or neuropathic bladder), then further investigation is indicated. In addition, daytime wetting may signal a structural or voiding abnormality that may require further evaluation. While the age of achievement of *daytime* continence is variable, children over age 6 years may be considered for further investigation, although specific causative pathology is rarely found. Further study usually begins with an excretory urogram and voiding cystourethrogram, but may also include urodynamic studies.

HEMATURIA. Microscopic hematuria in children is most commonly renal in origin (Chan); however, any child with gross hematuria must have an excretory urogram. If the hematuria is associated with infection, the child needs to be evaluated with both an excretory urogram and a voiding cystourethrogram, the same way any child with a urinary tract infection is evaluated. If the hematuria is associated with trauma, even seemingly minor trauma, an excretory urogram must be performed, in view of the increased risk that minor trauma may initiate bleeding in an already abnormal kidney (Campbell, 1970; Malek). If the trauma is to the pelvis, perineum, or external genitalia, a urethrogram and/or voiding cystourethrogram may also be needed. If casts are seen in the urine, then the child needs to be evaluated by a pediatric nephrologist. The role of cystoscopy in children with hematuria is extremely limited (Walther and Kaplan; Johnson et al). Indeed, if no radiographic abnormality is found in a child with hematuria, it is extremely rare to find an etiology by cystoscopy. Boys with post-void bloody urethral drainage or blood spotting on their undershorts (urethrorrhagia) should not undergo cystoscopy unless a radiographic lesion is identified (Kaplan and Brock).

FORESKIN. A common office referral is the boy with redundant foreskin and/or foreskin adherence. Many parents express concern about residual foreskin following neonatal circumcision. It must be explained that circumcision is rarely medically necessary and that it is highly unlikely that redundant foreskin will present a problem. Foreskin adherence represents normal or physiologic phimosis seen during the childhood and preadolescent years. The retraction of the foreskin or release of the adherence between foreskin and glans is gradual, spontaneous, and normal. It is common practice for some physicians to instruct parents to retract the foreskin daily to clean secretions. This should be discouraged, as it only promotes the development of a circumferential scar and true phimosis. The uncircumcised infant has physiologic phimosis which will spontaneously resolve in almost all. Parents may request circumcision because of thick, white "pus" that accumulates between the foreskin and glans. This "pus" is actually a collection of the shedding epithelial cells between the glans and the inner prepuce. These cells accumulate into thick white pearls that gradually separate the foreskin from the glans, and the parents can be assured that this is not infection. The foreskin should not be forcibly retracted to release these collections. They eventually work their way to the surface junction between the foreskin and glans (Wallerstein; Klauber et al).

CRYPTORCHIDISM. The pediatric urologist is often asked to evaluate a boy for cryptorchidism. The office examination is extremely important for accurate diagnosis. The boy should feel comfortable in the office surroundings, and the ambient temperature, as well as the examiner's hands, should be warm. The examiner should proceed in an organized fashion rather than immediately examining the scrotum. This will give the boy time to relax and will help the examiner to make the distinction between a retractile and a truly undescended testis. Examining the boy in the sitting cross-legged position or having him blow up a balloon may be helpful in allowing the cremasteric muscles to relax. The cremasteric reflex becomes more active a few months after birth and is most active through puberty. Retractile testes account for a high proportion of boys referred for supposedly undescended testes. The empty hemiscrotum is usually of normal size in boys with a retractile testis, whereas it is small and poorly rugated in those with the cryptorchidism. A retractile testis can be manipulated into the scrotum by gentle traction without immediate upward migration.

If one still cannot distinguish between a retractile and a true undescended testis, HCG stimulation will resolve this question. In the boy with bilateral nonpalpable testes, HCG stimulation studies can be diagnostic of the presence of testicular tissue when pre- and post-HCG testosterone, FSH, and LH studies are compared (Levitt et al). If cryptorchidism is associated with hypospadias, especially of severe degree, there is an increased incidence of an abnormality of sexual differentiation and chromosomal analysis is indicated (Rajfer and Walsh).

Office Procedures

As a general rule, few actual procedures are performed in the pediatric urologic office. Those that are performed must require no anesthesia or only local anesthesia and include meatal and post-hypospadias urethral dilation, meatotomy, release of foreskin adhesions and/or post-circumcision skin bridges, and lysis of labial adhesions.

MEATUS AND URETHRA. The boy referred with a diagnosis of "meatal stenosis" may indeed have a relatively small meatus, but observation of the urinary stream for deflection, straining, and pinpoint caliber is much more diagnostic. The correlation between the visual meatal size and the calibrated size is poor (Litvak et al). True meatal stenosis is the result of meatitis and is seen almost exclusively in boys circumcised in infancy. If there is significant meatal stenosis, management may be carried out in the office. A thin web of scarring over the meatus may be easily broken with the nozzle of a one-eighth ounce ophthalmic ointment tube or a small hemostat. Thick meatal scars that must be divided require a local anesthetic. This can be performed in some, but one must have the understanding and support of the parents and the child. Thus, an older child or adolescent or a baby will tolerate local anesthesia much better than a 2- to 4-year-old.

Boys who have recently undergone hypospadias repair may need meatal or urethral calibration with the nozzle tip of an ophthalmic ointment applicator or a metal sound. Here again, gentleness is of the utmost importance to retain the child's confidence.

FORESKIN. Adherence of the foreskin is generally best left alone, as it usually gradually lyses in time. Penile post-circumcision skin bridges, however, are commonly very thick and require incision. Often, the portion on the glans must be sutured for closure and hemostasis. Since this is rarely an urgent condition, one can usually wait until the boy is old enough to tolerate local anesthesia.

LABIAL ADHESIONS. Mild labial adhesions often need no treatment and will spontaneously lyse in time. Long adhesions that contribute to stasis of urine can be bluntly lysed with a cotton swab and lubricant. The application of estrogen cream may aid in keratinization of the denuded labial edges and prevent re-adhesion.

OUTPATIENT SURGERY

Ambulatory, outpatient, or day surgery programs have markedly expanded over the past few years to the extent that more than half of all surgical procedures can be performed in this fashion (AMA Socioeconomic Monitoring System). Ambulatory surgery is available in two thirds of all hospitals in the United States, and 16 per cent of all hospital surgery is performed on an ambulatory basis (American Medical News). Some insurance plans are now offering higher fees to the surgeon if certain procedures are carried out on an outpatient basis (Physicians' News Summary; Same-Day Surgery).

Historical Aspects

In ancient times, temples were used as houses of healing. The sick were administered to, often on an ambulatory basis, 5000 years ago. Most conditions then managed were lacerations and fractures. In the Middle Ages, while the number of hospitals were few, some had outpatient facilities (Schultz).

In the United States, the first outpatient department opened in 1818 at the Massachusetts General Hospital. There was little actual surgery performed, however, and the outpatient clinics were generally used as dispensaries (Schultz).

In 1909, early in the modern era of outpatient surgery, James Nicoll reported on more than 7000 pediatric surgical cases performed on an outpatient basis. He concluded that outpatient surgery in children was safe, successful, and cost effective. He stated ". . . I have no alternative to the opinion that the treatment of a large number of the cases at present treated indoor constitutes a waste of the resources of a children's hospital or a children's ward. The results obtained in the out-patient department at a tithe of the cost are equally good." Scattered reports of the success of outpatient surgical procedures appeared over the next half century, many dealing with outpatient hernia repairs and/or pediatric procedures (Herzfeld; Farquharson). In the mid to late 1960's, hospital-based outpatient surgery programs began springing up (Cohen and Dillon; Levy and Coakley), followed shortly thereafter by free-standing ambulatory surgery centers, the model of which is the Phoenix Surgicenter (Reed and Ford; Reed; Cloud et al). In addition to hospital-based and free-standing civilian ambulatory surgical facilities, this concept is also being utilized by the military (Lenneville and Steinbruckner).

Surgical Procedures

The list of surgical procedures performed on an outpatient basis has been progressively increasing. The list began with dilation and curettage, cystoscopy, vasectomy, circumcision, excision of skin lesions, myringotomy, hemorrhoidectomy, and herniorrhaphy, and now includes laparoscopy, tonsillectomy, varicose vein stripping, rhinoplasty, augmentation mammoplasty, strabismus repair, creation of arteriovenous fistulas for hemodialysis, varicocelectomy, unilateral and bilateral orchiopexy, and some hypospadias repairs (Reed and Dawson; Caldamone and Rabinowitz; Patterson et al; Nabatoff). A significant percentage of urologic procedures are amenable to ambulatory surgery facilities, and a significant percentage of the ambulatory surgery performed is urologic. Approximately one fourth of the utilization of pediatric outpatient units is for urologic procedures (Cohen et al; Kroovand and Perlmutter). During 1976 and 1977, Kroovand and Perlmutter performed 46 per cent of their urologic procedures on an outpatient basis. That percentage has remained relatively stable (48 per cent in 1981) (Kroovand), and is similar to the 58 per cent reported by Rabinowitz in Rochester, New York, and the 59 observed at the Children's Hospital of Philadelphia by one of the authors of this chapter (A.C.).

Patient Selection

In selecting children for outpatient surgery, pre-existing medical conditions, prior surgical history, simultaneous operative procedures, and family and social factors must all be considered (Caldamone and Rabinowitz). In the initial assessment, children with pre-existing medical conditions must have consultation regarding their condition, and anesthetic consultation to confirm that the condition is stable and does not represent an undue anesthetic risk. The length of time required for the procedure must also be considered. Even for outpatient orchiopexy, 9 per cent over a 4-year period had a major pre-existing medical condition (cardiac anomaly, stable seizures or other neurologic condition, stable asthma), and none had a postoperative complication (Rabinowitz). The personal or family history of anesthesia must be obtained, and any history of untoward reaction assessed. This often entails preoperative anesthetic consultation (Dimino).

The procedure best suited for an ambulatory center is a brief one with minimal trauma. Therefore, a history of a prior surgical procedure of the same nature or in the same area might mitigate against day surgery. The pediatric urologist is not infrequently asked to explore an inguinal area for a testis that has had a prior herniorrhaphy or failed orchiopexy. Nine (6 per cent) of 148 outpatient orchiopexies followed either a failed orchiopexy (6) or a prior inguinal herniorrhaphy (3) in which the previously descended testis was entrapped by scar and/or suture. While all of these were successfully managed as outpatients, these families were informed preoperatively of the possibility of extensive dissection and prolonged anesthesia and, thus, the increased probability of the child's requiring overnight hospitalization (Caldamone and Rabinowitz; Rabinowitz).

More than one operative procedure during the same period of anesthesia can be done on an outpatient basis. The same factors in selection hold (Caldamone and Rabinowitz).

The family and social circumstances must be accurately assessed in selecting children for ambulatory surgery. These factors include the distance that the family lives from the ambulatory facility, the assessed capability of the family to understand postoperative instructions and to handle minor postoperative problems, and the acceptance by the family that the quality of care and safety are not jeopardized by this method of treatment (Dimino; Caldamone and Rabinowitz).

Anesthesia

The anesthesiologist is an important partner in outpatient pediatric urologic surgery. The anesthesiologist must have prior knowledge of any anticipated surgical difficulties or chronic medical conditions. Ideally, the child should be in excellent health, the procedure should be relatively short, and recovery should be rapid, pain-free, and without physical limitation (Dawson). Most children are not premedicated (Steward, 1980) and their parents remain with them until they are taken to the operating room. The children are met by their parents as soon as they recover from the anesthetic. Many are ready for discharge within 2 hours of completion of the procedure and should be able to ambulate, retain oral fluids, and be relatively free of pain and nausea (Dawson). These ideals are easy to accomplish in children undergoing brief procedures (cystoscopy, circumcision, meatotomy, excision of skin lesions, and herniorrhaphy). However, we are beginning to perform longer and more extensive procedures (orchiopexy, hypospadias repair) on an ambulatory basis. For these children, the anesthetic may last 1½ hours and there is a higher incidence of postoperative nausea. Therefore, any child undergoing more than a 30-minute anesthetic period should have intraoperative and postoperative intravenous fluid hydration. The intravenous tube is commonly not removed until the time of discharge. This assures adequate hydration, yet does not force the child to take large volumes of oral fluids, which may contribute to nausea, vomiting, and increased discomfort.

The anesthetic technique is at the discretion of the anesthesiologist. While some are reluctant to intubate an outpatient (Cohen et al; Morse; Smith), many do use intubation during the procedure, and this has not affected the outcome or resulted in increased complications (Dawson; Steward, 1973; Caldamone and Rabinowitz; Jones and Smith). However, sore throat is much more frequent following use of an oropharyngeal airway (Steward, 1973). An analgesic can be administered during anesthesia to lessen the early postoperative pain. Alternatively, an ilioinguinal nerve block or caudal block using bupivacaine (Marcaine) administered prior to the termination of the general anesthetic can greatly relieve postoperative pain and quicken the early recovery.

Complications

Outpatient surgery has been highly successful from a complication standpoint. At the Surgicenter, over 50,000 patients have been treated with an overall hospitalization rate of 0.23 per cent. There were no deaths or cardiac arrests (Dawson). There was one postoperative death reported in a 5-year review of over 13,000 ambulatory surgery patients (Natof). Approximately 95 per cent of children who undergo ambulatory surgery are discharged the same day (Davenport et al; Caldamone and Rabinowitz; Kroovand and Perlmutter; Jones and Smith; Rabinowitz). The incidence of hospitalization is increased in certain procedures with a higher risk of postoperative bleeding (e.g., tonsillectomy), extensive dissection (e.g., umbilical herniorrhaphy), and longer anesthetic (e.g., orchiopexy) (Fahy and Marshall). Those children requiring hospitalization are almost invariably recognized prior to discharge. Fisher reported only a single instance in 10 years of a child being re-admitted after being sent home the day of outpatient surgery. Caldamone and Rabinowitz, and later Rabinowitz, reported no re-admissions in 4 years of outpatient orchiopexies. Likewise, Kroovand and Perlmutter reported no re-admissions in over 300 outpatient procedures during 1 year.

Advantages

The advantages of ambulatory pediatric surgery versus inpatient surgery are multiple and significant. Factors that must be considered are patient safety, surgical success, psychologic effects, and cost effectiveness.

The minimal risk and rapid recovery from modern pediatric anesthesia has permitted an increasing number of procedures in children to be performed on an outpatient basis. There has not been a noticeable increase in morbidity with endotracheal intubation.

From a surgical standpoint, the success rate has not been diminished by ambulatory surgery. If anything, the surgeon must be even more careful to be certain that hemostasis is secure and that tissue is handled gently. The shorter the time spent in the hospital and the fewer people the child comes in contact with, the lesser the risk of acquisition of nosocomial infection (Othersen and Clatworthy). Early mobilization has not affected results of herniorrhaphy (Othersen and Clatworthy) or orchiopexy (Caldamone and Rabinowitz).

The more brief the hospitalization and the shorter the separation from parents, the less the psychologic stress on the child. Children under 4 years of age appear to be more severely psychologically stressed by hospitalization (Vaughan). These younger children are more dependent on their mothers (Vernon et al), and there are significantly fewer postoperative behavioral disturbances when the parents spend more time with their hospitalized child (Prugh et al). Thus, ambulatory surgery reduces the psychologic stress by making the hospitalization as brief as possible and by minimizing the separation between parents and child.

Multiple studies have now confirmed the significant financial benefits of outpatient surgery (Reed and Dawson; Shah). The largest factor contributing to the increasing health care costs is the per diem cost of hospital care (Schultz). Savings of 50 per cent per procedure are common (Hoffmann; Reed and Dawson; Caldamone and Rabinowitz). This, however, does not include the additional savings of reduction in hospital bed usage, decreased requirement for hospital personnel, and savings in laboratory fees.

Ambulatory pediatric surgery is safe, surgically successful, psychologically less detrimental than inpatient surgery, and cost effective. The benefits of outpatient surgery touted in 1909 by Nicoll are still valid today. "Infants and young children in a ward are noisy, and not infrequently malodorous. The main idea in their admission is the supposed benefit of 'trained' nursing. That benefit is largely wasted on them . . . continuous quiet rest on the back on the part of a young child in pain is a pretty idea, rarely obtainable, and not specially necessary after such operations. After operation in the outpatient room, such young children with their wounds closed by collodion or rubber plaster are easily carried home in their mothers' arms, and rest there more quietly, on the whole, than anywhere else.''

BIBLIOGRAPHY

American Medical Association Socioeconomic Monitoring System, 1982.

American Medical News, October 1, 1982, p 10.

Belman AB: Office pediatric urology. Urol Clin North Am 7:64, 1980.

Bicknell FB: Pediatric urology. *In* American Urological Association—Roche Series: The History of Urology, 1980.

Bueschen AJ, Witten DM: Radionuclide evaluation of renal function. Urol Clin North Am 6:307, 1979.

Caldamone AA, Rabinowitz R: Outpatient orchiopexy. J Urol 127:286, 1982.

Campbell MF: Methods of examination and diagnosis. *In* Clinical Pediatric Urology. Philadelphia, WB Saunders Co., 1951, pp 1–102.

Campbell MF: Urogenital injuries. *In* Urology. Third ed. Edited by MF Campbell, JH Harrison. Philadelphia, WB Saunders Co., 1970, pp 1890–1895.

Chan JCM: Hematuria and proteinuria in pediatric patient. Diagnostic approach. Urology 11:205, 1978.

Cloud DT, Reed WA, Ford JL, et al: The Surgicenter: a fresh concept in outpatient pediatric surgery. J Ped Surg 7:206, 1972.

Cohen D, Keneally J, Black A, et al: Experience with day stay surgery. J Ped Surg 15:21, 1980.

Cohen DD, Dillon JB: Anesthesia for outpatient surgery. JAMA 196:1114, 1966.

Davenport, HT, Shah CP, Robinson GC: Day surgery for children. Can Med Assoc J 105:498, 1971.

Dawson B: Anesthetic management. *In* Outpatient Surgery. Edited by RC Schultz. Philadelphia, Lea & Febiger, 1979, pp 29–44.

Dimino ER: Preparation of patients for short-stay surgery at CHNMC: assessment and recommendations. Clin Proc Child Hosp Nat Med Cent 38:310, 1979.

Edwards D, Normand ICS, Prescod N, et al: Disappearance of vesicoureteric reflux during long-term prophylaxis of urinary tract infection in children. Br Med J 2:285, 1977.

Fahy A, Marshall M: Postanaesthetic morbidity in outpatients. Br J Anaesth 41:433, 1969.

Fair WR, Govan DE, Friedland GW, et al: Urinary tract infections in children. Part 1. Young girls with non-refluxing ureters. West J Med 121:366, 1974.

Farquharson EL: Early ambulation with special reference to herniorrhaphy as an outpatient procedure. Lancet 2:517, 1955.

Fisher CG: Outpatient surgery. Dial Ped Urol 4(12):6, 1981.

Grana L, Kidd J, Idriss F, et al: Effect of chronic urinary tract infection on ureteral peristalsis. J Urol 94:652, 1965.

Herzfeld, G: Hernia in infancy. Am J Surg 39:422, 1938.

Hoffmann GL: Quality control in ambulatory surgery. Bull Am Coll Surg 66(11):6, 1981.

Hollerman CE: Urinary tract infection, reflux (nephropathy) and enuresis. *In* Pediatric Nephrology. New York, Medical Examination Publishing Company, Inc., 1979, p 238.

International Reflux Study Committee: Medical versus surgical treatment of primary vesicoureteral reflux. Pediatrics 67:392, 1981.

Johnson DK, Kroovand RL, Perlmutter AD: The changing role of cystoscopy in the pediatric patient. J Urol 123:232, 1980.

Jones SEF, Smith BAC: Anesthesia for pediatric day-surgery. J Ped Surg 15:31, 1980.

Kaplan GW, Brock WA: Idiopathic urethrorrhagia in boys. J Urol 128:1001, 1982.

Klauber GT, Mutter AZ, King LR, et al: Neonatal circumcision. Dial Ped Urol. 5(12):2, 1982.

Kroovand RL: Update on outpatient pediatric urology. Dial Ped Urol 5(8):2, 1982.

Kroovand RL, Perlmutter AD: Short stay surgery in pediatric urology. J Urol 120:483, 1978.

Kunin CM: The natural history of recurrent bacteriuria in schoolgirls. N Engl J Med 282:1443, 1970.

Lenaghan D, Whitaker JG, Jensen F, et al: The natural history of reflux and long-term effects of reflux on the kidney. J Urol 115:728, 1976.

Lenneville, MW, Steinbruckner KP: Marketing of a military ambulatory surgical center. Milit Med 147:963, 1982.

Levitt SB, Kogan SJ, Schneider KM, et al: Endocrine tests in phenotypic children with bilateral impalpable testes can reliably predict "congenital" anorchism. Urology 11:11, 1978.

Levy M-L, Coakley CS: Survey of "in and out surgery"—first year. South Med J 61:995, 1968.

Litvak AS, Morris JA, McRoberts JW: Normal size of the urethral meatus in boys. J Urol 115:736, 1976.

Majd M, Belman AB: Nuclear cystography in infants and children. Urol Clin North Am 6:395, 1979.

Malek RS: Renal trauma. Dial Ped Urol 3(5):6, 1980.

Morse TS: Pediatric outpatient surgery. J Ped Surg 7:283, 1972.

Nabatoff RA: Ambulatory surgery. Hosp Physician 18:15, 1982.

Natof HE: Complications associated with ambulatory surgery. JAMA 244:1116, 1980.

Nicoll JH: The surgery of infancy. Br Med J 2:753, 1909.

Normand C, Smellie J: Vesicoureteric reflux: the case for conservative management. *In* Reflux Nephropathy. Edited by J Hodson, P Kincaid-Smith. New York, Masson Publishing USA, Inc., 1979, pp 281–286.

Othersen HB Jr, Clatworthy HW Jr: Outpatient herniorrhaphy for infants. Am J Dis Child 116:78, 1968.

Pais VM, Retik AB: Reversible hydronephrosis in the neonate with urinary sepsis. N Engl J Med 292:465, 1975.

Parkkulainen KV, Kosunen TU: Follow-up of female children treated for chronic or recurrent urinary tract infection. Birth Defects 13:409, 1977.

Patterson JF Jr, Bechtoldt AA, Levin KJ: Ambulatory surgery in a university setting. JAMA 235:266, 1976.

Perlmutter AD: Enuresis. *In* Campbell's Urology. Edited by JH Harrison, RF Gittes, AD Perlmutter, et al. Philadelphia, WB Saunders Co., 1979, pp 1823–1834.

Physicians' News Summary, Blue Shield of the Rochester Area, December, 1982.

Prugh DG, Staub EM, Sands HH, et al: A study of the emotional reactions of children and families to hospitalization and illness. Am J Orthopsychiat 23:70, 1953.

Rabinowitz R: Update on outpatient pediatric urology. Dial Ped Urol 5(8):5, 1982.

Rajfer J, Walsh PC: The incidence of intersexuality in patients with hypospadias and cryptorchidism. J Urol 116:769, 1976.

Ransley PG: Vesicoureteric reflux: continuing surgical dilemma. Urology 12:246, 1978.

Ransley PG, Risdon RA: Reflux and renal scarring. Br J Radiol 14(Suppl):1, 1978.

Reed WA: The Surgicenter experience. Contemp Surg 20:66, 1982.

Reed WA, Dawson B: The ambulatory surgical facility. *In* Outpatient Surgery. Edited by RC Schultz. Philadelphia, Lea & Febiger, 1979, pp 15–24.

Reed WA, Ford JL: Development of an independent outpatient surgical center. Int Anesth Clin 14:113, 1976.

Rolleston GL, Maling TMJ, Hodson CJ: Intrarenal reflux and the scarred kidney. Arch Dis Child 49:531, 1974.

Same-Day Surgery, 3(8):93–96, 1979.

Savage DCL, Wilson MI, Ross EM, et al: Asymptomatic bacteriuria in girl entrants to Dundee primary schools. Br Med J 3:75, 1969.

Schultz RC: Outpatient surgery from antiquity to the present. In Outpatient Surgery. Edited by RC Schultz. Philadelphia, Lea & Febiger, 1979, pp 5–14.

Scott JES, Stansfeld JM: Ureteric reflux and renal scarring in children. Arch Dis Child 43:468, 1968.

Shah CP: Day-care surgery in Canada: evolution, policy and experience of provinces. Can Anaes Soc J 27:399, 1980.

Smellie J, Edwards D, Hunter N, et al: Vesico-ureteric reflux and renal scarring. Kidney Int 8(Suppl 4):s-65, 1975.

Smith RM: Anesthesia for outpatient and emergency surgery. In Anesthesia for Infants and Children. Fourth ed. St. Louis, CV Mosby Co., 1980, pp 510–521.

Steward DJ: Experiences with an outpatient anesthesia service for children. Anesth Analg 52:877, 1973.

Steward DJ: Anaesthesia for paediatric out-patients. Can Anaes Soc J 27:412, 1980.

Tudor JM, Carter OW, McClellen RE, et al: An analysis of 2403 consecutive pediatric urological consultations. J Urol 87:68, 1962.

van Gool J, and Tanagho EA: External sphincter activity and recurrent urinary tract infections in girls. Urology 10:348, 1977.

Vaughan GF: Children in hospital. Lancet 1:1117, 1957.

Vernon DTA, Schulman JL, Foley JM: Changes in children's behavior after hospitalization. Some dimensions of response and their correlates. Am J Dis Child 111:581, 1966.

Vlahakis E, Hartman GW, Kelalis PP: Comparison of voiding cystourethrography and expression cystourethrography. J Urol 106:414, 1971.

Wallerstein E: Circumcision: An American Health Fallacy. New York, Springer Publishing Co., 1980.

Walther PC, Kaplan GW: Cystoscopy in children: indications for its use in common urologic problems. J Urol 122:717, 1979.

Willscher MK, Bauer SB, Zammuto PJ, et al: Renal growth and urinary infection following antireflux surgery in infants and children. J Urol 115:722, 1976.

4

GENETICS AND DYSMORPHOLOGY

Kenneth N. Rosenbaum

In the last few years, the field of genetics, much like other specialties, has undergone a period of extremely rapid growth with development of clinical subspecialties, for example, dysmorphology, along with dramatic changes in laboratory techniques. The urologist and geneticist share important roles in the management of the pediatric patient with a urologic abnormality. Both are frequently consulted shortly after delivery to define structural abnormalities of the genitalia; both are often placed in the position of coordinator of care for the infant with multiple malformations; yet each brings a unique approach to the clinical problem that is complementary to the other.

It is the purpose of this chapter to establish a framework of basic principles in genetics and dysmorphology that the urologist may use when assessing the malformed or dysmorphic child. An understanding of these principles may aid the urologist in establishing etiology and answering questions related to prognosis, the need for investigation of other possible systemic malformations, and the risk of recurrence. More pressing, however, is the fact that the patient with a genetic disorder, especially the infant with a serious malformation, may require rapid decision-making in the form of delivery room or nursery intervention. It is for this reason that all physicians dealing with infants should have an awareness of some of the conditions detailed later in the chapter. Areas that will be covered include the process of genetic counseling, determination of risk figures for specific isolated urologic conditions, laboratory techniques, and, briefly, prenatal diagnosis.

Significance of Genetic Disorders in the Pediatric Population

Numerous studies have been published detailing the significance of genetic disorders in the population. Hall et al reviewed admission data from a large pediatric center over a 12-month period and classified patients into five categories by diagnosis: (1) single-gene or chromosomal disorders; (2) multifactorial/polygenic disorders; (3) developmental anomalies of unknown etiology and without figures for recurrence; (4) familial disorders without an otherwise well-known genetic basis; (5) nongenetic disorders. The frequency of admission in the various categories was 26.6 per cent for patients with a single-gene, chromosomal, or multifactorial condition, 13.6 per cent with a developmental anomaly, and an additional 13.2 per cent with a familial disorder. The authors demonstrated that the group of patients with genetic disorders were admitted more frequently, remained in the hospital for a longer period of time, and were less likely to have third-party coverage for their expenses. Comparable figures exist from other studies in the U.S., Canada, and Europe (Scriver et al; Day and Holmes).

PRINCIPLES OF GENETICS

Consideration of a possible genetic basis for many urologic disorders dates back at least to the mid 1800's, when Virchow described three siblings with hydronephrosis (Raffle). Reports of familial clustering in other types of

Table 4–1. Single-Gene Disorders

Autosomal Dominant	Autosomal Recessive	X-Linked	Total
934*	588*	115*	1637*
(893)†	(710)	(128)	(1731)
1827	1298	243	3368

Adapted from McKusick VA: Mendelian Inheritance in Man: Catalogs of Autosomal Dominant, Autosomal Recessive and X-Linked Phenotypes. Sixth ed. Baltimore, Johns Hopkins University Press, 1983.
* Denotes inheritance proved.
† Parentheses denote inheritance not proved, but suspected.

urologic abnormalities exist in the early to mid 1900's as well (Raffle). These observations, paralleling the growth of mendelian genetics, were initially explainable on the basis of single-gene inheritance. As new chromosomal abnormalities were identified and better understanding of multifactorial traits developed, the genetics of many malformations became less clear. The contribution of single-gene disorders in the production of human disease should not be underestimated, however. McKusick, in his most recent catalogue (Table 4–1), lists 3368 single-gene entries, with over 1800 autosomal dominant disorders alone. This number will certainly rise in the next edition, as new single-gene disorders continue to be recognized. It is also worth noting that this compilation does not include cytogenetic abnormalities or a number of dysmorphic syndromes of unknown etiology.

Dysmorphology

Fascination with malformations and genetic disorders is not a modern phenomenon. Ancient civilizations, even prior to recorded history, fashioned idols of their malformed offspring to protect the population from recurrence of the problem, which was thought to be supernatural in origin (Warkany). Many of the examples that remain represent varying types of conjoined twins, but other well-categorized conditions such as achondroplasia and other skeletal dysplasias have been found. The Egyptians, and later the Greeks, appreciated the "natural" origin of malformations. In the Middle Ages scholars still viewed the birth of a malformed infant as an omen, or the result of maternal impression, a concept that persists to the present. Credit for the foundation of modern human genetics is usually given to Gregor Mendel, an Austrian monk, whose experiments with garden peas

in the mid 1800's demonstrated that genetic characteristics were inherited independently rather than as a result of blending of traits as previously thought. Unfortunately, his work was poorly understood, at best, by his colleagues and its accuracy and impact remained unknown until 1900 when three other Europeans arrived at the same conclusions (Dewald). It is not practical here to list the innumerable landmarks of genetics since that time, except to emphasize the foresight Mendel had in his observations over 100 years ago.

Recognition of patterns of abnormal development termed *dysmorphology* by Smith in 1966 has lead to more objectivity in the evaluation of the malformed child. Acronyms such as "FLK syndrome" have given way to the term "dysmorphic child," which is more palatable to families and professionals. Numerous clinical centers now exist to provide for diagnosis and management of such children, and many excellent texts and journals on dysmorphology and syndromes are available (McKusick; Smith, 1982; Gorlin et al, 1976; Bergsma). Classification continues to be a problem, especially since the diagnostic rate in most centers is approximately 40 to 50 per cent. The dysmorphologist is also faced with the unusual scenario of having to decide (often daily) whether a given patient has a previously seen syndrome or represents a unique complex, a situation that is infrequent in other specialties (Cohen).

Classification

A recent report from an international group on errors of morphogenesis lists four categories of abnormal development with the following definitions (Spranger et al):

1. *Malformation:* A morphologic defect of an organ, part of an organ, or larger region of the body resulting from an intrinsically abnormal developmental process.

Table 4-2. Errors in Morphogenesis

Type of Error	Example	Urogenital Abnormality
Malformation (syndrome)	BBB syndrome	Hypospadias
Disruption	Fetal alcohol syndrome	Renal hypoplasia
Deformation	Oligohydramnios (Potter syndrome)	Renal agenesis
Dysplasia	Neurofibromatosis	Urogenital neurofibromatosis

2. *Disruption:* A morphologic defect of an organ, part of organ, or a larger region of the body resulting from the extrinsic breakdown of, or an interference with, an originally normal developmental process.

3. *Deformation:* An abnormal form, shape or position of part of the body caused by mechanical forces.

4. *Dysplasia:* Abnormal organization of cells into tissue(s) and its morphologic result(s).

Examples of these categories are shown in Table 4-2.

In this system, the term *syndrome* is used for a recurrent pattern of multiple malformations that are pathogenetically related. *Association* refers to a nonrandom occurrence of multiple anomalies, not part of a syndrome. Two additional concepts relating to morphogenesis are that of a field defect and sequence. A *field defect* is a pattern of anomalies derived from the disturbance of a single developmental field. Examples of field defects are numerous and are seen in the facial variations of the child with a cleft lip or those frequently seen in children with underlying structural malformations of the brain. *Sequence* is a pattern of multiple anomalies derived from a single known anomaly or mechanical factor. Obvious clinical examples include the infant with myelomeningocele who develops limb wasting, club foot, and secondary renal disease.

The prevalence of minor and major anomalies varies greatly between populations and from examiner to examiner. Holmes (1976) studied 7742 infants looking for the presence of specific minor anomalies and normal variations. He defined *major malformations* as those which were of medical, surgical, or cosmetic significance; 2 to 3 per cent of patients in the sample had such a malformation. *Minor malformations* were unusual morphologic features of no significance and were seen in less than 4 per cent of patients. *Normal variations,* much like minor malformations, were of little

significance but were found with a frequency of greater than 4 per cent. As seen in Table 4-3, wide differences in frequency were seen between race and sex. In an update of the study, he found 6.8 to 10.3 per cent of infants had three or more minor anomalies, with 39 to 47 per cent having one or more (Holmes, 1982).

A final group of definitions concerning the results of gene action are in order before moving on to a discussion of principles:

1. *Heterogeneity:* This term describes situations in which a similar clinical picture is produced by different genetic mechanisms. Many examples of genetic heterogeneity are encountered. Excellent examples can be found among the mucopolysaccharidoses, with eight distinct types producing similar phenotypes, all the result of different enzymatic deficiencies.

Table 4-3. Prevalence of Minor Malformations and Normal Variations

Feature	White (%)		Black (%)	
	Male	*Female*	*Male*	*Female*
Epicanthal folds	1.2	1.6	0.7	1.2
Brushfield spots	7.4	7.0	0.0	0.3
Preauricular sinus (unilateral)	0.4	1.3	4.5	6.1
Diastasis recti	32.3	32.9	41.4	40.1
Umbilical hernia	0.4	1.0	3.6	8.6
Clinodactyly (fifth finger), both	5.8	4.5	5.2	8.7
Simian crease				
Unilateral	2.5	1.1	1.7	1.1
Bilateral	1.0	0.3	0.5	0.5

Adapted from Holmes LB: The Malformed Newborn: Practical Perspectives. Unpublished, 1976.

2. *Variable expressivity:* Differences in clinical severity within the same condition. This is not synonymous with penetrance, which will be discussed next. This term does not apply if the observed clinical differences are the result of heterogeneity.

3. *Penetrance:* A population figure which states that a given gene manifests itself in a given percentage of individuals. Penetrance is an all-or-none phenomenon, *is never variable,* but is either incomplete or reduced.

4. *Pleiotropy:* Multiple phenotypic effects from a single mutant gene.

Chromosomal Disorders

Following confirmation of the chromosome number in man as 46 and description of Down syndrome as the first clinically identified cytogenetic syndrome in 1959, there has been a proliferation of information on many new cytogenetic abnormalities. The reason for this is related primarily to the development of chromosomal banding techniques that allow for the identification of small aberrations along the length of the chromosome not previously possible.

Prevalence studies performed on newborns prior to the availability of banding have consistently demonstrated that 0.5 to 0.6 per cent of live births have a significant chromosomal abnormality. This number is slightly greater when newer techniques are considered, but the impact of this group, as shown by Hall et al, is great.

Chromosome Nomenclature and Techniques

It is estimated that there are on the order of 50,000 structural genes in the human genome, with at least one gene mapped to each chromosome. Of the approximate 450 loci that have been definitely mapped, over 115 are on the X chromosome alone (McKusick, 1983). Recombinant DNA techniques should now allow for more rapid assignment of gene loci.

Chromosomes consist of two chromatids joined together at the centromere. Using standard nomenclature, the portion of the chromosome above the centromere is designated as the *p* or *short arm* and the portion below, the *q* or *long arm.* Proper notation for a normal male chromosome complement is 46,XY. If a + sign *precedes* a chromosome number,

then an entire additional chromosome is present as in Down syndrome (trisomy 21): 47,XY,+21. A chromosome number *followed* by a + or − sign denotes presence or absence of material on that particular chromosome: e.g., 46,XY,6p+ or 46,XY,6p−. These patients are said to have a partial trisomy or partial monosomy state. Lastly, with banding techniques, chromosomes can be seen to be a series of light- and dark-staining bands (Fig. 4–1). The dark-staining bands tend to be rich in adenine-thymine base pairs and contain heterochromatin, or nonstructural genetic material. Lighter-staining areas are rich in guanine-cytosine base pairs and are thought to represent areas of euchromatin, or structural gene areas. The chromosome is subdivided into *regions* which are numbered and then into *bands* within regions so that the example used above with deleted material on chromosome 6 may further be designated: 46,XY,del(6)(p23) to indicate the point at which chromosomal breakage and loss of material occurred. More sophisticated nomenclature systems have been developed to allow further subdivision of chromosomes as techniques progress.

Clinical Cytogenetic Syndromes

Urologic abnormalities are frequently seen in many classic cytogenetic syndromes (Table 4–4).

Recent additions to the list include some patients who have aniridia associated with Wilms' tumor, primarily those with the AGR triad (aniridia–genital abnormality–retardation) who have been shown to have a small deletion of 11p13 (Riccardi et al, 1978, 1980; Turleau et al, 1981). It is worth noting that this deletion has not been detected in patients with aniridia and Wilms' tumor only, without other somatic abnormalities. Two of these patients have also developed gonadoblastomas (Turleau et al, 1981).

An interstitial deletion of proximal chromosome 15q has been seen in a number of patients with the Prader-Willi syndrome (Ledbetter et al, 1981, 1982; Kousseff). The frequency of this chromosomal abnormality as determined by sophisticated techniques in Prader-Willi children is approximately 50 per cent. Other abnormalities (partial trisomy, tetrasomy for 15p) have also been seen, and the remaining cases may represent genetic heterogeneity or as yet undetectable deletion at the same point. A lengthier discussion of the

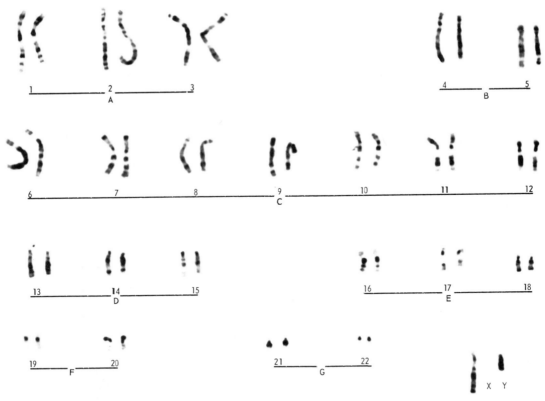

Figure 4–1. Banded karyotype from normal male.

Prader-Willi syndrome appears later in the chapter.

Single-Gene Disorders

This category includes those conditions which follow simple mendelian patterns of inheritance and are not secondary to an observable cytogenetic alteration.

Autosomal Dominant Traits

In this form of inheritance, a mutation at a single locus on a given pair of chromosomes is sufficient to allow for expression (Table 4–5). An affected individual is *heterozygous* for the trait, meaning that only one gene is abnormal. Autosomal dominant traits may be said to demonstrate the following characteristics:

1. Vertical transmission. The disorder may be seen in more than one generation.
2. Males and females are affected equally.
3. In a large population, 50 per cent of offspring born to affected individuals would have the condition.

4. Spontaneous mutation. Most dominant traits have a rate of spontaneous mutation in which the condition originates in a single ovum or sperm at or near the time of conception. Once established, a spontaneous mutation for a dominant trait will behave as expected.
5. The term *sporadic* is not synonymous with spontaneous mutation. It usually refers to the first affected individual within a family.
6. The risk of recurrence for an *affected* individual with a known dominant trait is, of course, ½ or 50 per cent with every pregnancy. For *unaffected* parents of a child with a dominant trait the risk of recurrence is extremely small and approaches the risk for the rest of the population. This assumes that the parents have been examined and are found to be unaffected, that pedigree data are negative, and that reduced penetrance is not a factor.

A common clinical example that is often perplexing is the neonate with polycystic kidney disease (discussed in more detail below). Despite early reports, the adult form of polycystic kidney disease may occur in infants, as discussed more fully in Chapter 25. Prior to

Table 4–4. Genitourinary Anomalies in Chromosomal Syndromes

	Malformations*
Autosomes	
Trisomies (duplication)	
4p	A,B,C,E
8(mosaic)	A
9p	A,B,C,E
9(mosaic)	A,C,E
10q	A,B,E
13	A,B,E
18	A,B,D,E
20p	A,C,E
21	A,C
22 (cat-eye syndrome)	E
Triploidy	A,C,E
Monosomies (deficiency)	
4p	A,B
5p	A,E
9p	A,C,D,E
11p	A,B,C,D
13q	A,B,E
15q (Prader-Willi syndrome)	A,C
18q	A,C,D,E
Sex Chromosomes	
XXY	A,B,C
XXXXY	A,B,C
XYY	A,B,C
X (Turner syndrome)	E

* Key: A, cryptorchidism; B, hypospadias; C, microphallus; D, ambiguous genitalia; E, renal abnormalities (including agenesis, dysplasia, horseshoe kidney, hydronephrosis, other).

counseling, along with a family history, renal ultrasonography should be conducted on the parents of such a child. If neither parent is affected, and they are old enough to have

Table 4–5. Single-Gene Inheritance

Autosomal Dominant
        Aa = affected heterozygote
        aa = normal
Parental genotypes   Aa × aa
Offspring genotypes   Aa($\frac{1}{2}$) or aa($\frac{1}{2}$)

Autosomal Recessive
        AA = normal
        Aa = heterozygote (carrier)
        aa = homozygote (affected)
Parental genotypes   Aa × Aa
Offspring genotypes   AA($\frac{1}{4}$); Aa($\frac{1}{2}$); aa($\frac{1}{4}$)

X-Linked Recessive
        XY = normal male
        X'Y = affected male (hemizygote)
        XX = normal female
        X'X = carrier female
Parental genotypes   X'X × XY
Offspring genotypes   X'X($\frac{1}{4}$); X'Y($\frac{1}{4}$); XX($\frac{1}{4}$); XY($\frac{1}{4}$)

manifested the disorder, then the infant probably represents a spontaneous mutation for autosomal dominant polycystic kidney (DPK) disease.

Autosomal Recessive Inheritance

In this form of inheritance, an affected individual has received two mutant genes (one from each parent) at corresponding points on a pair of chromosomes (Table 4–5). This individual is said to be *homozygous* for the trait. Here, spontaneous mutation is not a factor and both parents are *obligate carriers* for the mutant gene, despite a lack of findings either clinically or often biochemically. Characteristics that may be demonstrated with autosomal recessive inheritance are:

1. Horizontal transmission. Multiple siblings may be affected with unaffected parents. Since humans have small families, affected sibs are frequently lacking even with well-known recessive disorders, such as Tay-Sachs disease, sickle cell anemia, and cystic fibrosis.
2. Males and females are equally affected.
3. Consanguinity increases the risk of having an affected child, since first cousins share one in every eight genes.
4. Biochemical confirmation may be possible for certain recessive disorders, especially enzymopathies.
5. The risk of recurrence for two obligate carriers is $\frac{1}{4}$ (25 per cent with every pregnancy).
6. The offspring of an affected individual are *usually* unaffected, especially for rare recessive disorders, since the probability of meeting a carrier in the general population is low.

It is often necessary to calculate carrier frequencies for recessive disorders. Using the Hardy-Weinberg equilibrium

$$p^2 + 2pq + q^2 = 1,$$

where p represents the frequency of normal genes and q represents the frequency of mutant genes in the general population, the heterozygote frequency ($2pq$) is approximately equal to $2\sqrt{q^2}$ if p approaches 1. Thus, for example, if the frequency of cystic fibrosis in the population is 1 in 1600 births, then 1 in 20 individuals is a carrier for the gene ($2\sqrt{1/1600} = 1/20$).

A second important calculation relates to the risk of an *unaffected* child born to a family with a recessive disorder having a child with the same condition. This can be determined by the following:

risk of carrying mutant gene
$\times$ risk of transmitting gene
$\times$ risk of mate's having gene,

or $\frac{2}{3} \times \frac{1}{4} \times \frac{1}{20} = \frac{1}{120}$ for cystic fibrosis, using a carrier frequency of $\frac{1}{20}$.

X-Linked (Sex-Linked) Inheritance

Geneticists spent years debating the mechanism of X chromosome gene action (dosage compensation), since males have only one X chromosome whereas females have two. The Lyon hypothesis accounts for this paradox by stating that shortly after conception, one X chromosome is inactivated in all cells (Vogel and Motulsky). This process is theoretically random, with 50 per cent of cells having the paternal X chromosome as the active one and 50 per cent the maternal, and is usually irreversible. The inactivated X is identifiable as the Barr body in buccal smears, a densely staining body near the nuclear membrane. Females are, therefore, functional mosaics for genes located on the X chromosome.

X-linked inheritance may be either recessive or, in some instances, dominant. In X-linked recessive inheritance the following may be observed (Table 4–5):

1. In a large pedigree, males will be affected more frequently than females.
2. Lack of male-to-male transmission.
3. Detection of carrier females is often difficult.
4. For carrier females, the risk of having an *affected male* is 50 per cent with every pregnancy and 50 per cent for having a *carrier female* who will be clinically well. Spontaneous mutation does occur for X-linked traits. Although it has been suggested that one third of "lethal" X-linked traits arose as the result of spontaneous mutation, experience with conditions like hemophilia show a much lower rate of mutation, possibly 10 to 15 per cent of cases.
5. All daughters of an affected male are obligate carriers, as are sisters with more than one affected brother.

Calculation of probability for X-linked traits is based on Bayes' theorem, which takes into account the presence of additional historical information (such as numbers of male births) to develop a joint probability.

In X-linked dominant inheritance, females that have the mutant gene are more likely to express the trait than with X-linked recessive disorders but will be more mildly affected than males. Numerous dysmorphic syndromes (hypohydrotic ectodermal dysplasia, incontinentia pigmenti, Goltz syndrome) feature this mode of inheritance. The risk of recurrence in the male and female offspring of an *affected* woman with an X-linked dominant trait is 50 per cent with each pregnancy. For an *affected* male, all daughters and none of the sons will be affected.

Multifactorial Disorders

Multifactorial disorders are the result of the action of multiple genes with small additive effects in combination with environmental influences. Although often used interchangeably with the term *polygenic inheritance*, the term multifactorial allows for the role of environmental factors in the production of such traits. Multifactorial disorders are characterized by:

1. Increased frequency in close relatives. Twin studies on clefting, for example, have shown greater concordance for the defect than would be expected by chance but less than for a single-gene disorder.
2. Consanguinity increases the risk of multifactorial disorders, since relatives will have a greater share of common genes.
3. Most regional malformations and other ill-defined familial disorders are thought to have a multifactorial basis.

Multifactorial Model

Many measurable traits in the population, such as height, intelligence, blood pressure and even serum cholesterol levels, reflect hereditary factors that are multifactorial and define a normal distribution or bell-shaped curve. These traits are said to be continuous, with no interruptions in the curve. At first glance, malformations appear to be discontinuous (either unaffected or affected), although it has been proposed that they also follow a gaussian curve representing liability or likelihood of developing a given condition (Fig. 4–2). When the liability (genetic component) reaches a certain point (the threshold), the disorder becomes manifest. Environmental components, either extrauterine or intrauter-

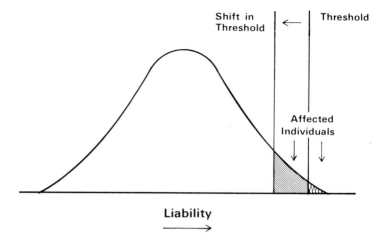

Figure 4-2. Liability curve representing model of multifactorial inheritance. (From Rosenbaum KN: The genetics of congenital heart disease. Clin Proc CHNMC 34:255–269, 1978.)

ine factors, theoretically may function by altering the position of the threshold, thereby increasing liability. Affected individuals have a mean liability near the tail of the curve, and first-degree relatives (siblings, parents, offspring) have a mean liability midway between the mean of the population and that of the affected group.

Calculation of Recurrence Risks

The multifactorial model has become the basis for the calculation of recurrence for most isolated regional malformations, including urologic abnormalities, congenital heart disease, and neural tube defects, to name a few. After exclusion of chromosomal and single-gene disorders, the theoretical risk of recurrence for a presumed multifactorial trait, as Falconer has suggested, can be expressed as:

$$\text{risk} = \sqrt{\text{frequency for specific lesion.}}$$

Observed risks in populations of at-risk individuals confirm the reliability of such calculations. Large amounts of data exist especially for congenital heart disease (Nora and Nora), but information is being accumulated for multifactorial urologic abnormalities and will be discussed below in the section on counseling for specific urologic conditions.

Caution must be exercised in the use of theoretical figures for counseling, however, since certain assumptions are made. The first is that a given family is of *average* liability and that they present with a *single* affected individual. Although figures are sparse for families with two affected children or an affected parent and child, the risk of recurrence appears to increase sharply and may approach mendelian risks. It has also been observed that the more severe the defect, as in perineo-

scrotal versus glanular hypospadias, the greater the risk.

EVALUATION OF THE DYSMORPHIC CHILD WITH UROGENITAL ABNORMALITIES

The process of evaluation for the malformed child must often, of necessity, be performed rapidly and under stressful conditions. Some isolated urologic abnormalities, such as penile agenesis or severe degrees of genital ambiguity, require responses in the delivery room in terms of gender identification. The same is true of the dysmorphic child who presents with a urologic abnormality as part of a more generalized disorder. Steps that should be carried out in the evaluation process are:

1. In-depth antenatal history, family history, and physical examination. Even in the delivery room, it may be possible to elicit important information related to prenatal drug exposure, fetal activity, maternal illness, and the presence or absence of urogenital or other malformations. A rapid physical exam should then be performed looking for nonurologic abnormalities and variations.

2. Measurements. Objective data on facial characteristics such as interpupillary distance (to determine whether the infant has hypertelorism), ear length, and philtrum (midline depression on upper lip) length among others are available to assist in assessment (Smith, 1982; Holmes, 1976). Often visual cues are misleading; therefore it is ideal to obtain objective measurement, if possible.

3. Know what is normal. As detailed in Table 4–3, many facial variations are seen so frequently in the general population that they

are of little significance. Conversely, many dysmorphic syndromes are characterized by a grouping of minor variations with few, if any, major malformations. The child with Down syndrome is an excellent example of a situation in which there are multiple minor malformations and variations that individually are of little significance but put together allow for diagnosis.

4. Interpretation of anomalies from the viewpoint of developmental anatomy. A good knowledge of fetal development is essential in understanding which anomaly came first and whether it was primary or secondary. Does the patient have a true malformation or is it explainable as a deformation or disruption?

5. Laboratory evaluation. Appropriate laboratory studies should be obtained early in the evaluation. For the child with an isolated urologic abnormality such as cryptorchidism or hypospadias, cytogenetic studies are not usually recommended because their yield is low. In cases of genital ambiguity, chromosomal analysis is mandatory. The buccal smear still has a role in the laboratory armamentarium, but its limitations should be recognized. Buccal smears are *screening tests only*, and decisions should not be made on buccal smear results. Falsely low percentages of Barr bodies are frequently seen in the normal newborn female, and some laboratories report low rates of false-positive Barr bodies in males. More specific is Y fluorescence, which intensely stains the heterochromatic area of the Y chromosome. Normal newborn males are 60 to 70 per cent Y-chromatin-positive in our laboratory, but again this procedure remains a screening test.

Preliminary chromosomal results can be obtained routinely in 72 hours; some laboratories harvest the sample as early as 48 hours if sex determination is the primary concern. Higher resolution using banding techniques to look for small additions or deletions will usually take an additional 3 to 4 days. *It should be stressed that the majority of children with a recognizable dysmorphic syndrome have normal chromosomes.* Thus, a negative result may be falsely reassuring to physicians and parents. The greatest diagnostic yield can be anticipated from examination by an experienced clinical geneticist or dysmorphologist.

Other laboratory studies should be obtained at this point depending on the specific abnormality. For the genetic female with genital ambiguity, serum 17-alpha hydroxyprogesterone and urinary 17-alpha hydroxysteroids and 17-ketosteroids are necessary. The

approach to the intersex child is detailed in Chapter 24.

6. Radiographic studies. Specific views of the urogenital system for the child with genital abnormalities are warranted. Depending on the clinical situation, ultrasound, genitogram, IVP, renal scan, or VCUG may be required.

7. Photographs. Documentation of physical differences is best performed with medical photos. This is especially true of the child with life-threatening malformations or the stillborn infant, since efforts to make diagnoses often cease after death and are anticlimactic. Many geneticists routinely provide consultation through the mail on malformed infants that were not able to be seen, although this is often suboptimal. Photographs also serve the purpose of reducing the "mystique" and fears that parents often develop about how malformed their infant was.

8. Overall diagnosis for appropriate counseling. Without a proper diagnosis little correct information about prognosis and the presence of related abnormalities can be given. Two of the primary considerations are whether the family is at risk for recurrence of the disorder and whether prenatal diagnosis is available.

GENETIC COUNSELING

The process of genetic counseling is one that should be implicit in all discussions with families who have a malformed child or one with a genetic disorder. The purpose of such counseling is manifold: to provide useful information in an understandable fashion, to reduce the often overwhelming stresses on the family, and to develop reproductive alternatives related to the risk of recurrence. Counseling is more art than science. Most genetic counselors provide nondirective counseling without making an actual decision for the family. The steps in counseling a family include:

1. Rapid diagnosis. As noted above, everything hinges on a rapid, accurate diagnosis after consideration of syndromic etiologies.

2. Counseling parents together. The reasons for this are obvious. Individuals hear selectively during counseling situations and are often unable to relay information correctly to one another. Also, feelings of guilt are more equally divided when both members of a couple are present.

3. Explanation of problems in biologic terms. This aids in reducing guilt by demonstrating that there is a scientific basis for why a malformation or genetic disorder occurred. Terms used should be understandable, but complex concepts like chromosomes and genes should not be avoided.

4. Discussion of recurrence risk. Parents should be told what the theoretical risk of recurrence is, and it should be placed in a real-life situation. A demonstration of the mechanical basis of inheritance is reasonable at this point.

5. Discussion of burden. As important as risk figures may be to a family, the burden or impact of a condition on a family emotionally, financially, and medically may be what makes the decision for them. Each family views burden differently, and the counselor should not bias the information with his own view of burden.

6. Consideration of reproductive options. The availability of prenatal diagnosis and other options including donor insemination and adoption should be introduced in an objective fashion.

7. Written summary. Throughout the counseling session, both visual and auditory cues are used. The pace of the session should be leisurely with periodic pauses where questions would be appropriate. If possible, some written material, either informal notes of the session highlighting key points or a more formal follow-up letter, should be provided.

8. Repetition. Much has been written on the imperfections of counseling. Although many families may retain risk figure information, the subtleties of what transpires in a counseling session are often lost. Repetition on the part of the urologist, geneticist, and other care providers is frequently necessary to insure a clear perception of transmitted information. Excellent reviews on the counseling process demonstrate well the inherent difficulties in transmitting information to families (Leonard et al; Targum).

SINGLE-GENE DISORDERS AND DYSMORPHIC SYNDROMES WITH UROLOGIC ANOMALIES

Autosomal Dominant Disorders

ALPORT SYNDROME (HEREDITARY NEPHRITIS). A number of single-gene disorders and dysmorphic syndromes feature the association of ocular and renal abnormalities, either functional or structural. One of the best known in pediatric populations is the association of nephritis with hearing loss. Although the condition is named after Alport's description of the entity in 1927, investigators prior to this time were aware of the association (Kenya et al; O'Neill et al; Gubler et al). Significant debate has gone on regarding the genetics of this condition, with autosomal dominant inheritance accepted as the most likely means of transmission for this gene (Gubler et al). Heterogeneity, however, of Alport syndrome is possible, given the increased numbers of affected females, the increased severity and progression in males, and a lack of male-to-male transmission in a number of pedigrees (Gubler et al; Tishler). O'Neill et al, in looking at 150 patients with hereditary nephritis in two large pedigrees, found no examples of male-to-male transmission. In addition, there was almost a 2 : 1 female : male ratio, and the risk of affected offspring born to affected females was approximately 50 per cent. O'Neill et al felt that these findings were more compatible with X-linked dominant inheritance in their pedigrees. Diagnosis rested on the demonstration of microscopic hematuria. Recently, Gubler et al reviewed the clinical experience in 58 pediatric patients with Alport syndrome. The most common presentations were microscopic hematuria and proteinuria. In regard to the auditory deficit in patients, 37 of 58 tested (63.8 per cent) had hearing loss, with males affected more than females, and a variety of ocular abnormalities were also seen, including anterior lenticonus and macular abnormalities.

BOR SYNDROME (BRANCHIO-OTO-RENAL SYNDROME, MELNICK-FRASER SYNDROME). This syndrome features the association of branchial arch anomalies with hearing loss and structural renal disease (Melnick et al; Fraser et al, 1978). As expected, marked variability of expressivity is noted in most affected patients. Auricular and branchial abnormalities include cupped ears with unusual helices, preauricular sinuses, branchial cleft sinuses, and ossicular abnormalities. Similarly, the renal anomalies have included renal agenesis, hypoplasia, polycystic disease, and calyceal dysplasia. The inheritance of the BOR syndrome is as an autosomal dominant trait. The prevalence has been estimated at 1 in 40,000 births (Smith, 1982).

HYPERTELORISM-HYPOSPADIAS SYNDROMES (BBB AND G SYNDROMES, OPITZ AND OPITZ-FRIAS

SYNDROMES). These two conditions will be discussed together, since recent data raise the question as to whether they represent variable manifestations of the same syndrome. The genetics of this group of syndromes is also uncertain, with many investigators believing that the entities are autosomal dominant with sex-limited inheritance and others suggesting that this is an X-linked dominant trait (Gonzalez et al; Funderburk and Stewart; Cordero and Holmes). Because of the ascertainment bias (finding that leads to investigation) with

the hypospadias, females may be underdiagnosed. There have been some instances of male-to-male transmission as well (Cordero and Holmes; Rosenbaum).

BBB Syndrome (Opitz Syndrome). Clinical findings seen most frequently in BBB syndrome include telecanthus, hypertelorism, and coarse facial features with a widow's peak, a large tongue, and clefting of the lip and palate (Fig. 4–3A). Eighty-six per cent of affected males in a recent report had hypospadias, with mental retardation and central

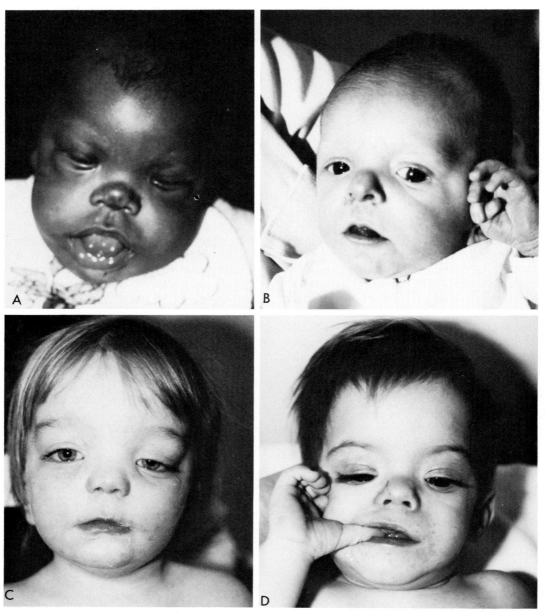

Figure 4–3. Selected dysmorphic syndromes. A, Hypertelorism-hypospadias syndrome. B, Noonan syndrome. C, Aarskog-Scott syndrome. D, Russell-Silver syndrome.

nervous system abnormalities in approximately half (Funderburk and Stewart). Cryptorchidism has also been described in approximately 33 per cent of patients. A variety of other malformations, including congenital heart disease, imperforate anus, and ocular abnormalities, can be seen.

G Syndrome (Opitz-Frias Syndrome). As noted above, because of phenotypic similarities, some investigators have questioned whether this entity is distinct from the BBB syndrome. Patients with G syndrome were originally described because of swallowing dysfunction leading to recurrent aspiration. The clinical findings in the two syndromes are quite similar, with a decreased frequency of clefting in the G syndrome as compared with the BBB syndrome.

NAIL-PATELLA SYNDROME (HEREDITARY OSTEO-ONYCHODYSPLASIA, HOOD SYNDROME). This autosomal dominant disorder may represent a connective tissue disorder, with patients manifesting a variety of skeletal and renal abnormalities. Linkage to the ABO blood group on chromosome 9 has been demonstrated in a number of pedigrees (Smith, 1982; Silverman et al; Bennett et al). Clinical findings seen with high frequency include nail hypoplasia (especially of the thumb), hypoplasia of the patellae, radial head abnormalities, unusual iliac bones, and a number of eye findings such as unusual iris pigmentation, microcornea, and keratoconus. In addition, approximately 30 per cent of patients have a glomerulonephropathy with proteinuria and, at times, hematuria. A characteristic appearance of the glomerular basement membrane has been suggested (Silverman et al; Bennett et al).

NOONAN SYNDROME. This is one of the more common dysmorphic syndromes featuring autosomal dominant inheritance with an estimated incidence of 1 in 3000 live births (Nora et al). Previously, this condition has been called the Turner-like syndrome with normal chromosomes and, on occasion, the male Turner syndrome despite the fact that males and females are affected with equal frequency. Clinical findings include craniofacial dysmorphism with frequent ptosis and epicanthal folds (Fig. 4–3B), a low hairline with webbed neck, broad chest, and congenital heart disease (pulmonary stenosis in 40 to 50 per cent of patients) (Nora et al). Cryptorchidism is common in affected males.

POLYCYSTIC KIDNEY DISEASE. Much has been written in the urologic, nephrologic, and genetic literature about polycystic kidney disease. Classification on the basis of age of onset is fraught with difficulties, since infants may have "adult type" disease (Shokeir; Anton and Abramowsky) and adults may have the "infantile" type (Piering et al). Distinction, however, on a genetic basis is still warranted, since most previously classified infantile forms are autosomal recessive and most adult forms are autosomal dominant. Variability even within specific genetic forms of polycystic kidney disease is to be expected. These considerations are also important in regard to prenatal diagnosis of polycystic kidney disease.

"Adult" or Autosomal Dominant Polycystic Kidney (DPK) Disease. The penetrance of the gene for this disease is higher with increasing age of the patient. The majority of patients come to attention because of renal failure or hypertension in the fourth decade. Visceral cysts in a number of organs are well described, and cerebral aneurysms have been found in 20 per cent of patients (Anton and Abramowsky; Sahney et al; Milutinovic et al; Rosenfield et al). The reliability of ultrasonography alone in screening at-risk individuals is now well documented (Rosenfield et al).

"Infantile" or Autosomal Recessive Polycystic Kidney (RPK) Disease. Presentation within this subgroup is also variable, with some patients manifesting oligohydramnios and pulmonary hypoplasia and dying in the perinatal period, and other patients surviving only to develop significant infantile hypertension leading to dialysis and transplantation (Lieberman et al). In survivors, hepatic fibrosis, cirrhosis, and portal hypertension may become manifest (Lieberman et al).

Prenatal diagnosis for structural renal abnormalities has been performed accurately in the second trimester (Kaffe et al; Shenker and Anderson; Hadlock et al). Caution, however, should be exercised, especially when trying to exclude infantile polycystic kidney disease, because of the small cyst size and natural history of the disease.

ROBINOW SYNDROME (FETAL FACE SYNDROME). This disorder produces a wide spectrum of malformations, including mild shortness of stature, relative macrocephaly with a large anterior fontanelle, hypertelorism with unusual palpebral fissures, and, frequently, short forearms and other extremity variations (Smith, 1982). Genital abnormalities include microphallus and cryptorchidism and, often, hypoplasia of the clitoris and labia majora in affected females (Smith, 1982). Lee et al have recently shown evidence for partial primary hypogonadism as evidenced by elevated serum FSH levels in adult males with the Robinow syndrome.

Autosomal Recessive Disorders

ASPHYXIATING THORACIC DYSTROPHY (JEUNE SYNDROME). This is an infrequent disorder producing short stature and often leading to death in the perinatal period because of a constricted chest. Renal abnormalities include dysplasia and, in survivors, chronic nephritis leading to renal failure (Smith, 1982; Shah, 1980).

BARDET-BIEDL SYNDROME (LAURENCE-MOON-BIEDL SYNDROME). This syndrome features some combination of obesity, mental retardation, and polydactyly of the hands, along with retinitis pigmentosa and genital hypoplasia or hypogonadism (Schachat and Maumenee). The hypogonadism is usually hypogonadotropic. Testicular failure has also been described (Smith, 1982).

CRYPTOPHTHALMOS SYNDROME (FRASER SYNDROME). This is an uncommon disorder featuring cryptophthalmos (eyes covered by skin) in association with an unusual facial appearance involving hypoplastic nares and auricular abnormalities. Affected males have been described with hypospadias and cryptorchidism, whereas affected females have hypoplastic external genitalia and may have müllerian abnormalities (Smith, 1982; Fraser).

MECKEL-GRUBER SYNDROME. This is a well-known disorder involving neural tube formation presenting primarily with encephalocele in association with cleft lip and palate and polydactyly. Survival is unlikely in this condition. A variety of visceral anomalies have been seen including hepatic cysts and renal dysplasia (Hsia et al; Seller; Fraser and Lytwyn). Cryptorchidism and ambiguity of external genitalia have been encountered as well.

POLYCYSTIC KIDNEY DISEASE. Autosomal recessive as well as autosomal dominant forms of polycystic kidney disease are discussed under Autosomal Dominant Disorders.

SMITH-LEMLI-OPITZ SYNDROME. This is an infrequent disorder with characteristic facies secondary to scaphocephaly, ptosis of the eyelids with epicanthal folds, and a number of extremity variations. Affected individuals are profoundly mentally retarded and survival is poor. Genital abnormalities reported in males include cryptorchidism, hypospadias, genital ambiguity, and, recently, focal renal hypoplasia. Females have been noted to have fewer genital abnormalities (Smith, 1982; Akl et al). We have recently had occasion to see a genetic female with apparent sex reversal secondary to the Smith-Lemli-Opitz syndrome (Patterson et al).

CEREBROHEPATORENAL SYNDROME (ZELLWEGER SYNDROME). This is another uncommon syndrome that is frequently lethal in early infancy. Craniofacial findings include a flat face with sloping forehead, upslanting palpebral fissures, and a large anterior fontanelle. Affected infants usually have hepatomegaly and, on autopsy, have renal dysplasia and microcysts (Smith, 1982; Danks et al, 1975). Resemblance of patients to those with other dysmorphic and chromosomal syndromes like Down syndrome is well established.

X-Linked Disorders

AARSKOG-SCOTT SYNDROME. Affected individuals demonstrate some degree of short stature with a broad, relatively large cranium, downslanting palpebral fissures and, often, ptosis (Fig. 4–3C). Other craniofacial findings include a long philtrum. The genital abnormalities typically are that of a "shawl scrotum" representing a mild degree of penoscrotal transposition and cryptorchidism (Smith, 1982; Fryns et al; Escobar and Weaver). In addition, in our own series and in the literature, absence or atrophy of a testis has been seen (Fryns et al). The inheritance of the Aarskog-Scott syndrome is uncertain at this time. In one of our families, the mother of the affected child demonstrates manifestations of the Aarskog-Scott syndrome, as did her father. This would be suggestive of X-linked dominant or possibly X-linked recessive inheritance. Escobar and Weaver, in a review of 10 pedigrees, felt that X-linked recessive inheritance was more likely since they found a paucity of affected daughters from affected men. Other investigators have suggested an autosomal dominant sex-limited mode of inheritance (Escobar and Weaver). The syndrome resembles in some ways Noonan syndrome and Robinow syndrome.

OCULOCEREBRORENAL SYNDROME (LOWE SYNDROME). This uncommon disorder features renal tubular acidosis leading to progressive dysfunction in association with mental retardation and severe ocular handicap, usually caused by cataracts or glaucoma or both (Smith, 1982; Abbassi et al). Affected infants at birth may appear relatively normal until the generalized aminoaciduria is detected. Carrier females may be discovered occasionally on the basis of their ocular abnormalities.

MENKES SYNDROME (KINKY HAIR SYNDROME). This is also an uncommon disorder characterized by sparse, kinky hair along with severe central nervous system abnormalities (primarily mental retardation and seizures) usually progressing to death (Danks et al, 1972). It appears that Menkes syndrome is a disorder of elastogenesis secondary to copper deficiency. A number of urinary tract findings have been described in patients with Menkes syndrome including urinary tract infection, hydronephrosis, ureteropelvic junction obstruction, vesicoureteral reflux, and cryptorchidism. Recently, Daly and Rabinovitch described bladder diverticula in three of four patients studied. One of their patients was managed with intravenous copper infusions and was alive at age 7. His bladder diverticulum on radiologic examination showed progressive enlargement, although the upper tracts were normal. The patient was also placed on intermittent catheterization. During therapy, calculi developed and a vesicostomy was then performed.

DYSMORPHIC SYNDROMES OF UNCERTAIN OR UNKNOWN CAUSE

CHARGE ASSOCIATION. This is a recently described entity which is likely to be heterogeneous in etiology. The acronym CHARGE stands for coloboma of the iris and/or retina, heart lesions, atresia choanae, retardation of growth and/or development, genital abnormalities, and ear abnormalities and/or deafness. Pagon et al (1981) reviewed a number of patients with the CHARGE association. The majority of patients were ascertained on the basis of their ocular and choanal abnormalities. However, a high frequency of genital abnormalities was noted in these patients. The CHARGE association is one of the more frequent colobomatous syndromes.

FACIOAURICULOVERTEBRAL DYSPLASIA (GOLDENHAR SYNDROME, HEMIFACIAL MICROSOMIA). This disorder of unknown etiology is a relatively prevalent malformation syndrome with an estimated frequency of 1 in 5000 births (Smith, 1982; Gorlin et al, 1963). Although this syndrome is classically described in patients with ocular dermoids, many patients have much milder manifestations of the syndrome. Overall, 50 per cent of affected patients have vertebral anomalies with 30 per cent of patients exhibiting cardiac malformations and a similar frequency having urogenital abnormalities. The structural abnormalities are varied and may include unilateral renal agenesis, hypoplasia, or dysplasia. The management of patients with the facioauriculovertebral syndrome is dependent on the spectrum of abnormalities. Patients with sufficient craniofacial abnormalities to make the diagnosis should at least have renal ultrasonography.

MURCS ASSOCIATION. The MURCS association was described by Duncan et al in their review of 28 patients with vaginal atresia. In their study, they found a high frequency of cervicothoracic vertebral anomalies and renal abnormalities. They therefore coined the acronym MURCS (müllerian duct aplasia, renal aplasia, cervicothoracic somite dysplasia) for this group of patients. They proposed that the etiology of the MURCS association was an early embryologic event that involved the developing renal blastema and cervical somites.

The clinical findings in these patients is quite similar to those of the VATER association (vertebral defects, anal atresia, tracheoesophageal fistula, renal and radial abnormalities) and may indicate that the MURCS association is a subgroup. Within the VATER association, which is a form of caudal regression, patients may have vaginal atresia and lower müllerian agenesis. The VATER association will be discussed in more detail below. The major reason for identifying patients with the MURCS and the VATER associations is to determine the need to search for renal anomalies in these patients.

PRADER-WILLI SYNDROME. This disorder was first described in 1956 by Prader in patients with short stature, obesity, and mental retardation. More males than females are recognized with the disorder because of the overt hypogonadism and hypogenitalism in boys. Typically, at birth a male presents with a small phallus and cryptorchidism (Hall and Smith, 1972). Despite a few reports of apparent autosomal recessive inheritance, the etiology of the Prader-Willi syndrome has been unknown until recently. As discussed earlier in this chapter under Chromosomal Disorders, Ledbetter et al (1981, 1982) have described a number of patients with an interstitial deletion of proximal 15q in the Prader-Willi syndrome. It would appear that this is a cause of this condition in at least some patients, although heterogeneity cannot be excluded since some patients with definite Prader-Willi syndrome have had normal chromosomes even on prophase banding (Ledbetter et al, 1982; Kousseff). The urogenital abnormalities seen in patients with the Prader-Willi syndrome have been discussed by a number of authors. In their review of 32 cases, Hall and Smith found cryptorchidism in 84 per cent of affected males and hypogenitalism in 100 per cent of males. More recently, Uehling studied 30 affected males with the Prader-Willi syndrome. Cryptorchidism was found in 21 of 30 patients (70 per cent), with 14 of 30 patients (47 per cent) having both testes maldescended. Testicular biopsies were performed on 4 patients ranging in age from 4 to 21 years of age. It was found that all the testes histologically had a Sertoli-cell-only appearance. Uehling used trials of gonadotropin therapy in an attempt to produce descent and was successful in 2 patients at 4 and 8 years of age and in a 5-year-old with unilateral cryptorchidism. Uehling recommended gonadotropin administration instead of immediate orchiopexy in patients with Prader-Willi syndrome.

PRUNE-BELLY SYNDROME. A historical review of the prune-belly syndrome (triad syndrome, Eagle-Barrett syndrome) is included in Chapter 20. It has been estimated that approximately 200 to 300 reports of this entity exist with the overwhelming majority of affected infant males. Rabinowitz and Schillinger reported their experience and reviewed the literature on 17 affected females and concluded that most were incomplete examples of the syndrome. There has been significant debate in the urologic and pediatric literature concerning the etiology of this syndrome. The prune-belly anomaly has been seen in association with fetal ascites, the Beckwith-Wiedemann syndrome, monosomy X (Turner syndrome), polycystic kidney disease, renal dysplasia, and anencephaly (Monie and Monie; Pagon et al, 1979; Lubinsky and Rapoport; Pramanik et al; Hodes et al). The perspective of the pediatric geneticist, who frequently deals with nonviable infants that have a prune belly, is often different from that of the urologist who sees a more homogeneous population. Two cases of twins

concordant for the prune-belly anomaly have been described (Garlinger and Ott), although there are a number of discordant presumed monozygotic twin pairs (Lubinsky and Rapoport; Garlinger and Ott; Ives). Garlinger and Ott reported a case with affected male siblings and male half-first cousins. Adeyokunnu and Familusi reported on the prune-belly syndrome in two male siblings and a male first cousin. One of the sisters had Turner syndrome.

The hypotheses that have been put forth to explain the prune-belly syndrome fall into two major categories: mesodermal dysgenesis and urethral dysgenesis (Pagon et al, 1979; King and Prescott; Kroovand et al, 1982). Pagon et al (1979) reviewed the sequence of events leading to the prune-belly syndrome ostensibly from urethral obstruction. It was their feeling that the developmental complexity of the prostatic urethra in males increased the risk for an abnormality and accounted for the large predominance of affected males. This would also account for manifestations of the prune-belly syndrome in the other conditions noted above. A genetic basis has been postulated by many authors as well (Garlinger and Ott; Ives; Adeyokunnu and Familusi; Riccardi and Grum). Riccardi and Grum suggested that the clinical data supported an unusual two-step autosomal dominant mutation with sex-limited expression partially mimicking X-linkage. Single-gene inheritance of a more conventional nature can be ruled out on the basis of the lack of affected monozygotic twins. It is likely that the prune-belly syndrome is multifactorially determined as are most of the other regional urogenital malformations. The other manifestations (musculoskeletal) of the prune-belly syndrome are probably secondary to the initiating factor and not additional primary malformations. Counseling should be directed toward identification of the *specific* urogenital lesion.

Prenatal diagnosis of the prune-belly syndrome is also possible (Bovicelli et al; Christopher et al). Pescia et al (1982) reported on a fetus that had elevations of maternal serum alpha-fetoprotein levels at 15 weeks and showed abnormalities at 17 weeks on sonography. Other investigators have made sonographic diagnosis of the prune-belly syndrome in the third trimester (Bovicelli et al; Christopher et al); however, some of these findings can be misleading.

RUSSELL-SILVER SYNDROME. This condition is associated with low birth weight and dwarfism in association with asymmetry of body parts in 75 per cent of patients, minor craniofacial dysmorphism with triangular facies, down-turned corners of the mouth (Fig. 4–3D), extremity variations including clinodactyly and syndactyly of the toes, and developmental delay and/or mental retardation in approximately 20 per cent of patients (Smith, 1982; Escobar et al; Marks and Bergeson). Marks and Bergeson reported on a case of Russell-Silver syndrome with ambiguous genitalia and reviewed 148 cases reported in the literature. They found 3 other examples of ambiguous genitalia, cryptorchidism in 22 patients, and hypospadias in 12 others. In addition, precocious sexual development was seen in 8 girls. The etiology of the Russell-Silver syndrome is unknown. The majority of affected patients have had normal chromosomes. Escobar et al reviewed the familial cases of Russell-Silver syndrome from a total sample of the 150 patients reported to date. Their findings were not conclusive for single-gene inheritance. There were a number of familial cases that did at least suggest the possibility of autosomal dominant inheritance. One problem in dealing with the Russell-Silver syndrome relates to the marked heterogeneity, with a number of disorders potentially mimicking the Russell-Silver syndrome. With otherwise unaffected family members, the risk of recurrence of the Russell-Silver syndrome is low.

VATER ASSOCIATION. As noted above in the discussion of the MURCS association, the VATER association, which was first formally described in 1973 (Quan and Smith), represents a defect in mesodermal development at the primitive streak level. The acronym VATER (*v*ertebral defects, *a*nal atresia, *t*racheo*e*sophageal fistula, *r*enal and *r*adial anomalies) reflects the physical manifestations, with most affected patients having three of the VATER components. Additional features frequently include congenital heart disease and a single umbilical artery. Other authors have suggested extending the acronym to include other limb abnormalities as well (Temtamy and Miller). Renal anomalies are seen in approximately 50 per cent of patients and include renal agenesis, dysplasia or hypoplasia (Smith, 1982; Temtamy and Miller). Abnormalities of the external genitalia have also been described. Uehling et al reviewed the data on 23 VATER patients and found 21 with significant genitourinary involvement. Seven patients had renal agenesis, 5 had ureteropelvic junction obstruction, 5

had crossed fused ectopia, and an additional 9 cases exhibited severe reflux. Complete evaluation of the urogenital system including both cystography and visualization of the upper tracts in patients that present with other components of the VATER association, especially imperforate anus and tracheoesophageal fistula, is likely to have a high yield.

COUNSELING FOR SELECTED ISOLATED UROLOGIC CONDITIONS

The situation that the urologist most often faces is the child with an isolated urogenital malformation and parents who are desirous of information on the risk of recurrence. As indicated throughout much of this chapter, it is presently thought that most regional malformations are multifactorially determined with both environmental and genetic components. Excellent reviews are available detailing the genetic basis of isolated urologic malformations (Burger and Burger; Klass; Mininberg).

HYPOSPADIAS. The largest body of data in regard to recurrence is found in the hypospadias literature (Burger and Burger; Klass; Mininberg; Editorial, British Medical Journal; Bauer et al; Czeizel et al; Page). Bauer et al reported their findings in 177 boys presenting with hypospadias. Forty-four of the 177 families (25 per cent) had a second affected family member in addition to the index case. Twelve families (7 per cent) had three affected members. When looking at the risk of recurrence, Bauer et al found that among the families of 150 patients, 14 recurrences occurred in 125 additional male children (Table 4–6). The overall risk factor was therefore 11 per cent. As expected, the risk of recurrence was proportionate to the severity of the hypospa-

Table 4–6. Risk of Recurrence of Hypospadias

	% Recurrence
Index case only affected	
Severity	
Coronal	0
Penile	12
Penoscrotal	19
Index case + second affected family member (excluding father)	15
Index case + father affected	27

Adapted from Bauer SB, Bull MJ, Retik AB: Hypospadias: a familial study. J Urol 121:474, 1979.

dias, with no recurrences among patients with a coronal meatus, 12 per cent risk in the penile hypospadias group, and 19 per cent risk in the penoscrotal group. Bauer et al also investigated the probabilities of recurrence when another family member was affected in addition to the index case. The risk was 15 per cent if an index child and another family member exclusive of the father was affected and 27 per cent if the father and the index child were the affected members. A large study conducted by Czeizel et al in Hungary demonstrated similar findings with 28 twin pairs that were affected among 907 patients with simple hypospadias. Four per cent of the first degree relatives of the index patients were affected with forms of hypospadias. Interestingly, there was a significant difference between sex hormone therapy in the mothers of index cases compared with controls (p < 0.01). Page reported evidence of presumed single gene inheritance of hypospadias. Two families were presented with multigenerational involvement. This, however, does not mitigate against multifactorial inheritance.

CRYPTORCHIDISM. It has been estimated that 4 per cent of term infants have cryptorchidism (Bartone and Schmidt). A number of factors need to be considered in counseling families with cryptorchid children, most importantly, exclusion of other genitourinary external anomalies or evidence of a generalized dysmorphic syndrome that would influence the risk of recurrence. Jones and Young, in looking at 51 males with cryptorchidism, found that 9.75 per cent of their male siblings were affected. In addition, 3.9 per cent of their fathers had cryptorchidism as well. In second degree relatives, the risk fell to 5 per cent overall.

A second important consideration in cryptorchidism is the frequency of associated chromosomal abnormalities. An early report by Mininberg and Bingol indicated that there was a high frequency of chromosomal abnormalities in cryptorchid patients. However, their data included syndromic causes and were obtained prior to the advent of advanced banding techniques. In addition, a number of what appear to be laboratory artifacts, such as random loss of chromosomes, were included as abnormalities. More recent studies, including those of Bartone and Schmidt, Dewald et al, and Waaler, have shown no increase in the frequency of chromosomal abnormalities in *isolated* cryptorchidism. It is our recommen-

dation that patients who have hypospadias or other genitourinary anomalies in addition to cryptorchidism should have a banded karyotype prior to gender assignment and naming.

POSTERIOR URETHRAL VALVES. As with other malformations, posterior urethral valves have been observed on occasion to be more frequent among siblings of affected children than in the general population. Hasen and Song described brothers with urethral valves, and Davidsohn and Newberger reported similar findings in twins. Kroovand et al (1977) documented the presence of valves in confirmed monozygotic twins as did Liune et al. Data for risk of recurrence are sparse but should be calculable using the equation given earlier in the chapter; the risk would be expected to be quite low.

RENAL AGENESIS. The incidence of bilateral renal agenesis is estimated to be approximately 1 in 3000 live births, with 1 in 1000 infants exhibiting unilateral agenesis (Burger and Burger; Schinzel et al). A number of reports exist of siblings with bilateral renal agenesis, as do instances of a parent with unilateral agenesis giving birth to a child with either unilateral or bilateral agenesis. Mauer first described renal agenesis in twins, and Schinzel et al found 14 families that had more than one affected child in a review of the literature. Pescia et al (1976) presented data to suggest a multifactorial cause in 2 of 91 siblings of male index cases and 2 of 20 siblings of female index cases and established an empirical recurrence risk of 2 to 5 per cent. Following the birth of a child with renal agenesis, sonography should be performed on the parents looking for unilateral or bilateral abnormalities. Sonography may be helpful in prenatal diagnosis as well.

VESICOURETERAL REFLUX AND OTHER UROPATHOLOGY. Numerous examples of familial reflux and other forms of uropathology have been described (Raffle; Burger and Burger; Simpson and German; Mulcahy et al; Burger and Smith; Mobley; Zel and Retik; Middleton et al; Dwoskin; Sengar et al; Jerkins and Noe). Raffle described four cases of hydronephrosis in two generations of a family. All affected patients were females. The etiology of the apparent ureteropelvic junction obstruction was not identified in his cases except for one individual with aberrant vessels.

Mulcahy et al reviewed 211 Mayo Clinic patients with reflux and found a positive family history of urinary tract symptomatology (dysuria) or proven infection in 13.2 per cent of parents and siblings. The frequency of finding affected relatives with reflux has ranged from approximately 2 per cent to as much as 60 per cent (Burger and Smith; Mobley; Zel and Retik). Burger and Burger found that in screening the siblings of patients with reflux, 60 per cent were also found to have reflux (Mininberg). After two affected members, 33 per cent of the remaining asymptomatic sibs had reflux. Dwoskin found that 47.6 per cent of sibships had uropathology when reflux was the primary problem in the proband and that 26.5 per cent of these patients also had reflux. When the uropathology was other than reflux, the number decreased to 13.2 per cent. Jerkins and Noe looked at the problem prospectively and found an incidence of reflux of 32 per cent in the siblings of index cases; 73 per cent of the siblings with reflux were asymptomatic. Lewy and Belman reported father-to-son transmission of reflux suggesting autosomal dominant inheritance.

The genetic basis of reflux would seem to be multifactorial, although sex-linked sibships have been described (Middleton et al). One group of investigators has also looked at HLA linkage and association (Sengar et al). In four families at risk for reflux and one with ureteropelvic junction obstruction the urogenital abnormalities segregated with a particular HLA haplotype, suggesting linkage of reflux to the HLA complex. This is currently unconfirmed by other investigators.

TERATOGENIC INFLUENCES

Available literature on the effect of teratogens on the male genital system is concentrated in two areas: the effects of diethylstilbestrol (DES) and other estrogens on male genitalia and the relationship of progestin exposure to the production of hypospadias. The latter question may be easier to answer than the former. Reports noting an increased association between fetuses exposed to progestins during pregnancy and hypospadias have existed for a number of years (Czeizel et al; Aarskog; Svensson; Mau; Kallen and Winberg; Schardein). Aarskog, in reviewing the problem, found that of 130 patients with hypospadias, 11 had early progestin exposure. However, this report does not include an estimate of the population at risk, and the significance of his findings is unknown. He also

referred to the United States Collaborative Perinatal Project, which examined 50,282 mother-child pairs. Here again there was a greater than expected rate of hypospadias among progestin-exposed infants, but no significant statistical differences existed between the exposed and unexposed groups. Other negative studies include that of Mau in West Germany and Kallen and Winberg's report from Sweden, which showed no statistical increase in the risk of hypospadias following progestin exposure. If there is any statistical association between progestin exposure and hypospadias, it is likely to be small.

Stillman has reviewed nicely the effects of in-utero DES exposure on male offspring. Most of his discussion is based on the data of Gill et al. These authors found a 31.5 per cent incidence of epididymal cysts and/or hypoplastic testes in men exposed to DES in utero, compared with 7.8 per cent in placebo-exposed controls. There were also a large number of patients with abnormalities of spermatozoa function and formation. Sixty-five per cent of exposed men with testicular hypoplasia had a history of cryptorchidism. Since DES is no longer used to any great extent, continued problems related to this drug should decrease.

The teratogenic influences of both estrogens and progestins in male fetuses are, therefore, unresolved. It is possible that the action of these agents is to increase the genetic susceptibility in at-risk families through a multifactorial means.

CONCLUSION

We have reached a point where technological advances are occurring so rapidly that they frequently outstrip one's ability to incorporate advances into a reasonable plan of management. Prenatal sonographic recognition of urinary tract abnormalities in the second trimester is now routine, and a number of centers are experimenting with the possibilities of prenatal intervention for fetal urologic abnormalities (Harrison et al; Berkowitz et al; Duckett). This topic has been reviewed recently by a panel of pediatric urologists, and at the present time it appears that there are no firm indications for fetal urologic intervention. Still, in the early 1950's the actual chromosomal number in man was unknown, and in the mid 1960's amniocentesis was regarded as a research technique with little idea of its practical applications. The desire to learn more about the fetus has heightened complex ethical issues that are also difficult to resolve. Fletcher defines four areas that are at the center of the problem: (1) possible conflicts of interest between fetus, parents, and physicians; (2) the inconsistency of fetal intervention on one hand and termination of a pregnancy on the other; (3) the development of research guidelines for fetal therapy; and (4) the social and economic priorities that should be given to fetal therapy. All of these factors will demand that the urologist become a better geneticist.

BIBLIOGRAPHY

Aarskog D: Maternal progestins as a possible cause of hypospadias. N Engl J Med 300:75, 1979.

Abbassi V, Lowe CU, Calcagno PL: Oculo-cerebral-renal syndrome—a review. Am J Dis Child 115:145, 1968.

Adeyokunnu AA, Familusi JB: Prune belly syndrome in two siblings and a first cousin—possible genetic implications. Am J Dis Child 136:23, 1982.

Akl KF, Khudr GS, Der Kaloustian VM, et al: The Smith-Lemli-Opitz syndrome—report of a consanguineous Arab infant with bilateral focal renal dysplasia. Clin Pediatr 16:665, 1977.

Anton PA, Abramowsky CR: Adult polycystic renal disease presenting in infancy: a report emphasizing the bilateral involvement. J Urol 128:1290, 1982.

Bartone FF, Schmidt MA: Cryptochidism: incidence of chromosomal anomalies in 50 cases. J Urol 127:1105, 1982.

Bauer SB, Bull MJ, Retik AB: Hypospadias: a familial study. J Urol 121:474, 1979.

Bennett WM, Musgrave JE, Campbell RA, et al: The nephropathy of the nail-patella syndrome—a clinicopathologic analysis of 11 kindred. Am J Med 54:304, 1973.

Bergsma D (editor): Birth Defects Compendium. Second ed. New York, Alan R. Liss, Inc., 1979.

Berkowitz RL, Glickman MG, Smith GJ, et al: Fetal urinary tract obstruction: what is the role of surgical intervention in utero? Am J Obstet Gynecol 144:367, 1982.

Bovicelli L, Rizzo N, Orsini LF, et al: Prenatal diagnosis of the prune belly syndrome. Clin Genet 18:79, 1980.

Burger RH, Burger SE: Genetic determinants of urologic disease. Urol Clin North Am 1:419, 1974.

Burger RH, Smith C: Hereditary and familial vesicoureteral reflux. J Urol 106:845, 1971.

Christopher CR, Spinelli A, Severt D: Ultrasonic diagnosis of prune belly syndrome. Obstet Gynecol 59:391, 1982.

Cohen MM: The Child with Multiple Birth Defects. New York, Raven Press, 1982.

Cordero JF, Holmes LB: Phenotypic overlap of the BBB and G syndromes. Am J Med Genet 2:145, 1978.

Czeizel A, Toth J, Erodi E: Aetiological studies of hypospadias in Hungary. Hum Hered 29:166, 1979.

Daly WJ, Rabinovitch HH: Urologic abnormalities in Menkes' syndrome. J Urol 126:262, 1981.

Danks DM, Campbell PE, Stevens BJ, et al: Menkes' kinky hair syndrome. An inherited defect in copper absorption with widespread effects. Pediatrics 50:188, 1972.

Danks DM, Tippett P, Adams C, et al: Cerebro-hepato-renal syndrome of Zellweger—a report of eight cases with comments upon the incidence, the liver lesion, and a fault in pipecolic acid metabolism. J Pediatr 86:382, 1975.

Davidsohn I, Newberger C: Congenital valves of the posterior urethra in twins. Arch Pathol 16:57, 1933.

Day N, Holmes LB: The incidence of genetic disease in a university hospital population. Am J Hum Genet 25:237, 1973.

Dewald GW: Gregor Johann Mendel and the beginning of genetics. Mayo Clin Proc 52:513, 1977.

Dewald GW, Kelalis PP, Gordon H: Chromosomal studies in cryptorchidism. J Urol 117:110, 1977.

Duckett JW (editor): Fetal intervention for obstructive uropathy. Dialog Ped Urol 5:1, 1982.

Duncan PA, Shapiro LR, Stangel JJ, et al: The MURCS association: müllerian duct aplasia, renal aplasia and cervicothoracic somite dysplasia. J Pediatr 95:399, 1979.

Dwoskin JY: Sibling uropathology. J Urol 115:726, 1976.

Editorial: Genetics of hypospadias. Brit Med J 2:189, 1972.

Escobar V, Gleiser S, Weaver DD: Phenotypic and genetic analysis of the Silver-Russell syndrome. Clin Genet 13:278, 1978.

Escobar V, Weaver DD: Aarskog syndrome—new findings and genetic analysis. JAMA 240:2638, 1978.

Falconer DS: The inheritance of liability to certain diseases, estimated from the incidence among relatives. Ann Hum Genet 29:51, 1965.

Fletcher JC: The fetus as patient: ethical issues. JAMA 246:772, 1981.

Fraser FC, Ling D, Clogg D, et al: Genetic aspects of the BOR syndrome—branchial fistulas, ear pits, hearing loss, and renal anomalies. Am J Med Genet 2:241, 1978.

Fraser FC, Lytwyn A: Spectrum of anomalies in the Meckel syndrome or: "Maybe there is a malformation syndrome with at least one constant anomaly." Am J Med Gen 9:67, 1981.

Fraser GR: Our genetical "load." A review of some aspects of genetical variation. Ann Hum Genet 25:387, 1962.

Fryns JP, Macken J, Vinken L, et al: The Aarskog syndrome. Hum Genet 42:129, 1978.

Funderburk SJ, Stewart R: The G and BBB syndromes: case presentations, genetics and nosology. Am J Med Genet 2:131, 1978.

Garlinger P, Ott J: Prune belly syndrome—possible genetic implications. Birth Defects 10:173, 1974.

Gill WB, Schumacher GF, Bibbo M, et al: Association of diethylstilbestrol exposure in utero with cryptorchidism, testicular hypoplasia and semen abnormalities. J Urol 122:36, 1979.

Gonzalez CH, Herrmann J, Opitz JM: Studies of malformation syndromes of man VB: The hypertelorism-hypospadias (BBB) syndrome. Eur J Pediatr 125:1, 1977.

Gorlin RJ, Jue KL, Jacobsen U, et al: Oculoauriculovertebral dysplasia. J Pediatr 63:991, 1963.

Gorlin RJ, Pindborg JJ, Cohen MM: Syndromes of the Head and Neck. Second ed. New York, McGraw-Hill Book Company, 1976.

Gubler M, Levy M, Broyer M, et al: Alport's syndrome—a report of 58 cases and a review of the literature. Am J Med 70:493, 1981.

Hadlock FP, Deter RL, Carpenter R, et al: Sonography of

fetal urinary tract anomalies. Am J Roentgen 137:261, 1981.

Hall BD, Smith DW: Prader-Willi syndrome—a resume of 32 cases including an instance of affected first cousins, one of whom is of normal stature and intelligence. J Pediatr 81:286, 1972.

Hall JG, Powers EK, McIlvaine RT, et al: The frequency and financial burden of genetic disease in a pediatric hospital. Am J Med Genet 1:417, 1978.

Harrison MR, Golbus MS, Filly RA, et al: Fetal surgery for congenital hydronephrosis. N Engl J Med 306:591, 1982.

Hasen HB, Song YS: Congenital valvular obstruction of the posterior urethra in two brothers. J Pediatr 47:207, 1955.

Hodes ME, Butler MG, Keitges EA, et al: Prune belly syndrome in an anencephalic male. Am J Med Genet 14:37, 1983.

Holmes LB: The Malformed Newborn: Practical Perspectives. Unpublished, 1976.

Holmes LB: Minor anomalies in newborn infants (abstract). Am J Hum Genet 34:94A, 1982.

Hsia YE, Bratu M, Herbordt A: Genetics of the Meckel syndrome (dysencephalia splanchnocystica). Pediatrics 48:237, 1971.

Ives EJ: The abdominal muscle deficiency triad syndrome —experience with 10 cases. Birth Defects 10:127, 1974.

Jerkins GR, Noe HN: Familial vesicoureteral reflux: a prospective study. J Urol 128:774, 1982.

Jones IR, Young ID: Familial incidence of cryptorchidism. J Urol 127:508, 1982.

Kaffe S, Rose JS, Godmilow L, et al: Prenatal diagnosis of renal anomalies. Am J Med Genet 1:241, 1977.

Kallen B, Winberg J: An epidemiological study of hypospadias in Sweden. Acta Paediatr Scand (Suppl) 293:1, 1982.

Kenya PR, Asal NR, Pederson JA, et al: Hereditary (familial) renal disease: clinical and genetic studies. South Med J 70:1049, 1977.

King CR, Prescott G: Pathogenesis of the prune belly anomalad. J Pediatr 93:273, 1978.

Klass P: Hereditary factors in urogenital disease. Ped Annals 4:87, 1975.

Kousseff BG: The cytogenetic controversy in the Prader-Labhart-Willi syndrome. Am J Med Genet 13:431, 1982.

Kroovand RL, Al-Ansari RM, Perlmutter AD: Urethral and genital malformations in prune belly syndrome. J Urol 127:94, 1982.

Kroovand RL, Weinberg N, Emami A: Posterior urethral valves in identical twins. Pediatrics 60:748, 1977.

Ledbetter DH, Mascarello JT, Riccardi VM, et al: Chromosome 15 abnormalities and the Prader-Willi syndrome: A follow-up report of 40 cases. Am J Hum Genet 34:278, 1982.

Ledbetter DH, Riccardi VM, Airhart SD, et al: Deletions of chromosome 15 as a cause of the Prader-Willi syndrome. N Engl J Med 304:325, 1981.

Lee PA, Migeon CJ, Brown TR, et al: Robinow's syndrome—partial primary hypogonadism in pubertal boys, with persistence of micropenis. Am J Dis Child 136:327, 1982.

Leonard CO, Chase GA, Childs B: Genetic counseling: a consumer's view. N Engl J Med 287:433, 1972.

Lewy PR, Belman AB: Familial occurrence of nonobstructive, noninfectious vesicoureteral reflux with renal scarring. J Pediatr 86:851, 1975.

Lieberman E, Salinas-Madrigal L, Gwinn JL, et al: Infantile polycystic disease of the kidneys and liver: clinical,

pathological and radiological correlations and comparison with congenital hepatic fibrosis. Medicine 50:277, 1971.

Liune DM, Delaune J, Gonzales EJ Jr: Genetic etiology of posterior urethral valves. J Urol 130:178, 1983.

Lubinsky M, Rapoport P: Transient fetal hydrops and "prune belly" in one identical female twin. N Engl J Med 308:256, 1983.

Marks LJ, Bergeson PS: The Silver-Russell syndrome—a case with sexual ambiguity, and a review of the literature. Am J Dis Child 131:447, 1977.

Mau G: Progestins during pregnancy and hypospadias. Teratology 24:285, 1981.

Mauer SM, Dobrin RS, Vermier RL: Unilateral and bilateral renal agenesis in monoamniotic twins. J Pediatr 84:236, 1974.

McKusick VA: Mendelian Inheritance in Man: Catalogs of Autosomal Dominant, Autosomal Recessive and X-Linked Phenotypes. Sixth ed. Baltimore, Johns Hopkins University Press, 1983.

Melnick M, Bixler D, Nance WE, et al: Familial branchio-oto-renal dysplasia: a new addition to the branchial arch syndromes. Clin Genet 9:25, 1976.

Middleton GW, Howards SS, Gillenwater JY: Sex-linked familial reflux. J Urol 114:36, 1975.

Milutinovic J, Fialkow PJ, Rudd TG, et al: Liver cysts in patients with autosomal dominant polycystic kidney disease. Am J Med 68:741, 1980.

Mininberg DT (editor): Genetics in urology. Dialog Ped Urol 2:1, 1979.

Mininberg DT, Bingol N: Chromosomal abnormalities in undescended testes. Urology 1:98, 1973.

Mobley DF: Familial vesicoureteral reflux. Urology 2:514, 1973.

Monie IW, Monie BJ: Prune belly syndrome and fetal ascites. Teratology 19:111, 1979.

Mulcahy JJ, Kelalis PP, Stickler GB, et al: Familial vesicoureteral reflux. J Urol 104:762, 1970.

Nora JJ, Nora AH: The evolution of specific genetic and environmental counseling in congenital heart diseases. Circulation 57:205, 1978.

Nora JJ, Nora AH, Sinha AK, et al: The Ullrich-Noonan syndrome (Turner phenotype). Am J Dis Child 127:48, 1974.

O'Neill WM, Atkin CL, Bloomer HA: Hereditary nephritis: a re-examination of its clinical and genetic features. Ann Intern Med 88:176, 1978.

Page LA: Inheritance of uncomplicated hypospadias. Pediatrics 63:788, 1979.

Pagon RA, Graham JM, Zonana J, et al: Coloboma, congenital heart disease, and choanal atresia with multiple anomalies: CHARGE association. J Pediatr 99:223, 1981.

Pagon RA, Smith DW, Shepard TH: Urethral obstruction malformation complex: a cause of abdominal muscle deficiency and the "prune belly." J Pediatr 96:900, 1979.

Patterson K, Toomey, KE, Chandra RF: Hirschsprung disease in an 46,XY phenotypic female with Smith-Lemli-Opitz syndrome. J Pediatr 103:425, 1983.

Pescia G, Cruz JM, Weihs D: Prenatal diagnosis of prune belly syndrome by means of raised maternal AFP levels. J Genet Hum 30:271, 1982.

Pescia G, Evans KA, Carter CO: The risk of recurrence for renal agenesis (abstract). Fifth Internat Cong Hum Gen, Mexico City, 1976.

Piering WF, Hebert LA, Lemann J: Infantile polycystic kidney disease in the adult. Arch Intern Med 137:1625, 1977.

Pramanik AK, Altshuler G, Light IJ, et al: Prune-belly syndrome associated with Potter (renal nonfunction) syndrome. Am J Dis Child 131:672, 1977.

Quan L, Smith DW: The VATER association–vertebral defects, anal atresia, TE fistula with esophageal atresia, radial and renal dysplasia: a spectrum of associated defects. J Pediatr 82:104, 1973.

Rabinowitz R, Schillinger JF: Prune belly syndrome in the female subject. J Urol 118:454, 1977.

Raffle RB: Familial hydronephrosis. Brit Med J 1:580, 1955.

Riccardi VM, Grum CM: The prune belly anomaly. Heterogeneity and superficial X-linkage mimicry. J Med Genet 14:266, 1977.

Riccardi VM, Hittner HM, Francke U, et al: The aniridia–Wilms' tumor association: the critical role of chromosome band 11p13. Cancer Genet Cytogenet 2:131, 1980.

Riccardi VM, Sujansky E, Smith AC, et al: Chromosomal imbalance in the aniridia–Wilms' tumor association: 11p interstitial deletion. Pediatrics 61:604, 1978.

Rosenbaum, KN: Unpublished observations, 1979.

Rosenfield AT, Lipson MH, Wolf B, et al: Ultrasonography and nephrotomography in the presymptomatic diagnosis of dominantly inherited (adult-onset) polycystic kidney disease. Radiology 135:423, 1980.

Sahney S, Weiss L, Levin NW: Genetic counseling in adult polycystic kidney disease. Am J Med Genet 11:461, 1982.

Schachat AP, Maumenee IH: The Bardet-Biedl syndrome and related disorders. Arch Ophthalmol 100:285, 1982.

Schardein JL: Congenital abnormalities and hormones during pregnancy: a clinical review. Teratology 22:251, 1980.

Schinzel A, Homberger C, Sigrist T: Case report: bilateral renal agenesis in male sibs born to consanguineous parents. J Med Genet 15:314, 1978.

Scriver CR, Neal JL, Saginur R, et al: The frequency of genetic disease and congenital malformation among patients in a pediatric hospital. Can Med Assoc J 108:1111, 1973.

Seller MJ: Phenotypic variation in Meckel syndrome. Clin Gen 20:74, 1981.

Sengar DP, Rashid A, Wolfish NM: Familial urinary tract anomalies: association with the major histocompatibility complex in man. J Urol 121:194, 1979.

Shah KJ: Renal lesion in Jeune's syndrome. Brit J Radiol 53:432, 1980.

Shenker L, Anderson C: Intrauterine diagnosis and management of fetal polycystic kidney disease. Obstet Gynecol 59:385, 1982.

Shokeir MH: Expression of "adult" polycystic renal disease in the fetus and newborn. Clin Genet 14:61, 1978.

Silverman ME, Goodman RM, Cuppage FE: The nail-patella syndrome—clinical findings and ultrastructural observations in the kidney. Arch Intern Med 120:68, 1967.

Simpson JL, German J: Familial urinary tract anomalies. JAMA 212:2264, 1970.

Smith DW: Dysmorphology (teratology). J Pediatr 69:1150, 1966.

Smith DW: Recognizable Patterns of Human Malformation. Third ed. Philadelphia, WB Saunders Co., 1982.

Spranger J, Benirschke K, Hall JG, et al: Errors of morphogenesis: concepts and terms. J Pediatr 100:160, 1982.

Stillman RJ: In utero exposure to diethylstilbestrol: adverse effects on the reproductive tract and reproductive performance in male and female offspring. Am J Obstet Gynecol 142:905, 1982.

Svensson J: Male hypospadias, 625 cases, associated malformations and possible etiologic factors. Acta Paediatr Scand 68:587, 1979.

Targum SD: Psychotherapeutic considerations in genetic counseling. Am J Med Genet 8:281, 1981.

Temtamy SA, Miller JD: Extending the scope of the VATER association: definition of the VATER syndrome. J Pediatr 85:345, 1974.

Tishler PV: Healthy female carriers of a gene for the Alport syndrome: importance for genetic counseling. Clin Genet 16:291, 1979.

Turleau C, de Grouchy J, Dufier JL, et al: Aniridia, male pseudohermaphroditism, gonadoblastoma, mental retardation, and del 11p13. Hum Genet 57:300, 1981.

Uehling D: Cryptorchidism in the Prader-Willi syndrome. J Urol 124:103, 1980.

Uehling DT, Gilbert E, Chesney R: Urologic implications of the VATER association. J Urol 129:352, 1983.

Vogel F, Motulsky AG: Human Genetics: Problems and Approaches. Berlin, Springer-Verlag, 1979, pp 69–70.

Waaler PE: Clinical and cytogenetic studies in undescended testes. Acta Paediatr Scand 65:553, 1976.

Warkany J: Congenital Malformations: Notes and Comments. Chicago, Year Book Medical Publishers, 1971.

Zel G, Retik AB: Familial vesicoureteral reflux. Urology 2:249, 1973.

5

ABDOMINAL MASSES

GEORGE W. KAPLAN AND WILLIAM A. BROCK

The infant or child who presents with a palpable abdominal mass represents one of the more challenging diagnostic problems facing the pediatric urologist. Blind adherence to the once sacrosanct dictum that "the sun should never set on an abdominal tumor in a child" has resulted in many ill-conceived and consequently unsuccessful operations. The foregoing is not meant in any way to imply that one should "watch" a child with a mass, but rather that each case should be given sufficient study to ensure a relatively accurate preoperative diagnosis. Surgical correction, if undertaken, can then be carefully planned and integrated into an overall therapeutic approach.

It is virtually axiomatic that proper therapy follows directly from accurate diagnosis. Choosing one's diagnostic approach to the problem of abdominal masses in infants and children is therefore of vital importance. Tailoring that approach to the individual patient requires knowledge of both the diagnostic possibilities and probabilities and the limitations of the diagnostic studies available.

INCIDENCE

Abdominal Masses

It is difficult to state with any degree of certainty how often abdominal masses occur in infants and children. The literature contains reports of multiple series that present skewed data and arbitrarily selected experiences, and it is from this type of material that many opinions have been formed. After reviewing the literature, one must conclude that no consistent data are available to indicate how often abdominal masses in infants and children might be encountered by the practic-

ing pediatrician or the average hospital admitting department. Yet there is no question that the condition arises often enough to be a diagnostic problem of genuine importance.

Groves and Wolfman reported 42 pediatric patients with abdominal masses seen over a 5-year period. They excluded infants and patients with hydronephrosis or cystic disease. Consequently, their data showed 75 per cent of their patients to have Wilms' tumor, splenomegaly, or neuroblastoma. Wedge et al reported 63 infants with abdominal masses seen over a 10-year period and noted an entirely different spectrum of lesions.

There are three series that report the incidence of renal anomalies detected by abdominal palpation in the newborn. During a 4-year period, Sherwood et al examined 12,160 neonates and uncovered abdominal masses in 24. Museles et al examined 10,000 consecutive newborns and found 55 renal anomalies; the majority of these anomalies were ectopia, agenesis, or fusion anomalies. Perlman and Williams noted 53 renal anomalies in over 11,000 otherwise normal infants examined. All of these studies underestimate the true incidence of abdominal masses in infants because they deal only with those detected by palpation and all of these series exclude older children.

Medical versus Surgical Masses

Abdominal masses in several reported series have been divided into medical and surgical masses (Fig. 5–1). Lee at the University of Singapore reported 341 children with abdominal masses seen over a 5-year period. Two thirds of the masses in his series were believed to be medical.

Melicow and Uson retrospectively re-

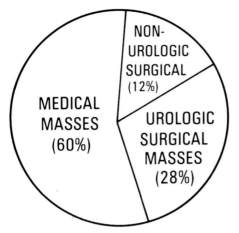

Figure 5–1. Medical versus surgical masses. Data are approximations from several series.

viewed 653 patients who presented with abdominal masses at Babies Hospital in New York over a 32-year period. In their series, medical conditions accounted for 60 per cent of the masses. Kasper et al reported their experience with 450 children with abdominal masses and noted that 55 per cent of the masses were medical.

Genitourinary Masses

Fortunately, more reliable data are available to indicate how often the urinary tract is the source of such abdominal masses as do occur in infants and children.

In Lee's series, in the one third of patients with abdominal masses classified as surgical in nature, 30 per cent were renal; of the renal masses, hydronephrosis accounted for over half. However, Lee classified as medical conditions cases of distended bladder and of prune-belly syndrome, both of which would preferably be categorized as surgical.

In Melicow and Uson's series, 50 per cent of the surgical masses arose in the urinary tract; of these, hydronephrosis was the problem encountered most often. Kasper et al classified 80 per cent of their surgical masses as urologic in origin and further noted that 45 per cent were neoplasms, 32 per cent hydronephroses, and 13 per cent cystic diseases.

Effect of Age on Nature of Mass

The nature of the urologic lesions seen varies depending on the age group one is considering. In an infant, a mass is especially likely to have a urinary source (Fig. 5–2). In Wedge's series of 63 infants with a palpable mass, 47 of the masses were renal in origin; two thirds of the renal masses were hydronephrosis. Raffensperger and Abousleiman reported 31 infants operated upon for abdominal masses; the genitourinary tract was the source of the mass lesions in 24 (77 per cent). Multicystic (cystic dysplastic) kidney was most common, followed closely by hydronephrosis. Parrott and Woodard noted that 8.4 per cent of 603 major operations in neonates at their institution were for urologic disease. Obstruction accounted for 56 per cent of these procedures, cystic disease for 16 per cent, and tumors for only 6 per cent. Emanuel and White reviewed 52 neonates with abdominal masses. Excluded from the study were cases of distended bladder, abdominal distention, hepatosplenomegaly, pyloric stenosis, and intestinal obstruction, as well as pelvic tumors that were not palpable abdominally. When these conditions were excluded from consideration, 44 of the remaining 52 masses (nearly 85 per cent) proved to be renal in origin. Hydronephrosis was slightly more common than multicystic kidney. Longino and Martin reported 32 infants who underwent surgery for abdominal masses discovered during the first day of life. In this series, 16 of the 32 masses (50 per cent) proved to be renal in origin. Multicystic kidney was the most frequent lesion. Kasper et al reported that hydronephrosis was observed in 50 per cent of the neonates in their series and cystic disease accounted for 37.5 per cent of lesions seen in this age group. *Hence, in the neonate one can*

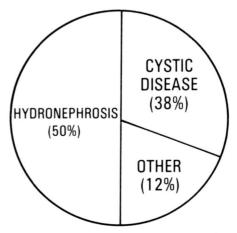

Figure 5–2. Distribution of urologic masses in newborns.

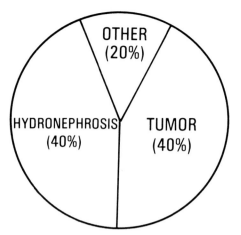

Figure 5-3. Distribution of urologic masses in children between 1 month and 1 year of age.

state with certainty that most abdominal masses are renal in origin. The frequency with which hydronephrosis and cystic dysplasia will be seen is probably equal.

The nature of the lesions seen after 1 month of age changes markedly from that seen in the neonate. Kasper et al noted that between 1 month and 1 year of age, hydronephrosis and neoplasm each accounted for 40 per cent of the masses seen (Fig. 5-3). After 1 year of age neoplasms account for almost 70 per cent of masses seen but the type of neoplasm differs (Fig. 5-4). Neuroblastoma is more common under 2 years of age, whereas Wilms' tumor is more common after that time.

Even when one surveys only series reporting solid abdominal tumors it becomes obvious that a genitourinary source is common. In the series of Slim et al, among 59 children with abdominal malignant neoplasms seen over a period of 11 years, only lymphoma was more common than Wilms' tumor. Lymphoma, Wilms' tumor, and neuroblastoma accounted for 55 patients in this series (93 per cent). Schultz et al reported 22 children presenting to Children's Memorial Hospital, Omaha, with solid abdominal tumors. Two thirds of these tumors were retroperitoneal (mostly Wilms' tumor or neuroblastoma).

The above statistics are enumerated to emphasize that a significant number of abdominal masses in infants and children arise within the urinary tract, and that many of these are benign lesions. If tragedies such as the extirpation of a solitary kidney or the loss of renal function due to hastily conceived or improperly performed operation are to be avoided, the approach to abdominal masses must be thoughtfully and meticulously planned. However, avoiding undue haste does not mean wasting time in the process of diagnosis. Most of the studies to be discussed can be completed within 24 to 48 hours of the patient's admission to the hospital.

DIAGNOSIS OF ABDOMINAL MASSES

In Utero

The first opportunity to detect an abdominal mass may come before the child is born. Ultrasonography is now utilized frequently in obstetric practice to determine fetal age and placental position and as a guide for diagnostic amniocentesis. The fetus is routinely visualized in the course of such studies, and abdominal masses are occasionally noted (Mendoza et al). Hydronephrosis, multicystic kidneys, and distended bladders have all been correctly identified in utero (Fig. 5-5).

History

An infant or child presenting with an abdominal mass will frequently be asymptomatic, the mass having been detected by the pediatrician during a routine examination, or by the mother while bathing the child. In some cases, the mass may have been discovered in the course of a search for the cause of fever or some indefinite complaint such as malaise, anorexia, or weight loss. When

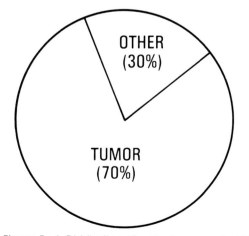

Figure 5-4. Distribution of urologic masses in children after 1 year of age.

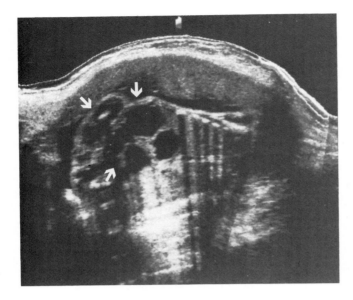

Figure 5–5. Maternal (fetal) ultrasound examinations demonstrating a cystic renal mass (*arrows*) subsequently proved to be cystic dysplasia.

present, pain is usually vague and diffuse, although it can be quite prominent if produced by torsion or rupture of an ovarian cyst or acute obstruction of the urinary tract. Gastrointestinal symptoms such as vomiting or diarrhea can be misleading, since obstructive uropathy or urinary infection also may present with these symptoms.

The lack of specificity of the symptoms presents pitfalls that make a carefully taken history especially crucial in guiding the investigation of an abdominal mass. For example, Figure 5–6*A* is an excretory urogram of a 1-year-old noted to have an abdominal mass. He was referred with a diagnosis of Wilms' tumor. His history revealed several unexplained episodes of fever and a hospitalization for *Pseudomonas* septicemia at age 1 week. Voiding cystourethrography demonstrated that the mass was a lower-pole hydronephrosis in a duplicated system (Fig. 5–6*B* and C). However, the history can also be misleading. One example is the case of a 3-month-old infant who had suffered a 3-foot fall from his crib and developed gross hematuria. An abdominal mass was palpable, and the parents insisted that it had not been present previously. The urogram suggested a renal tumor (Fig. 5–7). At exploration, a mesonephric blastoma, without any gross evidence of bleeding around or into the tumor, was found.

Physical Examination

A multitude of such anecdotes could be recounted by any practicing urologist that would only further strengthen the validity of

the following axioms: (1) Many diagnostic clues are furnished by a well-taken history alone, and (2) there is no diagnostic modality that equals a comprehensive physical examination by a knowledgeable, observant, conscientious examiner. The impressive diagnostic tools afforded the surgeon by modern medical science are of little use in the absence of an astute determination as to when—or even whether—these modalities should be employed.

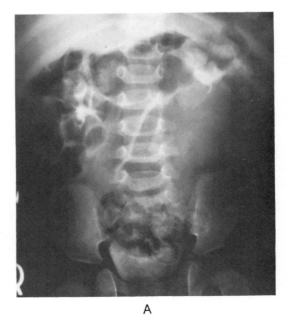

A

Figure 5–6. *A*, Excretory urogram demonstrating a large left-sided mass with distortion of calyces of the left kidney.

Illustration continued on opposite page

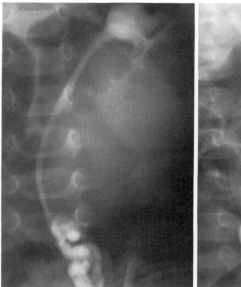

Figure 5–6 *Continued. B* and *C,* Voiding cystourethrogram in the same patient. (See text.)

B   C

Associated Abnormalities

Abnormal formation and position of the external ear may indicate the presence of renal anomalies. Microcephaly is sometimes associated with posterior urethral valves. An-

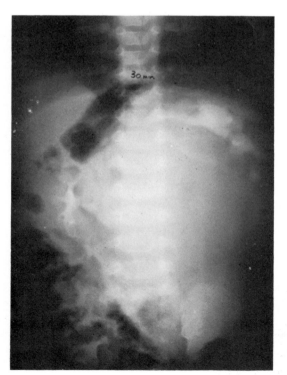

Figure 5–7. Excretory urogram demonstrating a large left renal mass that proved to be a mesonephric blastoma.

iridia can be associated with Wilms' tumor (Miller et al), as is hemihypertrophy (Björklund). Macroglossia is suggestive of Beckwith's syndrome, which has a known association with renal or adrenal tumors or hydronephrosis. Webbing of the neck is found in Turner's syndrome, as are coarctation of the aorta and fusion anomalies of the kidney. Hypertension may occur with Wilms' tumor; it occurs less often with neuroblastoma, and rarely with hydronephrosis. On the other hand, congenital heart disease is more likely to be associated with hydronephrosis. Respiratory distress in a neonate may be caused by any large mass in the upper abdomen, but is especially common with renal masses. Similarly, pneumomediastinum at birth may be associated with obstructive uropathy, as may ascites. Bright pink or bluish subcutaneous nodules in a newborn infant indicate the presence of disseminated neuroblastoma, whereas multiple neurofibromas in an older child might suggest the presence of a pheochromocytoma or an intra-abdominal neurofibroma.

Genitalia

Examination of the genitalia is similarly important. According to Bailey, failure to observe a phimosis as the sole cause for obstructive uropathy in an elderly man has resulted in the failure of more than one candidate for fellowship in the Royal College of Surgeons. To any list of such oversights one might add

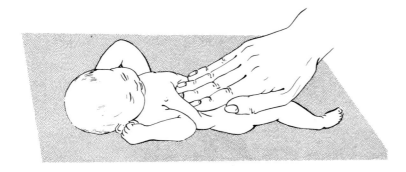

Figure 5–8. Abdominal palpation in an infant using the flat portion of the fingertips.

failure to observe a bulging hydrocolpos in a female infant with a lower abdominal mass. Sexual precocity might suggest an adrenal, ovarian, or testicular tumor. An imperforate anus or myelomeningocele should certainly direct attention to the urinary tract as the site of origin of a mass.

Abdomen

INSPECTION, PERCUSSION, PALPATION. Once the general examination has been carefully completed and relevant general observations noted, one can proceed to specific examination of the abdomen. Visual inspection and percussion are two modes of abdominal examination that are frequently underutilized. Visual inspection, especially when performed in a tangential light, may reveal a mass that might otherwise be missed in cursory palpation, especially when the abdomen is tense. Percussion of a distended abdomen will help to outline masses. By searching for any shifting dullness, one may find that percussion also can suggest the presence of fluid.

It should be emphasized that the normal infant's kidneys lie slightly lower in the lumbar area than the adult's. Consequently, the kidney is readily palpable (after some practice) in most normal infants until approximately 6 weeks of age. In the older child the kidney is less easily felt, but with good cooperation from the patient, one can usually discern the lower pole of the right kidney. An ectopic kidney is often palpable, as is the isthmus of a horseshoe kidney where it crosses the midline.

There are two generally accepted methods of renal palpation. No matter what method is utilized, the examiner's hands must be warm. For the infant, deep bimanual palpation, using the flat portion of the fingers rather than the fingertips, is preferred. When the left kidney is palpated, the left hand supports the flank while the right hand explores it. To palpate the right kidney the left hand supports the flank while the right hand explores it. Some physicians prefer to flex the patient's knees with one hand while deeply palpating the abdomen with the other. Methods of intra-abdominal palpation in an infant are depicted in Figures 5–8, 5–9, and 5–10.

The position and character of any palpable abdominal mass are important. The size of a mass, however, is of little diagnostic significance, as tumors can be small and hydronephroses can be huge (Brock et al) (Fig. 5–11).

Figure 5–9. Left renal palpation in an infant.

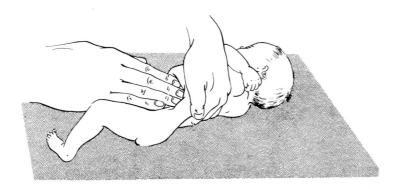

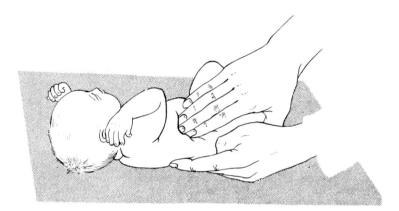

Figure 5–10. Right renal palpation in an infant.

In general, abdominal masses tend to lie in the region of their organ of origin (Fig. 5–12). Renal masses tend to be smooth and to move with respiration; they may be resonant on percussion because of overlying colon. The position of renal masses in infants frequently seems much farther forward than one might expect. A bulge in the loin suggests perinephric abscess or neuroblastoma rather than a renal mass. Splenic masses are usually identifiable by their position, as are hepatic masses. Neuroblastoma frequently tends to be more midline than Wilms' tumor, and also is more often fixed than mobile. Masses in the ovaries, mesentery, and intestine are frequently extremely mobile; this mobility sometimes causes ovarian masses to be present in the upper abdomen (Fig. 5–13). Masses in the lower abdomen are most often masses of the bladder or ovaries, or hydrocolpos. Most neoplasms are very firm, but hydronephrosis can seem very firm, also. The multicystic kidney often feels lumpy, but this lumpiness may be confused with that caused by persistent fetal lobulation in a hydronephrotic kidney.

TRANSILLUMINATION. Another helpful technique of physical examination is transillumination. This technique is quite informative when used for examining the infant, and will frequently demonstrate the cystic nature of a mass that has been palpated. For transillumination a dark room and a strong light source (e.g., a fiberoptic cystoscopic light cable and source) are essential. The baby is held supine, and the end of the light cord is placed behind the mass. Transillumination is seen as a reddish glow (Fig. 5–14). The majority of hydronephoses and approximately two thirds of multicystic kidneys are easily transilluminated.

Laboratory Studies

Laboratory studies are often ancillary aids in the differential diagnosis of abdominal masses in children. In the diagnosis of obstructive urinary lesions, the routine urinalysis helps by identifying hyposthenuria, albuminuria, pyuria, and bacteriuria. Gross hematuria, although frequently suggestive of renal tumor in adults, more commonly is a concomitant of obstruction or trauma in children. In newborns one should also consider the possibility of renal vein thrombosis. In patients with a mass in the left upper quadrant, the presence of anemia may suggest splenomegaly. Remember, however, that anemia often accompanies chronic urinary infection and renal insufficiency, problems that may accompany obstructive uropathy. Anemia may also occur with advanced tumors. Leukocytosis usually suggests an inflammatory process such as an infected hydronephrosis, or intra-abdominal torsion such as that from a twisted ovarian cyst. Thrombocytopenia may accompany renal vein thrombosis or gram-negative septicemia. Azotemia in neonates suggests renal dysplasia or obstructive uropathy, whereas in older children it is usually the result of a glomerulopathy, long-standing obstruction, or reflux nephropathy.

In patients thought to have neuroblastoma, a bone marrow aspirate for tumor cells is often of great value in establishing the diagnosis preoperatively. Similarly, urine testing for catecholamines or vanillylmandelic acid (VMA) can be a valuable supplementary aid in diagnosing neuroblastoma, since up to 80 per cent of patients with neuroblastoma display elevated urinary levels of one or the

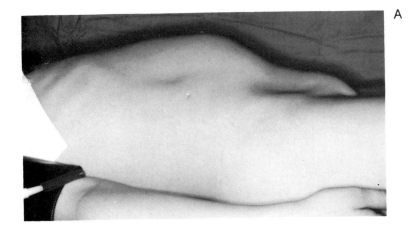

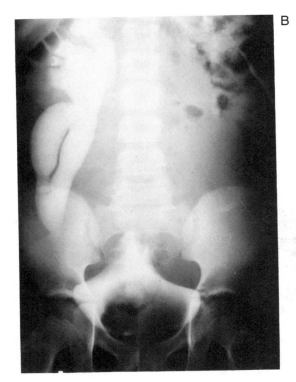

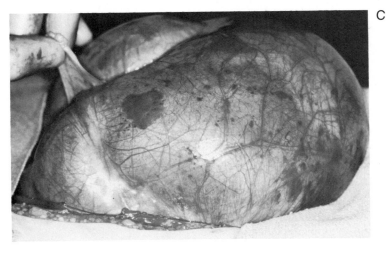

Figure 5–11. *A*, Lateral view of an abdominal mass in an 8-year-old girl. *B*, Excretory urogram of the same patient. *C*, Operative findings in this patient. The mass is an enlarged redundant ureter behind an ectopic ureterocele. Note the ovary and fallopian tube for comparative size.

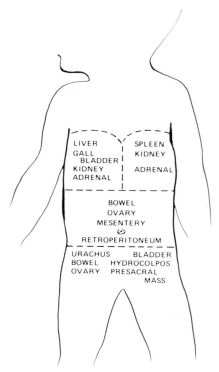

Figure 5–12. Expected organ of origin of an abdominal mass in any given location in the abdomen.

masses because images do not depend upon renal function, whereas urographic imaging does.

Cystic masses (including hydronephrosis) produce an image that is devoid of internal echoes (Fig. 5–15). Because there is no attenuation of energy within the mass, the far wall of the mass is precisely defined. Additionally, there will be strong echogenicity in the tissue interfaces immediately posterior to the mass. Solid masses (e.g., tumors) usually consist of heterogeneous tissues with many tissue interfaces and consequently are echogenic (Fig. 5–16). Because energy is lost at each of these interfaces, there will be relatively poor definition of the posterior wall of the mass. With current equipment it is possible to accurately identify solid masses as small as 2 cm in diameter.

A cystic dysplastic kidney will ultrasonographically appear as a multiseptated cystic mass usually without a definable renal pelvis. The cysts are of varying sizes that do not appear to communicate with each other or with the renal pelvis (Fig. 5–17). Ureteropelvic junction obstruction produces a cystic mass characterized by calyceal dilatation and a distended renal pelvis without ureteral dila-

other of these substances. One major drawback of ascertaining VMA and catecholamine levels has been the necessity of collecting urine for 24 hours.

Ultrasound

The advent of ultrasonography for abdominal and retroperitoneal imaging has markedly altered the diagnostic approach to abdominal masses in children over the past decades. Where radiography was once the preferred initial step in diagnostic imaging, ultrasonography is now preferable as the first test in almost all instances. It is noninvasive and painless. No special patient preparation is required (e.g., dehydration). The image obtained is not dependent on function. Radiation and contrast agents with their attendant hazards are not necessary to produce an image (Shkolnik).

Diagnostic ultrasound can confirm or refute the presence of a suspected mass. If present, it can identify its site (organ) of origin, its extent, and its consistency. In the neonate in whom renal concentrating ability is low, ultrasound is especially helpful with suspected renal

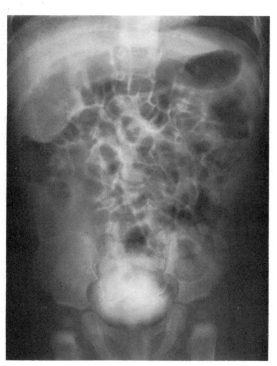

Figure 5–13. Excretory urogram of a 4-month-old girl who presented with a *right*-sided mass that proved to be a *left* ovarian cyst on a 15-cm pedicle.

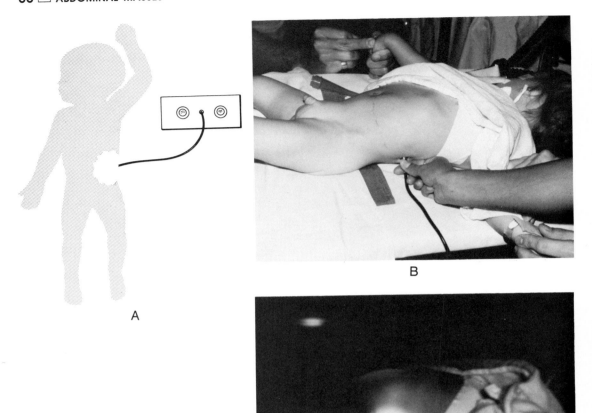

Figure 5–14. *A*, Schematic of abdominal transillumination using a fiberoptic light source and cable. *B*, A mass has been outlined in the left upper quadrant and the fiberoptic cable has been placed posteriorly. *C*, In a darkened room the mass transmits light.

Figure 5–15. Abdominal ultrasound image of a ureteropelvic junction obstruction in an infant (*arrows*).

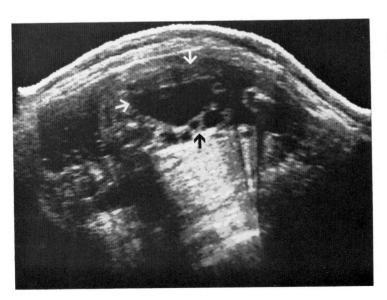

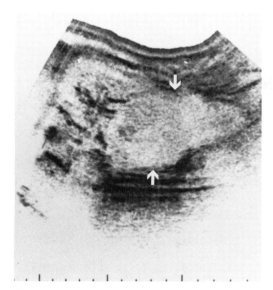

Figure 5–16. Abdominal ultrasound image of a Wilms' tumor (*arrows*) arising from the lower pole of the kidney.

with obstruction of the upper-pole moiety (e.g., ectopic ureterocele) may be difficult to differentiate from cystic lesions of the adrenal (e.g., adrenal hemorrhage) unless the associated dilated ureter is searched for and identified.

Solid lesions (Wilms' tumor and neuroblastoma) are usually highly echogenic. With Wilms' tumor multiple or bilateral lesions may be identified. Ultrasound is also capable of detecting extension of tumor thrombi into the inferior vena cava. Renal vein thrombosis presents as an enlarged kidney with disorganization of the internal renal echo pattern. Mesoblastic nephroma may ultrasonographically resemble renal vein thrombosis or a cystic lesion depending on the homogeneity of the histologic composition of the tumor. Infantile polycystic disease appears as bilateral diffuse renal enlargement with increased echogenicity and indistinct calyces and renal enlargement. In only some cases will small cysts be identified (Boal and Teele). However, cysts in the liver have been demonstrated ultrasonographically in some cases and may aid in diagnosis (Thomas et al.).

In urinary ascites, in addition to finding free fluid in the abdomen, hydronephrosis should be demonstrable. Ultrasonography can also be used to differentiate pelvic masses. A distended bladder appears as an anteriorly placed midline cystic mass. Intravesical masses (e.g., tumor, ureterocele) can be identified only if the bladder is full. Similarly, it is necessary to fill the bladder to identify correctly lesions such as ovarian cysts, urachal cysts, and hydrocolpos.

tation. This may be confused with a multicystic kidney, but the orderly arrangement of the calyces, the smaller number of calyces, and communication with a renal pelvis in hydronephrosis, compared with the random arrangement of cysts in a multicystic kidney, usually differentiates them. Megaureter of various types is differentiated from ureteropelvic obstruction by the identification of a dilated ureter. Vesicoureteral reflux has been diagnosed ultrasonographically so that it may be possible to separate refluxing from obstructed megaureters. Duplication anomalies

Figure 5–17. Abdominal ultrasound image of a cystic dysplastic (multicystic) kidney.

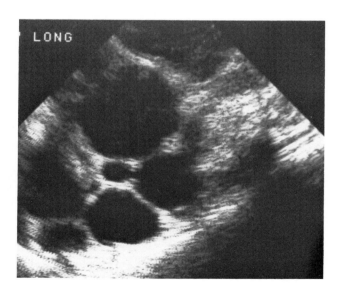

The diagnostic accuracy of ultrasound in experienced hands is excellent. In one series of 36 neonates with suspected abdominal masses, ultrasound was completely accurate in ruling out a mass in 7 patients and was 96 per cent accurate in predicting the final diagnosis in the 29 patients with a mass (Wilson).

Plain Film (KUB)

Once the presence of a mass is demonstrated ultrasonographically, excretory urography is usually the next step in diagnosis. Before considering the films themselves, it is necessary to consider briefly the effect of a mass lesion on its surrounding structures, for interpreting the films with these interrelationships in mind enhances the possibility of correct radiographic diagnosis.

Displacement of Organs

Intraperitoneal masses such as intestinal duplications tend to displace other intraperitoneal structures only. Retroperitoneal structures are usually unaffected. In contrast, retroperitoneal masses often displace not only other retroperitoneal structures but intraperitoneal structures as well.

Enlargement of the liver may displace the right hemidiaphragm cephalad and the right kidney caudad. The second portion of the duodenum is frequently displaced medially, and the colon may be displaced inferiorly. Enlargement of the right adrenal gland will depress the kidney and rotate its upper pole laterally and its lower pole anteriorly. The descending portion of the duodenum and the transverse colon may be displaced anteriorly. Lesions of the upper portion of the right kidney may displace the colon inferiorly and anteriorly, and simultaneously may displace the second portion of the duodenum anteriorly. Lesions of the lower third of the right kidney will tend to elevate the transverse colon and push it anteriorly (Whalen et al, 1972).

Enlargement of the spleen usually does not affect the left kidney, but may push the stomach medially. Lesions of the left adrenal gland push the left kidney down and laterally, while lesions of the left kidney deviate the spleen upward and laterally. Lesions of the lower two thirds of the left kidney may push the duodenojejunal junction inferiorly. Enlargement of the head of the pancreas widens the

"C" loop of the duodenum, but lesions of the tail of the pancreas may push the left kidney laterally and posteriorly (Whalen et al, 1971).

Midline structures in the retroperitoneum tend to deviate the ureters laterally, whereas structures arising in the lateral portions of the retroperitoneum tend to deviate the ureters medially. Enlargement of the bladder tends to elevate the intestines.

By keeping these "displacement factors" in mind, the urologist can more often accurately interpret urographic images.

Bony Structures

A plain film of the abdomen (KUB) is first obtained and surveyed. The bony structures should be scrutinized first for congenital abnormalities, inflammation, or metastatic lesions. The size and position of any abdominal masses should be noted.

Intestinal Gas

The pattern of intestinal gas should be inspected for the presence of intestinal obstruction, which usually indicates that any mass that is identified has a gastrointestinal origin. Medial displacement of the intestine bilaterally often indicates the presence of ascites. Most intra-abdominal mass lesions shift the intestine to the side of the abdomen opposite the mass. Retroperitoneal structures do the same, as well as shifting the intestine anteriorly. Elevation of the right hemidiaphragm often signals the presence of a hepatoblastoma or metastatic neuroblastoma. The presence of radiolucency in a mass prior to the injection of contrast material often indicates a high fat content, as in lipomas, dermoids, and chylous cysts.

Calcifications

One of the more striking features one might distinguish on the KUB film is calcification within a mass. The differential diagnosis of calcified intraperitoneal masses includes meconium peritonitis, intestinal atresia, and calcified lymph nodes. Retroperitoneal calcification, especially in the area of the adrenals, may indicate the presence of neuroblastoma. Finely stippled calcification in the adrenal area is found in 50 per cent of patients with neuroblastoma (Jarvis and Seaman). A triangular rim of calcium in the adrenal area suggests previous neonatal adrenal hemorrhage

(Rose et al). Wolman's disease, a rare lipid storage problem, may also result in adrenal calcification (Ellis and Patrick).

Eight to 12 per cent of Wilms' tumors present with calcification. Rarely, a renal cyst in a child is calcified. Pancreatic lesions may calcify on occasion. Intrahepatic calcification is usually indicative of hepatoblastoma or intrahepatic portal vein thromboemboli (Blanc et al). Calcification appearing in the lower abdomen suggests teratoma, in which calcification usually takes the shape of trabeculae or teeth. In the presacral area, one may occasionally encounter a calcified chordoma. The presence of calcification in rhabdomyosarcoma has been reported, but it is rare indeed.

Excretory Urography

The technique of excretory urography for infants and children is fully described in Chapter 7; therefore only those details pertinent to diagnosing abdominal masses are mentioned here.

Total Body Opacification

The dosage of contrast medium utilized in infants and children is quite large compared with adult dosages. These large dosages have, however, proved beneficial in the total body opacification phase of urographic study. The benefit of using high dosage rates in pediatric urography was originally described by O'Connor and Neuhauser, who were using a dosage of 4 mg per kg of body weight. They noted that relative radiolucencies that were discernible in early films would often be invisible on the 5-minute film. This phenomenon occurs because shortly after injection the contrast material opacifies all the vascular spaces of the abdominal and retroperitoneal viscera, which become comparatively radiodense, leaving avascular structures relatively radiolucent.

Such lesions as multicystic kidneys, adrenal hemorrhage, and choledochal cysts often appear initially as radiolucencies. Similarly, poorly functioning hydronephrosis may be radiolucent initially only to become radiopaque on later films as the contrast material enters the collecting system. Whereas avascular tumors may appear radiolucent in the early phases, vascular tumors such as hemangiomas may "blush" on total body opacification. Therefore, this study may be of value as a screening study but is being replaced by other more definitive tests.

Intestinal Gas

In infants, visualization of the pyelocalyceal system is often obscured by overlying intestinal gas. This problem can be combatted by using prone films, in which the gas has been displaced laterally, or by nephrotomography. Carbonated beverages may also be used to distend the stomach, but this method has its disadvantages: The stomach does distend at first, allowing good visualization, especially of the left kidney; however, after a few minutes the gas dissipates throughout the intestinal tract, and the pyelocalyceal system may become even more obscured than it was at the start.

Delayed Filming

Another useful technique in urographic study of children is delayed filming. Hydronephroses in young children will often take a long time to visualize — often as much as 24 hours. In the series of neonatal infants reported by Emanuel and White, 8 out of 10 patients with proven hydronephrosis showed delay in visualization of contrast material.

The incidence figures cited earlier in this chapter indicate that excretory urography should be useful in the diagnosis of masses of the abdomen, because a large percentage of abdominal masses arise from the urinary tract. Even in the case of masses arising outside the urinary tract, the effect of the mass upon the urinary tract may give a definite clue about the organ of origin if one keeps the effect of mass lesions on other organs in mind while interpreting films.

Interpretation

The size and position of the kidneys should be evaluated. Bilateral renal enlargement in children suggests polycystic renal disease, lymphomas, bilateral tumors such as Wilms' tumor or hamartomas, hemoglobinopathies, glomerulonephritis, glycogen storage diseases (principally von Gierke's disease), and Beckwith's syndrome. To the contrary, unilateral renal enlargement usually indicates the presence of a cystic dysplastic kidney, tumor, or hydronephrosis.

The classic concept of renal cystic dysplasia suggests that the kidney is totally function-

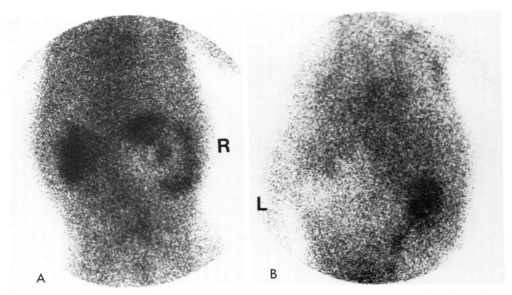

Figure 5–18. *A,* DTPA radionuclide scan demonstrating right hydronephrosis secondary to ureteropelvic junction obstruction. *B,* DTPA radionuclide scan demonstrating nonfunction in a multicystic left kidney.

less. Consequently, one would expect to find a radiolucent area in the renal fossa during the total body opacification phase of the excretory urogram. Rarely there may be sufficient numbers of normal glomeruli in the septa of a multicystic kidney to produce visualization of these septa (Emanuel and White, Warshawsky et al).

As a hydronephrotic kidney begins to visualize, one frequently in early films sees rims of contrast material about the margins of the calyces. This rim or crescent sign subsequently disappears as the contrast agent is excreted into the dilated collecting system. With intrarenal tumors, there is rarely complete nonvisualization and usually no true hydronephrosis, even though there is distortion of the pyelocalyceal system. True nonfunction of the kidney is most likely to be caused by polycystic disease, cystic dysplasia, hydronephrosis, or renal vascular occlusion. Neuroblastoma may occasionally distort the pyelocalyceal system by mass effect or by renal invasion.

Voiding Cystourethrography

An ancillary radiographic technique of inestimable value in the management of lesions originating in the urinary tract is voiding cystourethrography. When vesicoureteral reflux is present, this modality may allow diagnosis of a poorly functioning kidney by reflux of

contrast material from the bladder to the kidney. Sometimes an unsuspected duplication anomaly is uncovered by this method. Voiding cystourography should precede excretory urography when both studies are done on the same day.

Radionuclide Imaging

Advances in nuclear medicine have provided the urologist with another diagnostic tool that often has a role in the management of the child with an abdominal mass. Technetium-99–labeled diethylenetriamine penta-acetic acid (DTPA) and dimercaptosuccinic acid (DMSA) are the agents currently of greatest use. DTPA is excreted by the kidney and thus provides functional as well as anatomic information. In the neonate urography may not provide optimal information because of poor renal concentrating ability. DTPA, however, is excreted by the neonatal kidney and can provide evidence of obstruction (as in ureteropelvic obstruction) or nonfunction (as in cystic dysplasia) (Fig. 5–18). Additionally, one can reliably calculate differential renal function from the accumulation of isotope in each kidney during the early vascular phase shortly after injection. Lastly, by calculating the half-time of washout of DTPA from a dilated system after the administration of furosemide one can usually differentiate stasis from true obstruction. On the other hand,

DMSA is bound to tubular cells. In children with abdominal masses it is of greatest value in differentiating pseudotumors (dilated columns of Bertin) from true tumors. This is of specific utility in cases of Wilms' tumor suspected of being bilateral.

Liver and spleen scans and bone scans may be helpful in the detection of metastatic disease in patients with solid tumors. Gallium scans have been successful in demonstrating abscesses and other inflammatory mass lesions. Combining renal and liver scans can assist in those rare instances in which it is difficult to differentiate a primary hepatic tumor from a primary renal tumor (Samuels).

Retrograde Pyelography

Although largely supplanted by other modalities, retrograde pyelography does still have a role in the diagnosis of some abdominal masses. It is most helpful in establishing the normalcy of the ureter distal to an obstruction at the ureteropelvic junction. Because general anesthesia is required for retrograde pyelography, this examination, if used at all, is usually deferred until the time of definitive treatment of an abdominal mass.

Antegrade Pyelography

Although first developed in 1955 by Casey and Goodwin, percutaneous antegrade pyelography has only recently gained acceptance in the diagnosis and management of abdominal masses. Formerly, this study necessitated blindly inserting a needle into the collecting system through the flank to inject contrast material. The development of ultrasonic or fluoroscopic guidance of the needle has removed the "blind" aspect from this procedure. Additionally, it is now possible using a Seldinger technique to introduce a catheter percutaneously for drainage of an obstructed renal unit. In selected instances, antegrade pyelography is definitive in demonstrating hydronephrosis, the site of obstruction, or a nonvisualizing duplication anomaly. Percutaneous drainage may prove life-saving in cases of obstruction with sepsis or azotemia (Fig. 5 – 19).

Computed Tomography (CT Scanning)

While CT scanning has found a major role in the diagnostic imaging of abdominal

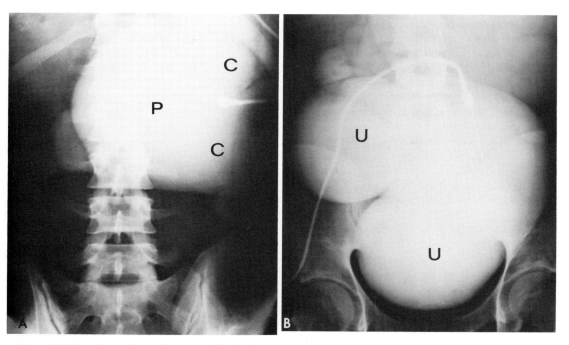

Figure 5 – 19. Antegrade pyelogram. *A*, Posterior puncture through the left flank filled only the dilated pelvis (P) and calyces (C). The lower portion of the mass failed to fill with the patient prone. *B*, Transabdominal puncture of the lower segment outlining the dilated ureter (U). (Reproduced with permission from Brock WA, et al: Congenital giant hydroureteronephrosis. Urol Radiol *1*:67 – 75, 1979. © 1979 Springer-Verlag New York, Inc.)

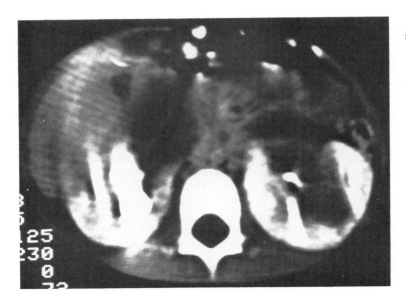

Figure 5–20. CT scan demonstrating bilateral Wilms' tumors.

tumors in adults, its place in the evaluation of an abdominal mass in a child is less secure. In neonates and small children there are many disadvantages that limit its utility. Contrast agents must be employed. Patient motion will decrease organ definition and resolution so that scanners with short scanning times are essential. However, sedation often is necessary. Radiation doses are high (skin doses up to 10 times those of excretory urography). The major limiting factor, however, derives from the fact that organ definition and resolution depend largely on retroperitoneal and perivisceral fat, both of which are lacking in small children (Kuhn and Berger).

Nevertheless, CT scans may prove quite helpful in solid tumors by defining the extent of disease. Intracaval tumor extension can be identified, as can the presence of multiple tumors (Fig. 5–20). In renal hamartomas, because of their high fat content, a pathognomonic picture may be obtained. This latter is of special utility in the patient with tuberous sclerosis in whom a renal mass is found.

Angiography

Arteriography

When the diagnosis of an abdominal mass lesion is in serious question, one occasionally needs to resort to arteriography. It was once felt that the hazards of this procedure in infants and children were such that the study should be avoided virtually at all costs. This attitude is slowly changing. Admittedly there is a slightly higher incidence of complications following arteriography in children than in adults. Yet, the complication rate is now at an acceptable level, and in selected instances the information provided can be quite useful. Occasionally, general anesthesia is required for arteriography, but more often it can be satisfactorily performed with sedation and local anesthesia. The Seldinger technique is generally used with aortic access gained through a

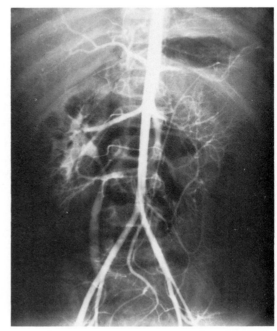

Figure 5–21. Percutaneous femoral aortogram in an 18-month-old demonstrating left renal artery obstruction.

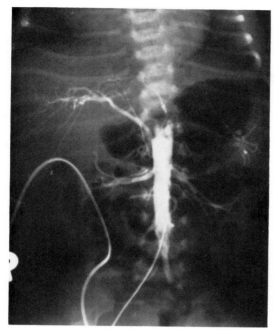

Figure 5-22. Aortography via the umbilical artery in a newborn with right renal vein thrombosis.

percutaneous puncture of the femoral artery (Fig. 5-21). In newborns, the umbilical artery is often used (Fig. 5-22). Once the artery has been punctured, a guidewire is passed, and a catheter is inserted. Contrast medium is injected directly by hand rather than by infusion, and a rapid film changer is employed. Selective renal angiography is utilized when necessary.

The exact rate of complications resulting from arteriography in children is not known. There have been occasional reports of decreased blood flow to the involved extremity following this procedure. This symptom usually disappears spontaneously, but arteriotomy and thrombectomy have been required in a few cases.

Wilms' tumor and neuroblastoma cannot always be differentiated on arteriography. The distinguishing characteristics (McDonald and Hiller) are:

1. Neuroblastoma.
   a. The structures adjacent to the lesion are displaced.
   b. Tumor vessels are present in approximately half the instances.
   c. The renal substance is usually intact.
2. Wilms' tumor.
   a. The aorta and the branches of the renal artery are usually displaced.

b. The intrarenal branches are markedly displaced and stretched.
   c. Tumor vessels are almost always seen.

In Moes and Burrington's series of 25 patients ranging in age from 3 weeks to 14 years, the site of origin and the nature of an abdominal mass were confirmed arteriographically in 20 patients. Five erroneous diagnoses were made: four in patients who subsequently proved to have neuroblastoma, and one in a patient who subsequently proved to have Wilms' tumor. It is this lack of specificity that limits the usefulness of arteriography in abdominal masses in children.

Inferior Venacavography

Another radiographic adjunct useful in diagnosing abdominal masses is inferior venacavography. By obtaining a venacavogram prior to injecting the contrast material for an excretory urogram, one can perform this additional test using only a single extra film. The contrast agent chosen for urography is injected into the greater saphenous vein at the ankle, and a film is taken immediately upon completion of the bolus injection (Fig. 5-23) (Tank et al).

Allen et al reported a large series of patients so handled who ranged in age from birth to 14 years. Of these patients, 35 were found to have normal cavography. Thirteen other patients had displacement of the vena cava without obstruction; 27 patients had obstructions of the vena cava.

Digital Subtraction Angiography

Digital subtraction angiography (DSA) is a newer modality that has some appeal in vascular imaging in children in that it combines principles of both intravenous angiography and photographic subtraction techniques. In DSA, analogue signals from an image-intensifier television screen are converted into digital signals that are subtracted from background signals, electronically amplified, and reconverted to analogue signals, which are viewed in real time on a monitor. DSA is less invasive than catheter angiography but requires special equipment to perform. Motion during the study (especially intestinal peristalsis) is a particular problem in children. Nonetheless, DSA does allow for better visualization of the inferior vena cava following foot vein injection (Fig. 5-24) than conven-

Nuclear Magnetic Resonance

Imaging utilizing nuclear magnetic resonance (NMR) is, as yet, an experimental modality that may have great utility in abdominal masses in children. Body tissues placed in a strong electromagnetic field release energy produced by the resonance of protons (hydrogen ions). With computer-assisted data integration, this energy can be measured and displayed in a cross-sectional fashion similar to computed tomography. Neither radiation nor contrast agents are required. Imaging of hydronephrosis (because of its high water content) seems particularly suited to study with NMR (Williams et al).

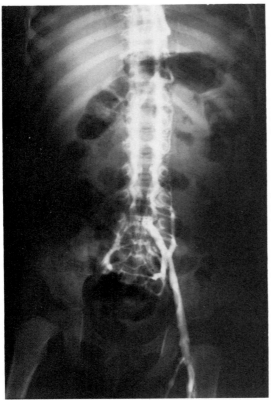

Figure 5–23. Inferior venacavogram in a 15-month-old with caval obstruction caused by neuroblastoma.

tional radiography. Additionally, gross abnormalities of the renal arterial anatomy can be identified noninvasively, although fine detail is still best displayed with intra-arterial catheter techniques (Hillman et al).

BIBLIOGRAPHY

Allen JE, Morse TS, Frye TR, et al: Vena cavagrams in infants and children. Ann Surg 160:568, 1964.

Bailey H: Demonstrations of Physical Signs in Clinical Surgery. Twelfth ed. Bristol, John Wright & Sons, 1954.

Björklund SI: Hemihypertrophy and Wilm's tumour. Acta Paediatr Scand 44:287, 1955.

Blanc WA, Berdon WE, Baker DH, et al: Calcified portal vein thromboemboli in newborn and stillborn infants. Radiology 88:287, 1967.

Boal DK, Teele RL: Sonography of infantile polycystic kidney disease. AJR 135:575, 1980.

Brock WA, Nachtsheim DA, Kaplan GW, et al: Congenital giant hydroureteronephrosis. Urol Radiol 1:67, 1979.

Casey WL, Goodwin WE: Percutaneous antegrade pyelography and hydronephrosis: direct intrapelvic injection of urographic contrast material to secure pyeloureterogram after percutaneous needle puncture and aspiration of hydronephrosis. J Urol 74:164, 1955.

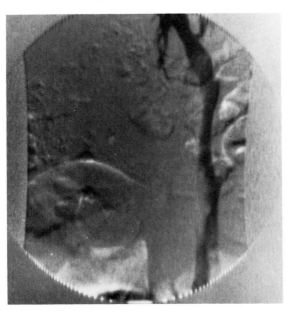

Figure 5–24. Inferior venacavogram using digital subtraction angiography demonstrating a normal inferior vena cava in a child with a Wilms' tumor.

Ellis JE, Patrick D: Wolman's disease in a Pakistani infant. Am J Dis Child 130:545, 1977.

Emanuel B, White H: Intravenous pyelography in the differential diagnosis of renal masses in the neonatal period. Clin Pediatr (Phila) 7:529, 1968.

Groves FB, Wolfman EF Jr: Problems in the management of abdominal tumors in infancy and childhood. Surg Clin North Am 41:1295, 1961.

Hillman BJ, Ovitt TW, Christenson PC, et al: Diagnosis of vascular disease by photoelectric intravenous angiography. JAMA 246:2853, 1981.

Jarvis JL, Seaman WB: Idiopathic adrenal calcification in infants and children. Am J Roentgenol 82:510, 1959.

Kasper TE, Osborne RW Jr, Smerdjian HS, et al: Urologic abdominal masses in infants and children. J Urol 116:629, 1976.

Kuhn JP, Berger PE: Computed tomographic imaging of abdominal abnormalities in infancy and childhood. Ped Ann 9:44, 1980.

Lee SL: Childhood abdominal masses. J Singapore Pediatr Soc 14:107, 1972.

Longino LA, Martin LW: Abdominal masses in the newborn infant. Pediatrics 21:596, 1958.

McDonald P, Hiller HG: Angiography in abdominal tumours in childhood with particular reference to neuroblastoma and Wilms' tumour. Clin Radiol 19:1, 1968.

Melicow MM, Uson AC: Palpable abdominal masses in infants and children: a report based on a review of 653 cases. J Urol 81:705, 1959.

Mendoza SA, Griswold WR, Leopold GR, et al: Intrauterine diagnosis of renal anomalies by ultrasonography. Am J Dis Child 133:1042, 1979.

Miller RW, Fraumeni JF Jr, Manning MD: Association of Wilms's tumor with aniridia, hemihypertrophy and other congenital malformations. N Engl J Med 270:922, 1964.

Moes CAF, Burrington JD: The use of aortography in the diagnosis of abdominal masses in children. Radiology 98:59, 1971.

Museles M, Gaudry CL, Bason WM: Renal anomalies in the newborn found by deep palpation. Pediatrics 47:97, 1971.

O'Connor JF, Neuhauser EB: Total body opacification in conventional and high dose intravenous urography in infancy. Am J Roentgenol 90:63, 1963.

Parrott TS, Woodard JR: Urologic surgery in the neonate. J Urol 116:506, 1976.

Perlman M, Williams J: Detection of renal anomalies by abdominal palpation in newborn infants. Brit Med J 2:347, 1976.

Raffensperger J, Abousleiman A: Abdominal masses in children under one year of age. Surgery 63:514, 1968.

Rose J, Berdon WE, Sullivan T, et al: Prolonged jaundice as the presenting sign of massive adrenal hemorrhage in the newborn. Radiology 98:263, 1971.

Samuels LD: Organ scan diagnosis of abdominal masses in children. J Pediatr Surg 6:124, 1971.

Schultz LR, Calvert TD, Lemon HM: Solid abdominal tumors in childhood. Nebr Med J 48:547, 1963.

Sherwood DW, Smith RC, Lemmon RH, et al: Abnormalities of the genitourinary tract discovered by palpation of the abdomen of the newborn. Pediatrics 18:782, 1956.

Shkolnik A: The role of ultrasound in pediatrics. Ped Ann 9:27, 1980.

Slim MS, Dabbons I, Frayha F, et al: Malignant abdominal neoplasms in childhood. Am J Surg 118:75, 1969.

Tank ES, Poznanski AK, Holt JF: The radiologic discrimination of abdominal masses in infants. J Urol 109:128, 1973.

Thomas JL, Sumner TE, Crowe JE: Neonatal detection and evaluation of infantile polycystic disease by gray scale echography. JCU 6:295, 1978.

Warshawsky AB, Miller KE, Kaplan GW: Urographic visualization of multicystic kidney. J Urol 117:94, 1977.

Wedge JJ, Grosfeld JL, Smith JP: Abdominal masses in the newborn. 63 cases. J Urol 106:770, 1971.

Whalen JP, Evans JA, Meyers MA: Vector principle in the differential diagnosis of abdominal masses. II. Right upper quadrant. Am J Roentgenol 115:318, 1972.

Whalen JP, Evans JA, Shanser J: Vector principle in the differential diagnosis of abdominal masses: the left upper quadrant. Am J Roentgenol 113:104, 1971.

Williams RD, London DA, Dombrovskis S, et al: Nuclear magnetic resonance (NMR) imaging: pre-clinical study in obstructed kidneys. Presented at American Urological Association Annual Meeting, Kansas City, Missouri, May 16–20, 1982.

Wilson DA: Ultrasound screening for abdominal masses in the neonatal period. Am J Dis Child 136:147, 1982.

6

URINALYSIS, INVESTIGATION OF HEMATURIA, AND RENAL BIOPSY

DONALD I. MOEL

URINALYSIS

Until Van Helmont devised a method of examining the urine by weight during the 17th century, the diagnosis of disease (both renal and nonrenal) was accomplished by macroscopic visual examination of the urine (uroscopy). Van Helmont accurately determined the specific gravity of urine by weighing it in a glass vessel with a narrow neck that was known to hold a certain weight of rainwater. In the 16th and 17th centuries, as the older science of alchemy began gradually to develop into a modern science of chemistry, discoveries of the constituents of urine were made. While it is known that Hippocrates noted the presence of urine cloudiness in patients with kidney disease, which in all probability was due to albumin, it was not until 1582 that Willichins noted clouding of the urine after it was heated. Lionel Beale stressed the importance of microscopic examination of the urine in 1861. His investigations placed the analysis of urine on a truly scientific basis for the first time (Wershub).

The modern version of this test is simple and inexpensive to perform. Despite the development of sophisticated techniques that allow the clinician to make specific renal and urinary tract diagnoses, the urinalysis still serves as an important screening test and its result forms the basis for further diagnostic procedures. In the vast majority of instances a normal urinalysis suggests the presence of normally functioning kidneys and urinary tract, but unfortunately, in a few instances, this is an erroneous conclusion. Examples of this have been reported in both children and adults with systemic lupus erythematosus or acute poststreptococcal glomerulonephritis who have had normal urinalyses but in whom renal biopsy revealed significant renal abnormalities (Woolf et al; Albert et al; Cohen and Levitt; Goorno et al; Kandall et al).

Simplified methods now available for the detection of protein, glucose, ketones, and pH, utilizing dipsticks of one kind or another, require little time and effort. Microscopic examination of the centrifuged specimen is also quick and easy to perform if the clinician is experienced in such an examination. Finally, the use of a refractometer to determine specific gravity using only a drop of urine, in contrast to a hydrometer requiring several milliliters of urine, facilitates specific gravity determination in patients who are severely oliguric or infants whose urinary volumes are small. Very recently a reagent strip for measuring specific gravity has been described (Burkhardt et al); it contains a polyacid whose acidity is sensitive to the ionic concentration in the urine in which it is immersed.

In older children and adolescents the ideal urine specimen should be obtained from the first void of the day, after overnight fluid restriction. This specimen is likely to have a high specific gravity, demonstrating intact concentrating ability, and is less likely to contain small amounts of protein that may be present in urine samples obtained after the subject is ambulatory. In boys, cleansing of the glans penis and collecting a midstream specimen is the most desirable method for routine urinalysis and culture. In girls, proper cleansing of the periurethral area is necessary to obtain a clean specimen.

Table 6-1. Normal Urine Values

Components	Quantity/24 Hours
Amino acids	1 to 5 mg/kg
Titratable acidity	20 to 30 mEq
Ammonia	20 to 70 mEq/liter
Calcium	100 to 150 mg
Potassium	40 to 65 mEq
Sodium	130 to 200 mEq
Phosphorus	1100 mg
Protein	400 mg

Obtaining an uncontaminated urine sample from an infant or toddler that also demonstrates normal concentrating ability is more difficult. A polyethylene bag with adhesive is attached to the perineum over the external genitalia (see Fig. 11-1). If the perineum is cleansed properly before the bag is applied and is removed soon after voiding, an uncontaminated sample can be obtained for routine urinalysis and culture.

To obtain the most reliable sample for examination of the sediment, the clean-catch concentrated specimen should be obtained and examined within 1 hour after excretion. A urine sample obtained for culture should be immediately refrigerated at 4 to 6° C until plated in order to prevent the growth of contaminating organisms.

Normal values for various components of urine are listed in Table 6-1.

Color

The normal amber color of urine is due to the pigment urochrome, the excretion of which is relatively constant each day. On standing, normal urine may become cloudy or turbid. Urates, which are of little clinical significance, often precipitate in acid urine as the specimen cools to room temperature and redissolve upon heating. These may give the sediment a pink color. The action of urea-splitting organisms in standing urine will release ammonia with precipitation of phosphates. Precipitated phosphates dissolve with the addition of acid.

Urine that appears very dark yellow is most likely highly concentrated and is frequently seen in dehydrated patients. Another cause of dark yellow urine is the presence of urobilin or bilirubin. Urine that is dark yellow or orangish in color is frequently seen in infants who ingest large amounts of carotene-containing foods.

The presence of red urine is an alarming sign that requires immediate clarification. Red urine that is orthotolidine positive (dipstick reaction) indicates the presence of free hemoglobin, myoglobin, or erythrocytes. Free hemoglobin in the urine is usually dark brown in color and is accompanied by a pink color in plasma. Patients with myoglobinuria have a clear, red to brown urine, and the serum appears grossly normal in color. The presence of red blood cells in the urine is confirmed by microscopic examination.

Other common and benign conditions that cause red urine include beeturia, in which excessive beet ingestion leads to coloration caused by a pigment called anthocyanin; heavy urate excretion, which turns the urine brick red; drugs, such as phenolphthalein (a laxative) and phenazopyridine (a urinary analgesic); and the red diaper syndrome associated with *Serratia marcescens* allowed to incubate in a diaper receptacle at 25 to 30° C for 24 to 36 hours (Waisman and Stone). The "Monday morning disorder of children" is usually noted a day after children have attended a birthday party at which sweets and drinks were consumed that were dyed red by rhodamine B, a food coloring.

Table 6-2 lists some of the agents and causes of reddish colored urines. The monograph by Cone discusses in detail colored urine syndromes.

Concentrating Ability

Normally, the concentration of the urine sample is determined by measuring the specific gravity with either a hydrometer or a refractometer. The total number of osmotically active particles is measured more accurately with an osmometer utilizing the

Table 6-2. Causes of Reddish Urine

Red blood cells

Hemoglobin

Myoglobin

Beets and berries (anthocyanin)

Urates

Red diaper syndrome (*Serratia marcescens*)

Monday morning disorder (rhodamine B)

Laxatives (phenolphthalein)

Urinary tract analgesics (phenazopyridine)

Porphyrias (congenital erythropoietic or intermittent acute)

method of freezing-point depression. It should be emphasized that a urine specimen which is clear yellow in color and free of protein, glucose, ketones, and significant cellular elements should not be considered normal until a specific gravity of at least 1.020 has been demonstrated. Patients with diseases that primarily affect the renal tubules and/or interstitium may lose concentrating ability before there is other biochemical evidence of renal disease. Often a history of polyuria and polydipsia can be elicited. For example, juvenile nephronophthisis, a disease that results in end-stage renal disease during the first two decades of life, is characterized in early childhood by polydipsia, polyuria, and hyposthenuria.

The ability to maximally concentrate the urine depends on normal secretion of antidiuretic hormone (ADH), end-organ responsiveness to ADH, and medullary osmolar gradients. Premature infants and young infants are unable to concentrate to levels of osmolality observed in older children and adults because of low protein intake, decreased secretion of ADH, and water or osmotic diuresis (Rubin and Baliah, 1971).

Conditions that markedly increase urinary osmolality but do not reflect intrinsic concentrating ability occur in patients soon after intravenous urography using contrast media with an osmolality between 1400 and 1500 mOsm/kg and in patients with glycosuria, each 1 per cent glucose adding 0.004 to the specific gravity. Protein, which is a high-molecular-weight substance, contributes very little to the urinary specific gravity. One per cent protein in urine contributes 0.003 to the specific gravity. One can appreciate how little 4 g of protein per 1000 ml contributes to specific gravity.

pH

The normal pH of urine is approximately 6.0. Urine with a pH above 6.5 is considered alkaline and that below 6.0 is considered acid. Urinary pH is most easily determined by the use of nitrazine paper, which is accurate to 0.5 pH unit. More accurate determinations are made in a laboratory with a pH meter. Acid urine is of little significance, but when freshly voided urine is alkaline it may signify urinary infection with urea-splitting organisms or renal tubular acidosis.

Under normal circumstances, the urine and serum pH both fall during metabolic acidosis and rise during metabolic alkalosis. When a discrepancy occurs, an explanation must be sought. For example, a patient with distal renal tubular acidosis is unable to actively transport hydrogen ions across the distal tubule and cannot elaborate an acid urine (pH less than 6.5) despite a plasma pH that is acid. A similar discrepancy is observed in patients with proximal renal tubular acidosis in which there is a defect in bicarbonate reabsorption in the proximal tubule. In these patients the threshold for maximal bicarbonate reabsorption is subnormal; when the serum total bicarbonate level is below threshold, the patient can elaborate an acid urine because distal tubular function is intact. Patients with chronic tubular/interstitial disease such as renal dysplasia, obstructive uropathy, or juvenile nephronophthisis often manifest decreased acidifying ability, but generally, unless end-stage renal disease is imminent, these patients are able to elaborate an acid urine.

Glucose

Under normal circumstances, urine does not contain detectable amounts of sugar. Two tests are used for detection of sugar in urine. The first, the copper reduction test (Benedict's test and Clinitest), which measures all reducing substances, is excellent for semiquantitation of sugar in the urine. The second test, the glucose-oxidase method, is specific for glucose (Clinistix, Testape) but is less suitable for quantitation. Among the reducing substances that give a positive copper reduction reaction are fructose, lactose, galactose, homogentisic acid, pentose, maltose, and glucuronic acid. Any infant with a negative glucose oxidase test and a positive copper reduction test should be suspected of having galactosemia until proved otherwise.

Mild transient glycosuria may occur in children after a heavy glucose intake. This condition is easily differentiated from diabetes mellitus in which hyperglycemia is demonstrated and glycosuria is not transient. Because diabetes mellitus is a serious chronic illness and not uncommon, the workup should be completed without delay.

Glucose may appear in urine in patients who are normoglycemic but have a proximal renal tubule defect in glucose reabsorption. Renal glycosuria without evidence of other proximal tubular dysfunctions (phosphaturia, aminoaciduria, or acidosis) is a benign condition that may be hereditary in nature. Any patient with renal glycosuria and any other component of Fanconi's syndrome (the signs of proximal tubular dysfunction listed above) must be investigated. One of the more common childhood conditions causing Fanconi's syndrome is cystinosis, a serious inborn error of metabolism.

Proteinuria

One of the more common referrals to the pediatric nephrologist is an asymptomatic child with proteinuria. Significant proteinuria indicates the presence of intrinsic renal disease. The qualitative test for proteinuria by the dipstick method utilizes an indicator color (bromophenol blue). A time-honored and more accurate method for protein determination is the sulfosalicylic acid method (8 drops of 20 per cent sulfosalicylic acid is added to 2 ml of urine). Protein is normally found in small amounts in the urine. A protein excretion rate of less than 100 mg per 24 hours is normal.

If a qualitative test for protein is positive, a search for orthostatic proteinuria should be made. By instructing the child to bring a first morning-voided sample to the office and comparing its protein content to that of a specimen obtained in the office, one can clarify the significance of the proteinuria. If the first voided sample has a significant protein : creatinine ratio (>1.0), then a 24-hour urine sample should be analyzed for protein. Certainly the diagnosis of nephrotic syndrome is readily apparent in any child with edema and 3+ or 4+ proteinuria. The cause of the nephrotic syndrome must then be investigated, even though 85 per cent of children with nephrotic syndrome have minimal change nephrotic syndrome.

Febrile proteinuria is transient and disappears with cessation of the fever; hyaline casts may also be present.

It has previously been thought that proteinuria in neonates is so common as to be considered physiological. Doxiadis et al have demonstrated that "physiological proteinuria" is an artifact resulting from the presence of urates. After treatment of urine with trichloroacetic acid, which removes urates, only 1 of 97 infants had a positive test for protein.

Sediment

Examination of the urinary sediment, unlike the simply performed qualitative biochemical tests, requires familiarity with the microscopic recognition of the various cellular and amorphous elements. A fresh (less than 1 hour old) clean-catch or midstream sample should be obtained. Preferably one should examine a first voided sample of the day; since most children are seen on an outpatient basis this is usually not done. Centrifugation of 5 to 10 ml of urine for 10 minutes in a standard countertop centrifuge is sufficient. After the supernatant is decanted a drop of sediment is placed on a slide under a cover slip and examined, first under low power using reduced light and later under high power, again with reduced light. This method reveals the basic elements of the sediment, both cellular and noncellular, in a qualitative manner. A more quantitative approach utilizes a standard counting chamber in the shaken, fresh, uncentrifuged specimen. This approach provides the possibility of quantitation but sacrifices cellular and noncellular detail.

The Addis test, a 12- or 24-hour quantitation of red and white blood cells, casts, and epithelial cells, is rarely used today. Its use should be limited to patients with chronic glomerulopathies, in which the excretion of cellular elements is used to monitor the activity of the renal disease.

Red Blood Cells

Blood in the urine may occur with many diseases of the urinary tract and, although often benign, should always be investigated. A formal discussion of hematuria in childhood is presented later in this chapter.

It is not unusual to find one red cell in every two or three high-power fields of a centrifuged specimen. Red blood cells originating from the renal parenchyma are subjected to intense osmotic and pH changes in their environment, so that their appearance may be altered. In children with acute poststreptococcal glomerulonephritis the hematuria produces an appearance of smoky or "Coke-colored" urine. Microscopically, the red blood cells appear in various forms: some swollen with fluid; some laked, appearing only as "ghost" cells; and some crenated as though they were in hypertonic solution (Lippman).

Sometimes other sedimentary elements of no particular significance are confused with red blood cells. The most common of these are yeast cells and urates. Yeast cells have a doubly refractile border which simulates the doughnut appearance of red blood cells (Fig. 6–1). However, yeast cells are ovoid rather than round and colorless, since they do not contain hemoglobin. Also, yeast cells some-

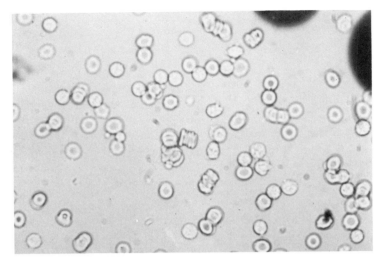

Figure 6–1. Erythrocytes (×45).

times bud. Urate crystals may be red or red-brown, but usually appear in large numbers and exhibit a high degree of variability and size, some being smaller than red blood cells, others being many times larger. Urates give a negative orthotolidine reaction.

If urinary tract infection is suspected by symptomatology or by the presence of red and white blood cells, a Gram's stain should be made of uncentrifuged urine. The presence of bacteria is good evidence of bacteriuria. More recently, using a drop of fresh unspun and unstained urine placed on a hemacytometer with a glass cover slip, Foshee et al examined the center grid under high dry magnification with subdued light. They found that there was excellent correlation between finding more than 10 bacteria within the grid and a urine culture of more than 10^5 colonies.

White Blood Cells

White blood cells are easy to distinguish from red blood cells in the urine because the former are larger and colorless. However, the distinction between a white cell and an epithelial cell may be more difficult. The distinction is easily made in a patient with pus cells

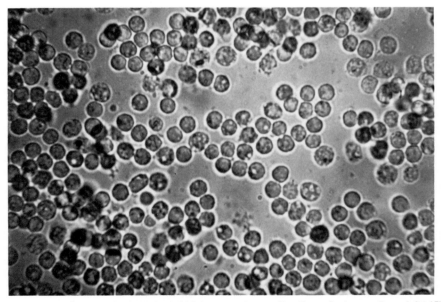

Figure 6–2. Numerous leukocytes at high-power magnification of urine sediment (×45).

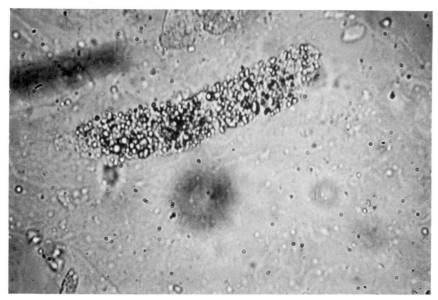

Figure 6-3. Oval fat body cast (×45).

associated with bacterial infection. Although the presence of many white cells in the urine (Fig. 6-2) is a cardinal sign of urinary tract infection, it is important to point out that noninfectious inflammatory glomerular and interstitial disease may be associated with significant leukocyturia. For example, acute poststreptococcal glomerulonephritis is a proliferative and exudative lesion of glomeruli, and although the hallmark of the disease is hematuria, the finding of significant leukocyturia with minimal hematuria is well described also.

Tradition requires the mention of special white cells referred to as "glitter cells," polymorphonuclear leukocytes with refractile granules which show brownian movement. The presence of glitter cells was once thought to be diagnostic of pyelonephritis, but glitter cells occasionally occur with any type of urinary infection.

Finally, an unusual type of cell that is some-

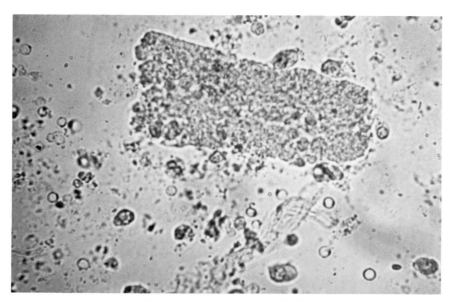

Figure 6-4. Granular cast (×45).

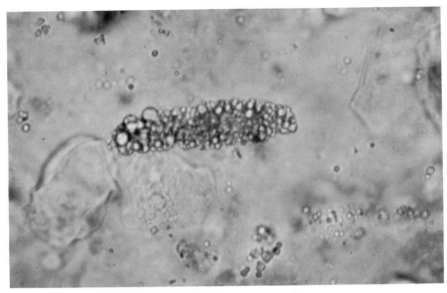

Figure 6–5. Fatty cast (×45).

times confused with white blood cells is the oval fat body, which is actually a renal tubular epithelial cell that is fat-filled and is often seen in patients with the nephrotic syndrome. At high magnification it is seen as a cell with an intact cell border stuffed with droplets of highly refractile fat. It must be viewed with subdued light.

Casts

Casts are thin, cylindrically shaped elements of the sediment that are the diameter and shape of the lumen of the distal tubule or collecting duct (Figs. 6–3 to 6–9). Since the origin of the cast is the kidney, its constituents are therefore localized to the kidney. Casts may be composed of cellular elements such as erythrocytes, leukocytes, or renal epithelial cells, serum proteins (granular casts), or fat bodies (hyaline casts that contain oval fat bodies in patients with the nephrotic syndrome). The elements that predominate are molded in a matrix of Tamm-Horsfall mucoprotein, a substance secreted by renal tubular cells or the interstitium.

Hyaline casts in small numbers are often seen in normal children but may be increased

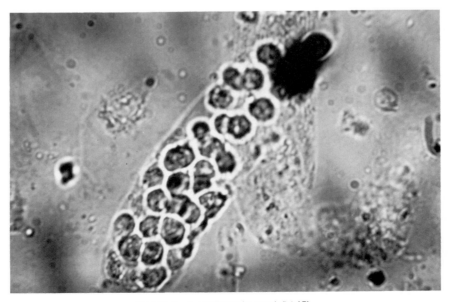

Figure 6–6. Leukocyte cast (×45).

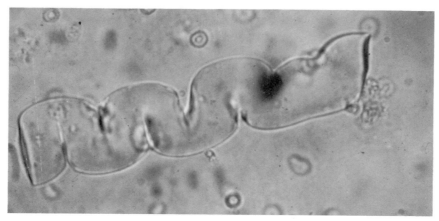

Figure 6–7. Waxy cast (×45).

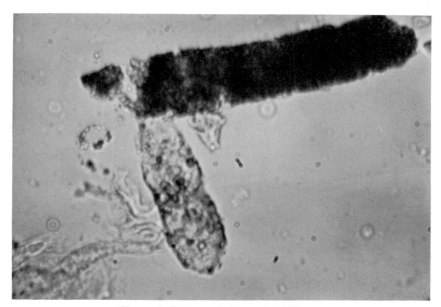

Figure 6–8. Hemoglobin cast (×45).

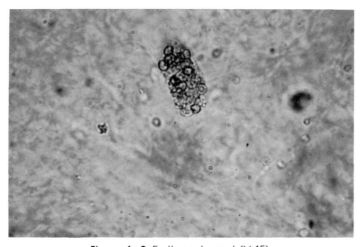

Figure 6–9. Erythrocyte cast (×45).

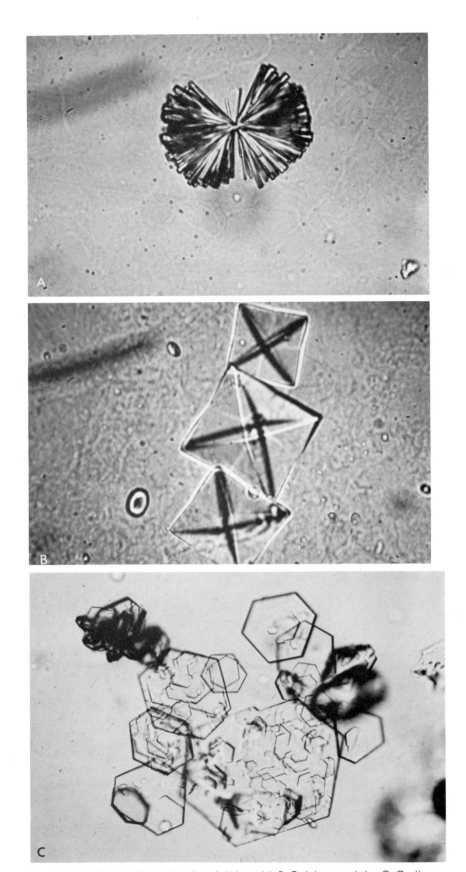

Figure 6–10. Crystals found in urine. *A*, Uric acid. *B*, Calcium oxalate. *C*, Cystine.

Illustration continued on opposite page

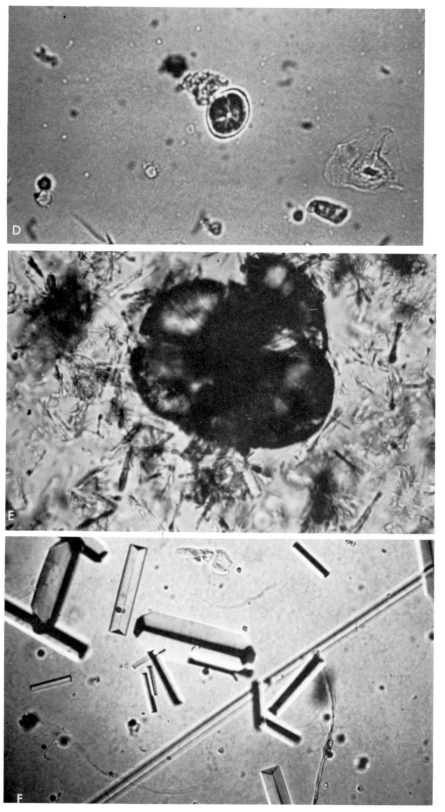

Figure 6–10 *Continued. D*, Leucine. *E*, Sulfa. *F*, Struvite.

during states of dehydration. If seen in large numbers on repeated urine samples, the likelihood of renal disease is great. The presence of cellular casts unequivocally indicates the existence of renal parenchymal disease. Epithelial casts are seen in inflammatory diseases of the kidney, erythrocytic casts with glomerular disease, and leukocyte casts with pyelonephritis. The term "telescoped sediment" refers to finding all types of casts including broadcasts (those derived from atrophic or dilated nephrons), red cell casts, and white cell casts in a single urine specimen. The telescoped sediment is frequently seen in patients with the nephritis of systemic lupus erythematosus.

Using a centrifuged urine specimen under reduced light and stained with Sternheimer-Malbin eosin stain increases the likelihood of finding casts. Hyaline and red cell casts readily dissolve in dilute and alkaline urine. White blood cells also dissolve in alkaline urine. Again, it is important to emphasize the advantages of analyzing a fresh, concentrated acid urine.

Crystals

Importance was once placed on the finding of crystals in the urinary sediment. However, the occurrence of crystals is of minor clinical significance except in special instances such as certain metabolic stone diseases, e.g., cystinuria and oxalosis. Under ordinary circumstances the positive identification of crystals is not a worthwhile endeavor.

In acid urine the most frequent crystals observed are those of uric acid and calcium oxalate (Fig. 6–10). Uric acid crystals are yellow and dissolve in sodium hydroxide. Calcium oxalate crystals are colorless and dissolve in hydrochloric acid. In acid urine, urates may also be precipitated in the amorphous form. Amorphous urates dissolve with heat.

In alkaline urine the most common crystalline deposits are those of the various phosphates. Phosphate crystals are colorless and dissolve in acetic acid. Phosphates may also precipitate in the amorphous form.

INVESTIGATION OF HEMATURIA

One can fully understand the concern of a parent who notices that his/her child is passing red or "Coke-colored" urine. As described below, not all urine that is red contains red blood cells. The physician who initially sees a child with red urine should certainly consider these causes. Once it is established that the patient has red blood cells in the urine, it is important to attempt to localize the source of the cells in the urinary tract. Table 6–3 divides the urinary tract into several anatomical

Table 6–3. Sources of Urinary Tract Bleeding

Ureters, Bladder, and Urethra	Nonglomerular Renal Bleeding	Glomerulopathies
Urolithiasis Metabolic Infectious and obstructive	Systemic diseases Sickle cell trait and disease Bleeding diathesis	Primary Acute poststreptococcal glomerulonephritis Acute postinfectious
Cystitis Infectious Bacterial Viral Parasitic Chemical	Vascular Renal venous thrombosis Renal artery thrombosis Renal cortical necrosis Arteriovenous malformation	glomerulonephritis Familial nephritis (Alport's syndrome) Rapidly progressive glomerulonephritis IgA nephropathy
Trauma Foreign body	Parenchymal Infectious — pyelonephritis Obstructive Ureteropelvic junction Ureterovesical reflux Nephrolithiasis Neoplastic — nephroblastoma (Wilms' tumor) Traumatic — blunt	Membranoproliferative glomerulonephritis Benign familial hematuria Sporadic hematuria
	Miscellaneous Idiopathic — unilateral Factitious Idiopathic hypercalciuria Hypertrophy of column of Bertin	Systemic diseases Hemolytic-uremic syndrome Systemic lupus erythematosus Schönlein-Henoch syndrome Subacute bacterial endocarditis Shunt nephritis

divisions and lists the causes of hematuria unique to that anatomical division. Most significant causes of glomerular bleeding are associated not only with hematuria but also with proteinuria.

The most common cause of gross hematuria in children is nephritis (Rubin and Baliah, 1975). Hemorrhagic cystitis is a relatively uncommon cause of hematuria in young children but is more common in adolescent females. However, hemorrhagic cystitis does occur in children and is an occasional cause of gross hematuria. A study examining the causes of gross hematuria in the general pediatric outpatient population showed that documented urinary tract infections accounted for 26 per cent of the patients; in only 9 per cent of the patients was glomerular disease apparent (Ingelfinger et al).

The practitioner may be faced with a patient who has either gross or microscopic hematuria, and this sign may be either persistent or intermittent. A careful medical history is essential. For example, a recent history of pharyngitis or impetigo would raise the suspicion of acute poststreptococcal glomerulonephritis. Recent immigration from such areas of the world as Africa and the Middle East might implicate *Schistosoma haematobium* (Jones). Treatment with such drugs as methicillin (London; Bracis et al), piperacillin (Joy), cyclophosphamide, and anticoagulants may be associated with urinary tract bleeding. An important aspect of the medical history is the family history. Familial conditions associated with hematuria are nephrolithiasis, sickle cell disease and trait, and hereditary nephritis with renal failure occurring during the second decade of life.

Once urinary tract infection has been satisfactorily eliminated, pediatricians and pediatric nephrologists generally will focus attention on glomerulopathy as the possible cause of the renal bleeding. If a patient has both hematuria and proteinuria, it is crucial that a thorough evaluation be completed and a diagnosis made. If the total hemolytic complement level or C_3 level is depressed and a rising titer of antistreptococcal antibodies (antistreptolysin O, antihyaluronidase, or antideoxyribonuclease B) is demonstrated, the diagnosis of acute poststreptococcal glomerulonephritis can be made. However, if the complement level is depressed but rising titers of antistreptococcal antibodies cannot be demonstrated, then other renal diseases such as systemic lupus erythematosus (SLE), sub-

acute bacterial endocarditis, shunt nephritis, and membranoproliferative glomerulonephritis must be considered. Positive serologic tests, such as for the antinuclear antibody or the anti-DNA antibody, are helpful in diagnosing SLE. A heart murmur accompanied by a positive blood culture is diagnostic of subacute bacterial endocarditis, and an infected ventriculoatrial or ventriculoperitoneal shunt is associated with shunt nephritis. However, in most cases the diagnosis can be confirmed only with a percutaneous renal biopsy.

The diagnosis of the hemolytic-uremic syndrome is made in a young child who has hematuria, proteinuria, microangiopathic hemolytic anemia, thrombocytopenia, and uremia. Any child with a family history of end-stage renal disease, presenting with microscopic hematuria, with or without high-pitched neurosensory hearing deficits, should be suspected of familial nephritis (Alport's syndrome). Benign familial hematuria is a diagnosis reserved for children who have microscopic hematuria without proteinuria and whose siblings or parents have hematuria; the condition should be considered benign if there is no family history of renal failure. Nevertheless, these patients should be followed yearly because some may develop renal failure several years later (Piel et al). Schönlein-Henoch syndrome is frequently associated with microscopic hematuria, which usually remits in several months. This syndrome is characterized by a characteristic purpuric rash, symmetrically distributed over the extensor surfaces of the lower legs and arms and over the sides of the buttocks, painful swollen joints, and colicky abdominal pain. Usually the renal involvement is mild, but it is more severe when hematuria is associated with the nephrotic syndrome. Finally, an interesting disorder characterized by intermittent gross hematuria occurring during upper respiratory infections is IgA nephropathy or Berger's disease. This is usually a benign condition, but in a significant number of cases it may lead to chronic renal insufficiency or hypertension (Joshua et al; Droz). The diagnosis is made only by a renal biopsy demonstrating the presence of mesangial granular deposits of IgA on immunofluorescence microscopy.

Renal bleeding without proteinuria is unlikely to indicate significant renal disease. Small amounts of protein may be detected when the hematuria is heavy, and this is related to the protein content of red blood cells. Table 6–3 divides the causes of nonglomerular renal bleeding into several major categories. The specific entities listed under these major categories do not by any means constitute all causes; many of these are exceedingly rare. However, approaching the problem of nonglomerular renal bleeding in a well-organized manner will help the practitioner in focusing on the broad categories.

A systemic disorder that frequently causes nonglomerular renal bleeding is sickle cell trait and disease. It should be mentioned that sickle cell trait has been described in patients who are not black (Crane et al; Richie and Kerr). A sickle cell preparation should therefore be considered in all patients with unexplained hematuria. Systemic diseases that predispose to bleeding, such as acute leukemia or hemophilia, do not often present with urinary tract bleeding as the sole manifestation of the disease.

Renal vascular disease as a cause of hematuria is rather unusual in a patient with no other signs or symptoms. Both renal venous thrombosis and renal arterial thrombosis occur primarily in the neonatal period and often are associated with perinatal asphyxia, sepsis, and use of umbilical artery or vein catheters; thrombosis of renal blood vessels is also frequently seen in infants of diabetic mothers (see Chapter 30).

Bleeding from the renal parenchyma may be caused by infection, obstruction, and neoplasia. However, less than 25 per cent of patients with Wilms' tumor have even microscopic hematuria (Jones and Campbell). There are three entities in the miscellaneous category that are of interest. Many patients have been described who have unilateral renal bleeding of undetermined origin, despite extensive evaluation including renal arteriography and biopsy (Lano et al).

Situations have also been described in which the blood in the urine is not from the patient being studied; the blood, often from another family member, has been intentionally introduced into the urine specimen (Outwater et al). So-called factitious hematuria is an example of a psychological disorder.

A more common cause of hematuria is idiopathic hypercalciuria. Recent reports have shown that patients who later develop signs and symptoms of nephrolithiasis may initially present with unexplained episodes of painless gross hematuria (Kalia et al; Roy et al). Most of these patients have a family history of nephrolithiasis. Diseases of the bladder and ureters may be the source of urinary tract bleeding. Stones may occur anywhere throughout the urinary tract, and despite the importance of searching for a metabolic cause such as oxalosis, hypercalciuria, or cystinuria, most stones occurring during childhood are caused by a combination of obstruction and infection (Gages et al).

Hemorrhagic cystitis is a very common cause of hematuria. Not all cystitis is the result of bacterial infection. Viruses such as adenovirus types 2 and 21 (Numazaki et al; Mufson et al) and parasites such as *Schistosoma haematobium* (Jones) may cause hemorrhagic cystitis. Finally, chemical cystitis may be a side effect of drugs. Cyclophosphamide, an im-

Table 6–4. Evaluation of Children with Hematuria

Hematuria (Microscopic) without Proteinuria	Hematuria (Gross) without Proteinuria	Hematuria and Proteinuria
Urinalysis (parents and siblings)	Perform tests for microscopic hematuria	Serology Complement — C_3 or CH_{50} Antinuclear antibody Antistreptococcal antibodies
Urine culture		
Sickle cell test	If gross hematuria is persistent: Cystoscopy	
Serum creatinine	Renal angiography — if unilateral bleeding	Serum creatinine
Audiogram		Quantitate protein excretion
Spot urine for calcium and creatinine		Serum total protein and albumin
Serology Complement — C_3 or CH_{50} Antinuclear antibody Antistreptococcal antibodies		Renal biopsy, if acute poststreptococcal glomerulonephritis is not proved
Intravenous urogram		
Cystogram		

If all normal, follow patient yearly: blood pressure, serum creatinine, and urinalysis.

munosuppressive and antineoplastic agent, can cause very severe bladder hemorrhage.

Postmicturition blood spotting in boys originating from the urethra may be caused by a dorsal urethral diverticulum. Sommer and Stephens suggest that this may be a common cause of urethral bleeding in boys, since they found this diverticulum in the urethrae of one third of male cadavers studied. Surgical treatment of the diverticulum relieved symptoms in the four patients reported. Kaplan and Brock, however, found no underlying cause in the patients that they studied.

The laboratory investigation of children with hematuria is easily conducted on an outpatient basis. Renal angiography, cystoscopy, and percutaneous renal biopsy, which are seldom indicated when the urogram is normal, require 1 or 2 days' hospitalization. In Table 6–4 are listed three major categories of hematuria. Patients with isolated microscopic hematuria require a rather brief evaluation emphasizing familial factors; a careful family history should be taken and a urinalysis should be performed on parents and siblings. The workup is usually concluded with an intravenous urogram and voiding film or with a formal voiding cystourethrogram to rule out urethral polyps in males. Since one cannot be certain that patients with isolated microscopic hematuria will maintain normal function, it is recommended that the family be given the encouraging news that the condition appears benign but that yearly urinalysis, serum creatinine determination, and blood pressure reading be performed.

Children who have gross hematuria should receive a workup similar to that for children with microscopic hematuria. If the hematuria is persistent, severe, or frequently intermittent, cystoscopy should be considered. One may then determine whether the bleeding is bilateral or unilateral, and, rarely, an isolated bladder lesion responsible for the bleeding is found. If the bleeding is unilateral, renal angiography is indicated in order to exclude a vascular or developmental malformation. Persistent or intermittent bilateral renal bleeding even in the absence of proteinuria is an indication for percutaneous renal biopsy.

Any patient with significant hematuria and proteinuria who does not unequivocally have acute poststreptococcal glomerulonephritis is a candidate for a percutaneous renal biopsy in order to determine the precise histologic diagnosis. The diagnosis is important not only for possible therapeutic implications but also from a prognostic standpoint.

PERCUTANEOUS RENAL BIOPSY

The overwhelming majority of renal biopsies performed in children are done percutaneously. Table 6–5 is an outline of the indications for renal biopsy in children. Most children with the nephrotic syndrome do not require a biopsy unless they (1) fail to respond to daily steroid therapy, (2) frequently relapse and become steroid-toxic, (3) become steroid-resistant after initially being steroid-responsive, (4) have gross hematuria, or (5) have a depressed C_3 level. Most patients with minimal change nephrotic syndrome (85 per cent of all children with the nephrotic syndrome) (International Study of Kidney Disease in

Table 6–5. Indications for Percutaneous Renal Biopsy

Nephrotic Syndrome

Proteinuria unresponsive to 4 to 5 weeks of daily therapy (either initially or any time subsequently)

Frequently relapsing patients in whom therapy in addition to prednisone is being considered

Patients with (1) onset beyond 10 years of age, (2) gross hematuria, or (3) reduced C_3.

Patients who present with triad of microhematuria, hypertension, and decreased renal function

Nephrotic syndrome associated with systemic disease — e.g., systemic lupus erythematosus or Schönlein-Henoch syndrome.

Hematuria

Significant hematuria and proteinuria not resulting from acute poststreptococcal glomerulonephritis

Significant hematuria and proteinuria associated with systemic disease such as systemic lupus erythematosus or polyarteritis nodosa

Rapidly progressive glomerulonephritis — any acute nephritic syndrome with significant renal functional deterioration observed over 2-week period

Asymptomatic microscopic hematuria with definite family history of renal disease (or neurosensory high-frequency hearing loss)

Recurrent or persistent bilateral macroscopic renal bleeding of unknown cause

Miscellaneous

Unexplained renal failure associated with normal or near normal kidney size; if renal failure severe, open renal biopsy should be considered because of risk of bleeding

Unexplained significant fixed proteinuria (after intravenous urogram and voiding cystourethrogram)

Children) become protein-free after daily prednisone. Other forms of the nephrotic syndrome seen in childhood, such as focal segmental glomerulosclerosis, membranous nephropathy, and membranous proliferative glomerulonephritis, are often unresponsive to adrenal steroids, and biopsy therefore should be considered in any patient who is resistant to steroid therapy.

A renal biopsy is indicated in patients with hematuria and significant proteinuria. Most cases of acute poststreptococcal glomerulonephritis can be diagnosed correctly with history, physical examination, and appropriate serologic tests; these patients do not require a renal biopsy unless the diagnosis is uncertain or they demonstrate a rapid deterioration of renal function over a period of 1 to 2 weeks after onset. Patients with other nephritides, whether isolated or part of a generalized disease, should undergo kidney biopsy.

The renal biopsy is usually unrewarding from a diagnostic point of view in patients with isolated microscopic hematuria without proteinuria and no family history of renal disease. Often electron microscopy in these patients reveals minimal alterations in the basement membrane, but its prognostic value is yet to be demonstrated (Piel et al).

Percutaneous renal biopsy can be performed with minimal risk in most children. However, patients with an underlying bleeding diathesis or far advanced chronic renal insufficiency who have abnormal platelet adhesiveness and small contracted kidneys are most likely to bleed after the procedure. In these patients and in infants with small diseased kidneys, it is safer to perform an open renal biopsy if a tissue diagnosis is of great importance.

Each pediatric nephrologist has his or her own method for performing a percutaneous renal biopsy. Some nephrologists prefer a blind approach. Localization of the kidney for biopsy can be done with landmarks from an excretory urogram. The urogram will confirm the presence of two functioning kidneys, a prerequisite for percutaneous renal biopsy, and at least one film in the series should be taken with the patient prone.

A site at the lower pole of one kidney is selected on the radiograph (Fig. 6–11). The horizontal distance from this site to the midline (usually over a vertebral body) is measured on the AP film and the spinous process is noted. Similarly, the distance from the

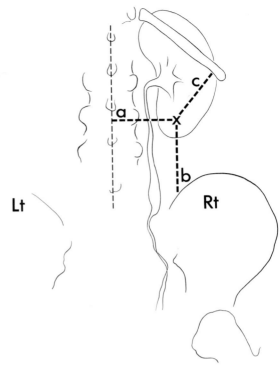

Figure 6–11. Artist's sketch, from excretory urogram, depicting manner by which lower pole of the kidney is located. The distances a–x, b–x, and c–x are marked on the patient's back. (From Burke EC: Procedure for needle biopsy of the kidney. Clin Pediatr (Phila) *10*:328, 1971. Reproduced by permission of JB Lippincott Company.)

lower-pole site to the posterior superior iliac crest is measured.

The spinous process and iliac crest are identified on the patient. The appropriate distances are measured and the site for biopsy is selected. The site should be lateral to the paraspinal muscles (to minimize bleeding) and should be at the correct spinous process (usually L3 in children).

Most nephrologists, however, use a form of visualization of the kidneys. During an infusion excretory urogram and conventional fluoroscopic imaging, the nephrologist can direct the tip of the biopsy needle into the superficial cortex of the lower pole of either kidney. The disadvantages of such a procedure are the relatively high radiation exposure, the need for the intravenous infusion of contrast media, the need to have a radiologist in attendance, and the unpleasantness of a darkened room and cumbersome lead apron.

More recently, localization of the kidneys with ultrasound provides accurate needle guidance. This method allows the procedure to be performed in a well-lit room without the infusion of intravenous solutions and other paraphernalia.

If sedation is required, the patient is premedicated 1 hour before the biopsy with intramuscular meperidine 2 mg/kg and promethazine 1 mg/kg and an oral dose of chloral hydrate 50 mg/kg (maximum dose is 1 gram). The patient is positioned prone on a stretcher and a rolled-up sheet is placed under the upper abdomen; the hard roll flattens the lordotic curve and limits movement of the kidneys in the posteroanterior direction.

Ultrasonic localization is done with a standard 13-mm, 3.5-megahertz transducer. The

B-scan is used to outline the lower pole of the kidney, which is marked on the skin surface with gentian violet. The calyceal echoes of the lower pole are identified, and a point midway between the lower margin of the kidney and the calyceal echoes is selected as the entry site and is marked with a dot. Renal depth at this point is determined and the axis of the transducer is noted. Needles used in renal biopsy are shown in Figure 6–12.

A successful biopsy, regardless of the method, requires a cooperative patient. A very young patient should be well sedated, but an older child can cooperate without sedation if the procedure is carefully and patiently explained to him or her on the previous day. The patient needs to feel comfortable with the doctor performing the procedure.

If done by a skilled physician, the test rarely leads to complications, and while post-biopsy microscopic hematuria is common, significant renal bleeding requiring blood transfusion is exceedingly rare (Altebarmakian et al). Most patients admitted for a percutaneous renal biopsy do not require more than 48 hours' hospitalization.

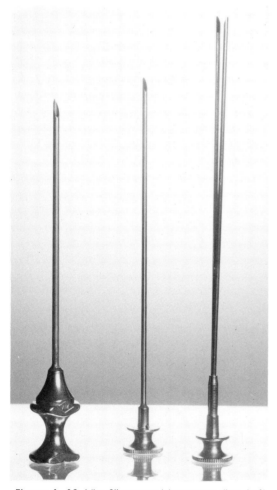

Figure 6–12. Vim-Silverman biopsy needles. *Left,* Outer needle. *Center,* Obturator. *Right,* Sampling needle. (From Burke EC: Procedure for needle biopsy of the kidney. Clin Pediatr (Phila) *10:*328, 1971. Reproduced by permission of JB Lippincott Company.)

BIBLIOGRAPHY

Albert MS, Leeming JM, Scaglione PR: Acute glomerulonephritis without abnormality of the urine. J Pediatr *68:*525, 1966.

Altebarmakian, VK, Guthinger WP, Yakub YN, et al: Percutaneous renal biopsies: complications and their management. Urology *18:*118, 1981.

Bracis R, Sanders CV, Gilbert DN: Methicillin hemorrhagic cystitis. Chemother *12:*438, 1977.

Burkhardt AE, Johnston KG, Waszak CE, et al: A reagent strip for measuring the specific gravity of urine. Clin Chem *28:*2068, 1982.

Cohen JA, Levitt MF: Acute glomerulonephritis with few urinary abnormalities: report of two cases proven by renal biopsy. N Engl J Med *268:*749, 1963.

Cone TE: Diagnosis and treatment: some syndromes, diseases, and conditions associated with abnormal coloration of the urine or diaper. Pediatrics *41:*654, 1968.

Crane DB, Hackler RT, Fischer LM: Significant hematuria secondary to sickle cell trait in a white female. South Med J *70:*750, 1977.

Doxiadis SA, Goldfinch NK, Cole A: Proteinuria in the newborn. Lancet *2:*1242, 1952.

Droz D: Natural history of primary glomerulonephritis with mesangial deposits of IgA. Contrib Nephrol *2:*150, 1973.

Foshee WS, Kotchmar GS, Harbison RW: Simplified urinary microscopy to detect significant bacteriuria. Pediatrics *70:*133, 1982.

Gages CGC, Gordon IRS, Shoare DF, et al: Urinary lithiasis in childhood in the Bristol clinical area. Science *188:*109, 1975.

Goorno W, Ashworth CT, Carter NW: Acute glomerulonephritis with absence of abnormal urinary findings. Diagnosis by light and electron microscopy. Ann Intern Med 66: 345, 1967.

Ingelfinger JR, Davis AE, Grupe WE: Frequency and etiology of gross hematuria in a general pediatric setting. Pediatrics 59:557, 1977.

International Study of Kidney Disease in Children: Prospective controlled trial of cyclophosphamide therapy in children with the nephrotic syndrome. Lancet 2:423, 1974.

Jones J: Schistosomiasis haematobium. JAMA 238:1275, 1977.

Jones PG, Campbell PE: Abdominal masses: tumors of the kidney. In Tumors of Infancy and Childhood. Oxford, Blackwell Scientific Publications, 1976, p 505.

Joshua H, Sharon Z, Gutglas E, et al: IgA-IgG nephropathy. A clinicopathologic entity with slow evolution and favorable prognosis. Am J Clin Pathol 67:289, 1977.

Joy VA: Piperacillin and hemorrhagic cystitis. Lancet 1:219, 1979.

Kalia A, Travis LB, Brouhard BH: The association of idiopathic hypercalciuria and asymptomatic gross hematuria in children. J Pediatr 99:716, 1981.

Kandall S, Edelmann CM, Bernstein J: Acute post-streptococcal glomerulonephritis. Am J Dis Child 118:426, 1969.

Kaplan GW, Brock WA: Idiopathic urethrorrhagia in boys. J Urol 128:1001, 1982.

Lano MD, Wagoner RD, Leary FJ: Unilateral essential hematuria. Mayo Clin Proc 54:88, 1979.

Lippman RW: Urine and the Urinary Sediment. Springfield, Ill., Charles C Thomas, 1952.

London RD: Hematuria associated with methicillin therapy. J Pediatr 70:285, 1967.

Mufson MA, Zallar LM, Mankad VN, et al: Adenovirus infection in acute hemorrhagic cystitis. Am J Dis Child 121:281, 1971.

Numazaki Y, Shigeta A, Kumasaka K, et al: Acute hemorrhagic cystitis in children. Isolation of adenovirus II. N Engl J Med 278:700, 1968.

Outwater KM, Lipnick RN, Luban NLC, et al: Factitious hematuria: diagnosis by minor blood group typing. J Pediatr 98:95, 1981.

Piel CF, Biava CG, Goodman JR: Glomerular basement membrane attenuation in familial nephritis and "benign hematuria." J Pediatr 101:358, 1982.

Richie JP, Kerr WS: Sickle cell trait: forgotten cause of hematuria in white patients. J Urol 122:134, 1979.

Roy S, Stapleton FB, Noe HN, et al: Hematuria preceding renal calculus formation in children with hypercalciuria. J Pediatr 99:712, 1981.

Rubin MI, Baliah T: Urinalysis and its clinical interpretation. Pediatr Clin North Am 18:246, 1971.

Rubin MI, Baliah T: Urine and urinalysis. In Pediatric Nephrology. Edited by MI Rubin, TM Barratt. Baltimore, Williams & Wilkins Co., 1975, p 97.

Sommer JT, Stephens FD: Dorsal diverticulum of the fossa navicularis: symptoms, diagnosis and treatment. J Urol 124:94, 1980.

Waisman HA, Stone WH: The presence of Serratia marcescens as the predominating organism in the intestinal tract of the newborn: the occurrence of the "red diaper syndrome." Pediatrics 21:8, 1958.

Wershub LP: Urology: From Antiquity to the 20th Century. St. Louis, Warren H. Green, Inc., 1980, pp 127–144.

Woolf A, Crocker B, Osofsky SG, et al: Nephritis in children and young adults with systemic lupus erythematosus and normal urinary sediment. Pediatrics 74:678, 1979.

7

URORADIOLOGY: PROCEDURES AND ANATOMY

ALAN D. HOFFMAN

The methods for imaging the urinary tract in children have proliferated significantly in recent years. Nuclear imaging, ultrasonography, and computed tomography have been added to the more traditional armamentarium of radiographic exams. In view of their impact on diagnosis and management, it is important that the indications, limitations, and complications of these procedures be familiar to urologists, pediatricians, and radiologists who deal with urinary tract disease in children. In various settings the availability of the newer modalities as well as the experience and interest of the radiologists involved in the per-

formance and interpretation of exams will have a significant influence upon the question of which exam should be done. More than ever before, the radiologist should be utilized in a consultative role prior to the evaluation of the child with problems involving the urinary tract. It is the appropriate role of the radiologist to direct the imaging workup of such patients. With this approach, the number of exams, the expense, the irradiation and patient discomfort are minimized while the useful clinical information is maximized.

Excretory urography and image-intensified, fluoroscopically monitored voiding cys-

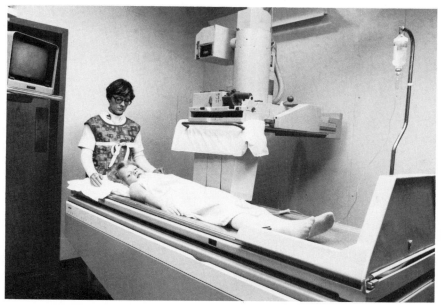

Figure 7–1. The fluoroscopic room used for pediatric radiology and voiding cystourethrography should be equipped with an image intensifier and spot film device capable of instantaneous recording of significant findings. In addition, television video recording can be useful for restudy and teaching.

93

tourethrography are still the roentgenographic procedures most frequently employed for the evaluation of the urinary tract in the practice of pediatric urology and nephrology (Figs. 7–1 and 7–2). They will be the major emphasis of this chapter. Nuclear imaging and ultrasonography are discussed in detail in Chapters 8 and 9, respectively. The diagnostic usefulness of the information about genitourinary anatomy and urinary tract disease that these techniques provide depends upon the manner in which the examination is conducted. The high-quality excretory urogram or voiding cystourethrogram expected as a matter of course in adult urography can certainly be achieved in pediatric urography. However, unnecessarily extensive roentgenographic examinations with an excessive number of films are sometimes performed to diagnose problems that could have been evaluated adequately on a high-quality excretory urogram monitored by a physician experienced in problem-solving pediatric uroradiology. With a knowledge of the usual pathologic processes, a fairly simple routine examination is generally possible using only a few films. Often appropriate tailoring of the examination by the radiologist is necessary.

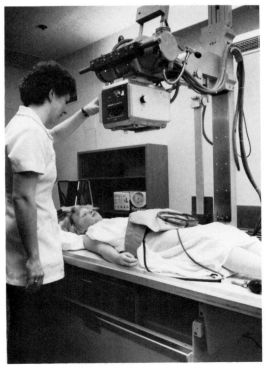

Figure 7–2. The modern excretory urography table is equipped for tomography; a ureteral compression device is shown in place.

EXCRETORY UROGRAPHY

Intravenous excretory urography is the fundamental roentgenographic examination used to evaluate the urinary tract in infants and children. An initial radiograph prior to the intravenous injection of contrast material is an important baseline for the evaluation of the urinary tract and the entire visualized abdomen. Following the injection of contrast material intravenously, the renal parenchyma, intrarenal collecting system, ureters, and bladder can be sequentially evaluated.

Many technical details of the procedure are variable, offering the examiner opportunities for critical choices. Peak kilovoltage and milliamperage; duration and timing of exposures; dosage of contrast medium; filming technique, including choice of x-ray film and screen combinations; positioning of the patient; and use or omission of tomography, ureteral compression, and catheter drainage of the bladder are all crucial to achieving the desired accuracy of diagnosis. Careful selection among these technical variables is of utmost importance in excretory urography and voiding cystourethrography.

Indications

With the addition of new methods of imaging the urinary tract, the indications for an initial excretory urogram have recently undergone some change. Urinary tract infection remains the most common clinical indication for excretory urography in children. Often, a voiding cystourethrogram is done immediately preceding the urogram. Other indications for excretory urography include hematuria, suspicious abdominal pain, and abnormal findings on a renal ultrasonogram. Patients with failure to thrive and an elevation of serum creatinine may also have a screening excretory urogram. In the investigation of urinary incontinence, excretory urography is likely to be diagnostic only in females (Stannard and Lebowitz). Depending upon the availability of high-quality ultrasonography and isotopic scanning, these exams may replace initial excretory urography in certain situations. Screening for congenital renal anomalies, investigating an abdominal mass or abdominal pain, or searching for renal vascular causes of hypertension might best be initially evaluated by these modalities. A considerable number of excretory urograms are done as postoperative or follow-up examinations when the primary diagnosis is known. Not infrequently, the number of radiographs in such exams might be reduced below the number routinely used.

Contraindications

There are a number of contraindications to the performance of excretory urography in children. Dehydration, particularly in a neonate, is a relative contraindication because of the hyperosmolarity of current contrast materials. Shock is an invariable contraindication to such exams. Hyperuricemia seen in children in a hypercatabolic state secondary to primary tumor breakdown or as a response to therapy of malignancy is also a contraindication to urography. In such patients, uric acid may be precipitated in renal tubules as a result of a normal dose of contrast material (Kelly; Poslethwaithe and Kelly).

It has long been known that neonates in the first days of life have a low glomerular filtration rate, and as a result, excretory urography attempted on these infants often has limited usefulness because of poor visualization. If urography is done, markedly delayed films may be of use. Generally, unless there are overwhelming clinical considerations, it is advantageous to delay excretory urography until at least the second week of life. When evaluation is necessary in the very young child, radionuclide renal scanning and ultrasonography are reliable means of evaluating the urinary tract.

Personnel and Equipment

More vital to successful diagnosis than any technical detail of equipment design is the participation of interested personnel — radiographers, nursing personnel, and radiologists — involved in the performance of the examination. People choosing to work in the area where children are seen must be empathetic and skilled in the art of blending the proper degree of gentleness and occasional firmness required to achieve excellent technical results while keeping the patient reasonably happy. Technologists must be dedicated to the concept of high-quality genitourinary radiography while keeping the radiation exposure to the patient to a minimum. Nursing personnel must have an understanding of their role in the performance of examinations, and the radiologists involved must be knowledgeable and interested in the normal anat-

omy and pathology involved in urinary tract problems of children.

The roentgenographic systems intended for the evaluation of pediatric patients must have capability for fast exposure times, since patient motion is one of the prime causes of poor results in any roentgenographic procedure. There are several acceptable systems that might be adaptable to the requirements of a given department or individual physician.

GONADAL PROTECTION. It must be emphasized that it is the responsibility of the radiologic technologist and the physician to insist that gonadal shielding and the basic fundamental techniques of radiation protection be applied to all pediatric patients, as well as to paramedical personnel and physicians involved in the use of ionizing radiation.

Gonadal protection should be used on all pediatric patients whenever it is feasible to do so without obscuring the part of the genitourinary system being evaluated. The male gonads can be shielded on all films taken for an excretory urogram, and the female gonads can be shielded on all films centered and coned for the kidneys.

A simple and practical shielding method consists of using vinyl-covered lead sheeting (0.5 mm of lead) cut into various sizes to shield the male gonads without obscuring the pelvis. The female gonads can be protected with a vinyl-lead sheet placed over the pelvis, but the shield must be removed when films of the lower ureters and bladder are taken. Triangular pieces of vinyl-lead sheeting, cut into various sizes so that they will not obscure the bones of the pelvis or hips, also can be used to shield female gonads for other roentgenographic procedures (Fig. 7–3) (Godderidge). Alternatively, a lead "shadow shield" can be attached to the x-ray tube. With a full field light localizing system, such a shield can be positioned to block radiation to either the male or female gonads (Fig. 7–4).

Preparation of Patient

FEEDING. Food and fluids are not withheld from infants except for the feeding just prior to the excretory urogram. Preschoolers and older children usually have a liquid meal in the evening prior to the exam and are restricted from fluids on the morning of the exam to avoid aspiration of gastric contents in the occasional patient who vomits after the injection of contrast material. It is emphasized that no attempt at dehydration is made in

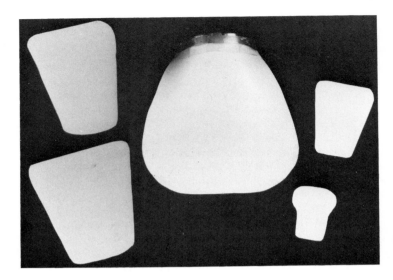

Figure 7–3. A variety of sizes of lead gonadal shields are shown that can be used for both males and females.

pediatric patients; this is particularly important in infants or in any patient who may already be dehydrated. In the past, dehydration has been implicated in renal failure occurring after excretory urography. One possible explanation for renal failure following excretory urography is tubular obstruction by a "gel" formed by contrast medium in combi-

nation with the Tamm-Horsfall urinary mucoprotein (Fig. 7–5) (Berdon et al, 1969).

BOWEL PREPARATION. Preparation of the gastrointestinal tract prior to excretory urography may be varied according to the patient's age. Infants do not require any type of bowel preparation. In preschoolers and older children, bisacodyl suppositories (Dulcolax)

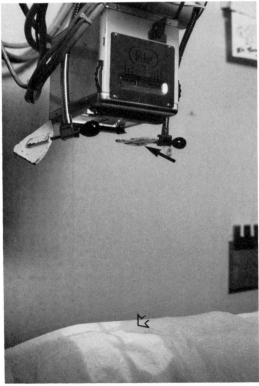

Figure 7–4. A shadow shield (*solid arrow*) casting a shadow over the gonadal region (*open arrow*) is shown with the collimator light on.

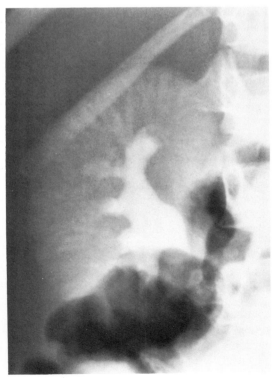

Figure 7–5. Excretory urogram, showing typical striated nephrogram usually attributed to interaction of contrast medium and Tamm-Horsfall mucoprotein.

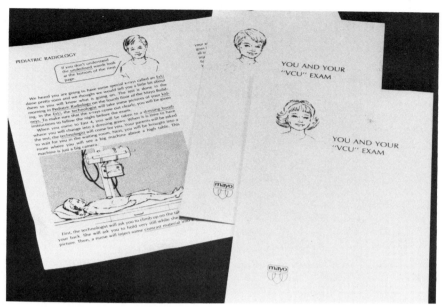

Figure 7–6. Educational pamphlets that explain the excretory urogram (*left*) and voiding cystourethrogram (*right*) in language that is understandable for parents and children.

administered in the morning a few hours before the exam is often helpful in eliminating excess amounts of fecal material from the colon. Adolescents will generally tolerate a normal adult preparation. Some radiologists, however, prefer to avoid bowel preparations altogether and rely upon tomography for proper visualization of the kidneys. Enemas are not usually used, since they may actually interfere with the examination if air is introduced into the colon during administration.

PATIENT EDUCATION. An important consideration in the preparation of the patient for urographic or any radiographic exam that is frightening or uncomfortable for a child is patient education. A successful method of educating young patients and also their parents about such exams may be provided by using patient education materials that can be made available to the parent at the time that the examination is initially requested. If this occurs a day or more before the time the exam is actually done, it is likely that both parent and child will have a reasonable idea of what to expect and overall anxiety will be reduced. These patient education materials can be written in simplified language with cartoonlike pictures which will appeal to young children. Frequently children as young as 4 or 5 years will have reasonable understanding of these exams and be more fully cooperative during the performance of the exams. Figure

7–6 shows pamphlets based on those originally devised by Haas and Solomon.

POSSIBILITY OF PREGNANCY. Adolescent females should be asked for the time of their last menstrual period prior to a radiographic exam of the abdomen. If pregnancy is a likely consideration, such examinations should be delayed unless there is a major, acute clinical indication. Alternatively, ultrasonography might be done.

Contrast Media

Numerous reports suggest theoretical advantages in using certain contrast agents for excretory urography (Benness; Dacie and Frie). However, no significant differences among various types of modern contrast media in regard to density of nephrogram, opacification, distention of collecting systems, or incidence of hypersensitivity reactions have been established in practice (McClennan and Becker; de Langen and Hermans).

DOSAGE. The dosage of contrast medium to be used can be determined by several guidelines. At our institution, we utilize 1.0 ml/lb up to a dose of 50 ml, which is our standard adult dose. In children with renal failure or urinary tract obstruction and in newborn infants, the dosage of contrast medium may be increased up to a maximum of 1.5 to 2.0 ml/lb.

Table 7–1. Summary of Dosages of Contrast Medium
Used in Major Pediatric Centers

Age of Patient	Dosage Used at Babies Hospital (ml)	Number of Centers Using This Dosage*
Neonate, full term	10	60
Less than 6 months	12 to 15	50
6 months to 2 years	15 to 25	42
2 to 5 years	25 to 30	40
5 to 10 years	30 to 45	40

Data from Baker DH, Berdon WE: The use and safety of "high" dosage in pediatric urography: a survey of the Society for Pediatric Radiology. Radiology 103:371, 1972.

* Out of total of 72 institutions surveyed. Remainder used slightly lower dosages.

The dosages used at the majority of pediatric centers are summarized in Table 7–1. The dosages recommended by manufacturers of contrast media are usually considerably smaller than those suggested above. Nonetheless, increasing the dose of contrast material has substantially improved the quality of the urogram without increasing the incidence or severity of hypersensitivity reactions. There is a dose beyond which improvement of the image does not occur, which is probably related to the diuretic effect of the contrast medium itself (Fischer et al).

Nonionic contrast materials for intravenous use may soon be available. Such substances may allow higher dose schedules with greater safety.

ADMINISTRATION. Contrast media should always be injected intravenously. Any one of a number of injection sites may be selected. Although an antecubital vein is most often used in adults and older children, it may be difficult to maintain a needle in this location in infants and young children. As a result, the most apparent superficial vein of any extremity may be utilized. Occasionally, an external jugular vein may be used by one experienced with the use of this route. In infants, scalp veins are occasionally used, but the femoral vein route is not appropriate because of the danger of a septic hip joint as a complication of a misdirected injection. Successful venipuncture requires careful immobilization, especially in the uncooperative patient. Butterfly needles or conventional needles may be used, depending upon the experience of the person performing the venipuncture.

The total amount of iodine injected is the important determinant in renal parenchyma and collecting system opacification. Since maximal opacification is achieved by presenting to the renal filtration apparatus the highest concentration of contrast material, the injection is done as a single bolus rather than a drip infusion (Dure-Smith et al). In patients who are thought to be predisposed to contrast media reactions, access to an intravenous route is maintained by leaving the needle in the vein and keeping it open with a slow infusion of saline for the duration of the examination.

REACTIONS. Gooding et al suggest that the incidence of hypersensitivity reactions to contrast media is lower in children than in adults, but the full range of reactions including death do occur rarely (Dunbar and Nogrady). Testing for hypersensitivity has been tried but does not seem to be predictive and could potentially give a false sense of security. A history of allergy to iodine and prior reactions to iodinated contrast material may be helpful in predicting an increased risk for subsequent examinations (Witten et al). There is renewed interest in the allergic, antibody-mediated hypothesis for contrast media reactions (Brasch). However, some of the most severe reactions reported have occurred in patients with no history of allergy or prior exposure to contrast media.

Fortunately, most reactions to contrast media are not serious. Nausea and vomiting occur occasionally but are not considered true hypersensitivity reactions. Erythema and urticaria are relatively common, but if mild will usually disappear after a short period. When these cutaneous reactions are irritating to the patient, treatment with oral or parenteral antihistamines such as diphenhydramine hydrochloride (Benadryl), a histamine H_1 receptor antagonist, will usually provide relief. Recent work (Philbin et al) suggests that cimetidine, a histamine H_2 receptor antagonist, may supplement the action of a histamine H_1 receptor antagonist. Such cutaneous reactions may occur even after only the retrograde instillation of contrast material into the bladder for voiding cystourethrography (Currarino et al). A previous cutaneous reaction to contrast material generally is not a contraindication to a future examination utilizing contrast material. Serious reactions are uncommon, but an appropriately equipped emergency cart like that shown in Figure 7–7 and a physician who is trained in the treatment of hypotension, cardiovascular collapse, cardiac arrest, and bronchospasm or laryngospasm must be immediately available in the uroradiology area when such exams are done. Medications that may be needed on such an emergency cart are listed in Table 7–2. Appropriate therapy depends upon the predominant symptoms, and each serious reaction has its unique characteristics; therefore, the personnel and equipment must be available to respond to any of the above clinical situations. It should be noted that the medications listed include several appropriate in the resuscitation of

Table 7–2. Medications on Emergency Cart

Aminophylline	Hydrocortisone sodium succinate
Atropine	
Calcium gluconate	Intravenous fluids
Chlorpheniramine	Lidocaine
Diazepam	Mephentermine
Diphenhydramine	Metaraminol
Dopamine	Nitroglycerin
Ephedrine	Oxygen
Epinephrine, 1 : 1000	Sodium bicarbonate

adults. Certainly an anxious parent or grandparent accompanying a pediatric patient might, in a rare instance, undergo a cardiorespiratory emergency, and it is for that possibility that a departmental emergency cart is so stocked.

General Technique

After arriving in the radiology department for an excretory urogram, the patient is asked to void prior to the examination. If the patient generally empties his or her bladder by performance of the Credé maneuver or self-catheterization, these methods should be employed. Occasionally a bladder catheter open to drainage is necessary during the exam.

In the routine excretory urogram, an abdominal film is obtained prior to the intravenous injection of contrast media. This film, often referred to as a KUB (kidneys, ureters, and bladder), is done with the patient in the supine position. It is coned to include the area between the diaphragm and symphysis pubis from flank to flank. Evaluation of this film before contrast medium is administered affords the radiologist and technologist the opportunity to check radiographic quality. Furthermore, the findings on this exam may suggest the need for a variety of actions other than the anticipated routine exam. Additional preparation of the patient, supplementary preliminary films, or performance of an exam other than an excretory urogram may be the result of careful evaluation of the KUB. This evaluation also is an opportunity to evaluate the lumbosacral spine for abnormalities prior to its being obscured by contrast material.

If a significant amount of barium is in the bowel from a prior examination, a cleansing enema may be necessary or the excretory urogram may be postponed. Densities that might represent renal calculi might lead to further filming prior to injection of contrast material.

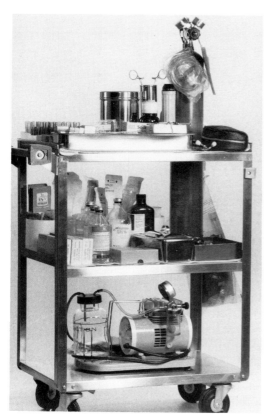

Figure 7–7. Emergency cart with ventilatory equipment, suction apparatus, sphygmomanometer, stethoscope, oxygen, fluids, and various medications.

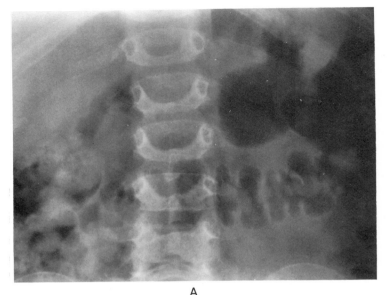

A

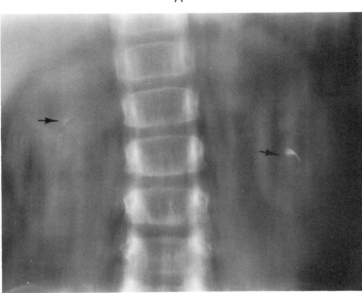

B

Figure 7–8. *A,* Both kidneys are largely obscured by overlying bowel content on the plain film. *B,* Tomogram obtained before injection of contrast medium clearly delineates dense calculus in lower pole of left kidney and poorly opacified calculus in upper pole of right kidney (*arrows*).

Overlying bowel and its contents may make the precise definition of small renal stones difficult. Linear tomography frequently will overcome this difficulty (Fig. 7–8). Additionally, this technique significantly helps in the differentiation of intrarenal from extrarenal location of calcific densities. Tomographic evaluation generally obviates the necessity for oblique radiographs of this area. Other plain radiographs, including prone or cross-table lateral views, may be of use in the evaluation of poorly defined soft tissue densities.

In the case of a clinically palpable abdominal mass, careful examination of the KUB may indicate continuing the evaluation with an exam other than an excretory urogram. If the mass is clearly extrarenal or has particular radiographic characteristics, other imaging modalities such as ultrasound, computed tomography, or isotope scanning may be the best approach.

After the KUB is completed and monitored, the appropriate dose of contrast medium is injected. The number and timing of the films should be varied according to the history and clinical indications for the excretory urogram. Monitoring should be performed from a problem-solving point of view, with several factors kept in mind. The number of films should be limited to those required to identify the clinical problem and to visualize adequately the anatomy of the genitourinary system. Radiation exposure should be closely monitored and restricted to the minimum required to produce a high-quality examination.

Our routine urogram consists of only three films taken after the injection of contrast medium. The first film, properly coned and localized to the renal area, is taken 3 to 5 minutes after the injection. A single tomogram also coned to the renal area is taken immediately after the first film. At this early period the density of the nephrogram is greatest and the renal collecting systems are most often ade-

quately filled. The use of tomography will commonly overcome the obscuring effect of the considerable amounts of overlying bowel and its contents common in infants and children. The third film, centered to include the entire urinary tract, is taken at 10 minutes and the upper collecting systems, ureters, and bladder usually are adequately demonstrated (Fig. 7–9).

Although these routine films are sufficient in 85 to 90 per cent of our pediatric excretory urograms, careful on-line evaluation of exams by the radiologist will reveal the need for additional radiographs in some patients. Further tomography or prone, lateral, upright, or delayed filming may be indicated. A post-

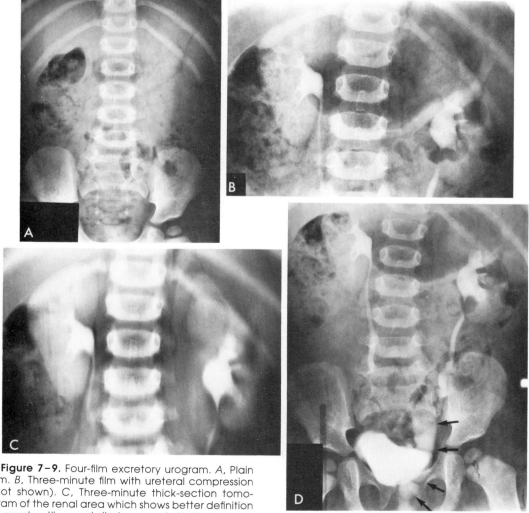

Figure 7–9. Four-film excretory urogram. *A,* Plain film. *B,* Three-minute film with ureteral compression (not shown). *C,* Three-minute thick-section tomogram of the renal area which shows better definition of renal outline and displays an obstructed upper-pole collecting system on the left. *D,* Ten-minute film obtained shortly after the release of ureteral compression. The dilated ureter draining the upper pole of the left kidney is shown emptying below the bladder (*arrows*).

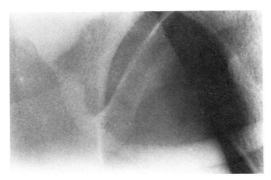

Figure 7–10. Antegrade (excretory) urethrogram done following excretory urogram in a 14-year-old male. This additional film was done to exclude posterior urethral valves.

void film of the bladder is rarely of use, since the significance of "residual" urine (contrast material) after voiding is questionable unless the bladder empties completely. Actually, detailed analysis of the bladder is often not possible with excretory urography because of the variable amount and concentration of contrast material reaching the bladder at any given point during the excretory urogram. On rare occasions, we will attempt to visualize the male urethra utilizing the contrast material that has reached the bladder. This extension of the excretory urogram is best made using fluoroscopically obtained spot films in a fashion similar to the voiding phase of a voiding cystourethrogram. The concentration, and consequently the density of the contrast medium, is generally only fair, but gross lesions such as partial obstruction of the urethra can often be excluded (Fig. 7–10). Improved visualization of the posterior urethra is often

achieved by the use of a Zipser penile clamp (Fitts et al).

Ureteral compression is used routinely during excretory urography in adults. The procedure is extremely helpful in enhancing distention and adequate filling of the pelvicalyceal systems and upper ureters. This technique can also be used in children, resulting in improvement of the quality of urograms. There are, however, several situations in which ureteral compression is not used in children, either because it cannot be easily applied or because it may potentially obscure a diagnosis. In the former category, it is not used for infants or very young children up to about age 18 months, on patients with external urine collecting devices, or on those who have just had abdominal surgery. Patients in whom ureteral compression may be detrimental in diagnosis include those with an abdominal mass or possible obstructive uropathy.

When ureteral compression is not contraindicated, it is applied using a band with two inflatable bags. The band is placed around the upper pelvis and the bags are positioned so that when inflated, the ureters will be compressed between the device anteriorly and the upper pelvis posteriorly (Fig. 7–11). The compression is applied just after the contrast material has been injected so that its effect is seen on the early view of the renal area and on the tomogram. These films are evaluated immediately after they are developed, and if no further tomography is necessary, the compression is released immediately prior to exposure of the full length film. In this way, the entire ureter may be shown on this film. If it is

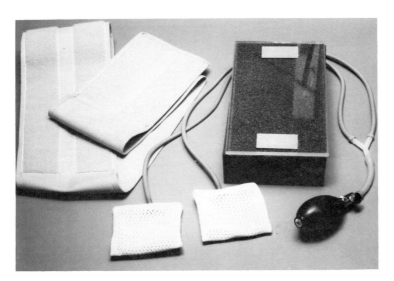

Figure 7–11. Compression device used to temporarily partially obstruct the ureters to better delineate the upper collecting system.

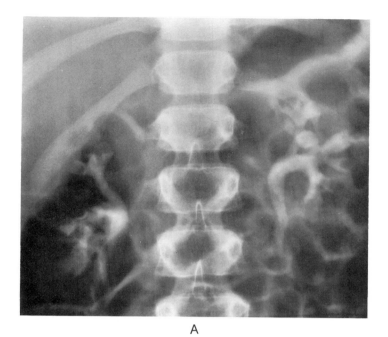

A

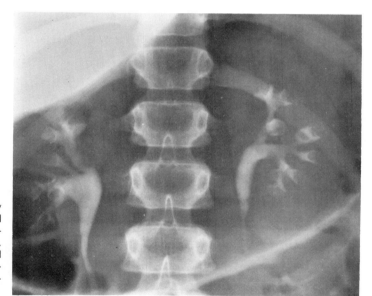

B

Figure 7–12. *A*, Kidneys are largely obscured by overlying gas in the small intestine. *B*, Immediately after administration of carbonated beverage, the stomach is noticeably distended with gas, displacing loops of small intestine inferiorly and allowing unobscured view of both kidneys.

not appreciated that this is an immediate post-decompression film, one might inadvertently assume that there is some degree of distal obstruction, reflux, or atony based upon the principle that a ureter fully outlined with contrast material on one film is usually abnormal.

The most common cause for inadequate visualization of the renal parenchyma and upper collecting system is overlying bowel content. Several techniques have been used to overcome this difficulty. Administration of a carbonated beverage will distend the stomach with gas, displacing the overlying bowel away from the kidneys (Fig. 7–12). Distention of the stomach is especially helpful if the left kidney is obscured, but it can also be of help in visualizing the right kidney, especially if a right posterior oblique film is obtained. However, if this gas passes through the pylorus and into the small bowel, it may obscure renal detail. Oblique films taken without administration of a carbonated beverage may help to visualize kidneys that are obscured by bowel content on conventional films.

Another method to better define the renal outlines in infants is achieved by nasogastric administration of noncarbonated fluid so that the stomach is distended by a homogeneous water-density material through which the kidneys might be visualized (Lutzker and Goldman). Alternatively, it may be helpful to obtain a film in the prone position because displacement of loops of bowel may result in better visualization of the kidneys. A compression paddle may be used as a further aid in the displacement of bowel loops in infants and small children in either the supine or prone position.

All of these methods suffer from a lack of reliability and reproducibility. In recent years, it has become increasingly apparent that tomography is technically feasible even in infants and young children and surpasses these other methods for defining renal outlines. Thin-section tomograms used for urography in adults require long tube travel distance and proportionately long exposure times. Such exposure times are unacceptable for infants and young children, since respiratory motion would blur the films in most cases. Consequently, decreased-amplitude (thick-section)

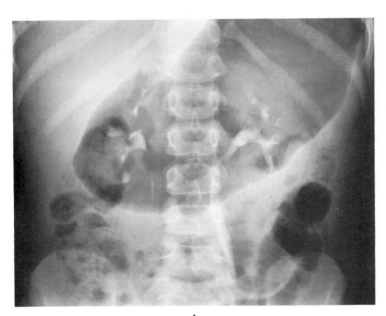

A

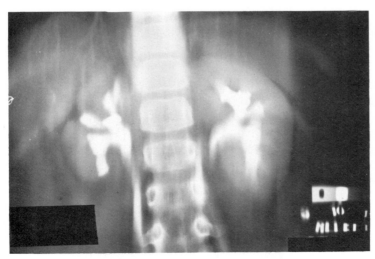

B

Figure 7–13. *A,* After administration of carbonated beverage, both kidneys remain partially obscured by overlying bowel content. *B,* Linear tomography provides excellent visualization of both kidneys, revealing multiple areas of scarring of the right kidney and compensatory hypertrophy of the left kidney.

tomography is used, and generally exposure times are short enough to minimize patient motion and allow adequate visualization of renal parenchyma and renal outlines. Thick-section tomograms or zonograms have the additional advantage of permitting a reduction in the number of films exposed. Generally, a single properly executed tomogram is sufficient; with consideration of all three post-injection films routinely obtained, we find that adequate definition of both renal outlines can generally be satisfactorily accomplished (Fig. 7 – 13). In older children who can cooperate and hold their breath and in situations where finer detail is necessary, increased-amplitude (thin-section) tomography can be done in the same manner as in adult urography.

Thick-section renal tomograms in young children are done using high milliamperage, low kilovoltage, and a short arc (20 degrees). The focus of the tomogram is at one third of the distance from the back of the patient to the front. Our routinely obtained tomogram is taken 3 to 5 minutes following injection of the contrast medium, when the nephrographic effect is greatest. Additional tomograms are occasionally ordered after the initial film is viewed.

The timing of filming is a critical factor in obtaining an optimal urogram. In the majority of patients, the schedule outlined above provides the appropriate diagnostic information with a minimum number of films.

In the neonate, however, delayed films are frequently required because of a combination of factors, including a lower glomerular filtration rate and a poorer concentrating ability. The excretion time for contrast medium is prolonged, and the concentration of contrast medium in the urinary tract is decreased. The peak excretion that occurs in older children and adults during the first 3 to 5 minutes may require from 30 minutes to as long as 3 hours in the neonate (Dunbar and Nogrady). Therefore, delayed films are advisable in infants when visualization of the kidneys and collecting systems is unsatisfactory on initial films. In patients with obstruction of the urinary tract, delayed films also are essential in order to demonstrate the degree of hydronephrosis and to identify the site of obstruction. Reinjection with an additional dose of contrast medium usually can be avoided by using ultrasonography in conjunction with excretory urography.

When a renal collecting system remains dilated following an operative procedure, it is often difficult subsequently to determine if obstruction is present on routine excretory urography. Augmentation of urinary flow can readily be accomplished by intravenous administration of a potent diuretic such as furosemide (Lasix). If this is injected at the end of a routine urogram, a radiograph of the abdomen exposed after an additional 10 or 20 minutes will show further dilatation if the renal collecting system is significantly obstructed. In such cases, the patient may experience colicky pain that simulates the symptoms that prompted the evaluation. The "Lasix test" can also be done in conjunction with an isotopic renal scan as described in Chapter 8.

Another technique for assessing possible partial obstruction of the urinary tract is the pressure-flow method of Whitaker. This requires placement of a percutaneous nephrostomy tube. If this test is done in the fluoroscopic suite, opaque contrast material is used so that a nephrostogram will show any areas of partial obstruction. This technique is described in detail in Chapter 16.

Anatomic Considerations

Accurate interpretation of the excretory urogram requires a knowledge of the normal renal anatomy and experience in recognizing the many anatomic variations found in the normal individual. No attempt is made in this chapter to discuss all possible variations, but some that cause diagnostic difficulty have been singled out for emphasis.

KIDNEY SIZE. The size of the normal kidney in children varies according to age and to length and weight of the body. Renal lengths are not only easy to obtain from high-grade urograms, but have been shown to correlate well with actual renal size (Ludin). The pole-to-pole measurement of the left kidney of infants is usually a few millimeters longer than the right; in older children, the difference in measurement may be as much as 0.5 to 1.5 cm.

Just as pediatricians use growth charts to mark the progress of their patients, so is it important that those involved with renal disease in children be aware of renal growth over a period of time in their patients. The acceptance of this principle has resulted in the development of a number of renal growth charts. Although height correlates more consistently with renal size and growth (Hodson

RENAL GROWTH AND HYPERTROPHY

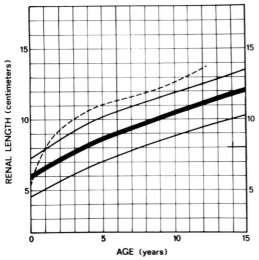

Figure 7–14. Renal growth chart showing renal length as a function of age. The bold line is the mean renal length; the thinner lines above and below show two standard deviations about the mean. The dotted line shows expected compensatory hypertrophy which does not begin to deviate from the mean until birth. (From Lebowitz RL, Hopkins T, Colodny AH: Measuring the kidneys—practical applications using a growth hypertrophy chart. Ped Radiol 4:37, 1975.)

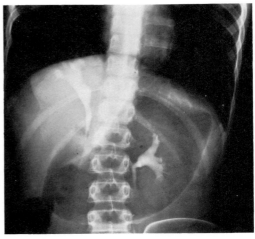

Figure 7–15. "Intrathoracic" right kidney demonstrated on excretory urography.

et al), we utilize a renal growth chart that relates renal length to the patient's chronologic age, since date of birth is readily obtained (Currarino). This chart has an additional tracing that represents the normal expected hypertrophy when only one kidney is present and functioning (Laufer and Griscom) (Fig. 7–14). In certain clinical circumstances, height or bone age may be the appropriate parameter to be related to renal length (Lebowitz et al).

Factors involved in the exam itself that might change the renal measurements include difference in centering, change in the axis of the kidneys with respiration, and swelling of the kidneys during the post-injection period as a result of the diuretic effect of the contrast medium. Hernandez et al feel that the first two factors are the more significant. Partly to obviate some of these factors, the films taken at the same stage on each exam should be used for the measurement of renal size.

Certain anatomic factors that may affect pole-to-pole measurement of the kidneys include anomalies of position such as ectopy or malrotation. Also, the normal kidney with a bifid collecting system has a pole-to-pole length longer than its nonduplicated mate. Bilateral duplication results in pole-to-pole measurements that appear as bilateral enlargements when compared with standard charts. Hydronephrosis or renal mass may also result in misleading renal measurements.

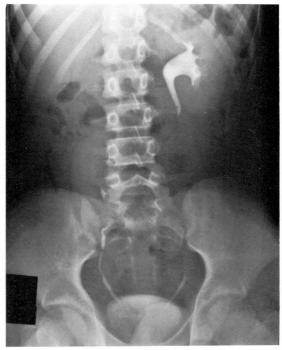

Figure 7–16. Patient with a palpable right abdominal mass which is shown on excretory urography to be a low-lying, normal right kidney.

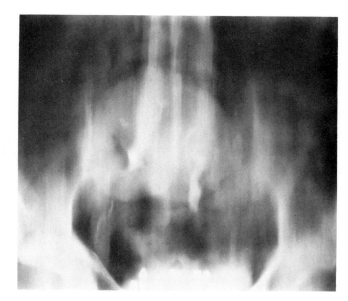

Figure 7-17. Fused pelvic kidney (pancake kidney) that was not visualized adequately on conventional films. Linear tomogram of the presacral region clearly demonstrates the anomalously fused pelvic kidney.

Severe dehydration rarely may cause a decrease in overall renal size due to diminished blood flow.

KIDNEY POSITION. The right kidney is lower than the left kidney under normal conditions in more than 90 percent of patients. Both kidneys tend to be mobile, and their positions relative to the spinal column will vary with different phases of respiration. The left kidney occasionally may be situated just beneath the diaphragm; the right kidney is seldom seen at this level because of the location of the liver in the right upper quadrant (Fig. 7-15). The lower pole of the right kidney will commonly descend over the iliac crest in adults; this position is only occasionally seen in children (Figs. 7-16 and 7-17).

The upper poles of the kidneys are normally situated 1 to 2 cm closer to the midline than the lower poles, resulting in a characteristic angulation such that the axis of the kidneys parallels the psoas shadow. Variations in the degree of angulation are common, especially in infants and young children in whom the axis normally parallels the longitudinal axis of the body. The lower pole of the kidney will, however, not normally be situated medial to the upper pole unless there is incomplete rotation or a horseshoe-shaped kidney (Fig. 7-18).

A mass in the suprarenal region or medial aspect of the upper pole of a kidney may result in a change in the axis of the kidney so that it is parallel to the spine or even reversed so that the upper pole lies lateral to the lower pole. When only the lower pole is being visu-

alized, the abnormal axis may be the first indication of an obstructed, nonvisualized upper pole.

The location of the kidneys varies with changes in body position. By convention, the

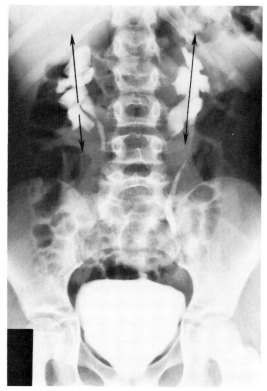

Figure 7-18. Horseshoe kidney in an 8-year-old female. *Arrows* indicate the abnormal orientation of the renal axes.

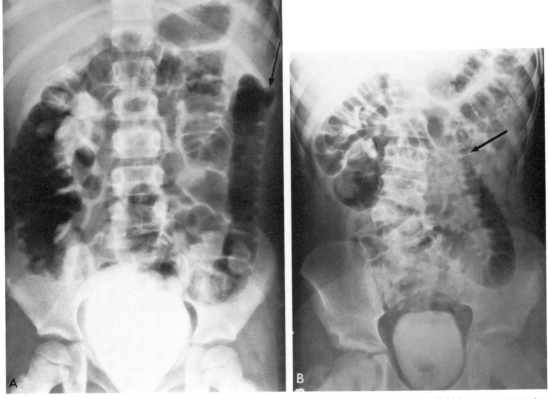

Figure 7–19. Air colograms on two patients who had nonvisualization of the left kidney on excretory urography. *A, Arrow* shows the normal position of the anatomic splenic flexure in this patient who had a multicystic dysplastic kidney shown at ultrasonography and subsequently at operation. *B,* Abnormal position of the anatomic splenic flexure in a patient who was shown not to have any renal tissue in the renal fossa.

routine urogram is obtained with the patient in the supine position. If the patient is positioned on his right side, the anterior movement of the left kidney is greater than that of the right, and vice versa. Both kidneys normally may descend several centimeters when the patient is upright or prone. These factors must be kept in mind when interpreting films taken in positions other than the supine; otherwise, normal variations may be misinterpreted.

When the left kidney is not visualized on an excretory urogram, its presence or absence may be further ascertained by appreciation of the "splenic flexure" sign (Mascatello and Lebowitz; Meyers et al). When a left kidney is present in the left renal fossa, the splenic flexure of the colon is normally attached to the posterolateral abdominal wall by the phrenicocolic ligament. Absence or ectopia of the left kidney is associated with nondevelopment of the phrenicocolic ligament and resultant malposition of the anatomic splenic flex-

ure of the colon so that it occupies the empty renal fossa (Fig. 7–19).

RENAL PARENCHYMA. Since the mid 1960's, use of improved roentgenographic techniques and larger intravenous doses of contrast medium has made it possible to visualize the renal parenchyma during the nephrographic phase of excretory urography. Previously, emphasis was placed on the pyelographic phase, and consequently on the secondary effects on the pelvicalyceal system produced by disease processes within the renal parenchyma. Other chapters in this book present detailed discussion of various disease processes whose parenchymal changes can be demonstrated on high-quality excretory urography.

It is the role of the radiology team to achieve the optimal demonstration of the renal parenchyma outline. However, as the clinical situation dictates, and in the interest of minimizing radiation exposure, there are cases, especially in infants, in which less than complete visualization of the renal border is accepted. Nonetheless, it is generally readily possible to demonstrate the renal outline clearly on the nephrographic phase permitting (1) accurate measurement of the pole-to-pole measurement of the kidneys, (2) determination of the relationship of the cortical margin to the calyceal tips, and (3) differentiation of anatomic variations that may mimic renal disease.

The simple technique of constructing the "interpapillary line" is often quite useful in establishing the relationship of the renal outline to the calyceal tips and in determining the thickness of the renal parenchyma (Fig. 7–20).

The relationship of abnormalities of the renal parenchyma to the calyces is often the key to the diagnosis. The thickness of the renal parenchyma at the upper and lower poles is usually symmetric and greater than the thickness of the parenchyma along the lateral margin of the kidney. The renal parenchyma is frequently prominent at the medial aspect of the upper pole of the kidney (Fig. 7–21).

The most common normal variation of renal parenchyma seen on an excretory urogram is persistent fetal lobulations. Fetal lobulations frequently persist during the first year of life and can be detected on high-quality urograms. In some persons, distinct indentations persist throughout life; these normal indentations should not be confused with scarring of the renal parenchyma or with a renal mass. Normal indentations are typically well demarcated and distinct and lie between minor calyces (Fig. 7–22).

Thin- or thick-section tomograms taken during the nephrographic phase of the excretory urogram are often of vital importance in demonstrating inflammatory scars, infarcts, renal masses, and perinephric abnormalities. Areas of persistent fetal lobulation, prominent but normal areas of renal parenchyma, localized areas of compensatory hypertrophy in a scarred kidney, and other "pseudotumors" that may be confused with a renal mass can usually be differentiated on good-quality excretory urograms (Fig. 7–23). Occasionally, isotopic scanning is required to differentiate the pseudotumor caused by septa of Bertin (Parker et al) from an intrarenal mass.

The technique of total body opacification during excretory urography is a method for the evaluation of abdominal masses in infants and children (Griscom and Neuhauser; O'Connor and Neuhauser). Cystic masses may thus be differentiated from solid ones. This technique depends upon administering the appropriate dose of contrast material intravenously as a bolus. A film of the renal area and the region of any known mass is obtained immediately. Total body opacification allows visualization of the contrast medium within the vascular compartment and the extracellular fluid compartment of the abdominal organs. A cystic avascular abnormality such as a multilocular cystic kidney, a multicystic dysplastic kidney, or hydronephrosis may be visualized as a radiolucent mass with walls that are enhanced by the contrast material (Fig. 7–24). Solid masses and other abdominal masses, on the other hand, may be visualized either as masses with a homogeneous increased density or as masses with a "mottled" opacity caused by alternating areas of increased and decreased density. Tomography also may be used to define the mass more

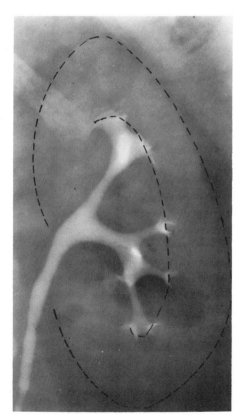

Figure 7–20. Localized view of left kidney with interpapillary line superimposed and renal margin outlined. Renal poles are equal in thickness, and there is slight thinning of upper lateral portion of kidney due to splenic impression.

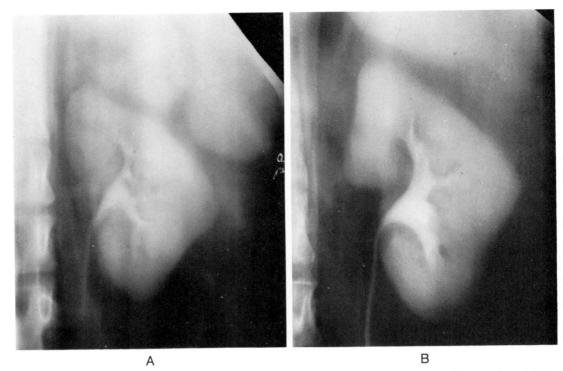

A   B

Figure 7–21. Tomograms of two kidneys with prominent areas of normal parenchyma that may be mistaken for renal tumor. *A,* Lower lateral aspect of left kidney (dromedary hump). *B,* Medial aspect of the upper pole of the left kidney adjacent and superior to the hilus (hilar lip) and at the lateral margin of the left kidney.

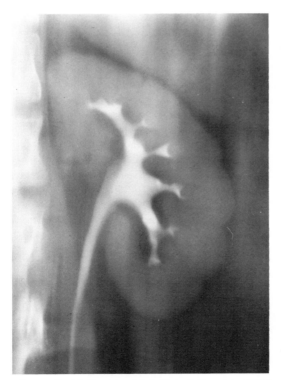

Figure 7–22. Persistent fetal lobulation, identified by classic appearance of sharp indentations of renal cortex between underlying calyces.

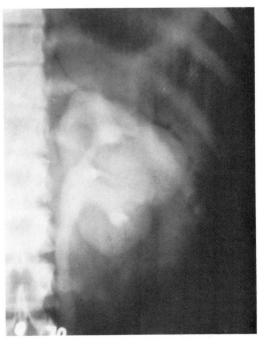

Figure 7–23. Localized compensatory hypertrophy resulting in pseudotumor in left kidney. Tomogram obtained during excretory urography reveals scarring of both poles. Localized compensatory hypertrophy on lateral aspect of the kidney simulates an intrarenal mass.

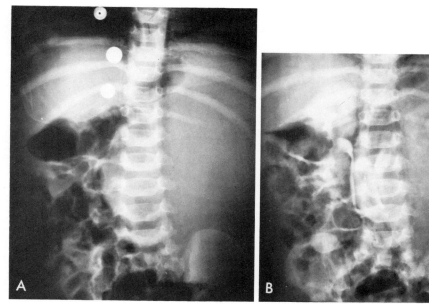

Figure 7-24. Total body opacification (TBO) effect. *A,* Preliminary film (KUB) demonstrates left abdominal mass displacing bowel to the right. *B,* Radiograph of renal areas 2 minutes after an IV injection of contrast media. Normal right kidney. Left kidney is markedly distorted. *Arrows* indicate enhancing septa in a multilocular cyst of the kidney.

clearly and to delineate the thickness of the mass wall (Fig. 7-25). After the early films, the routine excretory urogram is completed with delayed films obtained as required to visualize the collecting systems adequately. Currently, high-quality ultrasound or computed tomography (when done with intravenous contrast material utilizing the same prin-

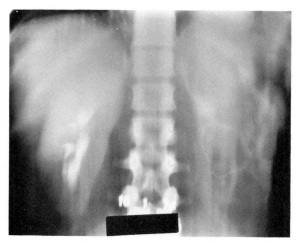

Figure 7-25. Total body opacification in a child with congenital hydronephrosis. Tomogram obtained shortly after injection of contrast material shows radiolucent cystic areas in the region of the left kidney with opacification of thin rims of remaining renal tissue.

ciples as total body opacification) allow better definition of most abdominal masses, either cystic or solid, than does excretory urography with total body opacification (Fig. 7-26). Nonetheless, because of its ease, if excretory urography is being done, an early film is often obtained because of the additional information that might thus be obtained.

PELVIS AND CALYCES. The pelvicalyceal system of human kidneys is extremely variable in appearance. The usual number of calyces varies from 6 to 8, but as many as 12 are often found. The calyces usually are arranged in two distinct rows, one projecting anteriorly and the other projecting posteriorly (Fig. 7-27). The anterior calyces drain the anterior portion of the kidney and, when seen in profile, are situated closer to the lateral margin of the kidney than are the posterior calyces. The relative positions of the anterior and posterior rows of calyces result from the normal rotation of the kidney on its axis. As a result of this calyceal deployment, minor changes in the papilla, fornices, and renal parenchyma are more readily recognized anteriorly than posteriorly. Anatomically, the area of renal parenchyma drained by the posterior row of calyces is usually smaller than that drained by the anterior row.

"Papillary blush," a vague cloudlike area of

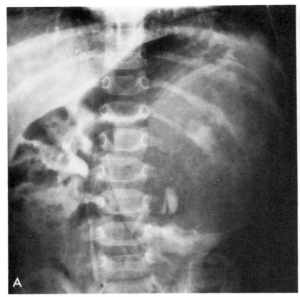

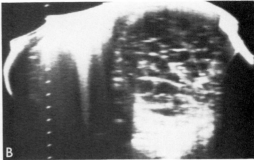

Figure 7–26. Multilocular cyst of the kidney presenting as a large left abdominal mass. *A*, Excretory urogram demonstrating a normal right kidney and a distorted left kidney largely replaced by a mass that appears relatively radiolucent. Distortion of the collecting system is noted. *B*, Transverse ultrasound graphically displays the cystic nature of the mass more readily than the excretory urogram. (From Hoffman AD: Pediatric case of the day. AJR *142*:1069, 1984. © 1984, American Roentgen Ray Society.)

increased density, is frequently observed at the papillary tips. It represents concentration of contrast medium in the collecting ducts. This "blush," which is enhanced when larger doses of contrast medium, high-quality films, and ureteral compression are employed, is a normal phenomenon; it should not be con- fused with ectasia or cystic dilatation of the collecting ducts (medullary sponge kidney) (Figs. 7–28 and 7–29).

Renal papillae are usually funnel-shaped, but they may be rounded or elongated. Multiple papillae frequently drain into compound calyces, particularly at the polar regions of the

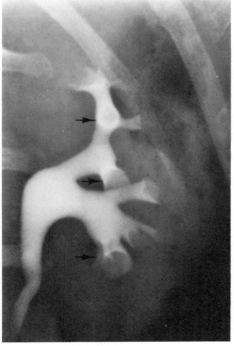

Figure 7–27. Localized view of left kidney. *Arrows* indicate three posterior calyces. The remaining calyces make up the anterior row.

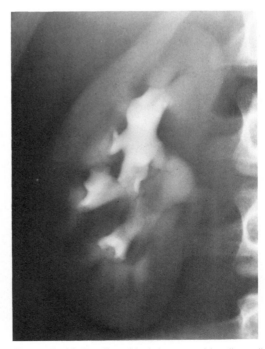

Figure 7–28. Papillary blush is present in all papillae of right kidney. This finding should not be confused with pathologic conditions such as papillary necrosis or medullary sponge kidney.

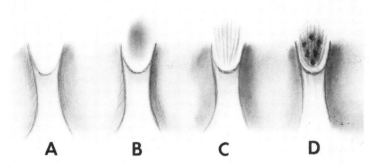

Figure 7–29. Drawings demonstrating possible appearances of renal papilla during excretory urography. *A*, Usually no contrast medium is identifiable within renal papilla. *B*, Papillary blush resulting in hazy, indistinct papillary opacification. *C*, Linear striations of the papilla, representing opacification of ectatic collecting tubules. *D*, Ectatic collecting tubules and tiny spherical collections of contrast medium as seen in medullary sponge kidney.

kidney (Fig. 7–30). Such compound calyces are of considerable significance, since it has now been shown that because of the anatomy of collecting tubule ostia of these papillae, the possibility of intrarenal reflux at these sites is enhanced. The phenomenon of intrarenal reflux is demonstrated on voiding cystourethrography (Ransley).

Multiple variations in the size, shape, and location of renal papillae are common (Fig. 7–31). A papilla associated with an ectopic calyx that drains into an infundibulum may be confused with a filling defect. In cases of

this normal anatomic variation, however, a dense rim of contrast medium within the fornix of the calyx usually can be seen around the papilla (Fig. 7–32).

The renal pelvis may be partially intrarenal and partially extrarenal in location, or it may be entirely intrarenal or extrarenal (Fig. 7–33). The renal pelvis commonly appears to vary in size and shape in response to changes in the position of the kidney. These variations may be observed fluoroscopically or on films made with the patient in various positions. Variations of this type do not indicate an ab-

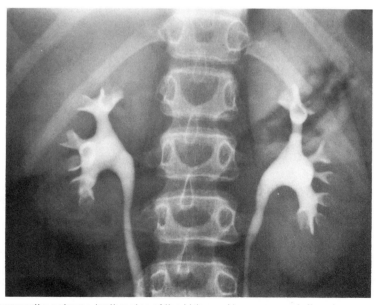

Figure 7–30. Composite calyces, both poles of the kidneys. Numerous variations in appearance of calyces are possible. Composite (multipapillary) calyx, most commonly seen at the poles of the kidney, predispose to intrarenal reflux and foci of reflux nephropathy.

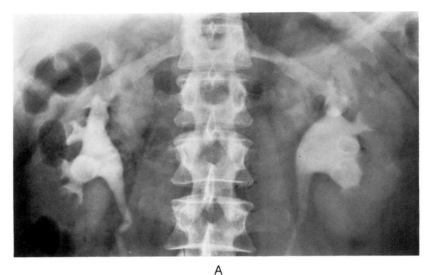

A

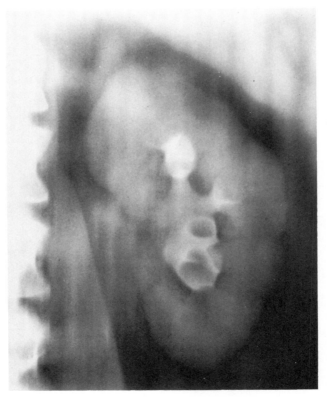

B

Figure 7-31. Variation of normal. *A*, Excretory urogram shows unusually large papillae in both kidneys. *B*, Tomogram of left kidney shows in detail persistent fetal lobulation and the size of papillae of lower pole.

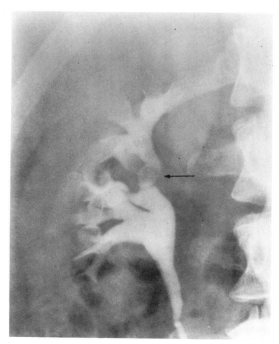

Figure 7–32. Localized view of right kidney reveals radiolucent filling defect in infundibulum of upper pole (*arrow*) due to ectopically located papilla.

normality and must not be mistaken for obstruction at the ureteral pelvic junction.

The size of the renal pelvis is volume-dependent; it can look normal on one examination but "ectatic" on an examination done during diuresis or when filled with refluxed urine.

URETERS. The anatomic course of the ureters is normally quite variable; therefore, any diagnosis of a retroperitoneal mass based only on an apparently unusual position of the ureter on the excretory urogram must be considered with caution. The ureters usually overlie the transverse processes of the lumbar vertebrae, and on rare occasions may project as far medially as the pedicles in normal persons (Fig. 7–34).

A cross-table lateral view of the kidneys, ureters, and bladder can be especially helpful when one suspects a retroperitoneal mass. Because the position of the kidneys shifts when the patient is on his side or prone, supine cross-table lateral films should be obtained. Alterations in the anteroposterior axis shown on these films will not be related to renal motion but will reflect instead the actual anatomic relationship of the kidneys to the

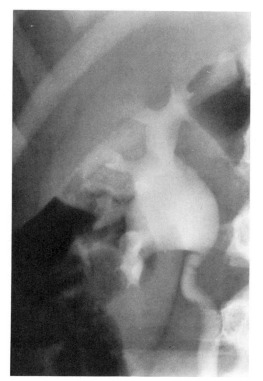

Figure 7–33. Right kidney showing prominent extrarenal pelvis, which is a variation of normal and should not be mistaken for ureteropelvic junction obstruction.

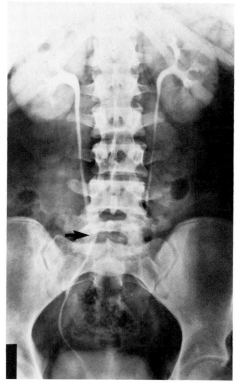

Figure 7–34. Normal amount of variation in ureteral course (*arrow*) on excretory urogram in a 16-year-old female.

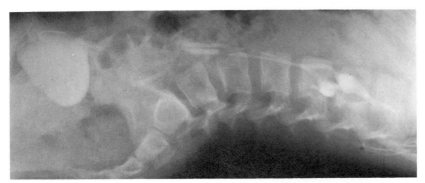

Figure 7–35. Cross-table lateral view, demonstrating normal relationship of kidneys and ureters to lumbar vertebrae.

retroperitoneal structures. On cross-table lateral views the kidneys normally are superimposed over the vertebral column and the ureters course along the anterior margin of the vertebral bodies to the level of the sacrum (Fig. 7–35).

Because of the para-aortic location of lymph nodes within the abdomen, enlarged nodes may be associated with lateral displacement of the upper ureters. The pelvic lymph nodes, on the other hand, are lateral to the lower ureters, and enlarged nodes in this location will produce medial displacement (Fig. 7–36).

The normal course of the ureters is oblique and anterior to the iliac vessels. Because of this relationship, extrinsic indentations and localized ureteral dilatation may be seen on an excretory urogram (Fig. 7–37). Such ureteral dilatation has been found in one third of pediatric patients' excretory urograms (Kaufman et al). This phenomenon was more commonly seen on the right than the left and is felt to be related to slight compression by the crossing iliac vessels. Infants showed this dilatation less commonly than older children.

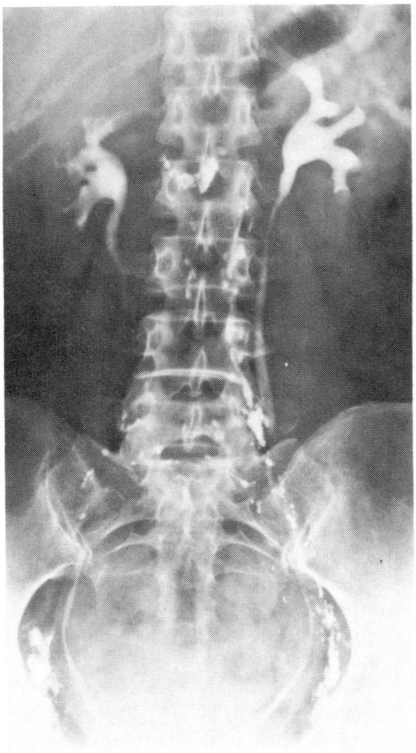

Figure 7–36. Excretory urogram made after lymphangiogram, showing relationship between iliac and para-aortic lymph nodes and ureters.

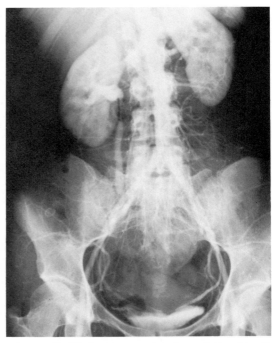

Figure 7–37. Aortogram showing relationship of ureters and iliac arteries.

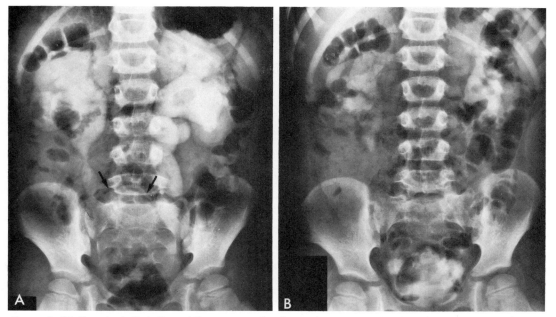

Figure 7–38. Transient dilatation of the upper collecting systems secondary to a full bladder. *A,* Prone film from an excretory urogram showing dilatation of the upper collecting systems. *Arrows* indicate the dome of the bladder, which is filled with only slightly opacified urine. *B,* Prone post-void film shows marked decrease of the apparent obstructive process, which was largely caused by a full bladder.

A normal variant sometimes noted on the excretory urograms of infants is transverse folds in the proximal ureter. Histologically, folds of tissue are seen projecting into the ureteric lumen and are thought to represent persistence of normal fetal structures (Kirks et al).

On urographic studies, ureteric filling is quite variable because of normal active peristalsis. Successive films in the course of a single excretory urogram will commonly show various parts of the ureters filled or empty. Generally, in a normal system an entire ureter is not filled with contrast material on a single film unless a ureteral compression device has just been released. If this method is utilized, complete visualization of the ureter will frequently be seen. A less commonly seen cause for dilatation of a ureter and even of the upper collecting system is a full bladder (Fig. 7–38). Because of this phenomenon, it is always appropriate to insist upon a film with an empty bladder before making the diagnosis of hydroureteronephrosis. If the patient is unable to void sufficiently, catheter drainage of the bladder should be employed.

Occasionally, reflux of contrast material into the ureter and upper collecting system of a nonfunctioning kidney may mimic excretion (Fig. 7–39), or reflux of nonopaque urine may make a well-functioning kidney appear to have diminished function. Errors may be avoided if such a situation is anticipated and if catheter drainage of the bladder is maintained while the excretory urogram is performed. Thus, contrast material or nonopaque urine is drained from the bladder instead of refluxing into the pelvicalyceal system.

BLADDER. The ability to recognize anatomic abnormalities of the bladder must not be overestimated on the excretory urogram. Generally, on the pediatric exam only a single view is available with the patient in a supine position, so that the amount of contrast medium seen in the bladder is variable. On the voiding cystourethrogram, on the other hand, there is the opportunity to visualize the bladder with various degrees of filling, and with the use of fluoroscopy, any degree of obliquity can be obtained.

On the single frontal view generally available on the excretory urogram, a common source of asymmetry is extrinsic compression by the feces-filled rectosigmoid (Fig. 7–40). The bichambered nature of the bladder may cause misinterpretation, particularly on prone films in which contrast material may be seen only in the superior portion of the bladder (Lebowitz and Avni). Significant pathologic lesions of the bladder, such as mass, divertic-

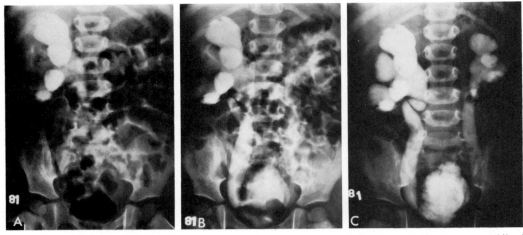

Figure 7–39. Reflux mimicking function. Evaluation of the changes during an excretory urogram (A) at 10 minutes, (B) at 40 minutes, and (C) at 2 hours shows progressively increasing opacification of the left collecting system after the bladder has filled from contrast material excreted on the right side. On an isotopic renal scan, there was essentially no function on the left.

ula, or the vertically oriented, trabeculated bladder seen with neuropathic disorders, can generally be shown on excretory urography.

CYSTOURETHROGRAPHY

After excretory urography, the imaging exam most often performed to define the pediatric urinary tract is the voiding cystourethrogram (VCU, VCUG). This examination has appropriately supplanted exams of the recent past including static retrograde cystography, expression cystourethrography, and excretory cystourethrography. The VCU is superior since it provides better anatomic detail while recording normal physiologic events. The VCU is superior to excretory urography in

the demonstration of bladder and urethral anatomy and abnormalities; additionally, vesicoureteral reflux and its precise extent are best defined with the VCU.

Voiding cystourethrography is most often done after a child has had a urinary tract infection and it becomes important to find out if that patient also has vesicoureteral reflux. Often, an excretory urogram is done later on the same day to appraise renal integrity. The voiding cystourethrogram should precede the excretory urogram so that a valid assessment for vesicoureteral reflux can be made. Similarly, the sequence of the voiding cystourethrogram and other diagnostic urologic exams is important. Since the decision to proceed with cystoscopy often depends on the findings on a voiding cystourethrogram, it is ap-

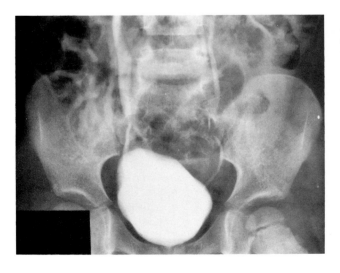

Figure 7–40. Impression on the dome of the bladder on the left is caused by a feces-filled sigmoid colon; this is a common appearance on pediatric excretory urograms.

propriate to perform the radiographic exam initially. However, when a VCU and a cystometrogram are to be performed, the chemical irritation resulting from the contrast medium of the VCU may distort the findings on the latter exam. Consequently, the cystometrogram should precede the voiding cystourethrogram or be performed a few days after it.

Voiding cystourethrography should not be performed routinely during an acute urinary tract infection, principally because bacteria in the lower urinary tract in the patient with vesicoureteral reflux may cause ureteral atony, which could exaggerate the grade of vesicoureteral reflux. It has not, however, been convincingly shown that urinary tract infection causes reflux through the otherwise normal vesicoureteral junction. The concern that bladder infection may result in reflux is not borne out by the recent study by Gross and Lebowitz, who showed an equal rate of vesicoureteral reflux in children with and without microscopic bacteria.

Contrast Media

The choice of contrast medium is of considerable importance. The medium must be non-irritating to the bladder in order to minimize spasm and edema of the vesical wall, which some believe may lead to transient reflux (Shopfner, 1967). Large volumes of high-concentration contrast material result in inflammatory changes in the bladder wall of animals (McAlister et al). Currently, commercially available 17.2 per cent iothalamate meglumine (8.1 per cent iodine) (Cysto Conray II) is suitable for voiding cystourethrography. Besides being less irritating than higher-concentration compounds, the decreased density allows visualization of filling defects in the bladder. The density of this contrast material is still great enough to define subtle grades of

vesicoureteral reflux and intrarenal reflux adequately and to show the detail necessary to define urethral lesions (Fig. 7–41).

Method of Exam

Voiding cystourethrography is done as a dynamic examination; that is, the events occurring during micturition are seen as they occur (Colodny and Lebowitz, 1974a). Image-intensified fluoroscopy allows monitoring during the exam and spot films obtained in the course of the exam provide a permanent record. A further adjunct is videotaping of the television fluoroscopic image for review and teaching. The advantages of camera films obtained from the output phosphor of the image intensifier in a 70, 90, 100, or 105 mm format include rapid filming sequence, good detail, and lower radiation than with conventional films.

Preparation of the patient for this exam is carried out in a fashion similar to that for excretory urography in that educational sheets explaining the voiding cystourethrogram are available for the parents and child at the time that the exam is scheduled (Fig. 7–6). However, for voiding cystourethrography, no bowel preparation is required. Neither anesthesia nor sedation should be used because they are not necessary and their use impedes normal voiding, which this exam is meant to simulate as closely as possible.

Using aseptic technique, the child is gently catheterized using a soft, straight catheter. Generally, an 8 F infant feeding tube with an opaque line is best. Occasionally it is necessary to utilize a 5 F feeding tube in premature patients, certain patients following urethral surgery, and those with urethral stricture. To minimize discomfort, lidocaine jelly may be introduced intraurethrally in older males prior to catheterization. Balloon catheters are not used. The urine obtained at the time of cathe-

Figure 7–41. Spot film of the urethra from a voiding cystourethrogram using a 17.2 per cent concentration of contrast material. The detail of reflux into Cowper's duct is well demonstrated (*arrows*).

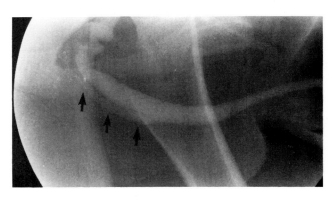

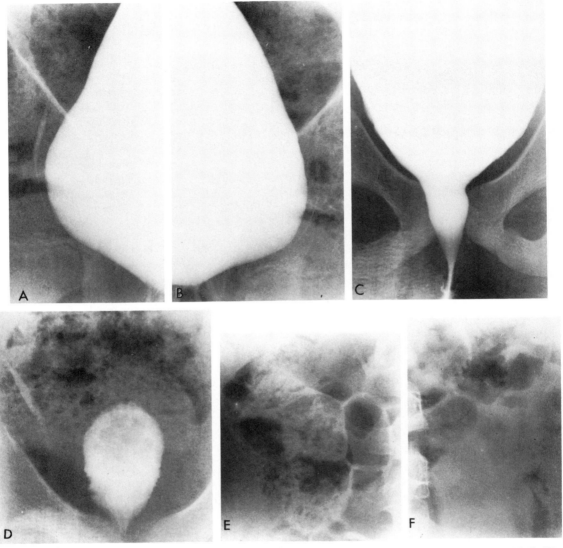

Figure 7–42. Voiding cystourethrogram. Usual spot films obtained in females: Right (*A*) and left (*B*) ureterovesical junctions at the end of filling; Anteroposterior view of urethra during voiding (*C*); bladder at the end of voiding (*D*); right (*E*) and left (*F*) renal fossae at the end of voiding. Bilateral Grade I vesicoureteral reflux is faintly seen on *A* and *B*.

terization may be used for urinalysis, culture, sensitivity testing, and colony count.

After successful catheterization, the catheter tip is attached to conventional intravenous tubing, and the contrast material is instilled into the bladder by a gravity drip from a container suspended from an IV pole. The height of the reservoir relative to the table top should not exceed 100 cm (Koff et al). In the rare instance when catheterization cannot be performed in infants, suprapubic needle insertion, a method frequently employed by pediatricians, may be used. A full bladder is

necessary and its presence can be ascertained by palpation or by ultrasound (Fletcher et al).

In the performance of voiding cystourethrography gross areas of pathology are defined on the fluoroscopic exam. More importantly, fluoroscopy allows appropriate position, timing, and collimation for spot films, which often define more subtle abnormalities. In this manner, a set of routine films are taken utilizing only a minimal amount of fluoroscopy time. Another way to decrease the radiation dose during this exam is to use low fluoroscopic milliamperage (Sane and

Worsing). This reduces the definition on the fluoroscopic exam, but as stated, the definitive diagnosis is usually based on the spot films.

Our routine films include (1) steep oblique views of each ureterovesical junction area in the filling phase, (2) urethral films during voiding, (3) a film of the bladder at the end of voiding, and (4) a film of each renal fossa at the end of voiding or, if vesicoureteral reflux is present, when it is maximal. Since radiographically definable pathology of the female urethra is exceedingly rare, only a single anteroposterior urethral view is exposed during voiding (Fig. 7–42). For the male, a steep oblique position is best to see the urethra in profile. Two films of the posterior urethra and one of the anterior segment are routinely obtained (Fig. 7–43). Modification of this routine may be required as a result of clinical information, abnormalities on previous exams, or findings noted at fluoroscopy during the current exam (Fig. 7–44).

To get the cooperation of a patient to initiate and continue the act of voiding under fluoroscopic visualization requires a carefully planned setting and what might be considered the "art" of radiology. A dimly lit room and a limited number of people in the fluoro-scopic room are helpful. Adolescents, particularly females, have the greatest difficult voiding during such examinations; the gender of the examiner does not seem to be as important as the experience and reassurance provided by the person performing the exam (Poznanski and Poznanski). Different positions, including supine, sitting, or standing, may be utilized. We find that most patients of any age will be able to void in a recumbent position — females supine and males in a steep oblique so that the urethra is seen in profile. Others may find the specialized potty-chairs or a variety of urine receptacles are more efficacious. A variety of measures are used to help the patient initiate the urinary stream, including repeated assurance, warm water poured over the perineum, and suprapubic pressure, particularly for those with a neurogenic bladder. However, the primary method to insure voiding is continued filling of the bladder until the contrast material stops dripping. The catheter should not be removed until the patient is producing a good urinary stream. This technique should be used particularly in infants, who often will require refilling before adequate filming can be done. There should be no concern that voiding is prevented by the presence of the catheter, since even very young patients can readily void around the small catheters used. Spot films of the urethra are taken just after the catheter is slipped out. In a small minority of patients, voiding is not initiated even after the methods suggested above are employed. It may then become appropriate to allow the patient to void in a nearby bathroom, and quickly return to the radiographic room for a post-void film. This maneuver compromises the exam in the male, in whom visualization of potential urethral pathology then is not obtained.

Anatomic Considerations

The definition of vesicoureteral reflux is the most common finding on the VCU. Many observers have noted that the degree of vesicoureteral reflux, and indeed, its absence or presence, can vary from one examination to the next or from one day to another. Therefore, the technique used for voiding cystourethrography should be rigidly standardized in order to minimize error introduced by the examination itself. The significance of transitory reflux and the effects of medical and surgical management are discussed elsewhere.

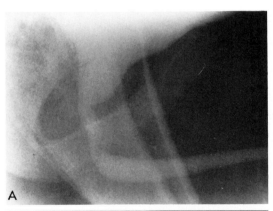
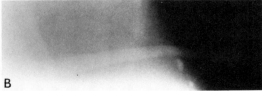

Figure 7–43. Male voiding cystourethrogram varies from the female voiding cystourethrogram in that oblique views of the urethra are obtained; *A*, Posterior urethra (usually two views are obtained); *B*, anterior urethra.

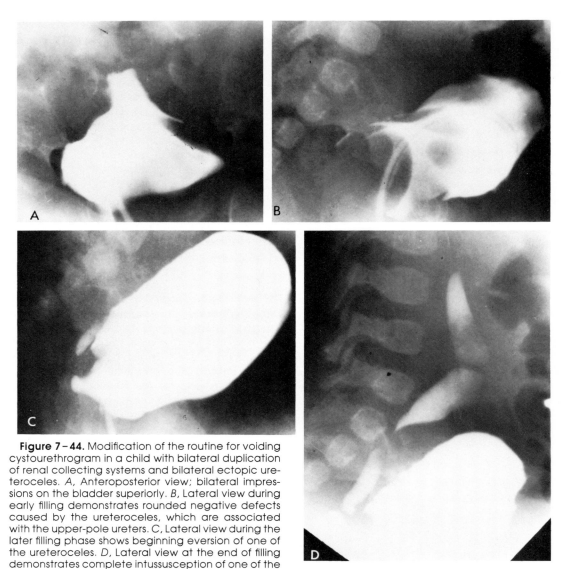

Figure 7–44. Modification of the routine for voiding cystourethrogram in a child with bilateral duplication of renal collecting systems and bilateral ectopic ureteroceles. A, Anteroposterior view; bilateral impressions on the bladder superiorly. B, Lateral view during early filling demonstrates rounded negative defects caused by the ureteroceles, which are associated with the upper-pole ureters. C, Lateral view during the later filling phase shows beginning eversion of one of the ureteroceles. D, Lateral view at the end of filling demonstrates complete intussusception of one of the ureteroceles into the ureter. Also noted is reflux into a lower-pole ureter.

The degree of reflux has a significant bearing on the prognosis for the resolution of reflux as well as the development of complications such as reflux nephropathy and, consequently, the therapy for each patient. As a result, a number of grading systems have been devised. One currently in use by the International Reflux Study Committee has five gradations (Fig. 7–45) (Levitt et al). Because of the significant implications regarding prognosis and treatment, this or one of the other systems of grading should be utilized.

Infrequently when vesicoureteral reflux into the upper collecting system is seen, detection of further extension of contrast material into collecting tubules is also demonstrated. Such intrarenal reflux most often occurs when reflux is severe in degree and when compound calyces, which are those draining more than a single papilla, are present (Fig. 7–46); these are most common in the polar regions of the kidney.

The position of the ureteral vesical junctions at the posterolateral aspects of the bladder determines the optimal patient position for filming to show vesicoureteral reflux and periureteric bladder diverticula. With a straight anteroposterior position, reflux into the lower ureter may be obscured by contrast material in the bladder. The right ureteral

I	II	III	IV	V

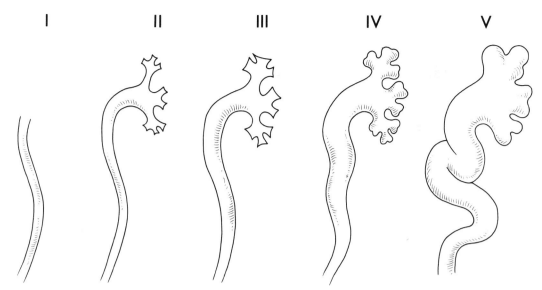

Figure 7–45. Radiographic grades of reflux (according to the International Reflux Study Committee): I, ureter only; II, ureter and upper collecting system without dilatation; III, mild or moderate dilatation of the ureter and mild or moderate dilatation of the renal pelvis, but no or slight blunting of the fornices; IV, moderate dilatation and/or tortuosity of the ureter with moderate dilatation of the renal pelvis and calyces and complete obliteration of the sharp angles of the fornices, but maintenance of papillary impressions in the majority of calyces; V, gross dilatation and tortuosity of ureters, renal pelves, and calyces; papillary impressions are not visible in the majority of calyces.

vesicle junction is therefore best demonstrated with right anterior oblique position, and the left ureterovesical junction is best seen in the left anterior oblique position. If the urethral catheter is shown on the oblique film and if the patient has vesicoureteral reflux, the relative position of the refluxing ureter to the urethra is established. Closer proximity than usual indicates ureteral ectopy (Fig. 7–47).

For (1) the followup of mild to moderate vesicoureteral reflux, (2) determination of whether reflux has been corrected by reimplantation of the ureter, or (3) initial detection when a positive family history is the indication, it is appropriate to do a radionuclide voiding cystogram. Although anatomic detail is reduced, there is a significant reduction in radiation dose. This subject is more fully covered in a subsequent chapter.

To evaluate a voiding cystourethrogram

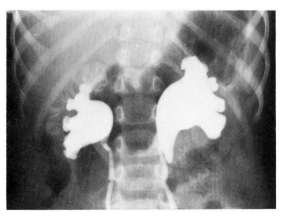

Figure 7–46. Bilateral vesicoureteral reflux resulting in complete filling of both collecting systems and associated with intrarenal reflux (IRR) on right.

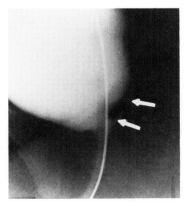

Figure 7–47. Ectopic ureter demonstrated on voiding cystourethrography during voiding. *Arrows* mark the left ureter, which drains into the urethra marked by the opaque line of the bladder catheter.

properly, it is important to assess patient position, filming sequence, variations of the appearance of the bladder and urethra, and changes in urethral caliber carefully during voiding. Correct interpretation of bladder and urethral findings depends on a clear, thorough comprehension of anatomic and physiologic variations that are normal in these organs (Fig. 7–48). For example, normal anatomic variations visualized in the region of the vesical neck and the prostatic urethra of males, and in the entire urethra of females, have been misinterpreted in the past as representations of lower urinary tract disease. Unusual configurations of the vesical neck may sometimes suggest abnormalities when viewed on a single film. Yet it has been clearly demonstrated that most such contours represent normal variations of the anatomy of the trigonal region or sphincteric mechanisms reflecting the dynamics of micturition.

The normal anatomic relationships of the

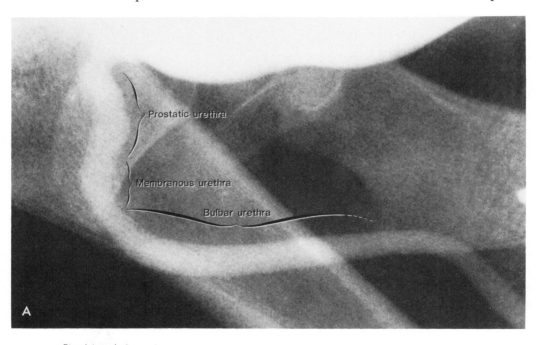

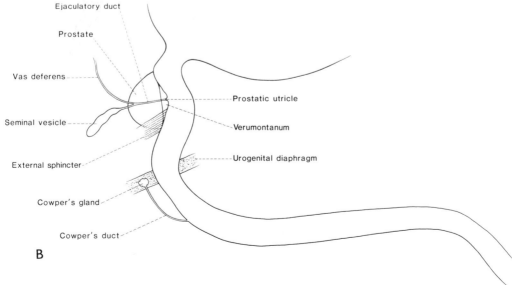

Figure 7–48. Normal male urethra, posterior portions, in a child. *A,* Spot film from the voiding phase of a VCU. The segments of the posterior urethra are indicated. *B,* Diagram drawn from the spot film indicating the various important structures immediately adjacent to the posterior urethra.

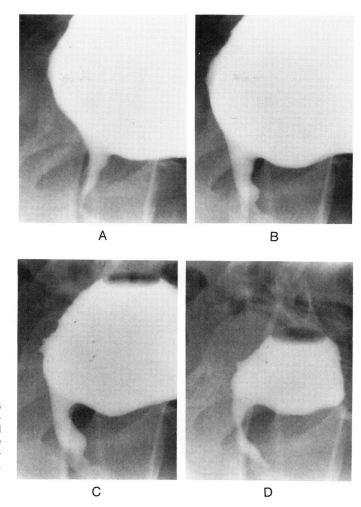

A   B

C   D

Figure 7–49. Sequence of spot films in steep oblique projection during voiding cystourethrography in a 5-year-old girl. The variation in appearance of the bladder base and urethra during voiding is shown. *A*, Early voiding. *B* and *C*, Mid voiding. *D*, Late voiding phase.

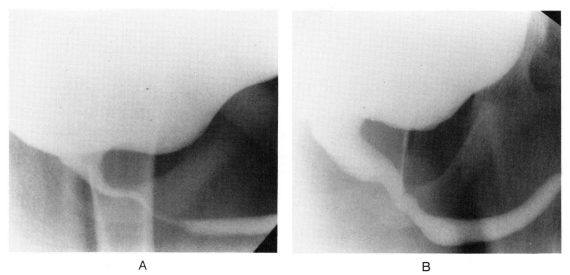

A   B

Figure 7–50. Voiding cystourethrogram spot films in an 8-year-old male. *A*, Early voiding with urethra incompletely distended. *B*, Later stage demonstrated normal urethral appearance with urethra distended by a good urine flow.

bladder base plate, the anterior and posterior trigonal plate, the trigonal canal, the bladder neck, the intermuscular incisura, and the urogenital diaphragm have been stressed by Shopfner and Hutch (Fig. 7–49). The roentgenographic appearances of these anatomic units of the bladder and urethra were elegantly illustrated by Shopfner (1971) in a monograph on cystourethrography.

Variations in the caliber and contour of the urethra are dependent on the volume and rate of flow during voiding; therefore, a roentgenographic diagnosis of stricture or other cause of urethral obstruction must be documented on more than one film during maximal distention of the urethra (Fig. 7–50). However, because of the extreme rarity of abnormalities in the female urethra, it is our policy routinely to obtain only a single spot film in the anteroposterior projection. A common finding is va-

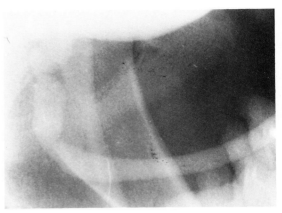

Figure 7–52. Voiding cystourethrogram spot film from a 4-year-old boy with prominent intramuscular incisura that could be mistaken for a urethral lesion.

ginal reflux (Kelalis et al) (Fig. 7–51). Vaginal reflux is accentuated in the presence of female hypospadias or labial adhesions but is usually due to voiding in the supine position. In males variations such as prominent muscular incisura (Fig. 7–52), or narrowing caused by constriction of the bulbocavernosus muscle (Currarino), must be differentiated from true stricture. External sphincter spasm or fibrosis (Mandell et al) (Fig. 7–53) is a feature commonly seen in patients with a neuropathic bladder. Irregularity of the urethra does not generally indicate an obstructing lesion without proximal dilation. Videotape recording of each exam permits restudy of changes in caliber and contour without repeat examination and further radiation exposure to the child. Evaluation by videotape is particularly important when a questionable abnormality has

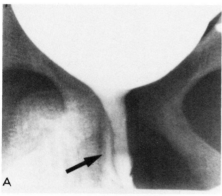

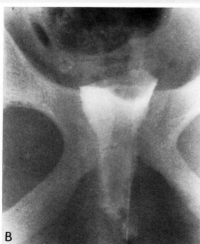

Figure 7–51. Vaginal reflux shown on voiding cystourethrogram in a 7-year-old female with dribbling after voiding. *A,* Urethra during voiding, anteroposterior view; vagina *(arrow)* is shown. *B,* Post-void anteroposterior view; vagina clearly outlined by contrast material.

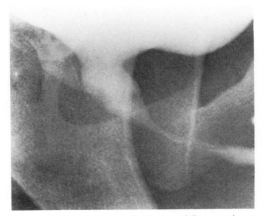

Figure 7–53. Spot film from a voiding cystourethrogram in a 14-year-old male with myelodysplasia. There is narrowing of the posterior urethra at the level of the external sphincter which was persistent on this exam.

been seen on the spot films taken during the procedure.

Adjunctive Examinations

Definition of abnormalities in the pelvis is often insufficiently accomplished by filling of the bladder alone. To define a tumor in this region adequately, it is often useful to obtain spot films or radiographs in the lateral projection after filling of the rectum and sigmoid with barium or air (Fig. 7–54). In this manner, a tumor is localized to a specific region in the pelvis (e.g., presacral, prerectal, or even prevesical), and depending upon the sex of the patient, the differential diagnostic possibilities are significantly reduced. Cross-sectional imaging by ultrasonography or computed tomography may also contribute to anatomic definition in these cases.

For children and particularly infants with ambiguous genitalia or intersex, another ad-

junct to voiding cystourethrography is often helpful in the definition of anatomy. *Genitography* is the term used to describe the radiographic examination in which an attempt is made to fill all genital cavities with opaque contrast material (Shopfner, 1964). The method of examination is similar to that used in cystourethrography. After filling of the bladder in the usual fashion, a second catheter is advanced into any other genital orifice and contrast material is again instilled. Fluoroscopy and spot films in frontal, lateral, and occasionally oblique projections are done. An alternative means for filling these structures is the "flush method," in which a leak-proof seal is attempted by the use of a tapering connector or syringe tip. This tip is gently inserted into the visualized genital orifice and contrast material is injected. Another method for performing genitography utilizes a feeding tube passed through a single-hole disposable nipple that is filled with cotton (Peck and

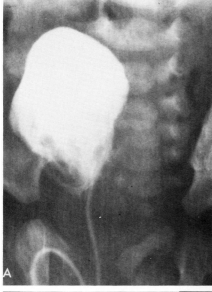

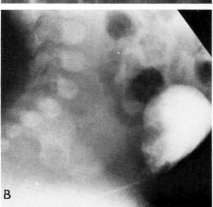

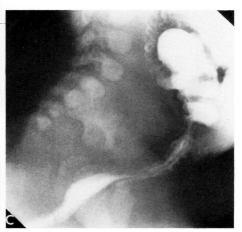

Figure 7–54. Sixteen-day-old female presented with a palpable abdominal mass and urinary retention. *A,* Cystogram in frontal projection shows the bladder to be displaced to the right and elevated. *B,* Lateral view shows that the bladder is also displaced anteriorly. However, better definition of the anatomic position of the mass is shown after barium has been introduced into the rectum, and the lateral spot film shows the retrorectal position of the mass which was a presacral teratoma (*C*).

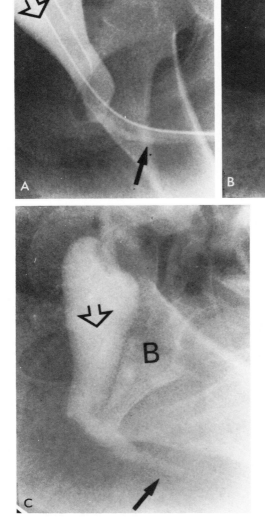

Figure 7–55. Genitogram in a 5-year-old female with adrenogenital syndrome. *A*, It was possible to catheterize only the vagina (*open arrow*). Partial drainage of the vagina was accomplished via the urethra (*closed arrow*). *B*, Following excretory urography the bladder (B) is filled. *C*, With voiding, some of the contrast material from the bladder refluxes into the vagina.

Poznanski). The nipple acts as an obturator and the tube can be passed the desired distance into the genital orifice. If the bladder cannot be catheterized, its position and anatomic connections can be determined after excretory urography (Fig. 7–55).

OTHER UROGRAPHIC EXAMS

Loopography

The kidneys and ureters draining into an ileal or sigmoid conduit should be evaluated periodically (yearly) by excretory urography,

radionuclide studies, or ultrasonography as long as the conduit is present (Shapiro et al; Hardy et al; Lebowitz). The approximate length, width, and peristaltic activity of the conduit also can be evaluated fluoroscopically during the excretory urogram. If elongation or dilatation of the ureters or intestinal segment is noted on any of these examinations, a retrograde study of the ileal or sigmoid conduit should be done.

A retrograde loopogram can be obtained by introducing a catheter into the stoma, occluding the stoma around the catheter, and instilling contrast medium into the conduit by gravity drip under fluoroscopic guidance.

Occlusion of the stomal lumen can be accomplished by inserting the tip of a Foley catheter into the stoma, with the balloon inflated outside the stoma. Alternatively, one end of a straight rubber catheter can be inserted through a predrilled hole into a small rubber ball, and the tip of the catheter can then be inserted into the stoma. The patient, if cooperative, presses the ball or balloon against the stoma with sufficient force to occlude the external opening. The examination should be combined with the use of fluoroscopy and spot filming so that proper positioning, sequential filming, adequate distention of the conduit, and the degree of reflux and peristalsis of the ureters and conduit can be observed and recorded.

Normal conduits are easily distended, and reflux is generally demonstrated during the examination of an ileal conduit with opacification of the ureters and pelvicalyceal system (Nogrady et al) (Fig. 7–56). Reflux should not occur with sigmoid conduits or ileal conduits in which an anti-reflux procedure has been done.

Obstruction of the stoma may be evaluated by removing the catheter and fluoroscopically observing the peristaltic activity and emptying of the conduit. Vigorous peristaltic waves and ineffectual emptying of the ileal loop may indicate stomal obstruction. In unobstructed systems, a drainage film 20 minutes after an exam will generally show almost complete drainage of contrast material from the collecting systems and the conduit.

Loopography for sigmoid or other conduits which have had anti-refluxing anastomoses need be done initially only to exclude the presence of ureteral reflux. Periodic followup is done by excretory urography, radionuclide studies, or ultrasonography, and if hydronephrosis develops, cutaneous antegrade pyelography can be helpful in defining ureteral sites of obstruction; intrinsic sigmoid conduit strictures have not yet been reported. Fluoroscopic evaluation of the sigmoid conduit is less informative because the colonic conduit behaves more like a conducting tube, with only minimal peristalsis, or even none at all.

Retrograde Urethrography in the Male

Visualization of the urethra is an integral part of voiding cystourethrography. Even though the entire urethral profile may be seen with the voiding method, the anatomy distal to a site of urethral obstruction often is not accurately depicted because urethral distention may be incomplete, and significant lesions may be missed. Therefore, retrograde urethrography may be employed for the evaluation of the urethra distal to a site of urethral obstruction.

Water-soluble contrast medium in a concentration of 17 per cent may be used for retrograde injection. A syringe fitted with an adapter of appropriate size may be inserted into the urethral meatus to inject the medium. Alternatively, a small, 8 or 10 F Foley catheter can be introduced into the urethra so that the balloon just passes through the meatus. If 0.5 to 1.0 ml. of fluid are injected into the balloon, it will seat in the fossa navicularis. As a result, the catheter will be maintained in position and leakage of contrast material will not occur (McCallum and Colapinto). The contrast material is then gently injected through the catheter, and the urethra is viewed fluoroscopically in a lateral or steep oblique projection. Appropriate spot films are obtained.

Retrograde urethrography is particularly applicable in the evaluation of strictures, diverticula, and urethral trauma when rupture of the urethra is suspected. However, caution must be exercised in interpreting the films, since the region of the membranous urethra is often incompletely distended because the ex-

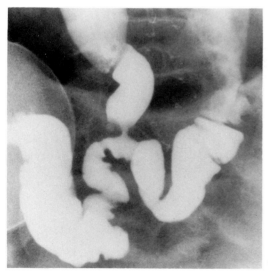

Figure 7–56. Loopogram. Spot film demonstrating filling and distention of the ileal conduit. A stricture is seen at the anastomosis between the right ureter and the ileal loop.

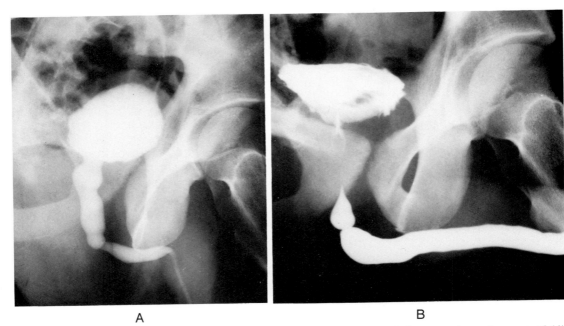

A

B

Figure 7–57. Lesions such as urethral strictures are well delineated with the complementary use of (*A*) voiding cystourethrogram and (*B*) retrograde urethrogram. A bulbar urethral stricture is shown to be of limited length with the addition of the retrograde study. Adequate filling of the area beyond the stricture frequently is not shown on the voiding exam alone.

ternal sphincter is not relaxed, and apparent narrowing in this region could be falsely interpreted as stricture (Fig. 7–57).

Retrograde Pyelography

The need for retrograde pyelography was greatly reduced with the advent of modern excretory urography. In recent years, the use of this exam has been reduced even further as other modalities, such as isotopic studies, ultrasound, and computed tomography have demonstrated renal anatomy when excretory urography is inadequate. Furthermore, percutaneous studies are increasingly employed in children with dilated collecting systems, and using catheters introduced in this manner, antegrade studies of the renal collecting systems can be done. Therefore, retrograde pyelography is infrequently necessary. However, in a small percentage of cases in which these other examinations are not available or will not show the ureter beyond an obstruction, retrograde pyelography may be appropriate (Fig. 7–58).

Combining retrograde pyelography with fluoroscopy in the cystoscopic suite eliminates the disadvantage of blind filling and filming

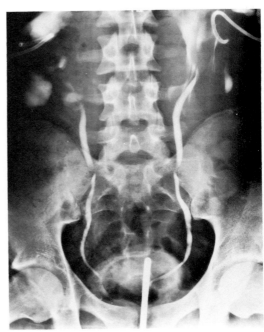

Figure 7–58. Retrograde pyelogram in an adolescent female with congenital ureteropelvic junction obstructions, bilaterally. Nephrostomy tubes previously placed percutaneously are present and have decompressed both upper renal collecting systems.

technique and allows the ureteral catheter to be positioned optimally at the site of the suspected lesion. With the use of fluoroscopy, overdistention of the renal pelvis and possible extravasation of contrast medium can be avoided. Also, questionable obstruction to the outflow of urine in the upper urinary tract is best evaluated with fluoroscopy.

Antegrade Pyelography and Percutaneous Nephrostomy

Operatively placed nephrostomy tubes or percutaneous nephrostomy needles or catheters allow ready access for the definition of the upper collecting system down to the bladder. The role of the radiologist in the percutaneous placement of needles and catheters into the renal pelvis has greatly expanded in the last few years. These techniques are now commonly utilized so that antegrade pyelography and ureteral perfusion studies (Whitaker test) can be performed (Fig. 7–59). Catheter placement via the percutaneous route allows temporary or long-term treatment of obstructive processes. In children such obstruction is most often on a congenital or postoperative basis. Other disorders that might be diagnosed and perhaps treated include leaks, fistulas, and stones.

The technique for performance of percutaneous needle or catheter placement varies. Mild sedation is useful for relieving anxiety, particularly in younger patients. Local anesthetic is initially injected at the puncture site. Although ultrasound, computed tomography, or reference to previous radiographic exams may be used for guidance, we generally use fluoroscopic monitoring to direct needle or catheter placement. Routine radiographs can then be obtained readily to document the pathologic changes and the final position of the needle or catheter.

One method for percutaneous placement of catheters includes a modified angiographic technique utilizing initial passage of a fine needle into the appropriate space, most often a dilated upper renal collecting system. Subsequently, successively larger dilators are introduced along the track with a guide wire, and eventually a 6 to 10 F angiographic pigtail catheter can be placed. Another method utilizes a trocar-cannula unit.

Percutaneous nephrostomy is successful in the majority of cases; failure is most often

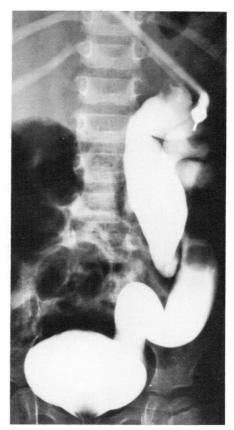

Figure 7–59. Antegrade pyelogram done as part of a Whitaker test showing a markedly dilated left ureter in a 2-year-old female with primary megaureter without obstruction.

likely to occur with nondilated or minimally dilated systems. Significant complications including bleeding or the introduction of infection are uncommon. Transient hematuria, however, is very common and should not cause alarm. The incidence of the introduction of new infection can be held to a minimum with adherence to sterile technique. Dislodgement or malfunction of a catheter also occurs. The occurrence of these latter problems has been reduced greatly with added experience and improvement in the design of equipment used.

Close communication between urologists and interventional radiologists is essential for optimal management of patients who require these procedures. Increasingly sophisticated endouroradiologic procedures have been performed, particularly in adults, including internal drainage of kidneys, stone removal, and lithotripsy.

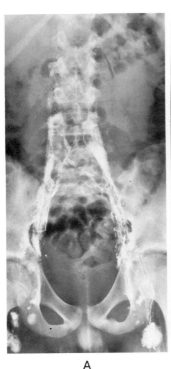 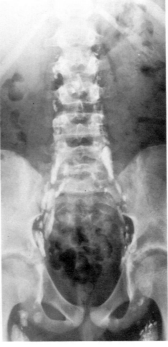

A   B

Figure 7-60. Selected films from a lymphangiogram. *A,* Anteroposterior film immediately after injection of contrast material demonstrating filling of lymph ducts and early filling of lymph nodes. *B,* Similar view 24 hours later shows lymph node architecture with some bilateral enlargement of femoral nodes and enlargement of left para-aortic node. Oblique projections are also routinely obtained.

VASCULAR STUDIES

Lymphangiography (Lymphography)

Newer imaging modalities such as computed tomography and ultrasonography have reduced the need for lymphangiography in children. Generally, lymphangiography has been technically more difficult to do in children than in adults. However, with modern techniques and experienced radiologists, success in accomplishing lymphangiography and diagnostic accuracy and interpretation in pediatric patients can be expected to equal the rates achieved with adults (Dunnick et al).

A 30- or 31-gauge needle, rather than a 29-gauge needle, should be used, and sedation or anesthesia is almost always required in younger children. Evans blue dye is injected into the webbing between the great and second toe to opacify the lymph channels. After cannulation, iodized oil (Ethiodol) is slowly infused until the contrast material reaches the L4, L5 interspace. The total average infusion is 0.2 ml of Ethiodol per kilogram of body weight. The relatively low dose results in decreased adverse effects from pulmonary embolism. Films are obtained after contrast material has reached the lumbar level and at 24 hours (Fig. 7-60).

The procedure is most often done in the evaluation of lymphoma, or of gonadal or other pelvic malignancies that may also require staging lymphangiography. Demonstration of abnormal lymph nodes acts as a guide to the surgeon when biopsy or lymphadenectomy is to be done. Furthermore, because the contrast material stays in the nodes for weeks to months, progress of therapy and the extent of disease may often be followed simply with plain x-rays of the abdomen. Since not all lymph nodes are opacified with lymphangiographic contrast material, some metastases may be missed. However, the recognition of the entity of reactive hyperplasia and the ability to distinguish it from malignant involvement has reduced the rate of false-positive interpretations (Castellino).

Angiography

INFERIOR VENACAVOGRAPHY. In the past, inferior venacavography in conjunction with excretory urography was the method most frequently used as the initial roentgenographic study in the evaluation of abdominal masses in infants and children. With this approach, preliminary films in frontal and lateral projections are obtained. Contrast material is then injected into a vein in the dorsum of one foot, preferably the right, with a tourniquet on the contralateral thigh. A frontal

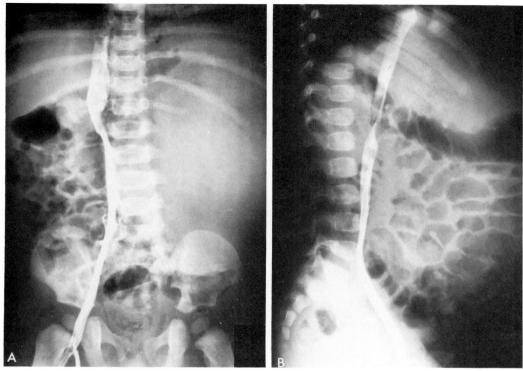

Figure 7–61. Inferior venacavogram in a 16-month-old male with a left renal mass. Contrast material is injected into a right foot vein after a tourniquet has been applied to the left thigh to decrease mixing of contrast material with nonopacified blood. "Streaming" of nonopacified blood is, however, shown especially at the renal vein level. *A,* Anteroposterior view after half of the contrast material has been injected. *B,* Lateral projection after the second half of the contrast material has been injected. No evidence is seen of thrombus or obstruction in the abdominal inferior vena cava.

abdominal film is obtained after half of the dose of contrast material has been injected, and a lateral radiograph is exposed at the end of the injection (Fig. 7–61). Subsequently, early "total body opacification" films and tailored films for excretory urography are obtained.

A significant technical problem occurs in the performance of the examination described above because the infant or child often will be crying when the radiographs are taken as a result of the injection, of being restrained, or of the warm sensation that is produced by the contrast material. The resultant Valsalva maneuver causes shunting of contrast material away from the inferior vena cava and into the ascending lumbar veins. Thus, nonfilling of the inferior vena cava cannot necessarily be interpreted as caval obstruction.

More reliable opacification of the inferior vena cava can be achieved by a formal inferior venacavogram using the Seldinger technique and a femoral vein route (Fig. 7–62). Even

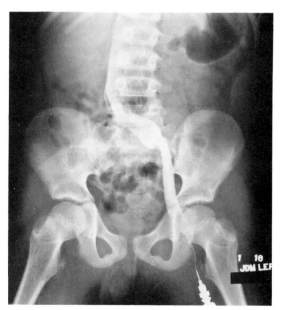

Figure 7–62. Normal inferior venacavogram (anteroposterior view) after left femoral vein injection.

with good opacification of the inferior vena cava, extrinsic compression deformities may be confused with tumor invasion, and interpretation therefore is often difficult.

Modern ultrasonography has largely supplanted contrast studies of the inferior venacavogram in the pediatric patient with an abdominal mass. The sonogram will not only give information about the mass, but usually will also readily demonstrate the inferior vena cava (Slovis et al).

One of the remaining roles for catheterization via the femoral vein is to gain access to the renal vein for sampling of renin levels in the evaluation of hypertension.

ARTERIOGRAPHY. Arteriography may be helpful in evaluating certain abdominal masses in children, but it is not indicated in most instances. The majority of such masses are best evaluated by other, less invasive imaging modalities, including excretory urography, ultrasonography, radionuclide studies, and computed tomography. Arteriography does have a role, however, in evaluation of certain tumors, for example, bilateral Wilms' tumor or a right-sided mass that may be hepatic in origin. Other indications for renal arteriography include childhood hypertension when renal vascular hypertension is suspected, renal trauma when vascular injury is suspected, and rarely inflammatory masses of the kidney. In the newborn with anuria, nonpalpable kidneys, or Potter facies, neonatal angiography by the transumbilical route may be indicated. Since hydronephrotic kidneys will best be shown by ultrasonography, this examination should usually be done first.

Transumbilical Neonatal Angiography. In infants during the first several days of life, the umbilical vessels provide an easily accessible site for performing rapid angiography. The lumen of the umbilical artery may be reopened and the recut ends expanded with forceps to allow the insertion of a catheter. A 5 F infant feeding tube with an opaque line is frequently used. The catheter is advanced under fluoroscopy to the level of the renal arteries for the injection of radiopaque medium (Fig. 7–63).

Percutaneous Transfemoral Retrograde Aortography and Selective Renal Arteriography. Percutaneous transfemoral introduction of the catheter by the Seldinger technique can be performed safely, providing diagnostic accuracy by those skilled in this technique. Certain risks are inherent in the procedure, however, and the referring physician as well

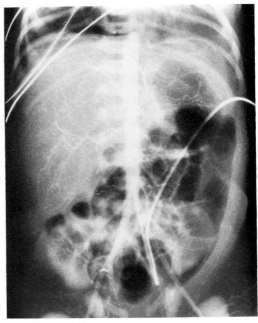

Figure 7–63. Single film from an arteriogram injected through an indwelling umbilical artery catheter. This neonate with Potter's syndrome demonstrates no filling of renal arteries. Patient shown to have renal agenesis at post mortem.

as the radiologist must be aware of these potential complications.

Bleeding may occur from the site of the arterial puncture after the catheter is removed. However, this may be avoided by applying continuous pressure over the arterial puncture site for a period of 10 minutes or more. Vascular occlusion in the legs due to clot formation on the catheter may occur, and arterial spasm can result in ischemia of the leg.

Arterial peak flow has been shown to be reduced in a percentage of children below the age of 8 years. For this reason, particularly in this age group, the smallest catheter that can deliver the necessary flow should be utilized (Kirks et al). Hypersensitivity reactions to the contrast material can occur, but the risk of such reactions is less than that incurred during intravenous excretory urography. The heightened incidence of hypersensitivity reactions to venous, as opposed to arterial, injections is thought to be due to the release of histamine from the lungs when contrast material is injected intravenously.

Patient preparation in regard to hydration and bowel status should be similar to that used for excretory urography. Combinations of meperidine (Demerol), promethazine

(Phenergan), and chlorpromazine (Thorazine) administered intramuscularly or a general anesthetic such as ketamine used without endotracheal intubation may be necessary to achieve the immobility necessary for optimal filming.

A detailed discussion of the technical aspects of angiography is not appropriate in this chapter. However, the physician in charge of pediatric angiography must thoroughly familiarize himself with the special considerations affecting examinations in infants and small children before attempting the procedure. Small catheters should be used to minimize intimal trauma, to prevent bleeding at the puncture site, and to increase the probability of successful arterial catheterization. In infants and children, the initial examination should be a midstream aortic injection (Fig. 7–64).

Several technical variations of the examination may be of significant value in children. In recent years magnification arteriography has been utilized, and this may be especially helpful in visualizing tiny normal and pathologic vessels. Methods of subtraction have been described, and most recently digital subtraction angiography (DSA) has been introduced. This latter method utilizes subtraction and a computer to digitize the information obtained radiographically. The improved resolution usually results in excellent visualization of arterial structures after only intravenous injections of contrast material.

BODY COMPUTED TOMOGRAPHY

One of the most revolutionary changes in radiologic imaging has occurred in the last

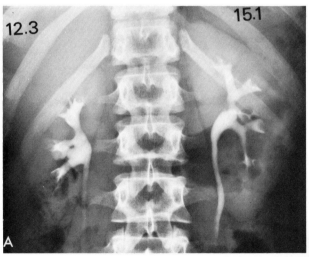
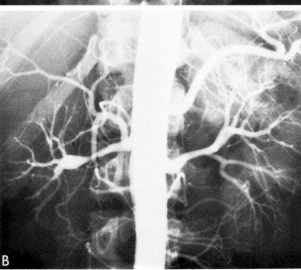
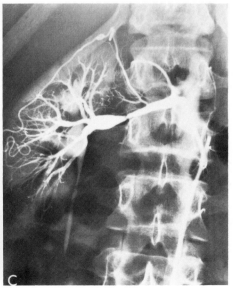

Figure 7–64. Fourteen-year-old female with renal vascular hypertension. *A,* Excretory urogram shows significant variation in renal size. Right renal length is 12.3 cm and left, 15.1 cm. Aortogram (*B*) and right selective renal arteriogram (*C*) show right renal artery stenosis.

decade with the advent and proliferation of computed tomography. This technique was first used for the evaluation of intracranial contents, but subsequently technology was quickly expanded to permit imaging of the entire body. Radiographic images are acquired from a number of angles in axial projection; slice thickness may be varied. Accurate measurement of attenuation coefficients (density) of each small volume (voxel) of tissue results in excellent anatomic detail. The large amount of data generated is collated by a computer, and the resultant images can be electronically manipulated to best define anatomy and pathology. Often intravenous or oral contrast materials are given to the patient to further define structures in the abdomen.

The advantages of body computed tomography are the remarkable image resolution displayed in full cross-sectional views and the relative noninvasiveness of the technique. Images obtained are not as dependent on function as in excretory urography, and they are not obscured by gas and bone as in ultrasound. However, the cost and limited availability of the examination can be disadvantages. Radiation dose, particularly compared with ultrasound, must be considered. In pediatric exams of the renal area and retroperitoneum, additional problems of resolution occur because of respiratory motion and lack of retroperitoneal fat. Faster, newer generations of computed tomographic machines can partially obviate respiratory motion, but refinements in other imaging modalities — ultrasound, radionuclide studies — have limited the use of computed tomography in urographic problems in children.

When body computed tomography is to be used in young children, sedation is often required, particularly for children between the ages of 1 month and approximately 5 years. Immobilization may be necessary, and attention to maintenance of body temperature during the exams in infants is particularly important.

A major role for body computed tomography in pediatric patients is the demonstration of extension of renal, other retroperitoneal, and pelvic masses. This is particularly important when excretory urography and ultrasound have failed to define these lesions adequately (Fig. 7–65). Recurrence of such tumors is often best shown on CT exams (Brasch et al). Computed tomography is occasionally used as a secondary exam in the evaluation of renal cystic disease, some inflammatory lesions, and severe hydronephrosis (Fig. 7–66). Body computed tomography has also been used early in the evaluation of trauma involving the kidneys and other intra-abdominal structures. Changes in renal transplants can also be shown well on computed tomography. To maximize diagnostic accuracy while minimizing excessive numbers of examinations and risk, it is critical to have an appreciation for not only which imaging modality is best for the presumptive diagnosis in the individual clinical situation, but which exam is best done in a particular setting or specific institution.

Acknowledgment

Doctors Glen W. Hartman and Robert R. Hattery were the authors of the chapter in the first edition

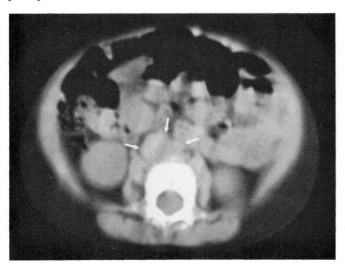

Figure 7–65. Computed tomographic slice demonstrates a mass (*arrows*) surrounding the aorta and inferior vena cava with a few small calcific densities within it. This was a neuroblastoma which was not visualized on either excretory urography or ultrasonography.

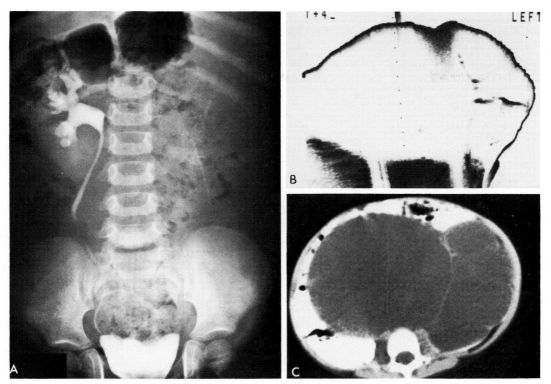

Figure 7–66. Hydronephrosis secondary to ureteropelvic junction obstruction in a 2-year-old female who presented with abdominal prominence. *A*, Excretory urogram, 10-minute film showing a normal right kidney and nonopacification of the left kidney. *B*, Transverse ultrasonogram showing large cystic structures in the abdomen which are not as well defined as on CT. *C*, Computed tomography slice with oral contrast material in the markedly displaced bowel; the massively dilated renal pelvis is seen centrally and calyces are displayed to the right (patient's left).

of this book, upon which this chapter is based. Doctor Robert L. Lebowitz kindly reviewed the current chapter. Their contributions are gratefully acknowledged.

BIBLIOGRAPHY

EXCRETORY UROGRAPHY

Baker DH, Berdon WE: The use and safety of "high" dosage in pediatric urography: a survey of the Society for Pediatric Radiology. Radiology 103:371, 1972.

Benness GT: Urographic contrast agents: a comparison of sodium and methylglucamine salts. Clin Radiol 21:150, 1970.

Berdon WE, Baker DH: The significance of a distended bladder in the interpretation of intravenous pyelograms obtained on patients with "hydronephrosis." Am J Roentgenol Radium Ther Nucl Med 120:402, 1974.

Berdon WE, Baker DH, Leonidas J: Advantages of prone positioning in gastrointestinal and genitourinary roentgenology studies in infants and children. Am J Roentgenol Radium Ther Nucl Med 103:444, 1968.

Berdon WE, Schwartz RH, Becker J, Baker DH: Tamm-Horsfall proteinuria: its relationship to prolonged nephrogram in infants and children and to renal failure

following intravenous urography in adults with multiple myeloma. Radiology 92:714, 1969.

Binder R, Korobkin M, Clark RE, et al: Aberrant papillae and other filling defects of the renal pelvis. Am J Roentgenol Radium Ther Nucl Med 114:746, 1972.

Brasch RC: Allergic reactions to contrast media: accumulated evidence. AJR 134:797, 1980.

Cook IK, Keats TE, Seale DL: Determination of the normal position of the upper urinary tract on the lateral abdominal urogram. Radiology 99:499, 1971.

Currarino G: Roentgenographic estimation of kidney size in normal individuals with emphasis on children. Am J Roentgenol Radium Ther Nucl Med 93:464, 1965.

Currarino G, Weinberg A, Putnam R: Resorption of contrast material from the bladder during a cystourethrography causing an excretory urogram. Radiology 123:149, 1977.

Dacie JE, Frie IK: A comparison of sodium and methylglucamine diatrizoate in clinical urography. Br J Radiol 44:51, 1971.

de Langen JE, Hermans J: Comparative multiclinical studies of iodamide and diatrizoate in excretory urography. Radiology 106:73, 1973.

Dunbar JS, Nogrady B: Excretory urography in the first year of life. Radiol Clin North Am 10:367, 1972.

Dure-Smith P, Simenhoff M, Zimsking PD, et al: The bolus effect of excretory urography. Radiology 101:24, 1971.

Fischer HW, Rothfield NJH, Carr JD: Optimum dose in excretory urography. Am J Roentgenol Radium Ther Nucl Med 113:423, 1971.

Fitts FB Jr, Mascatello VG, Mellins HZ: The value of compression during excretion voiding urethrography. Radiology 125:53, 1977.

Gill WB, Curtis GA: The influence of bladder fullness on upper urinary tract dimensions and renal excretory function. J Urol 117:573, 1977.

Godderidge C: Female gonadal shielding. Appl Radiol 8(2):65, 1979.

Gooding CA, Berdon WE, Brodeur AE, et al: Adverse reactions to intravenous pyelography in children. Am J Roentgenol Radium Ther Nucl Med 123:802, 1975.

Green WM, Pressman DB, McLennan BL, et al: "Column of Bertin": diagnosis by nephrotomography. Am J Roentgenol Radium Ther Nucl Med 116:714, 1972.

Griscom NT, Neuhauser EBD: Total body opacification. J Pediatr Surg 1:76, 1966.

Haas EA, Solomon DJ: Telling children about diagnostic radiology procedures. Radiology 124:521, 1977.

Hernandez RJ, Poznanski AK, Kuhns RL, et al: Factors affecting the measurement of renal length. Radiology 130:653, 1979.

Hodson CJ, Davies Z, Prescod A: Renal parenchymal radiographic measurement in infants and children. Pediatr Radiol 3:16, 1975.

Kassner EG, Elguezabal A, Pochaczevsky R: Death during intravenous urography: overdosage syndrome in young infants. NY State J Med 73:1958, 1973.

Kaufman RA, Dunbar JS, Gob DE: Normal dilatation of the proximal ureter in children. AJR 137:945, 1981.

Kelly WM: Uricosuria and x-ray contrast agents. N Engl J Med 284:975, 1971.

Kirks DR, Currarino G, Weinburg AG: Transverse folds in the proximal ureter: a normal variant in infants. AJR 130:463, 1978.

Kumar D, Cigtay OS, Klein LH: Case reports: aberrant renal papilla. Br J Radiol 50:141, 1977.

Laufer I, Griscom NT: Compensatory renal hypertrophy. Absence in utero and development in early life. Am J Roentgenol Radium Ther Nucl Med 113:646, 1971.

Lebowitz RL: Pediatric uroradiology 1982. Annual Meeting, American College of Radiology, Boston, 1982.

Lebowitz RL, Avni FE: Misleading appearances in pediatric uroradiology. Pediatr Radiol 10:15, 1980.

Lebowitz RL, Hopkins T, Colodny AH: Measuring the kidneys—practical applications using a growth hypertrophy chart. Pediatr Radiol 4:37, 1975.

Ludin H: Radiological estimation of kidney weight. Acta Radiol (Diagn) 6:651, 1967.

Lutzker LG, Goldman HS: A method for improved urographic visualization for children. Radiology 111:217, 1974.

Mascatello V, Lebowitz RL: Malposition of the colon in left renal agenesis and ectopia. Radiology 123:371, 1976.

McClennan BL, Becker JA: Excretory urography: choice of contrast material—clinical. Radiology 100:591, 1971.

Meyers MA, Whalen JP, Evans JA, et al: Malposition and displacement of the bowel in renal agenesis and ectopia: new observations. Am J Roentgenol Radium Ther Nucl Med 117:323, 1973.

Nogrady MB, Dunbar JS: The technique of roentgen investigation of the urinary tract in infants and children. Prog Pediatr Radiol 3:3, 1970.

O'Connor JF, Neuhauser EBD: Total body opacification in conventional and high dose intravenous urography in infancy. Am J Roentgenol Radium Ther Nucl Med 90:63, 1963.

Parker JA, Lebowitz RL, Mascatello V, et al: Magnification renal scintigraphy in the differential diagnosis of septa of Bertin. Pediatr Radiol 4:157, 1976.

Philbin DM, Moss J, Akins CW, et al: The use of H_1 and H_2 histamine antagonists with morphine anesthesia: a double-blind study. Anesthesiology 55:292, 1981.

Poslethwaithe AE, Kelly WN: Uricosuria effects of radio-contrast agents. A study in man of more commonly used preparations. Ann Intern Med 74:845, 1971.

Ransley PG: Opacification of the renal parenchyma in obstruction reflux. Pediatr Radiol 4:226, 1976.

Stannard M, Lebowitz RL: Urography in the child who wets. AJR 130:959, 1978.

Whitaker RH: Methods of assessing obstruction in dilated ureters. Br J Urol 45:15, 1973.

Witten DM, Hirsch FD, Hartman GW: Acute reactions to urographic contrast medium: incidence, clinical characteristics and relationship to hypersensitivity states. Am J Roentgenol Radium Ther Nucl Med 119:832, 1973.

CYSTOURETHROGRAPHY

Colodny AH, Lebowitz RL: The importance of voiding during cystourethrogram. J Urol 111:838, 1974a.

Colodny AH, Lebowitz RL: A plea for grading vesicoureteral reflux. Urology 4:357 1974b.

Currarino G: Narrowing of the male urethra caused by contractions or spasms of the bulbocavernosus muscle: cystourethrographic observations. Am J Roentgenol Radium Ther Nucl Med 108:641, 1970.

Fletcher EWL, Forbes WSC, Gough MH: Suprapubic micturating cystourethrography in infants. Clin Radiol 29:309, 1978.

Gross GW, Lebowitz RL: Infection does not cause reflux. AJR 137:929, 1981.

Kelalis PP, Burke EC, Stickler GB, et al: Urinary vaginal reflux in children. Pediatrics 51:941, 1973.

Koff SA, Fischer CP, Poznanski AK: Cystourethrography: the effect of reservoir height upon intravesical pressure. Pediatr Radiol 8:21, 1979.

Leibovic SJ, Lebowitz RL: Reducing patient dose in voiding cystourethrography. Urol Radiol 2:103, 1980.

Levitt SB, et al: Medical versus surgical treatment of primary vesicoureteral reflux. Pediatrics 67:392, 1981.

Lucaya J: A simple technique of retrograde urethrography in male infants. Radiology 102:402, 1972.

Mandell J, Lebowitz RL, Hallett M, et al: Urethral narrowing in region of external sphincter: radiologic-urodynamic correlations in boys with myelodysplasia. AJR 134:731, 1980

McAlister WH, Cacciarelli A, Shackelford GD: Complications associated with cystography in children. Radiology 111:167, 1974.

Peck AG, Poznanski AK: A simple device for genitography. Radiology 103:212, 1972.

Poznanski E, Poznanski AK: Psychogenic influences on voiding: observations from cystourethrography. Psychosomatics 10:339, 1969.

Sane SM, Worsing A Jr: Voiding cystourethrography. Recent advances. Minn Medicine 58:148, 1975.

Shopfner CE: Genitography in intersex states. Radiology 82:664, 1964.

Shopfner CE: Clinical evaluation of cystourethrographic contrast media. Radiology 88:491, 1967.

Shopfner CE: Cystourethrography. Med Radiogr Photogr 47:2, 1971.

Shopfner CE, Hutch JA: The trigonal canal. Radiology 88:209, 1967.

Vlahakis E, Hartman GW, Kelalis PP: Comparison of voiding cystourethrography and expression cystourethrography. J Urol 106:414, 1971.

OTHER UROGRAPHIC EXAMS

Hardy BE, Lebowitz RL, Baez A, et al: Strictures of the ileal loop. J Urol 117:358, 1977.

Hudson HC, Kramer SA, Anderson EE: Identification of uretero-ileal obstruction by retrograde loopography. Urology 17:147, 1981.

Lebowitz RL: Urinary diversion. In Postoperative Pediatric Uroradiology. New York, Appleton-Century-Crofts, 1981, pp 103–130.

McCallum RW, Colapinto V: Urologic radiology of the adult male lower urinary tract. Springfield, Ill., Charles C Thomas, 1976, p 43.

Nogrady MB, Peticlerc R, Moir JD: The roentgenologic evaluation of supravesical permanent urinary diversion in childhood (ileal and colonic conduit). J Canad Assoc Radiol 20:75, 1969.

Shapiro Sr, Lebowitz R, Colodny AH: Fate of 90 children with ileal conduit urinary diversion a decade later: analysis of complications, pyelography, renal function and bacteriology. J Urol 114:289, 1975.

VASCULAR STUDIES

Berdon WE, Baker DH, Santulli TV: Factors producing spurious obstruction of the inferior vena cava in infants and children with abdominal tumors. Radiology 88:111, 1967.

Berk RN, Wholey MH, Stockdale R: Angiographic diagnosis of splenic and hepatic trauma. J Canad Assoc Radiol 21:230, 1970.

Castellino RA: Observations in "reactive (follicular) hyperplasia" as encountered in repeat lymphography in the lymphomas. Cancer 34:2042, 1974.

Castellino RA, Bergeron C, Markovits P: Experience with 659 consecutive lymphograms in children. Cancer 40:1097, 1977.

Castellino RA, Markovits P, Musumeri R: Lymphography. In Pediatric Oncologic Radiology. Edited by Parker BR, Castellino RA. St. Louis, CV Mosby Co., 1977, pp 58–84.

Dunnick NR, Parker BA, Castellino RA: Pediatric lymphography: performance, interpretation, and accuracy in 193 consecutive children. AJR 129:639, 1977.

Fellows K: Angiography. In Pediatric Oncologic Radiology. Edited by Parker BR, Castellino RA. St. Louis, CV Mosby Co., 1977, pp 11–39.

Fellows KE Jr, Nebesar RA: Abdominal, hepatic and visceral angiography. In Angiography in Infants and Children. Edited by Gyepes MT. New York, Grune & Stratton, Inc., 1974, pp 193–232.

Fitz CR, Harwood-Nash DC: Special procedures and techniques in infants. Radiol Clin North Am 13:191, 1975.

Harper AP, Yune HY, Franken EA, Jr: Spectrum of angiographically demonstrable renal pathology in young hypertensive patients. Pediatr Radiol 123:141, 1977.

Kirks DR, Fitz CR, Harwood-Nash DC: Pediatric abdominal angiography: practical guide to catheter selection, flow rates and contrast dosage. Pediatr Radiol 5:19, 1976.

Korobkin M, Pick RA, Merten DF, et al: Etiologic radiographic findings in children and adolescents with nonuremic hypertension. Radiology 110:615, 1974.

Mortensson W, Hallbook T, Lundstrom N-R: Percutaneous catheterization of the femoral vessels in children. I. Influence on arterial peak flow and venous emptying rates in the calves. Pediatr Radiol 3:195, 1975.

Nebesar RA, Fleischli DJ, Pollard JJ, et al: Arteriography in infants and children with emphasis on the Seldinger technique and abdominal diseases. Am J Roentgenol Radium Ther Nucl Med 106:81, 1969.

Slovis TL, Philippart AI, Cushing B, et al: Evaluation of the inferior vena cava by sonography and venography in children with renal and hepatic tumors. Radiology 140:767, 1981.

Tucker AS: The roentgen diagnosis of abdominal masses in children: intravenous urography vs. inferior venacavography. Am J Roentgenol Radium Ther Nucl Med 95:76, 1965.

COMPUTED TOMOGRAPHY

Berger PE, Kuhn JP, Brusehaber J: Techniques for computed tomography in infants and children. Radiol Clin North Am 19:399, 1981.

Brasch RC, Randel SB, Gould RG: Follow-up of Wilms' tumor: comparison of CT with other imaging modalities. AJR 137:1005, 1981.

Kuhn JP, Berger PE: Computed tomography of the kidney in infancy and childhood. Radiol Clin North Am 19:445, 1981.

8

NUCLEAR MEDICINE

MASSOUD MAJD

The use of nuclear medicine in the diagnosis and follow-up of urologic problems in infants and children has dramatically increased over the past several years. Major factors that have contributed to this rapid growth include the introduction of better radiopharmaceuticals, the improvement in imaging devices (gamma cameras), and the use of computers in analysis of the functional parameters of the genitourinary system. The introduction of the mobile gamma camera–computer system has expanded the use of nuclear medicine studies to the intensive care unit, the operating room, and the patient's bedside.

Nuclear medicine procedures are generally noninvasive, require neither fasting nor bowel preparation, are performed without anesthesia or sedation, and do not require hospitalization. Radiopharmaceuticals have no systemic pharmacologic effects and do not cause any allergic reaction. Absorbed radiation doses from the radionuclide studies do not reach a harmful range and in some instances are much lower than the doses from comparable radiographic tests. Most importantly, radionuclide studies offer quantitative functional information currently not available with other imaging modalities. Many disorders of the genitourinary system in children are part of a dynamic process that requires serial assessment. Noninvasive radionuclide studies are the optimal means of evaluating and following the course of such disorders.

RENAL IMAGING AND FUNCTIONAL ANALYSIS

Radiopharmaceuticals

Radionuclide renal studies are used to assess renal perfusion and certain aspects of renal function and structure. The information gained depends upon which radiopharmaceutical is used. Currently, the following radiopharmaceuticals are used for the evaluation of the kidneys:

Technetium-99m DTPA (diethylenetriamine-pentaacetic acid) is the agent most commonly used for renal studies. Its initial transit through the kidney reflects renal perfusion, and the tracer accumulation in each kidney between 1 and 3 minutes after injection is proportional to the functioning renal mass. Renal clearance of DTPA is by glomerular filtration with no significant tubular secretion or cortical retention. Therefore, its rate of clearance provides an accurate measurement of the glomerular filtration rate (GFR). Because of rapid clearance, the high concentration of technetium-99m DTPA in the urine also provides excellent visualization of the pelvicalyceal systems, ureters, and bladder. Because of its low retention in the renal cortex, however, this agent may fail to demonstrate small cortical lesions.

Technetium-99m glucoheptonate is cleared by a combination of tubular secretion and glomerular filtration. Most is excreted in the urine, allowing moderately good visualization of the pelvicalyceal systems, ureters, and bladder. Approximately 12 per cent of the administered dose of glucoheptonate, however, remains in the renal cortex, firmly bound to the tubular cells. Therefore, delayed imaging at 2 to 4 hours provides visualization of the renal cortex. Glucoheptonate, owing to its complex mode of clearance, is not a suitable agent for measuring GFR. Its relative renal uptake, however, corresponds to relative functioning mass.

Technetium-99m DMSA (dimercaptosuccinic acid) is the best cortical imaging agent available. The majority is tightly bound to the cortical tubular cells, and only a small amount is excreted in the urine. DMSA allows excellent visualization of the renal parenchyma without interference from pelvicalyceal activity and is therefore recommended for detection of small cortical lesions such as masses, infarcts, or pyelonephritis. The relative uptake of technetium-99m DMSA is an accurate measure of relative functioning renal mass and in most situations correlates well with the relative GFR and other parameters of renal function (Taylor).

Iodine-131 orthoiodohippurate (Hippuran) is primarily a tubular agent. Almost 80 per cent of intravenously injected Hippuran is extracted from the blood and secreted by renal tubular cells. The remaining 20 per cent is

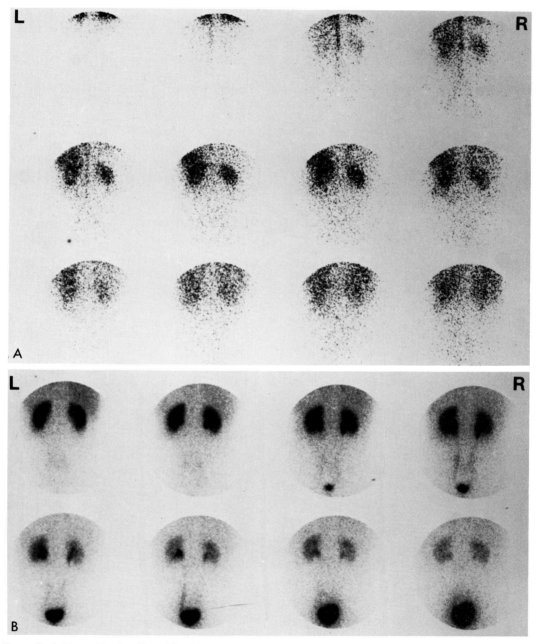

Figure 8–1. Normal technetium-99m DTPA dynamic renal function study. *A*, The perfusion phase or radionuclide renal angiogram demonstrates prompt and equal perfusion to both kidneys. *B*, The sequential static images show uniform distribution of the tracer in the cortex of both kidneys, early visualization of the collecting systems, and normal drainage.

excreted by passive glomerular filtration. Despite these excellent biologic properties of iodine-131 Hippuran and its early popularity, it currently has little place in pediatric nuclear medicine. The major disadvantages of this agent are poor characteristics of its radiation for imaging and high radiation dose due to the emission of beta particles. This necessitates the use of a low dose of the tracer, leading to a poor resolution image. Hippuran labeled with iodine-123, on the other hand, is an excellent imaging agent for the kidneys (Zielinski et al). Iodine-123 is a pure gamma emitter with an energy level suitable for imaging with the scintillation camera. It can be used in millicurie doses with a significantly lower radiation dose than would be received from microcuries of iodine-131 Hippuran. Radiochemically pure iodine-123 Hippuran, however, is not readily available.

Procedures

Renal Imaging

The conventional renal scan should consist of a radionuclide angiogram followed by sequential analogue and digital images of the kidneys, ureters, and bladder. After rapid intravenous injection of the appropriate amount of the tracer (100 microcuries [μCi] of technetium-99m DTPA or of technetium-99m glucoheptonate per kg of body weight), a series of 2 to 3 second dynamic posterior images of the kidneys is obtained during the first minute (angiographic phase) (Fig. 8–1A). This is followed by a series of static images of the kidneys for 20 to 30 minutes for the evaluation of renal excretion and drainage of the tracer (Fig. 8–1B). Further delayed images are obtained if necessary.

The digital images are acquired on a computer at the rate of 1 image per second for 60 seconds (angiographic phase) followed by a series of 10 second images for 3 to 4 minutes. These digital images are used to evaluate renal perfusion and calculate relative renal function.

Renal cortical imaging is accomplished by 2 to 4 hour delayed imaging after injection of either technetium-99m glucoheptonate (100 μCi/kg) or technetium-99m DMSA (50 μCi/kg). Magnified high resolution images obtained with a pinhole collimator are often essential for delineation of the cortical defects (Fig. 8–2).

Renal Perfusion

Although analogue images allow for a rough visual assessment of renal vascular perfusion (Fig. 8–1A), computer analysis is essential for a precise assessment. Areas of interest are flagged over the abdominal aorta and the kidneys. Time-activity curves are generated from these areas of interest. The renal

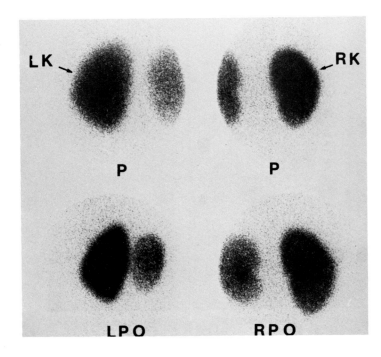

Figure 8–2. Normal renal cortical scan. Posterior and posterior oblique images obtained 3 hours after injection of technetium-99m DMSA demonstrate excellent visualization of the kidneys with no significant residual background activity. A pinhole collimator was used to obtain these magnified high resolution renal cortical images. LK, left kidney; RK, right kidney, P, posterior; LPO, left posterior oblique; RPO, right posterior oblique.

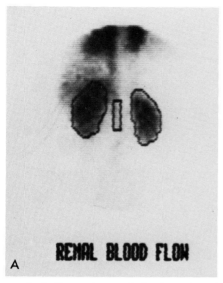

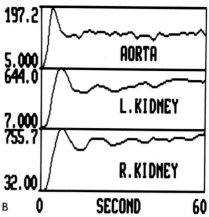

Figure 8–3. Computer analysis of renal perfusion. *A,* Regions of interest are flagged over the abdominal aorta and the kidneys. *B,* Time-activity curves of the first transit of the tracer through the abdominal aorta and the kidneys demonstrate similar slopes, indicating normal symmetrical renal blood flow.

slopes are then compared with each other and with the aortic slope (Fig. 8–3).

Relative Renal Function

The differential or relative function of each kidney can be calculated by determining the accumulation of the tracer in each kidney between 1 and 3 minutes after injection. During this period all the radioactivity within the kidney is confined to the vessels and functioning renal parenchyma, as the tracer has not yet reached the collecting system. Regions of interest are selected for each kidney and its background. Background activity is then subtracted from corresponding renal activity. The net counts within each kidney are expressed as a percentage of the total renal counts (Fig. 8–4*A*). The same principle can be used in calculating the relative contribution of different segments of a kidney to its total function. The pitfalls of the differential renal function analysis based on the 1 to 3 minute ratio of the counts in the kidneys are:

1. The technique is operator-dependent, and selection of the frames and the areas of interest affects the results. This is particularly critical for the background regions of interest, which may include a portion of the liver and spleen with high concentration of the tracer.
2. The results may be invalid in the presence of extreme hydronephrosis. When the

cortex is thin and poorly functioning, selecting an area of interest is difficult. Attenuation of the counts from the anterior parenchyma, which is widely displaced by the dilated urine-filled pelvicalyceal system, will result in inaccurate calculation of the total activity contained in the entire renal parenchyma.

The relative renal function can also be calculated on delayed images (2 to 3 hours) using technetium-99m DMSA or technetium-99m glucoheptonate. Advantages of this method are:

1. The background activity is negligible by that time, and thus one source of potential error is eliminated.
2. Both anterior and posterior images can be obtained from which a mean value can be calculated. The mean may be more reliable than the count ratios from posterior images alone as routinely obtained when using DTPA, particularly when the kidneys are at different depths.

Several investigators have confirmed the validity of these methods of calculating differential renal function by comparing results from DMSA, DTPA, and ureteral catheterization studies with split creatinine clearances (Powers et al; Price et al). The percentages calculated using DTPA and glucoheptonate are the same, in spite of their different modes of renal excretion. Futhermore, the glucohep-

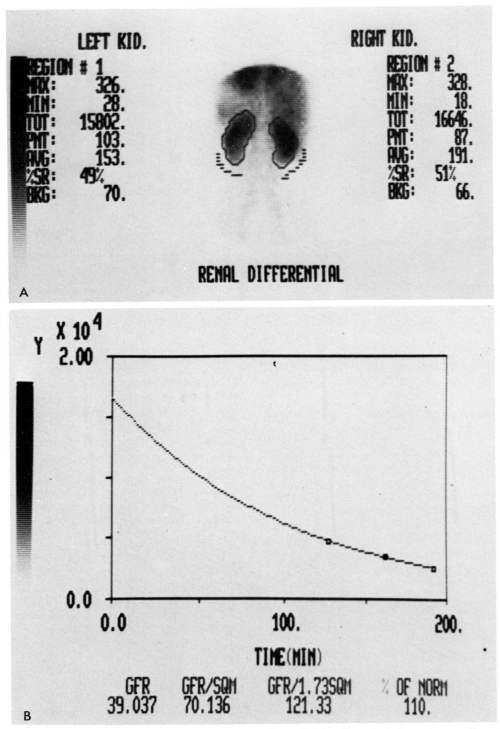

Figure 8–4. Total and separate GFR. *A,* The renal differential function study based upon the relative accumulation of the tracer in each kidney at the interval between 1 and 2 minutes post injection of technetium-99m DTPA shows that the kidneys function equally. *B,* The total GFR calculated on the basis of plasma clearance of technetium-99m DTPA is 121 ml/min/1.73 m². The GFR from each kidney, therefore, is about 60.5 ml/min/1.73 m².

tonate ratios calculated at 1 to 3 minutes, reflecting the amount of parenchyma perfused, and the calculated ratios at 4 to 6 hours, reflecting tubular binding, are similar.

The differential renal functional analysis is an index only of relative function of the kidneys and does not provide information about absolute function of each kidney.

Total and Separate GFR

Since technetium-99m DTPA is excreted almost exclusively by glomerular filtration, its rate of clearance from blood is an accurate measure of GFR. A variety of methods may be used to calculate GFR using technetium-99m DTPA (Dubovsky and Russell). The simplest method, which employs three blood samples drawn between 2 and 3 hours after injection, is based on single compartmental analysis of the DTPA clearance (Fig. 8–4B). There is excellent correlation between this technique and 24-hour urinary creatinine clearance (Braren et al). Absolute GFR of each kidney can then be calculated by multiplying the total calculated GFR in ml/min by the percentages obtained from the renal differential function. This method of GFR calculation is relatively noninvasive and obviates the need for 24 hour urine collection. Because of the need for multiple venous punctures, however, the test is unpleasant for children and their parents. Because of uncertainty about the effect of diuretics on the GFR in different pathologic states, the test cannot be performed in conjunction with diuretic renography.

Other methods of calculating GFR based on external counting without blood samples or with a single blood sample have been developed (Piepsz et al, 1978; Gates). These methods are becoming popular and may gain greater acceptance in their application to children.

Radionuclide Renography

The radionuclide renogram is a time-activity curve of renal extraction and excretion of a radiopharmaceutical. Conventional iodine-131 Hippuran renography is seldom used in children. A modification of iodine-131 Hippuran or technetium-99m DTPA renography using deconvolution analysis is used to measure renal parenchymal transit time of the tracer (Diffey et al; Whitfield et al, 1978, 1981). Parenchymal transit time is prolonged in patients with obstructive uropathy or renal

ischemia. Diuretic radionuclide renography is another modification of the conventional renography used in the evaluation of hydronephrosis. These procedures will be explained in detail later in this chapter.

Clinical Applications

Although the renal scan lacks the anatomic resolution of the excretory urogram, it has several advantages, including quantitative assessment of renal function, independence of image quality from overlying bowel contents and bony structures, and ability to visualize renal tissue with a very low level of function. These advantages are particularly important in neonates.

Neonatal Renal Evaluation

GFR at birth is about 21 per cent of the corrected adult value and reaches only to 44 per cent by 2 weeks of age (McCrory). The low GFR, together with overlying bowel gas, generally results in poor visualization of kidneys on the excretory urogram and often necessitates multiple radiographs and occasionally tomography. This may expose the child to an unacceptably high radiation dose. In addition, the urographic contrast media may have osmotic side effects (Wood and Smith). Radionuclide scanning, which is limited only by renal function, is superior to excretory urography for localization and functional analysis of the kidneys. In combination with ultrasound it is the procedure of choice in the evaluation of neonatal renal disorders.

Congenital Anomalies

Any functioning renal tissue, irrespective of its location, can be visualized on renal scan. Ectopic kidneys, which are often superimposed on bones and may remain obscure on an excretory urogram, can be easily demonstrated and differentiated from renal agenesis (Fig. 8–5). The horseshoe kidney and other variants of fused kidneys are also better evaluated on a renal scan than on an excretory urogram (Figs. 8–6 and 8–7).

The renal scan is frequently useful to confirm renal duplication suspected on excretory urogram or ultrasound, or even to diagnose unsuspected cases. The function of each moiety of a duplicated kidney relative to the other and to the opposite kidney can be as-

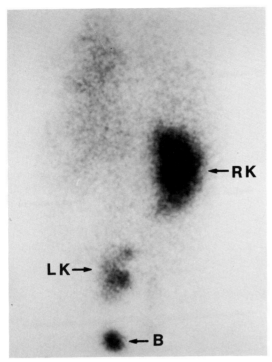

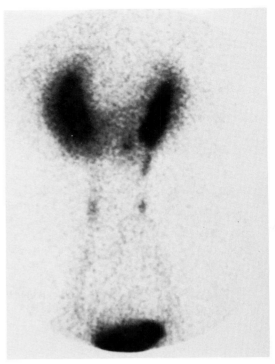

Figure 8–5. Ectopic kidney. Posterior image of a technetium-99m DTPA renal scan demonstrates ectopic (pelvic) left kidney. The right kidney is normal. RK, right kidney; LK, left kidney; B, bladder.

Figure 8–6. Horseshoe kidney. Anterior image of a technetium-99m DTPA renal scan demonstrates fusion of the lower poles of the kidneys.

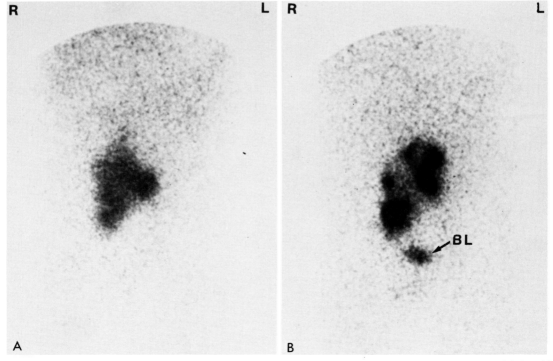

Figure 8–7. Crossed fused ectopia. *A,* The anterior image of a technetium-99m DTPA renal scan obtained 2 minutes after injection demonstrates a single irregular mass of functioning renal tissue located in the mid-lower abdomen. *B,* The image obtained at 10 minutes after injection shows two separate sets of pelvicalyceal systems. BL, bladder.

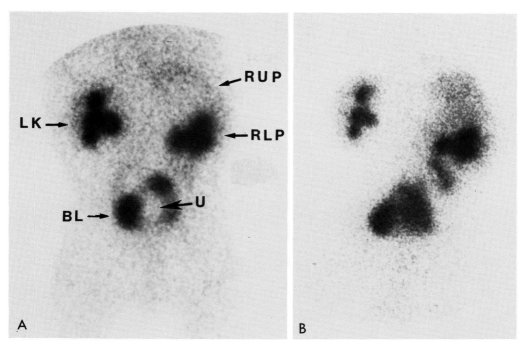

Figure 8–8. Ectopic ureterocele. The posterior images of a technetium-99m DTPA renal scan obtained at 10 minutes (*A*) and 30 minutes (*B*) after injection demonstrate duplication of the right renal collecting systems. The upper pole is hydronephrotic and shows delayed and decreased function. The collecting system of the lower pole of the right kidney is tilted. There is a filling defect in the bladder. This constellation is characteristic of ectopic ureterocele. The left kidney is normal. LK, left kidney; RUP, right upper pole; RLP, right lower pole; BL, bladder; U, ureterocele.

Figure 8–9. Dysgenetic nonfunctioning left kidney. Sequential 2 minute posterior images obtained from 2 to 14 minutes after injection of technetium-99m DTPA demonstrate a photon-deficient area in the left flank (*arrows*). The 14 to 20 minute images show appearance of the tracer in the distal left ureter (*arrowheads*). The 20 to 24 minute images show retrograde filling of a dilated left pelvicalyceal system and ureter (*open arrows*). The left kidney is nonfunctioning, and the sudden appearance of the tracer in the left ureter on the delayed images is due to reflux. The right kidney is normal.

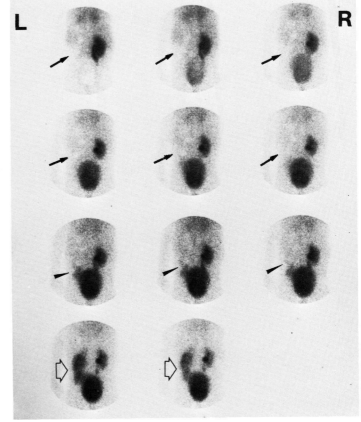

sessed. This may be important in deciding whether there is enough function to salvage the hydronephrotic, poorly functioning moiety (Fig. 8–8). Occasionally a dysgenetic, nonfunctioning whole kidney or one moiety of a duplicated kidney is visualized on renal scan by reflux of the tracer from the bladder into the corresponding ureter and pelvicalyceal system (Fig. 8–9).

The multicystic dysplastic kidney and

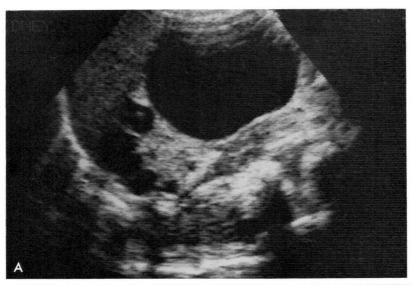

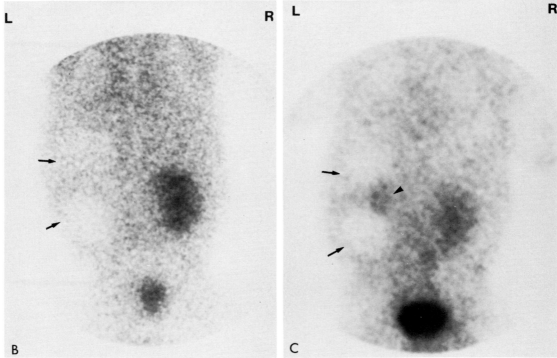

Figure 8–10. Multicystic dysplastic kidney in a newborn with a left flank mass. *A,* The renal sonogram demonstrates cystic lesions in the left kidney. *B,* The early image of a renal scan obtained at 4 minutes after injection of technetium-99m DTPA shows photon-deficient areas in the left flank *(arrows)* with no renal function on that side. *C,* The 3 hour delayed image shows persistence of the photon-deficient areas *(arrows)* and accumulation of a small amount of the tracer in the medial portion of the region between the photon-deficient areas *(arrowhead).*

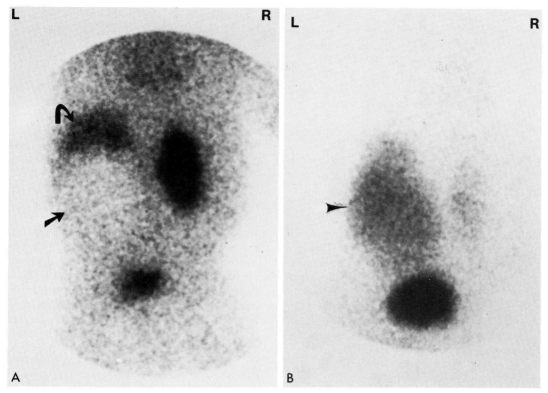

Figure 8–11. Hydronephrosis due to congenital UPJ obstruction in a newborn with a left flank mass. *A,* The early image of the renal scan obtained at 10 minutes after injection of technetium-99m DTPA demonstrates a large photon-deficient area in the left flank (*straight arrow*) with a cap of renal tissue (*curved arrow*). *B,* The delayed 60 minute image shows filling of the photon-deficient area, which represents a massively dilated pelvicalyceal system (*arrowhead*).

hydronephrosis due to congenital UPJ obstruction are the two most common flank masses in the neonatal period. The multicystic dysplastic kidney is caused by atresia of the ureter, renal pelvis, or both during the metanephric stage of renal development and is probably the end of the spectrum of ureteral obstruction (Felson and Cussen; Griscom et al). The continuing function of a few glomeruli and tubules creates hydronephrosis proximal to the obstruction. The altered excretory function inhibits cellular development, and the kidney becomes dysplastic. Depending on the number of functioning glomeruli remaining, the kidney may show minimal or no function. On the other hand, a kidney with congenital UPJ obstruction without dysplasia of the renal parenchyma usually retains significant function, unless prolonged obstruction has existed or infection has supervened. Therefore, management of the patient depends upon early recognition of the presence or absence of adequate renal cortex.

Ultrasound is the ideal first imaging procedure in the evaluation of neonatal abdominal masses. It shows whether the mass is of renal or extrarenal origin and establishes the tissue character of the mass (solid, cystic, mixed). The next step should be renal scintigraphy to evaluate renal function. Both multicystic kidney and severe hydronephrosis appear as an avascular mass on the angiographic phase of the examination. The static images in multicystic kidney show either no evidence of functioning renal tissue or only very minimal function on the delayed images (Fig. 8–10). In a salvageable hydronephrotic kidney the early static images demonstrate a cap of functioning cortex of varying thickness at the periphery of the hydronephrotic kidney, and the delayed images show significant accumulation of the tracer in the dilated pelvicalyceal system (Fig. 8–11).

Hydronephrosis

One of the common problems in pediatric urology is the differentiation between obstructive and nonobstructive hydronephrosis. The diagnostic procedures used in the evaluation of hydronephrosis include cystography, excretory urography with or without a diuretic, retrograde pyelography, renal scanning and renography with or without a diuretic, and pressure-perfusion studies (the Whitaker test).

Vesicoureteral reflux as the cause of hydronephrosis is readily diagnosed by radiographic or radionuclide cystography. It should be noted, however, that reflux and obstruction may coexist (Lebowitz and Blickman). The conventional excretory urogram is occasionally diagnostic of obstruction, but frequently does not differentiate between obstructive and nonobstructive hydronephrosis. A retrograde pyelogram may define the site of the change in ureteral caliber but does not provide any functional information. The conventional renal scan and renogram demonstrate the presence, extent, and severity of hydronephrosis and allow quantitative assessment of residual renal function. They do not, however, differentiate obstructive from nonobstructive hydronephrosis.

The pressure-perfusion study (the Whitaker test) is based on the hypothesis that if the dilated upper urinary tract can transport 10 ml/min without an inordinate increase in pressure, the hydrostatic pressure in the system under physiologic states should not cause deterioration of renal function, and the degree of obstruction, if any, is insignificant. The Whitaker test is generally accepted as the standard for distinguishing obstructive from nonobstructive hydronephrosis. Its invasive nature, however, makes it undesirable for screening purposes and particularly for serial assessments.

Diuretic excretory urography is based on the principle that, in the presence of significant obstruction, the urinary tract is unable to transport fluid over the physiologic range of flow rate, and diuresis produces significant increase in the dimensions of the pelvicalyceal system. A 20 to 22 per cent increase in the area of the pelvicalyceal system after furosemide-induced diuresis has been reported to indicate significant obstruction (Whitfield et al 1977; Nilson et al). Quantification by planimetry of the changes in the size of the pelvicalyceal system, however, is imprecise, and the test is not reliable. The following modifications of radionuclide renography offer more objective means of differentiating obstructed from nonobstructed dilatation.

DIURETIC-AUGMENTED RADIONUCLIDE RENOGRAPHY.

This provocative test is based on the hypothesis that the prolonged retention of the tracer in the nonobstructed dilated upper urinary tract is due to a reservoir effect, and that increased urine flow following diuretic administration should result in prompt washout of the tracer, whereas in obstructive hydronephrosis there should not be any significant washout. O'Reily et al and Thrall et al have described distinct patterns of diuretic renogram curves in normal, dilated obstructed, and dilated nonobstructed upper urinary tracts. These authors have used the shape of the curve to characterize four patterns but have not attempted to quantify the washout rate of the tracer in response to the diuretic (Fig. 8–12). The normal pattern consists of spontaneous washout of the tracer, which makes administration of furosemide unnecessary. The washout is, however, accelerated under furosemide-induced diuresis. The obstructed pattern consists of progressive accumulation of the tracer before furosemide injection with little or no washout after diuresis. The dilated nonobstructed pattern consists of gradual accumulation of the tracer in the dilated system with prompt washout following administration of furosemide. The equivocal pattern shows initial progressive accumulation of tracer with a minimal or

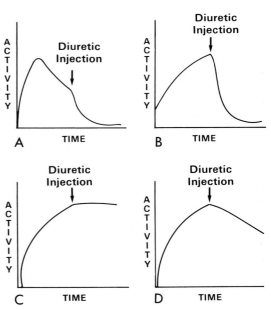

Figure 8–12. Patterns of response to diuretic in normal (A), dilated nonobstructed (B), and dilated obstructed (C) collecting systems. Pattern D is equivocal.

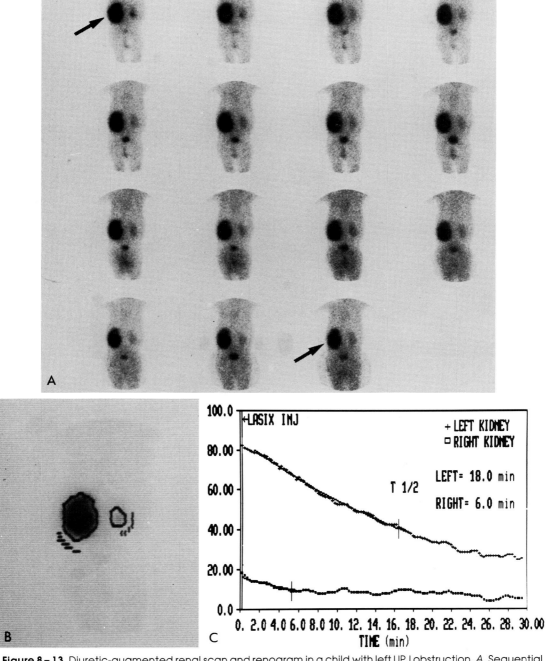

Figure 8–13. Diuretic-augmented renal scan and renogram in a child with left UPJ obstruction. *A*, Sequential 2 minute images obtained after injection of furosemide show marked retention of the tracer in the dilated left pelvicalyceal system (*arrow*). The tracer from the normal right pelvicalyceal system washes out rapidly. For quantitative analysis of washout of the tracer, regions of interest for the pelvicalyceal systems and the corresponding backgrounds are selected (*B*) and the renogram curves are generated (*C*). The washout half-time is 18 minutes on the left and 6 minutes on the right. The relative flatness of the lower curve in *C* is due to the rapid washout from the nonobstructed right side of the tracer before the diuretic was injected.

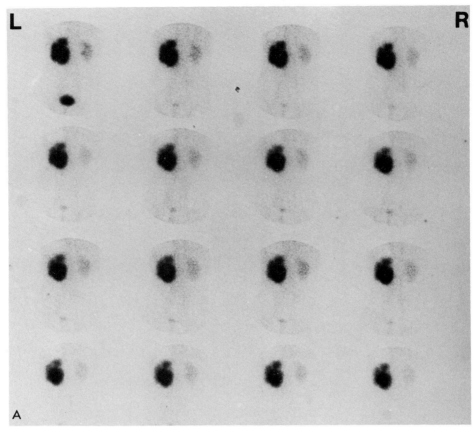

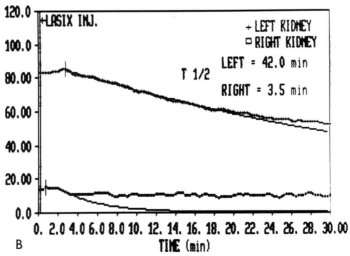

Figure 8–14. Diuretic-augmented renal scans and renograms in a patient with left UPJ obstruction before and after pyeloplasty. The initial study demonstrates poor drainage from a markedly dilated left pelvicalyceal system (*A*) with a washout half-time of 42 minutes (*B*).

Illustration continued on opposite page

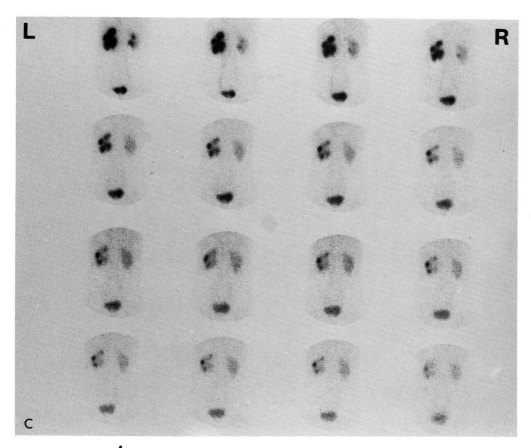

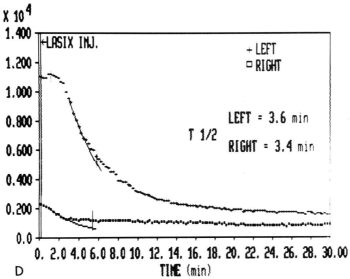

Figure 8–14 *Continued.* The follow-up study 3 months after pyeloplasty (C) demonstrates residual mild dilatation of the left pelvicalyceal system and improved drainage with a washout half-time of 3.6 minutes (D). In both B and D, the upper curve depicts the left kidney.

moderate washout under the effect of furosemide. The typical obstructed and nonobstructed patterns are usually diagnostic. Many dilated systems, however, show the intermediate or nondiagnostic response. Quantitative assessment of the slope of the washout curve eliminates some of the indeterminate results and improves the accuracy of the test. The following technique has evolved at the Children's Hospital National Medical Center.

The patient is positioned supine on the scanning table with the gamma camera underneath. A venous line is established and kept open with a slow infusion of 5 per cent dextrose in one-third normal saline. An indwelling bladder catheter is inserted. A standard technetium-99m DTPA renal scan is obtained. When the dilated system is entirely filled with tracer, furosemide is injected intravenously in a dose of 1 mg/kg up to 40 mg. Sequential analogue (15 images, taken one every 2 minutes) and digital (120 images, taken one every 15 seconds) images are obtained for 30 minutes. Intravenous fluid is infused rapidly in a dose of about 10 ml/kg during the 30 minutes immediately following furosemide injection, and the urine output during that period is measured. The computer data are then processed and clearance half-time of the tracer from the dilated upper urinary tract is calculated (Fig. 8–13).

In addition to the degree of obstruction, several factors influence the washout rate of the tracer. These factors include renal function, response to diuretic, distensibility and volume of the dilated system, fullness of the bladder, intravesical pressure, vesicoureteral reflux, and the patient's position at the time of examination. Administration of intravenous fluid assures adequate hydration and better diuresis and prevents dehydration under the effect of furosemide. The indwelling bladder catheter eliminates the effects of a full bladder, increased intravesical pressure, and vesicoureteral reflux on the drainage of the upper urinary tract. Preventing distention of the bladder during the examination also reduces the patient's discomfort and movement and obviates the need for interrupting the study for urination. Continuous drainage of the tracer from the bladder reduces the gonadal radiation dose and allows measurement of the urine output at desired intervals to assess the response to the diuretic.

Our experience with this technique in over 200 children indicates that most nonobstructed systems drain with a half-time of less than 15 minutes, whereas most obstructed systems drain with a half-time of over 20 minutes. The range between 15 and 20 minutes is equivocal. The results are unreliable in the presence of poor renal function, poor response to furosemide, or extreme dilatation of the upper urinary tract. The critical volume of the dilated system beyond which diuretic renography is not reliable has yet to be defined.

Improvement in the washout of the tracer after pyeloplasty varies greatly. In some, the half-time returns to the nonobstructed range in a short period of time (Fig. 8–14), whereas in others this may take significantly longer. In many instances the washout half-time remains in the obstructed or equivocal range for at least 6 months. Therefore, in post-pyeloplasty cases, particularly within the first 6 months, a gradual change in the half-time, rather than the absolute half-time, should be considered as the indicator of the result of surgery. Using these criteria, the accuracy of diuretic renography in our institution has been over 90 per cent. Only one false negative study, a mild ureteropelvic junction obstruction in a newborn, has been observed. All false positive studies and indeterminate results have occurred only in the presence of poor renal function, massively dilated collecting systems, or following recent reconstructive surgery. Pressure-perfusion studies have been performed in 37 of our patients. The diuretic renogram and the pressure-perfusion study agreed in 30 cases, disagreement was found in three cases, and the remaining pressure-perfusion studies were either indeterminate or technically deficient. Of the three cases in which there was disagreement, the pressure-perfusion study was wrong in two instances, one a false positive and the other a false negative. In the third case, the pressure-perfusion study correctly diagnosed obstruction that had been missed on the diuretic renogram (our only false negative diuretic study). There has not been a single individual in whom both studies were either falsely negative or falsely positive.

In summary, diuretic-augmented radionuclide renography appears to be a safe and accurate method for differentiating obstructive from nonobstructive hydronephrosis in children. The use of this test may eliminate many of the Whitaker tests. If the diuretic renogram unequivocally indicates presence or absence of obstruction the patient can be safely managed accordingly. The Whitaker test can then be used as a complementary test only in cases with indeterminate results.

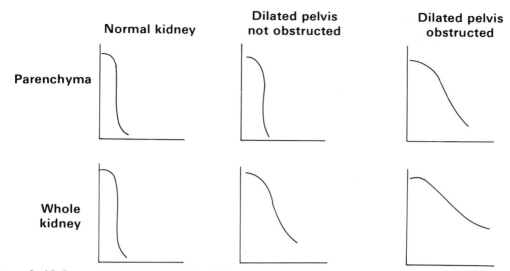

| Normal kidney | Dilated pelvis not obstructed | Dilated pelvis obstructed |

Parenchyma

Whole kidney

Figure 8–15. Deconvolution of the whole kidney and parenchymal renogram curves of normal, nonobstructed hydronephrotic, and obstructed hydronephrotic kidneys. In nonobstructed hydronephrosis the whole kidney renogram is abnormal but the renogram of the parenchyma alone is normal, whereas in obstructed hydronephrosis both are abnormal. (From Whitefield HN, Britton KE, Hendry WF, et al: The distinction between obstructive uropathy and nephropathy by radioisotope transit times. Br J Urol 50:433, 1978.)

DECONVOLUTION ANALYSIS OF RENOGRAM. Parenchymal transit time of technetium-99m DTPA based on deconvolution analysis of the cortical renogram curve has been advocated as a sensitive indicator of obstructive nephropathy (Diffey et al; Whitfield et al, 1978, 1981; Nawaz et al). This test is based on the principle that in the presence of renal outflow obstruction, the intratubular pressure is increased and reabsorption of salt and water is enhanced. The reabsorption of fluid from the tubular lumen leads to prolongation of the parenchymal transit time of nonreabsorbable tracers. Regions of interest are flagged over both the renal pelvis and the entire kidney, and time-activity curves are generated. The renal parenchymal time-activity curve is then derived by subtracting the pelvic curve from the whole kidney curve. Using the renal input function obtained by monitoring the cardiac blood pool activity, deconvolution analysis provides whole kidney and parenchymal curves corresponding to a theoretical instantaneous injection of the tracer into the renal artery (Fig. 8–15). Although deconvolution analysis appears

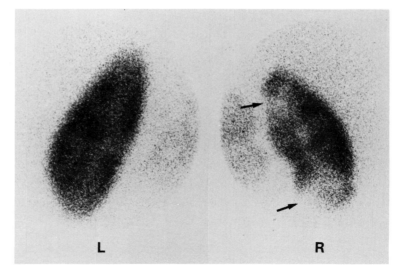

Figure 8–16. Acute pyelonephritis. The magnified posterior oblique views of the kidneys obtained 3 hours after injection of technetium-99m DMSA using a pinhole collimator demonstrate defects in the uptake of the tracer in the lower pole and the medial aspect of the upper pole of the right kidney (*arrows*). The left kidney is normal.

L   R

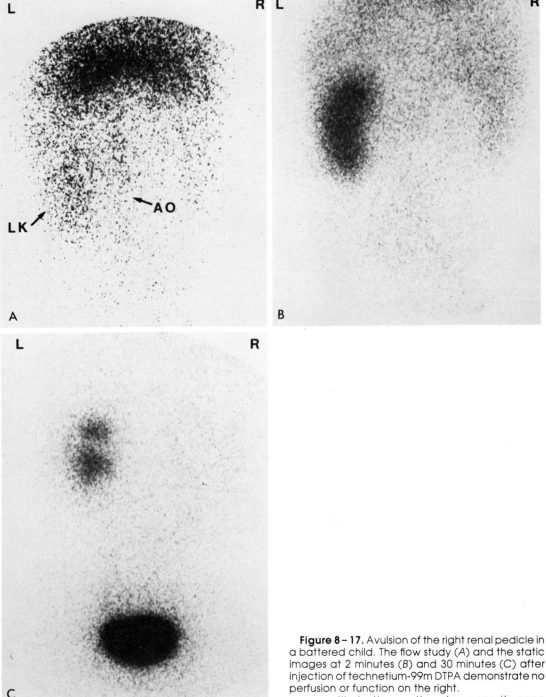

Figure 8 – 17. Avulsion of the right renal pedicle in a battered child. The flow study (*A*) and the static images at 2 minutes (*B*) and 30 minutes (*C*) after injection of technetium-99m DTPA demonstrate no perfusion or function on the right.

Illustration continued on opposite page

promising, it is technically complex and there is some doubt about its efficacy in children (Piepsz).

Inflammatory Disease

Acute pyelonephritis is usually diagnosed on the basis of clinical signs and symptoms. In certain cases, however, the clinical presentation is atypical and diagnostic imaging is necessary. Conventional radiographic examinations are of limited value in early detection of acute pyelonephritis. Excretory urograms suggestive of an acute inflammatory condition are found in less than 30 per cent of all cases (Silver et al). Ultrasound examination is useful in detection of renal or perirenal abscesses but is of little value in confirming acute pyelonephritis.

Renal cortical imaging using technetium-99m DMSA or technetium-99m glucoheptonate has been shown to be very sensitive in early detection of parenchymal abnormalities secondary to acute pyelonephritis. Handmaker found abnormal renal cortical scans in 10 of 60 patients suspected of having acute pyelonephritis and reported a sensitivity of 100 per cent. The cortical scan often shows one or more defects of varying size and shape

(Fig. 8–16). Occasionally a generalized decreased uptake of the tracer is seen. Cortical imaging also offers the quantitative evaluation of relative renal function and a noninvasive method of assessing response to treatment.

Renal cortical imaging has also been proven to be more accurate than excretory urography in detection of pyelonephritic scarring. Merrick et al (1980) compared renal cortical imaging and excretory urography in 79 children with proven urinary tract infection followed for a period of 1 to 4 years. Both techniques

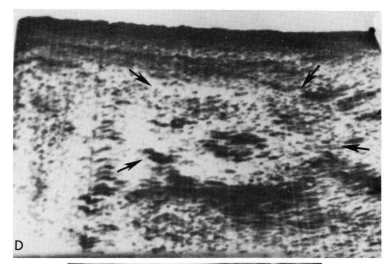

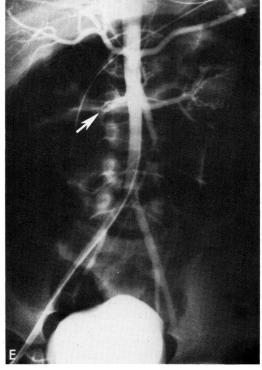

Figure 8–17 *Continued. D*, The renal sonogram shows presence of the right kidney in its normal location (*arrows*). *E*, The abdominal aortogram demonstrates abrupt cut-off of the right renal artery (*arrow*). At surgery avulsion of the right renal pedicle was found and the nonviable kidney was removed. AO, abdominal aorta; LK, left kidney.

were in agreement as to the presence or absence of scarring as well as to the extent of abnormality in 93.5 per cent of the kidneys studied. There was, however, discrepancy in 10 kidneys. Excretory urography had a sensitivity of 86 per cent and a specificity of 92 per cent in the detection of pyelonephritic scarring, whereas renal cortical imaging had a sensitivity of 96 per cent and a specificity of 98 per cent.

It should be noted that with technetium-99m DTPA there is no significant cortical retention of the tracer, and cases of acute pyelonephritis as well as pyelonephritic scarring may remain undetected. Therefore, technetium-99m glucoheptonate is the preferred renal scanning agent in the initial evaluation and follow-up assessments of renal changes following acute urinary tract infection. This agent, unlike technetium-99m DTPA, is not suitable for GFR measurement.

Trauma

Renal injuries are often due to blunt abdominal trauma or, less commonly, to penetration. Iatrogenic injuries may also occur as a result of surgical intervention, renal biopsy, retrograde pyelography, or interventional radiographic procedures. Diagnostic imaging procedures used in the evaluation of renal trauma include excretory urography with or without nephrotomography, sonography, computed tomography, radionuclide studies, and arteriography. The position of these imaging modalities in the diagnostic algorithm depends on the patient's condition and associated injuries as well as the availability of equipment and expertise.

Excretory urography, the most readily available procedure, is sensitive in the detection of renal pedicle injuries but underestimates minor renal injuries. It has a low sensitivity for the detection of urinary leakage and does not provide information about injury to the other organs.

Ultrasound is useful in the detection of subcapsular and perirenal hematomas, lacerations, blood clots in the renal pelvis, and urinary tract obstruction. However, it does not provide any information about the status of renal perfusion and function, which is the most critical factor in the acute management of the patient. Nonvisualization of a kidney on an excretory urogram or renal scan may be due to renal agenesis, and unless a renal silhouette is observed on the plain abdominal radiograph, ultrasound may be required to differentiate renal pedicle injury from renal agenesis.

Computed tomography (CT) of the abdomen with intravenous contrast enhancement provides superior anatomic detail, which allows accurate evaluation of the extent of renal trauma as well as simultaneous evaluation of other organs, the peritoneal cavity, and the retroperitoneum. It may be regarded as the single most informative imaging procedure in the evaluation of abdominal trauma. In a restless, injured child, however, motion artifacts may result in poor image quality.

Angiography is the best method of demonstrating vascular injury directly and also offers an opportunity to control active hemorrhage by selective arterial embolization (Chuang et al). It is, however, invasive and is not suitable for screening and serial evaluation. The role of digital subtraction angiography is yet to be defined.

Radionuclide renal imaging provides information about overall and regional perfusion and function of the kidneys. It is extremely sensitive in detecting renal pedicle injuries (Fig. 8–17), segmental infarctions, contusions (Fig. 8–18), lacerations, and urine extravasation (Fig. 8–19). Pre-existing congenital anomalies such as fusion, ectopia and hydronephrosis, which make the kidneys more susceptible to trauma, are easily detected. Radionuclide renal studies in conjunction with ultrasound are particularly useful in follow-up assessments of healing of traumatic injuries to the urinary tract and detection of secondary complications.

Renal Vascular Abnormalities

Renal artery stenosis is the cause of approximately 5 per cent of all cases of childhood hypertension (Hendren et al). The incidence is considerably higher when the hypertension occurs in association with neurofibromatosis or aortic anomalies (Stanley and Frey). Half of all hypertensive children less than 10 years old have a vascular cause for their disease (Lawson et al).

Renal arteriography and renal vein renin measurements are needed for definitive diagnosis and management of the renal vascular causes of hypertension. Renal arteriography, however, is an invasive procedure and is not suitable for screening. The role of less invasive digital subtraction angiography for this purpose has yet to be defined. The so-called

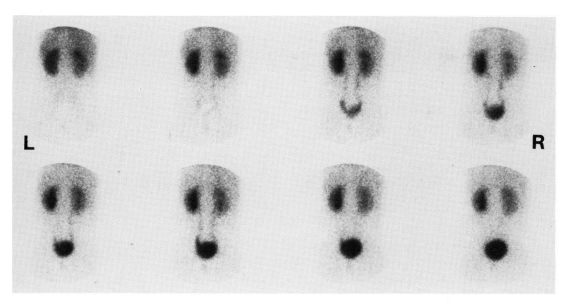

Figure 8–18. Mild right renal contusion in a child who presented with hematuria after trauma to the right flank. The posterior images obtained 2 to 30 minutes after injection of technetium-99m DTPA demonstrate minimal decrease in the right renal function with no evidence of laceration or extravasation.

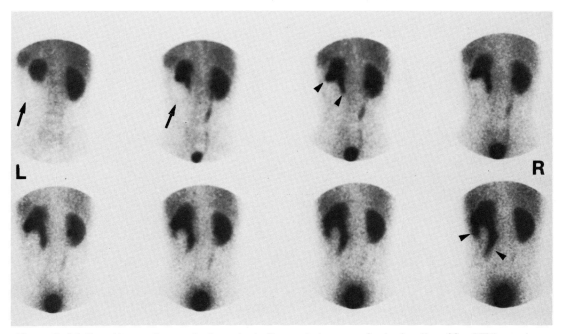

Figure 8–19. Renal laceration and urinary leak. The early images of a technetium-99m DTPA renal scan show a photon-deficient region below the functioning upper pole of the left kidney (*arrows*). This area is occupied by the nonfunctioning lacerated lower pole of the kidney and surrounding fluid collection. The subsequent images show gradual accumulation of the tracer in this area and along the left paravertebral region due to urinary leak (*arrowheads*).

hypertensive excretory urogram is not sensitive enough to be used as a screening procedure. Lawson et al, reporting a group of 107 hypertensive children, found abnormalities with rapid sequence excretory urography in all patients with renal parenchymal disease but in only 9 of 21 children (42 per cent) with renovascular disease. Stanley et al (1978) found abnormalities with rapid sequence excretory urography in 11 of 17 children (65 per cent) with unilateral renovascular disease.

Conventional radionuclide imaging and renography in the presence of unilateral renal artery stenosis may show evidence of decreased renal perfusion and function on the affected side. In the presence of hypertension, however, the kidney beyond a stenotic artery may remain adequately perfused and the renal scan and renogram may remain normal. Arlart et al, reporting a group of 105 patients with angiographically proven unilateral renal artery stenosis and 45 patients with essential hypertension, found 18 per cent false negative and 13 per cent false positive renal scans

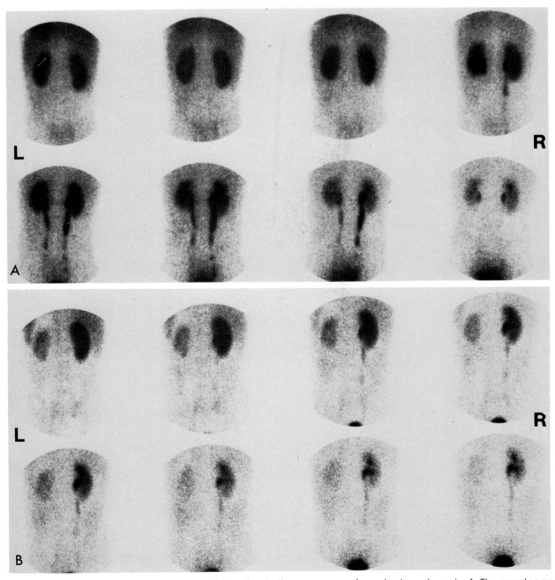

Figure 8–20. Effect of captopril on renal function in the presence of renal artery stenosis. *A,* The renal scan obtained as a part of the initial hypertensive workup was normal. *B,* The repeat study after 2 months of captopril therapy showed marked deterioration of the left renal function.

Illustration continued on opposite page

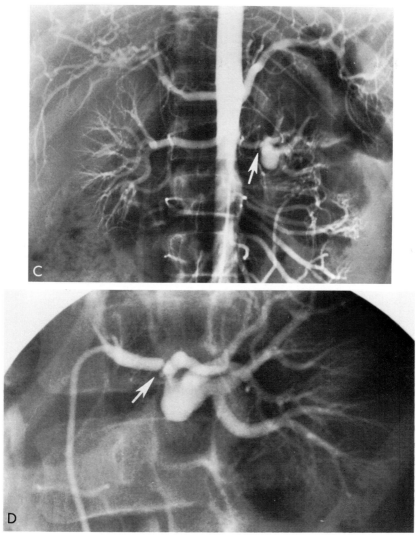

Figure 8-20 *Continued.* Abdominal aortogram (*C*) and a selective left renal arteriogram (*D*) showed stenosis of the left renal artery (*arrow*) with poststenotic aneurysmal dilatation.

for renal artery stenosis. The percentages for Hippuran renography were 17 and 26 per cent, respectively. Radionuclide studies are even less efficacious in the diagnosis of bilateral or segmental renal artery stenosis.

We have recently observed that captopril therapy in hypertensive children with renal artery stenosis causes dramatic but reversible deterioration of renal function that is easily detectable on renal scan (Fig. 8–20). We have proposed the use of captopril as a provocative test to increase the efficacy of renal scanning in the detection of renal artery stenosis (Majd et al, 1983b). Captopril is an orally active inhibitor of the angiotensin-converting enzyme, the enzyme responsible for converting

inactive angiotensin I to potent angiotensin II. The exact mechanism by which captopril, in the presence of renal artery stenosis, causes deterioration of renal function is not clear. Experimental studies have shown that autoregulation of the glomerular filtration rate in the presence of decreased renal blood flow is dependent on angiotensin II. Blockade of the renin-angiotensin system by captopril disturbs this autoregulation of GFR and, in the presence of low renal perfusion pressure, leads to decreased renal function.

Other vascular abnormalities of the kidney, such as thrombosis of the main or segmental renal veins or arteries, can often be diagnosed on the radionuclide studies. Renal vein thrombosis occurs most often in neonates and is usually secondary to hemoconcentration. The renal scan generally shows both decreased perfusion and function in an enlarged kidney. Renal artery thrombosis in the neonate occurs most commonly as a complication of an indwelling aortic catheter. Renal artery thrombosis also causes decreased perfusion and function of the kidney but, unlike renal vein thrombosis, usually does not cause enlargement of the kidney. Scintigraphic findings of renal vascular occlusion are nonspecific and should be interpreted in the clinical context.

Renal Masses

Most renal masses are adequately localized and characterized by excretory urography, sonography, or computed tomography. Radionuclide renal cortical imaging, however, may be of value in differentiating pseudotumors such as prominent columns of Bertin (Fig. 8–21), fetal lobulation, and dromedary humps from true pathology such as tumor, infarct, or hemorrhage (Mazer and Quaife).

The relative sensitivity of different diagnostic imaging modalities in early detection of Wilms' tumor in children with aniridia or he-

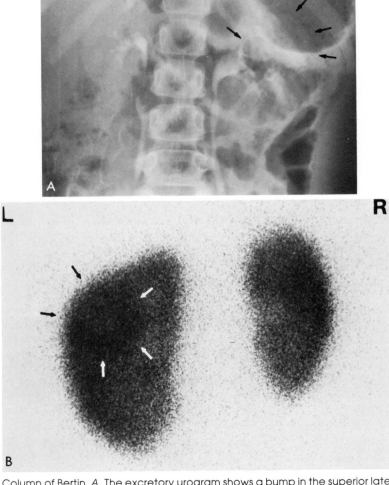

Figure 8–21. Column of Bertin. *A,* The excretory urogram shows a bump in the superior lateral aspect of the left kidney (*lateral arrows*) and an impression on the infundibulum of the upper calyx (*medial arrow*) suggestive of a space-occupying lesion. *B,* DMSA renal scan in posterior projection shows this area to be occupied by normal renal cortex (*arrows*).

mihypertrophy has not been defined. The combination of renal cortical imaging and sonography may prove to be the most effective approach to the periodic evaluation of these children during the risk period.

Renal Transplant

EVALUATION OF DONOR. Renal scan (including total and separate GFR determination) is often used in the evaluation of the living donor to ensure that he or she has two kidneys with normal function. This is usually followed by selective renal arteriography. When the use of the kidney of a "brain dead" patient is contemplated, a cerebral flow study may be performed as a part of technetium-99m DTPA renal scan both to confirm brain death and to evaluate renal function.

EVALUATION OF RECIPIENT. A variety of radionuclide studies have been used to evaluate perfusion and function of the transplanted kidney (Kirchner and Rosenthall; George). The most common procedure in children is technetium-99m DTPA renal scintigraphy, including quantitative analysis of the first transit of tracer from the aorta and iliac artery to the transplanted kidney. The renal time-activity curve is compared with that of the aorta or iliac artery. A normally perfused transplanted kidney shows a sharp rise and fall in the renal time-activity curve, which closely parallels the aortic curve (Fig. 8–22).

Possible complications following renal transplantation can be classified into two general categories: (1) those due to parenchymal failure, such as acute tubular necrosis (ATN), rejection, and infection; and (2) those due to mechanical injuries, including complete or partial obstruction of blood vessels, ureteral obstruction, urinary leak, and lymphocele.

In ATN, renal function decreases while renal perfusion remains relatively normal (Fig. 8–23), whereas in rejection both perfusion and function decrease proportionally (Fig. 8–24). Differentiation of rejection from ATN on the basis of a single study, however, is often difficult, and serial studies over several days or weeks may be necessary. A kidney injured by ATN generally displays its lowest level of perfusion and function by 24 to 48 hours after transplantation. Therefore, on the serial examinations the perfusion and function should improve or remain unchanged. By contrast, deterioration of renal perfusion and function due to rejection, if untreated, is generally progressive.

Complete renal arterial or venous occlusion as well as hyperacute rejection result in nonperfusion of the transplant and cannot be differentiated by radionuclide angiography alone. The scintigraphic finding of a "photon-deficient" zone (renal activity distinctly less than surrounding background activity) indicates a nonsalvageable transplant (Fig. 8–25).

Obstructive uropathy and urinary extravasation are readily detected on the renal scan, provided that renal function is adequate. A photon-deficient zone adjacent to the kidney on the early images may be due to urinary extravasation or lymphocele. In the case of urinary extravasation, delayed images demonstrate accumulation of tracer in the area, whereas a lymphocele remains photon-deficient. Sonography is complementary to scintigraphy in the detection of the urologic complications of renal transplantation.

RADIONUCLIDE CYSTOGRAPHY

The use of radionuclides for the detection of vesicoureteral reflux dates back to 1959 when Winter reported the appearance of radioactivity in the area of the kidneys after iodine-131 diodrast or iodine-131 rose bengal had been instilled into the bladder. For these studies scintillation probes were positioned over the kidneys. In 1964 Berne and Ekman reported the use of colloidal gold (gold 198) for cystography and emphasized the advantage of its low radiation dose as compared with that of retrograde x-ray cystography. With the advent of the gamma camera and technetium-99m compounds, retrograde radionuclide cystography with isotope directly instilled in the bladder was modified by Corriere et al (1967, 1970) and by Blaufox et al and popularized by Conway et al (1975). This technique is known as direct radionuclide cystography.

In 1963, Dodge reported his observation that a brisk rise in activity occurred in some patients with known reflux upon voiding at the end of a radionuclide renogram. This suggested a new technique for the detection of vesicoureteral reflux using intravenous injection of iodine-131 Hippuran and external scintillation counting over the renal area. This technique of indirect (intravenous) cystography was later modified by Handmaker et al.

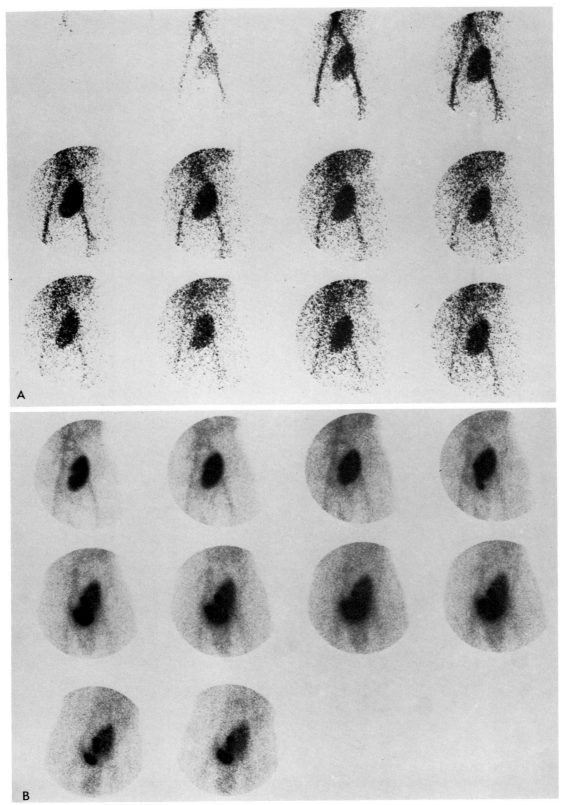

Figure 8–22. Renal transplant with normal function. *A,* The radionuclide angiogram shows prompt perfusion of the kidney. *B,* The static images from 2 to 35 minutes after injection of technetium-99m DTPA demonstrate prompt renal function and normal drainage.

Illustration continued on opposite page.

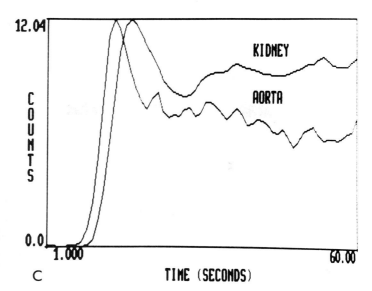

Figure 8–22 *Continued. C,* The time-activity curves of first transit of the tracer through the kidney parallels that of the aorta, confirming normal blood flow to the transplant.

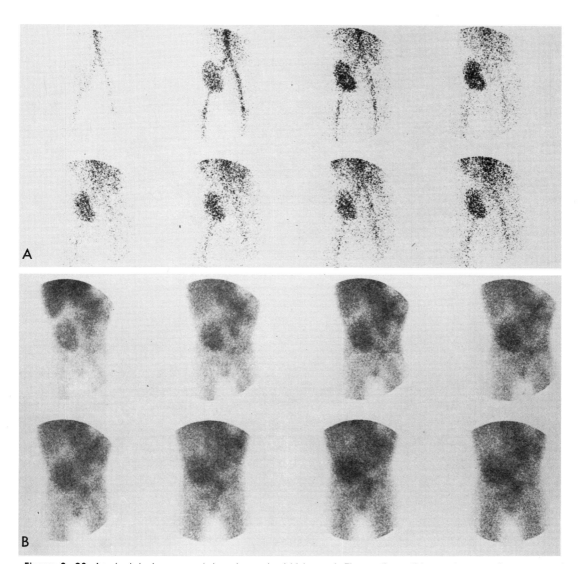

Figure 8–23. Acute tubular necrosis in a transplant kidney. *A,* The radionuclide angiogram shows normal blood flow to the kidney. *B,* The static images from 2 to 25 minutes after injection show decreased renal function.

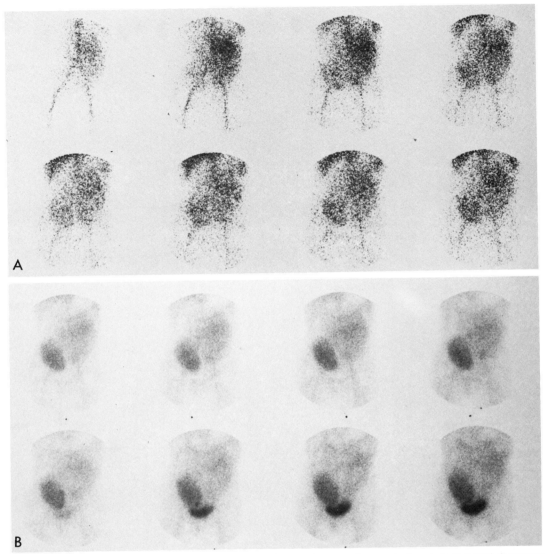

Figure 8–24. Transplant rejection. *A,* The radionuclide angiogram demonstrates delayed and decreased blood flow to the kidney. *B,* The static images from 2 to 35 minutes after injection show decreased renal function.

Direct (Retrograde) Radionuclide Cystography

Technique

No preparation or sedation is needed. The patient is supine with the gamma camera underneath. Following aseptic preparation, the urethra is catheterized with an 8 F Foley catheter or an infant feeding tube. The bladder is emptied and a urine sample is collected in a sterile bottle for culture. The catheter is connected to a bottle of normal saline by a regular intravenous infusion tubing set. The bottle of saline is placed 100 cm above the table top.

After the flow of normal saline is established, 1 mCi of technetium-99m pertechnetate is injected into the stream of saline through the rubber injection site of the infusion tube. The patient is positioned with the bladder on the lower edge of the field of view of the gamma camera. While the bladder is filling, it is continuously monitored on the persistence scope of the gamma camera, and multiple analogue and digital posterior images of the bladder and upper abdomen are obtained (Fig. 8–26). If bilateral reflux is observed, flow of normal saline is immediately discontinued. If no reflux is seen or only unilateral reflux occurs, the bladder is filled to capacity. In the major-

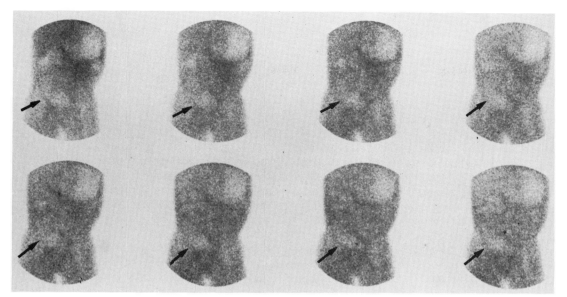

Figure 8-25. Nonsalvageable rejected transplant. Accumulation of the tracer in the region of the transplant (*arrows*) is less than in surrounding background.

ity of children bladder capacity ranges from 100 to 250 ml. The capacity of a hypertonic bladder, however, may be as low as 10 to 20 ml, whereas, in those who void infrequently, capacity may be as great as 500 ml. The signs of a full bladder include backup of saline in the tube, leakage around the catheter, upgoing toes, and crossing of the legs.

When reflux is seen, the volume of instilled saline is recorded. After adequate filling, the older patient is seated on a bedpan in front of the gamma camera, which has been placed in a vertical position. The catheter is removed and the patient is encouraged to void. Analogue and digital images are obtained before,

during, and after voiding (Majd and Belman) (Fig. 8-26). The number of counts on the pre-voiding and post-voiding images as well as total volume of instilled saline and the volume of the voided fluid are recorded. These values, together with the volume of instilled saline at the time of reflux, are used to calculate residual urine volume and the bladder volume at the time of reflux (Weiss and Conway). The volume of refluxed urine and the rate of its drainage back to the bladder can also be calculated. In infants, the voiding phase of the examination is carried on with the child in the supine position without measuring the voided urine volume. The volume

Figure 8-26. Selected images from the filling (F), voiding (V), and post-voiding (PV) phases of a direct radionuclide cystogram. Left vesicoureteral reflux is seen during filling and voiding phases.

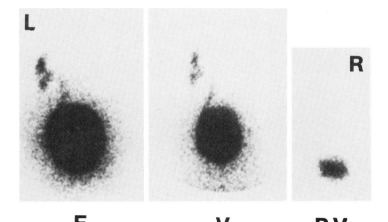

of instilled saline at the time of reflux is accepted as the total bladder volume at that time.

Advantages

LOW RADIATION DOSE. The most important advantage of direct radionuclide cystography is its extremely low radiation dose. With 1 mCi of technetium-99m pertechnetate in 200 ml of saline, the dose to the bladder wall during direct radionuclide cystography is about 1 mrad per minute of contact (Conway et al, 1972). In our experience, the average length of bladder exposure is only about 15 minutes, which results in a radiation dose of about 15 mrad to the bladder wall. The dose to the gonads, which in boys are at a considerable distance from the bladder wall, is probably less than 5 mrad. On the other hand, gonadal dose with standard x-ray voiding cystourethrography ranges from 75 mrad to several rads, depending on the fluoroscopy time and the number of films taken (Leibovic and Lebowitz). Therefore, on the average, the gonadal dose is about one one-hundredth that of standard x-ray studies. The total body radiation that may result from possible ab-

sorption of a minimal amount of technetium-99m pertechnetate is negligible (Blaufox et al; Conway et al, 1972).

SENSITIVITY. Reflux is a dynamic, intermittent phenomenon. A considerable amount of reflux may vanish within a matter of seconds (Fig. 8–27). With standard x-ray voiding cystourethrography, continuous extended observation under fluoroscopy is unacceptable because of excessive radiation. With direct radionuclide cystography, the urinary tract is monitored continuously during filling, during voiding, and after voiding with no increase in the amount of radiation. In addition, reflux is more easily detected because overlying bowel contents and bones do not interfere with detection as they may do during standard x-ray studies. The exception is minimal reflux to the distal ureter, which may be obscured by the isotope-filled bladder. Direct radionuclide cystography is more sensitive than x-ray cystography in detecting vesicoureteral reflux (Conway et al, 1972).

QUANTITATIVE ANALYSIS. Parameters such as residual urine volume, bladder volume at the time of reflux, volume of refluxed urine, and the rate of clearance of refluxed urine can be calculated. The clinical

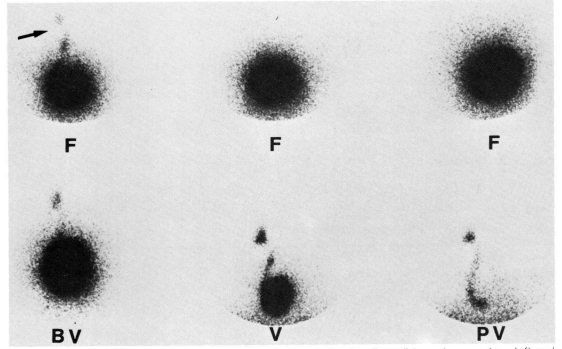

Figure 8–27. Intermittent reflux. Sequential images from a direct radionuclide cystogram show left vesicoureteral reflux in early filling phase (*arrow*), which disappears on the subsequent images but reappears just before and during voiding. F, filling phase; BV, before voiding; V, during voiding; PV, post-voiding.

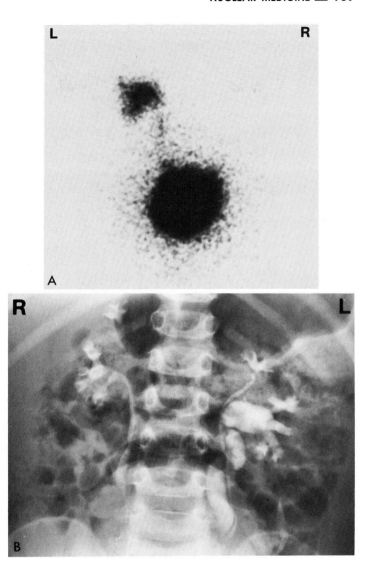

Figure 8-28. Reflux in a duplicated system. *A*, Posterior image of a direct radionuclide cystogram shows left vesicoureteral reflux. The "drooping lily" appearance of the collecting system is suggestive of duplication. *B*, Excretory urogram shows bilateral duplication with dilatation of the pelvicalyceal system and ureter of the lower pole of the left kidney.

significance of these functional parameters is not clear. Bladder volume at the time of reflux appears to have a prognostic significance. If the bladder volume at the time of demonstration of reflux increases on annual serial examinations, it may indicate a better prognosis for spontaneous cessation of reflux (Nasrallah et al). Maizels et al recorded intravesical pressures during the nuclear cystogram and reported that this combined information facilitates the management of children with vesicoureteral reflux and voiding abnormalities.

Disadvantages

The major disadvantage of direct radionuclide cystography is its unsuitability for evalu-ation of the male urethra. Therefore, its use for the initial study in boys with urinary tract infection is not advised unless the urethra is adequately evaluated on a voiding film obtained as part of an excretory urogram.

Because the anatomic resolution of direct radionuclide cystography is not as good as that of x-ray voiding cystourethrography, reflux cannot be graded accurately. The extremes of the spectrum (grades I, II, and V) can be differentiated, but grades III and IV cannot be accurately separated. Major abnormalities such as large filling defects in the bladder (ureterocele), distortion and displacement of the bladder, and most duplications associated with reflux can be appreciated (Fig. 8–28), but minor abnormalities of the bladder wall such as diverticula will be missed.

Indirect (Intravenous) Radionuclide Cystography

Technique

Indirect radionuclide cystography is a means of identifying reflux without urethral catheterization. It is based on the ideal condition of rapid and complete renal clearance of an intravenously injected radiopharmaceuti-

cal. The patient is normally hydrated (oral fluids). Following injection of 100 μCi/kg of technetium-99m DTPA a conventional renal scan is obtained. The patient is instructed not to void and is monitored intermittently. When the upper urinary tract is drained and most of the tracer is contained in the bladder, the child is placed before the gamma camera in a sitting or standing position, and analogue and digital

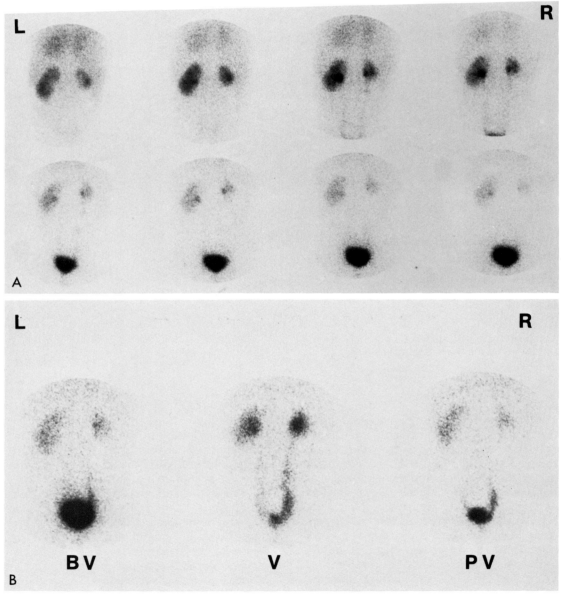

Figure 8–29. Indirect radionuclide cystogram. *A*, The sequential images from a conventional technetium-99m DTPA renal scan show prompt function and normal drainage bilaterally. The right kidney is small. *B*, The delayed images before (BV), during (V), and after (PV) voiding demonstrate bilateral vesicoureteral reflux, more severe on the right.

Illustration continued on opposite page

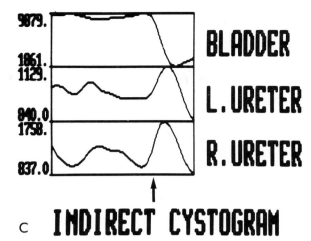

9879.
1861.
1123.
840.0
1758.
837.0

BLADDER

L. URETER

R. URETER

↑

C **INDIRECT CYSTOGRAM**

Figure 8–29 *Continued. C,* The time-activity curves of the regions of interest over the ureters and the bladder (C) demonstrate a rise in the activity over both ureters (*arrow*) as the bladder activity decreases during voiding. Slight terminal rise in the bladder activity curve is due to return of refluxed urine into the bladder during postvoiding phase.

images are obtained before, during, and after voiding. A sudden increase in radioactivity over a kidney or ureter indicates vesicoureteral reflux (Fig. 8–29).

Advantages

The theoretical advantages of indirect radionuclide cystography are that unpleasant catheterization is avoided, voiding may be more normal since the urethra is not irritated, and the study is performed without overdistending the bladder. A final advantage is that renal function and morphology as well as reflux may be evaluated simultaneously.

Disadvantages

Although some reports indicate good correlation between the indirect radionuclide cystography and x-ray voiding cystourethrography (Hedman et al; Merrick et al, 1977; Pollet et al), our recent review comparing the two methods in 120 children with known reflux showed that the indirect technique produced an overall false negative rate of 41 per cent (Majd et al, 1983a) (Fig. 8–30).

Other disadvantages of the indirect method include its dependence upon renal function and adequate drainage as well as upon cooperation by the patient, who must be able to void on request. The study is not practical in children who have a neuropathic bladder and in those who are not toilet trained. The radiation dose is higher than that of the direct cystogram and may become considerable if the child withholds urine for a protracted period.

Clinical Applications

Direct Cystography

1. Direct radionuclide cystography, because of its superior sensitivity and minimal radiation dose, is the method of choice for follow-up assessments of a child with known reflux and to ascertain that reflux has ceased following surgical correction.

2. In girls it can be used as the initial screening test for detection of reflux, since visualization of the urethra by and large serves no useful diagnostic purpose.

3. Direct radionuclide cystography in boys in conjunction with a voiding film as part of excretory urography may occasionally obviate the need for x-ray voiding cystourethrography for the initial screening.

Indirect Cystography

1. Indirect radionuclide cystography has a very low sensitivity for detection of reflux and should not be used as an initial screening test.

2. In children with known reflux, if renal scanning is part of the follow-up evaluation, an indirect cystogram may be obtained. A positive study is reliable, but the negative studies should be confirmed by direct cystography.

SCROTAL SCINTIGRAPHY

Diagnostic testicular scanning was first proposed by Nadel et al in 1973. Since then, radionuclide scrotal imaging has been refined

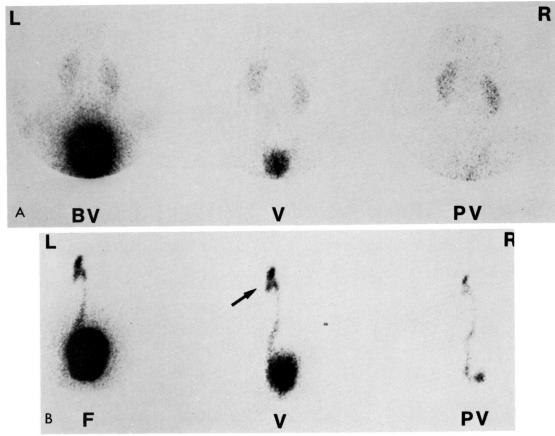

Figure 8–30. *A,* False negative indirect radionuclide cystogram. An indirect cystogram in a patient with known history of left vesicoureteral reflux shows no evidence of reflux. *B,* A direct radionuclide cystogram obtained 7 days later demonstrates persistence of the left vesicoureteral reflux (*arrow*). BV, before voiding; V, during voiding; PV, post-voiding; F, filling.

and has proved very useful in differentiating "surgical" from "nonsurgical" disorders of the scrotal contents. This study, if done properly in patients presenting with an acutely enlarged and painful hemiscrotum, may drastically decrease the number of unnecessary surgical explorations.

Technical Considerations

The patient's thyroid is blocked by oral administration of potassium perchlorate in a dose of 5 mg/kg immediately prior to the test. The child is positioned supine on the imaging table. The penis is taped up over the pubis. The scrotum is supported by towels positioned between the thighs or by a tape sling. Lead shielding under the scrotum is not recommended for the angiographic phase of the examination (Holder et al), but for the static images, particularly in younger children, a lead shield under the scrotum facilitates detection of areas of decreased blood flow. The scrotum is positioned under the center of a gamma camera equipped with a converging collimator.

After rapid intravenous injection of technetium-99m pertechnetate in a dose of 200 μCi/kg, multiple 3 second dynamic images (radionuclide angiogram) are obtained. Immediately after the angiographic phase, early static images ("blood pool" or "tissue phase") are obtained. This is usually followed by the use of a pinhole collimator to obtain high resolution magnified static images.

Physical examination of the scrotum and accurate localization of the testicles by the nuclear physician is crucial in correct interpretation of the scintigraphic findings.

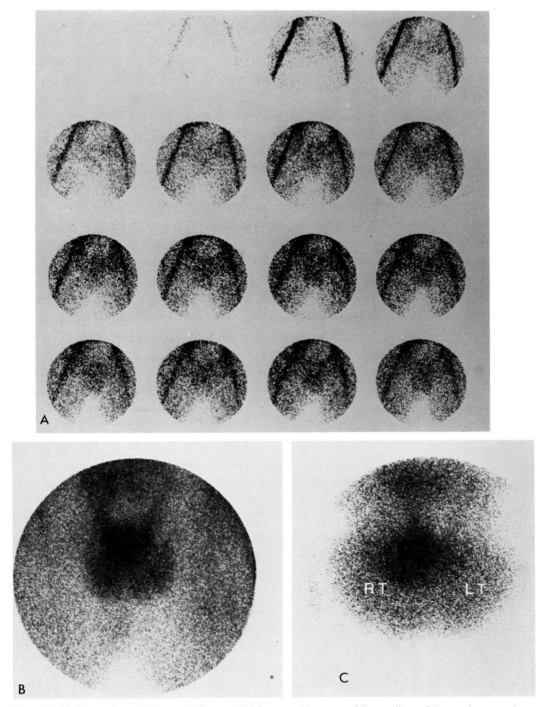

Figure 8-31. Normal scrotal scan. *A*, Sequential 3 second images of the radionuclide angiogram demonstrate excellent visualization of the iliac arteries. The vessels supplying the scrotum and its contents are not well defined. There is, however, homogeneous symmetrical accumulation of the tracer in the hemiscrotums. The unshielded static image (*B*) and the magnified image with the lead shield under the scrotum (*C*) also show symmetrical accumulation of the tracer in the testicles. RT, right testicle, LT, left testicle.

Scintigraphic Patterns

Basic knowledge of the vascular anatomy of the scrotal contents is essential for understanding the scintigraphic findings. The scrotal contents have a dual blood supply. The first pathway is composed of the vessels entering the spermatic cord: the testicular artery, which supplies the testicle, epididymis, and tunica vaginalis; the deferential artery; and the cremasteric artery. These three vessels enter the spermatic cord at different levels and usually anastomose at the testicular mediastinum. The cremasteric artery forms a network over the tunica vaginalis and also participates in anastomoses with vessels supplying the scrotal wall. The second pathway is composed of the vessels that do not enter the spermatic cord. These include the internal pudendal artery and the superficial and deep external pudendal arteries. These arteries supply the scrotum and penis.

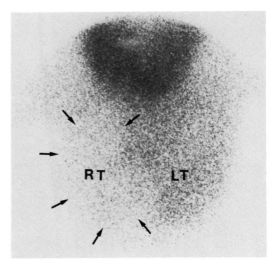

Figure 8–32. Acute testicular torsion in a 16-year-old boy with pain and swelling of the right testicle of 6 hours' duration. The static image using a pinhole collimator and lead shield under the scrotum shows decreased accumulation of the tracer in the right testicle (*arrows*). RT, right testicle; LT, left testicle.

Normal Scrotal Scintigram

In a normal scrotal scintigram the iliac arteries are well visualized, but owing to their size and the relatively small amount of blood flow, the vessels supplying the scrotal contents are ill-defined and the scrotum and its contents blur into a homogeneous area of tracer accumulation similar in intensity to the image of the thigh. Dartos activity cannot be separated from testicular or epididymal activity (Fig. 8–31).

Testicular Torsion

The scintigraphic pattern in testicular torsion depends on the duration of torsion.

EARLY PHASE (ACUTE TORSION). In the early phase (probably within the first 6 hours), the radionuclide angiogram may show decreased blood flow to the hemiscrotum or may appear normal. Blood flow to the hemiscrotum is never increased at this stage. The static images ("tissue phase") show decreased accumulation of the tracer in the testicle without the reactive surrounding halo of increased activity seen in the later phases (Fig. 8–32).

MIDPHASE. After a few hours, there is reactive hyperemia in the region supplied by the pudendal arteries. The radionuclide angiogram shows increased blood flow to the dartos, and the early static images show a halo of mildly increased activity around a cold center. The halo of increased activity gradually disappears on the subsequent images.

This pattern is usually seen in patients who have been symptomatic for 6 to 24 hours.

LATE PHASE (MISSED TORSION). If the patient with torsion does not seek immediate medical attention or is erroneously diagnosed, irreversible testicular infarction occurs. This late phase of torsion is termed "missed torsion." If the torsion persists, the pain and swelling will resolve in a few days to weeks with subsequent atrophy of the testicle. It is important to diagnose missed testicular torsion in order to remove the necrotic testicle and to perform orchiopexy on the contralateral side.

Missed torsion has a characteristic scintigraphic pattern. The angiographic phase shows marked increased blood flow to the dartos, and static images reveal a complete rim or "halo" of increased activity around a cold center. The halo persists throughout the examination, which usually takes about 15 to 20 minutes (Fig. 8–33).

SPONTANEOUS DETORSION. A spontaneously detorsed testicle may appear normal on the scans or may show slight diffuse increased scrotal activity (Fig. 8–34). The diagnosis is best made on the basis of clinical history if examination has not been carried out prior to the detorsion. Demonstration of an intact blood supply to the testicle obviates only the need for emergency surgery. If the history is typical of intermittent torsion, but

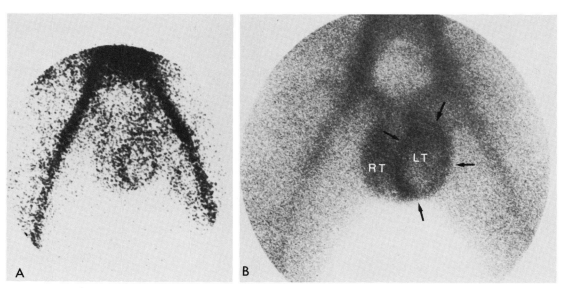

Figure 8 – 33. "Missed" testicular torsion in a 15-year-old boy who presented with a 2-day history of pain and swelling of the left hemiscrotum. *A,* A selected image of the radionuclide angiogram demonstrates increased blood flow *around* the left testicle. *B,* The static image shows decreased accumulation of the tracer in the left testicle associated with a surrounding rim or "halo" of increased accumulation of the tracer (arrows). RT, right testicle; LT, left testicle.

physical examination shows the testis to be normally positioned and the scrotal scan shows intact perfusion and slightly increased activity, elective orchiopexy may be indicated (Lutzker).

Acute Epididymitis

In acute epididymitis, the radionuclide angiogram and the static images show markedly increased blood flow and blood pool activity

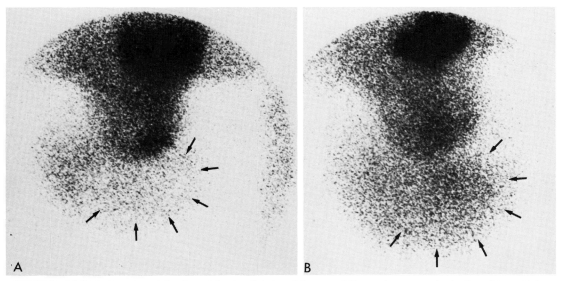

Figure 8 – 34. Spontaneous detorsion of the testicle in a 16-year-old boy who presented with a 4-hour history of pain and swelling of the left testicle. *A,* The magnified static image of the scrotum with a lead shield underneath shows decreased accumulation of the tracer in the left testicle (*arrows*) typical of an acute testicular torsion. Shortly after this image was obtained and while the patient was still on the scanning table, the pain abruptly subsided. *B,* Another image taken about 10 minutes after the image in *A* shows mild increased accumulation of the tracer in the left testicle (*arrows*). At surgery nonfixation of the testicle and evidence of spontaneous detorsion were found.

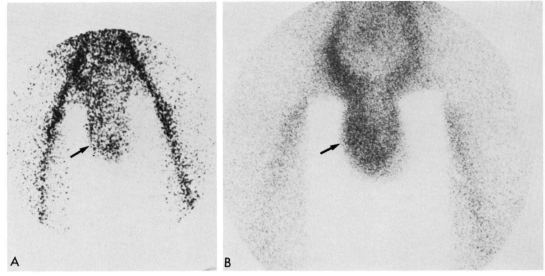

Figure 8–35. Acute epididymitis in a 15-year-old boy. The radionuclide angiogram (*A*) and the static image of the scrotum (*B*) show increased blood flow and accumulation of the tracer in the right hemiscrotum (*arrows*).

to the area corresponding to the epididymis, or diffusely in the scrotum, if epididymo-orchitis is present (Fig. 8–35). Intense increased activity in the epididymis may occasionally resemble the halo of missed torsion. But unlike the halo of missed torsion, the rim is incomplete and asymmetrical (Fig. 8–36). Epididymitis in infants and young children may be secondary to an underlying anatomic abnormality such as an ectopic ureter and warrants complete investigation of the genitourinary system.

Torsion of the Testicular Appendages

Torsion of the appendix testis or epididymis may be visualized as a focal area of increased blood flow and blood pool activity probably secondary to reactive hyperemia around the torsed appendix. The ischemic appendix itself is too small to be resolved on the images (Fig. 8–37). A more common scintigraphic pattern is that of mild generalized increased activity

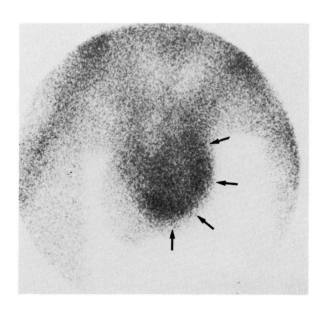

Figure 8–36. Acute epididymitis in a 17-year-old boy. The static image of the scrotum with a lead shield underneath demonstrates a semicircular area of increased accumulation of the tracer on the left corresponding to the epididymis (*arrows*).

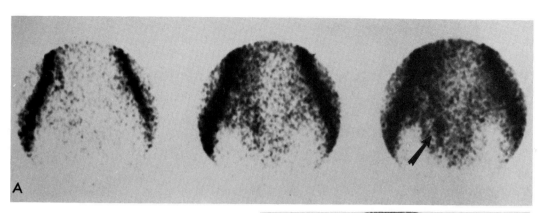

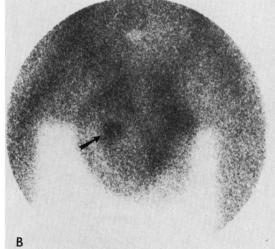

Figure 8–37. Torsion of the appendix testis in a 9-year-old boy who presented with a 2-day history of pain and swelling of the right hemiscrotum. The radionuclide angiogram (A) and the static image (B) of the scrotum demonstrate a small focal area of increased accumulation of the tracer on the right (arrows).

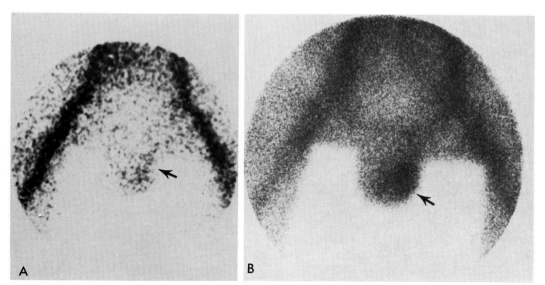

Figure 8–38. Torsion of the appendix testis in a 10-year-old boy who presented with a 3-day history of pain and swelling of the left hemiscrotum. The radionuclide angiogram (A) and the static image (B) demonstrate diffuse increased blood flow and accumulation of the tracer on the left (arrows) similar to the scintigraphic appearance of epididymitis.

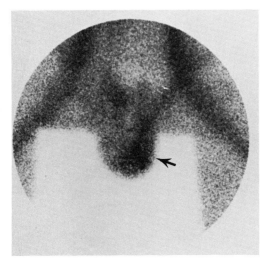

Figure 8–39. Scrotal trauma. This 16-year-old boy presented with a painful, swollen left testicle 2 days after direct trauma to his scrotum. The scan shows diffuse increased accumulation of the tracer on the left (*arrow*) similar to the scintigraphic pattern that may be seen in epididymitis or some cases of torsion of the appendix testis.

(vascularity) indistinguishable from epididymitis (Fig. 8–38). This differentiation is of no surgical significance, because both epididymitis and torsion of the appendix testis are generally considered to be nonsurgical problems. Radionuclide studies in the early phase

of torsion of the appendix testis, prior to a significant inflammatory response, may be normal (Holder et al).

Scrotal Trauma

The scintigraphic pattern following scrotal trauma depends on the extent of injury as well as the time elapsed between the trauma and the scan. Mild traumatic changes may appear as slightly to moderately diffuse increased tracer accumulation (Fig. 8–39). Intratesticular or intrascrotal hematoma may appear as a cold lesion with or without a surrounding halo of increased activity similar to testicular torsion (Fig. 8–40). Testicular rupture is also a surgical problem. Ultrasound may be a useful adjunct in localizing a hematoma in relation to the testicle.

Hydrocele

The diagnosis of a simple hydrocele is made by physical examination and transillumination. In secondary hydrocele, which is seen in association with torsion, epididymitis, trauma, or following herniorrhaphy, scintigraphic findings reflect the underlying condition. Hydroceles often appear as a horseshoe or a half-moon–shaped photon deficiency surrounding the testicle (Fig. 8–41).

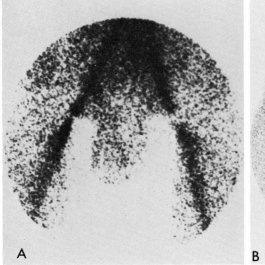
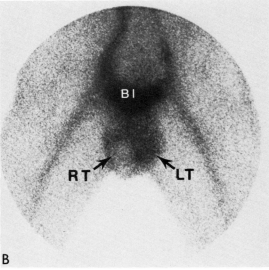

Figure 8–40. Testicular hematoma. This 12-year-old boy presented with painful swelling of the right testicle 14 hours after trauma to his scrotum. *A,* The radionuclide angiogram shows moderately increased blood flow around the right testicle. *B,* The static image shows decreased accumulation of the tracer in the right testicle with a "halo" of mildly increased activity. This scintigraphic pattern is similar to that of a missed torsion. Bl, bladder; RT, right testicle; LT, left testicle.

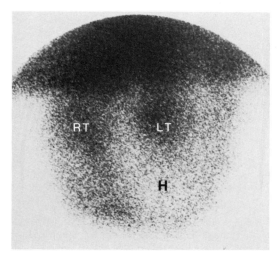

Figure 8-41. Hydrocele. There is a horseshoe-shaped area of decreased accumulation of the tracer surrounding the left testicle. RT, right testicle; LT, left testicle; H, hydrocele.

Abscess

Scans of testicular or intrascrotal abscesses demonstrate a cold center surrounded by a rim of increased activity similar to that of missed torsion. The diagnosis is usually made in the context of the clinical history.

Summary

The scintigraphic patterns in the acute hemiscrotum can be divided into two groups:

1. Diffuse or focal increased blood flow and blood pool activity without any cold component. This pattern is seen in patients with epididymitis, torsion of the appendix testis, and minor posttraumatic abnormalities, all of which are nonsurgical conditions. The problem of differentiation between these conditions and spontaneous detorsion is usually solved on the basis of clinical history.

2. Cold lesions with or without a surrounding rim of increased activity (excluding typical hydrocele). This pattern is seen in patients with testicular torsion, hematoma, and abscess, all of which are surgical conditions.

Clinical Applications

Acute Hemiscrotum

When the clinical presentation and physical findings are typical of the early phase of acute testicular torsion, surgery should be carried out immediately without delaying for a testicular scan.

When the clinical presentation suggests inflammatory disease or conditions other than acute torsion, or when the patient cannot be properly examined because of extreme swelling and tenderness, testicular scanning is indicated and can reliably differentiate the "surgical" from the "nonsurgical" conditions.

Nonacute Indications

Testicular scanning may also be helpful in the following conditions: (1) if there is any clinical doubt as to testicular viability after corrective detorsion and orchiopexy; and (2) in the occasional patient with suspected incompletely treated epididymo-orchitis when the question of abscess arises.

BIBLIOGRAPHY

Arlart I, Rosenthal J, Adam WE, et al: Predictive value of radionuclide methods in the diagnosis of unilateral renovascular hypertension. Cardiovascular Radiol 2: 115, 1979.

Berne E, Ekman H: Method for clinical studies of vesicoureteral reflux using colloidal 198 Au. Urol Int 18:335, 1964.

Blaufox MD, Gruskin A, Sandler P, et al: Radionuclide cystography for detection of vesicoureteral reflux in children. J Pediatr 79:239, 1971.

Braren V, Versage PN, Touya JJ, et al: Radioisotopic determination of glomerular filtration rate. J Urol 121:145, 1979.

Chuang VP, Reuter SR, Schmidt RW: Control of experimental renal hemorrhage by embolization with autogenous blood clot. Radiology 117:55, 1975.

Conway JJ, Belman AB, King LR, et al: Direct and indirect radionuclide cystography. J Urol 113:689, 1975.

Conway JJ, King LR, Belman AB, et al: Detection of vesicoureteral reflux with radionuclide cystography. A comparison study with roentgenographic cystography. Am J Roentgenol Radium Ther Nucl Med 115:720, 1972.

Corriere JN Jr, Kuhl DE, Murphy JJ: The use of 99mTc labeled sulfur colloid to study particle dynamics in the urinary tract. Vesicoureteral reflux. Invest Urol 4:570, 1967.

Corriere JN Jr, Sanders TP, Kuhl DE, et al: Urinary particle dynamics and vesicoureteral reflux in humans. J Urol 103:599, 1970.

Diffey BL, Hall FM, Corfield JR: The 99mTc-DTPA dynamic renal scan with deconvolution analysis. J Nucl Med 17:352, 1976.

Dodge EA: Vesicoureteral reflux: diagnosis with iodine-131 sodium ortho-iodohippurate. Lancet 1:303, 1963.

Dubovsky EV, Russell CD: Quantitation of renal function with glomerular and tubular agents. Semin Nucl Med 12:308, 1982.

Felson B, Cussen LJ: The hydronephrotic type of unilateral congenital multicystic disease of the kidney. Semin Roentgenol 10:113, 1975.

Gates GF: Glomerular filtration rate: estimation from fractional renal accumulation of 99mTC-DTPA (stannous). AJR 138:563, 1982.

George EA: Radionuclide diagnosis of allograft rejection. Semin Nucl Med 12:379, 1982.

Griscom NT, Wawter GF, Fellers FX: Pelvoinfundibular atresia: the usual form of multicystic kidney: 44 unilateral and two bilateral cases. Semin Roentgenol 10:125, 1975.

Handmaker H: Nuclear renal imaging in acute pyelonephritis. Semin Nucl Med 12:246, 1982.

Handmaker H, McRae J, Buck EG: Intravenous radionuclide voiding cystography (IRVC). An atraumatic method of demonstrating vesicoureteral reflux. Radiology 108:703, 1973.

Hedman PJK, Kempi V, Voss H: Measurement of vesicoureteral reflux with intravenous 99mTc-DTPA compared to radiographic cystography. Radiology 126:205, 1978.

Hendren WH, Kim SH, Herrin JT, et al: Surgically correctable hypertension of renal origin in childhood. Am J Surg 143:432, 1982.

Holder LE, Melloul M, Chen D: Current status of radionuclide scrotal imaging. Sem Nucl Med 11:232, 1981.

Kirchner PT, Rosenthall L: Renal transplant evaluation. Semin Nucl Med 12:370, 1982.

Lawson JD, Boerth R, Foster JH, et al: Diagnosis and management of renovascular hypertension in children. Arch Surg 112:1307, 1977.

Lebowitz RL, Blickman JG: The coexistence of ureteropelvic junction obstruction and reflux. AJR 140:231, 1983.

Leibovic SJ, Lebowitz RL: Reducing patient dose in voiding cystourethrography. Urol Radiol 2:103, 1980.

Lutzker LG: The fine points of scrotal scintigraphy. Semin Nucl Med 12:387, 1982.

Maizels M, Weiss S, Conway JJ, et al: The cystometric nuclear cystogram. J Urol 121:203, 1979.

Majd M, Belman AB: Nuclear cystography in infants and children. Urol Clin North Am 6:395, 1979.

Majd M, Kass EJ, Belman AB: The accuracy of the indirect (intravenous) radionuclide cystogram in children. J Nucl Med 24:23, 1983a.

Majd M, Potter BM, Guzzetta PC, et al: Effect of captopril on efficacy of renal scintigraphy in detection of renal artery stenosis. J Nucl Med 24:23, 1983b.

Mazer MJ, Quaife MA: Hypertrophied column of Bertin pseudotumors: radionuclide investigation (letter to the editor). Urology 14:210, 1979.

McCrory WW: Developmental Nephrology. Cambridge, Mass., Harvard University Press, 1972, p 96.

Merrick MV, Uttley WS, Wild SR: A comparison of two techniques of detecting vesico-ureteric reflux. Br J Radiol 52:792, 1977.

Merrick MV, Uttley WS, Wild SR: The detection of pyelonephritic scarring in children by radioisotope imaging. Br J Radiol 53:544, 1980.

Nadel NS, Gitter MH, Hahn LC, et al: Pre-operative diagnosis of testicular torsion. Urology 1:478, 1973.

Nasrallah PF, Conway JJ, King LR, et al: Quantitative nuclear cystogram. Aid in determining spontaneous resolution of vesicoureteral reflux. Urology 12:654, 1978.

Nawaz MK, Nimmon CC, Britton KE, et al: Obstructive nephropathy: a comparison of the parenchymal transit time index and furosemide diuresis. J Nucl Med 24:16, 1983.

Nilson AE, Aurell M, Bratt CG, et al: Diuretic urography in the assessment of obstruction of the pelvi-ureteric junction. Acta Radiol (Diagn) (Stockh) 21:499, 1980.

O'Reily PH, Lawson RS, Shields RA, et al: Idiopathic hydronephrosis — the diuresis renogram: a new non-invasive method of assessing equivocal pelvioureteral junction obstruction. J Urol 121:153, 1979.

Piepsz A, Denis R, Ham HR, et al: A simple method for measuring separate glomerular filtration rate using a single injection of 99mTc-DTPA and the scintillation camera. J Pediatr 93:769, 1978.

Piepsz A, Ham HR, Dobbeleir A, et al: How to exclude renal obstruction in children: comparison of intrarenal transit times, cortical times and furosemide test. In Radionuclides in Nephrology. Edited by AM Joekes, AR Constable, NJG Brown, et al. London, Academic Press, Inc., 1982, pp 199–204.

Pollet JE, Sharp PF, Smith FW: Radionuclide imaging for vesico-renal reflux using intravenous 99mTc-DTPA. Pediatr Radio 8:165, 1979.

Powers TA, Stone WJ, Grove RB, et al: Radionuclide measurement of differential glomerular filtration rate. Invest Radiol 16:59, 1981.

Price RR, Torn ML, Jones JP, et al: Comparison of differential renal function determination by Tc-99m DMSA, Tc-99m DTPA, I-131 Hippuran and ureteral catheterization. J Nucl Med 20:631, 1979.

Silver TM, Kass EJ, Thornbury JR, et al: The radiological spectrum of acute pyelonephritis in adults and adolescents. Radiology 118:65, 1976.

Stanley JC, Frey WJ: Pediatric renal artery occlusive disease and renovascular hypertension. Arch Surg 116:669, 1981.

Stanley P, Gyepes MT, Olson DL, et al: Renovascular hypertension in children and adolescents. Radiology 129:123, 1978.

Taylor A Jr: Quantitation of renal function with static imaging agents. Semin Nucl Med 12:330, 1982.

Thrall JH, Koff SA, Keyes JW Jr: Diuretic radionuclide urography and scintigraphy in the differential diagnosis of hydronephrosis. Semin Nucl Med 11:89, 1981.

Weiss S, Conway JJ: The technique of direct radionuclide cystography. Appl Radiol 4(3):133, 1975.

Whitfield HN, Britton KE, Fry IK, et al: The obstructed kidney: correlation between renal function and urodynamic assessment. Br J Urol 49:615, 1977.

Whitfield HN, Britton KE, Hendry WF, et al: The distinction between obstructive uropathy and nephropathy by radioisotope transit times. Br J Urology 50:433, 1978.

Whitfield HN, Britton KE, Nimmon CC, et al: Renal transit time measurements in the diagnosis of ureteric obstruction. Br J Urol 53:500, 1981.

Winter CC: A new test for vesicoureteral reflux: an external technique using radioisotopes. J Urol 81:105, 1959.

Wood BP, Smith WL: Pulmonary edema in infants following injection of contrast media for urography. Radiology 139:377, 1981.

Zielinski FW, Holly FE, Robinson GD Jr, et al: Total and individual kidney function assessment with iodine-123 ortho-iodohippurate. Radiology 125:753, 1977.

9

ULTRASONOGRAPHY OF THE UROGENITAL SYSTEM

Arnold Shkolnik

Ultrasonic imaging for medical diagnosis was initially developed in the 1940's, following the utilization of high-frequency sound in metal flaw detectors and sonar in World War II. Widespread clinical utilization of this modality, however, awaited the 1970's, when a dramatic improvement in ultrasonic image quality and detail was achieved through the technologic innovation of gray-scale sonography. The wide clinical applications of static gray-scale ultrasonography that subsequently evolved have been dramatically increased as a result of the recent development of real-time ultrasound. Real-time scanners have added the capability to display dynamic events, and mobile units have facilitated portable ultrasound examination. Both static and dynamic ultrasound are widely utilized for evaluation of the urogenital system of the pediatric patient (Waterhouse) and have been instrumental in the detection of abnormalities of the fetal urinary tract.

BASICS OF ULTRASONOGRAPHY

Audible sound ranges in frequency from 16,000 to 20,000 cycles per second. In contrast, frequencies of 3 million to 10 million cycles (megahertz) per second are utilized for diagnostic ultrasonography. Imaging is initiated with the transmission of sound into the patient's body, and is ultimately derived from the subsequent recording of increments of this sound that are reflected back to their source from successive tissue interfaces that lie in the path of and are essentially perpendicular to the sonic beam. A crystal with piezoelectric characteristics, housed in the scanning transducer, serves as both sonic sender and re-

ceiver. When subjected to a pulsed electrical current, the crystal periodically contracts, resulting in the production of sound waves, which are propagated into the patient's body via the scanning surface of the transducer. Conversely, when a returning echo strikes the crystal, its energy is converted to electricity, which is processed and displayed as a dot on a video screen, in an orientation that reflects the site of its origin within the body. It is noteworthy that during scanning, the transducer crystal is in a receiving mode more than 99 per cent of the time. The extremely brief period of actual induction of sonic energy into the patient during an examination is very likely a significant contributory factor in the apparent biologic safety of this imaging modality.

The interfaces that give rise to echo production are formed by adjacent tissues of differing acoustic impedances, a property that is primarily determined by tissue density. The greater the degree of impedance mismatch, the greater the increment of sound reflected back to the transducer. As an area is scanned, a cross-sectional image, termed a B-mode sonogram, is formed by the coalescence of multiple echo-dots. The "B" alludes to the brightness of each dot, which is displayed in a shade of gray relative to the amplitude of the echo. Thus, the kidney and other abdominal and pelvic organs, as well as solid mass lesions, produce a textural pattern of gray shades that reflects the heterogeneity of their tissues. A homogeneous fluid mass offers no internal acoustic interfaces and is therefore anechoic. An uncomplicated fluid mass is further characterized by precise definition of its deep wall, and strong echogenicity from tissues lying immediately posterior to the mass. The delineation of both free and compartmentalized fluid is a major forte of ultrasonography which contributes greatly to its clinical usefulness.

Both static and real-time ultrasonography are displayed in a B-mode format. Higher-frequency transducers provide better imaging resolution, but at the expense of decreased sound wave penetration. Thus, the choice of transducer frequency is primarily dependent on the depth of the area of interest. The thickness of tissue encompassed in the two-dimensional image corresponds to the diameter of the scanning transducer, which for pediatric usage varies from 6 to 13 mm.

STATIC SCANNING. This technique is also referred to as B-mode or articulated-arm scanning. The transducer is housed in a hinged arm that limits the transducer motion for a given scan to a single plane. The generation of a sonogram requires that the sonographer manually pass the transducer across the patient's skin, over the area of interest. The scanning arm can be mechanically driven in graduated increments, allowing multiplanar scans of the area of interest.

REAL-TIME SCANNING. Sector scanners are currently utilized in pediatric imaging. The scanning transducer, comparable to an electric shaver in size, shape, and weight, is freely movable, being attached to the scanning console only by an electric cord. In contrast to articulated-arm scanning, real-time scanning is achieved by maintaining the transducer in a fixed position on the patient's body over the desired plane of interest. B-mode sector sonograms, fanning out from the skin surface from 45 to 90 degrees, are regenerated from 15 to 30 or more times per second, resulting in a persistent image display comparable to fluoroscopy.

RECORDING THE SONOGRAM. Both static and real-time sonograms are displayed on a television monitor. Videotaping of real-time sonography can be highly advantageous for both diagnostic and teaching purposes. The real-time image can be "frozen," resulting in an image similar to that achieved with an articulated-arm scanner. This sonogram can be recorded on either Polaroid or radiographic film. Echo display, initially limited to grays on a white background, can now also be displayed in a white-on-black-background format. The preference for either format among sonographers is highly subjective, and examples of each are contained in this chapter.

There are a number of excellent texts available to the reader desiring in-depth information regarding the physical principles and instrumentation of diagnostic ultrasonography, several of which are listed in the bibliography (Bartrum and Crow; Kremkau; Rose and Goldberg).

ATTRIBUTES OF ULTRASONOGRAPHY

The variety and sophistication of diagnostic imaging procedures available to the clinician are continually increasing. Each modality possesses a variety of unique attributes that, in experienced hands, can justify its use either as a primary or as a complementary imaging tool. A review of the advantages of ultrasound and its capabilities relative to renal imaging is presented to aid the reader's perspective in regard to this modality.

Advantages

1. The scanning procedure is painless. Special patient preparation is not required, and the need for sedation is exceedingly rare.
2. No significant biologic damage has been noted as a result of pulsed diagnostic ultrasound (Baker and Dalrymple). This means of imaging is therefore highly desirable, where applicable, for primary investigations, and when repetitive examinations are necessary (Slovis and Perlmutter).
3. Imaging is not dependent on organ function. The functionally impaired kidney can therefore be rapidly delineated (Shkolnik, 1977). Thus, for example, the diagnosis of severe hydronephrosis can be made literally within seconds. The relative benefit of such rapid information can be extremely meaningful to parents, who often deeply fear that the recently discovered flank mass in their child represents a neoplasm.
4. The examination is extremely flexible. Scanning can be accomplished in multiple planes and with the patient in virtually any position. Portable real-time scanning can be performed anywhere in the hospital, including the surgical suite.
5. Real-time scanning has facilitated imaging of the cardiovascular system and the visualization of other dynamic events such as bowel peristalsis and respiratory excursions. In addition, the urodynamics of bladder emptying, the ureteral jet (Kremer et al), and the more pronounced degrees of vesicoureteral reflux (Kessler and Altman) can be observed.

Capabilities

1. Kidney location and size (Brandt et al) can be determined. Three-dimensional measurement through a combination of transverse and longitudinal scanning provides a means for volumetric assessment of the kidneys (Moskowitz et al).
2. The renal sinus, medullary pyramids, and cortex can be distinguished, and the cortical thickness can be measured. Definition of the arcuate blood vessels provides a general demarcation of the corticomedullary junction. The renal arteries and veins can often be visualized via real-time scanning.
3. The presence and magnitude of dilatation of the collecting system can be determined.
4. The presence and consistency of space-occupying intrarenal masses can be documented.
5. The intrarenal echo pattern can be assessed. Variations from the normal pattern can aid in the recognition of parenchymal abnormalities, inflammatory conditions, and infiltrative disorders.

NORMAL KIDNEY

The renal cortex, including the islands of Bertin, is normally less echogenic than normal liver parenchyma. However, in infants up to 6 months of age, cortical echogenicity may be equal to that of the liver; in contrast, the medullary pyramids are hypoechoic, and it is important that they are not mistaken for dilated calyces or cysts (Haller et al). The arcuate blood vessels are seen as strongly echogenic foci (Cook et al). The renal sinus, composed of the pelvis, parapelvic fat, connective tissue, and blood vessels, is characteristically strongly echogenic; however, a paucity of parapelvic fat in the neonate and young infant can result in a less distinguishable renal sinus. In the neonate and young infant, the renal cortex is quite thin, whereas the medullary pyramids are relatively large in size (Figs. 9–1 and 9–2). Transient dilatation of the renal pelvis during the phase of rapid diuresis following oral intake of a large volume of fluid can simulate hydronephrosis; repeat scanning after a brief interval can serve to document this occurrence (Fig. 9–3). Also, a suggestion of mild pelvic dilatation may be seen in the normal extrarenal pelvis.

IMAGING OF THE FETAL URINARY TRACT

Altered fetal growth, as well as a wide variety of fetal abnormalities, can now be diagnosed by maternal sonography (Sabbagha and Shkolnik). The great majority of such abnormalities await treatment following term delivery. However, the intrauterine detection of a severe abnormality offers the options of termination of pregnancy, or preterm delivery in order to initiate treatment. More recently,

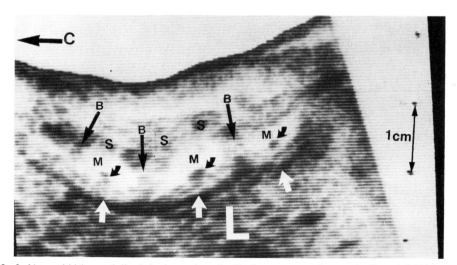

Figure 9–1. Normal kidney. Articulated-arm longitudinal sonogram demonstrating right kidney of prone neonate. Lowly echogenic cortex is seen between arcuate blood vessels (*curved arrows*) and anterior surface of kidney (*white arrows*). C, cephalad; B, island of Bertin; M, medullary pyramid; S, renal sinus. Note greater echogenicity of normal liver (L).

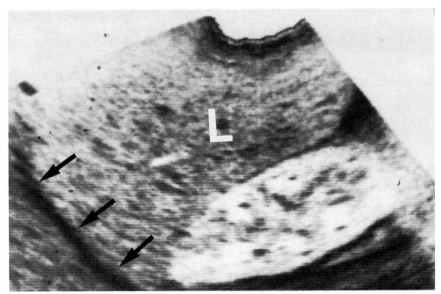

Figure 9–2. Intrarenal architecture of normal right kidney and liver (L) is shown on longitudinal sonogram of supine infant. The diaphragm is indicated (*arrows*).

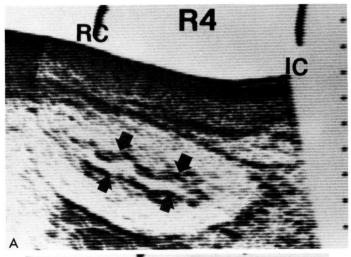

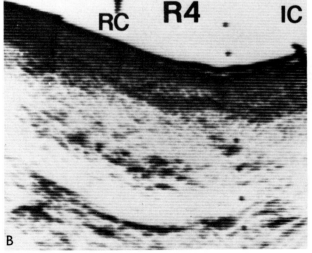

Figure 9–3. *A,* Prone longitudinal sonogram of 6-year-old boy, 4 cm to right of midline, taken 15 minutes after copious oral fluid intake. There is mild separation of the walls of the renal pelvis (*arrows*). RC, base of rib cage; IC, posterior-superior iliac crest. *B,* Repeat sonogram 15 minutes later shows no evidence of a dilated pelvis.

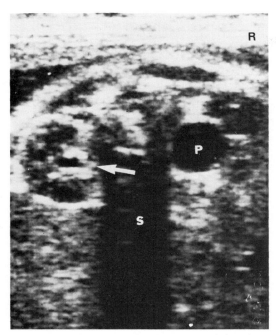

Figure 9–4. Transverse fetal sonogram taken from linear real-time scan displays white echoes on black background. Right renal pelvis (P) is markedly dilated. Note mild dilatation of left renal pelvis (*arrow*), considered within normal limits, and the acoustic shadow (S). (Courtesy of Dr. Carlos Reynes, Loyola University Medical Center, Maywood, Illinois.)

intrauterine interventional procedures for decompression of fetal hydrocephalus and for severe bilateral obstructive uropathy have been undertaken.

Normal Fetal Urinary Tract

The fetal kidneys can be identified initially by the 15th week of gestation. However, the definition of internal renal architecture is generally not feasible until after the 20th week

(Hadlock et al), following which one or both kidneys can be identified approximately 95 per cent of the time (Lawson et al). The parameters of fetal kidney size and volume have been correlated with gestational age (Jeanty et al). The fetal bladder is also identifiable early in the second trimester, and changes in volume, reflecting fetal urination, can be noted with both static and real-time scanning.

Abnormalities of the Urogenital Tract

Hydronephrosis can be identified. An example of ureteropelvic junction obstruction in a 35-week-old fetus is shown in Figure 9–4. The intrauterine detection of multicystic kidney (Friedberg et al) and infantile polycystic kidneys (Habif et al) has been reported, as well as dilatation of the urinary tract in relation to prune-belly syndrome (Shih et al). The presence of megacystis and megaureter, as well as hydrocele (Conrad and Rao) and ovarian cysts (Rumack et al), has also been detected.

Oligohydramnios is a consistent manifestation of severe bilateral renal compromise in the fetus. Bilateral renal agenesis is additionally characterized by absence of bladder filling. The reniform outline of the fetal adrenal glands may simulate the kidneys; therefore, the diagnosis of renal agenesis is best confirmed by establishing that the bladder is never visualized (Dubbins et al). Failure of recognizable fetal bladder distention within a 2-hour period following the intravenous administration of 60 mg of furosemide to the mother is considered a confirmatory test of bilateral renal agenesis (Wladimiroff).

Bladder distention and bilateral hydronephrosis is demonstrated in Figure 9–5 in a

Figure 9–5. Articulated-arm fetal sonogram demonstrating marked hydronephrosis of each kidney (K) and a distended urinary bladder (B). (Courtesy of Dr. Carlos Reynes, Loyola University Medical Center, Maywood, Illinois.)

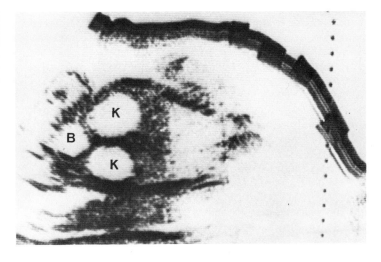

26-week-old fetus that proved to be a male with posterior urethral valves. Confirmation of this diagnosis has been achieved in utero by means of antegrade pyelography effected under ultrasonic guidance (Gore et al). Decompression of bilaterally obstructed kidneys in utero by means of ultrasonically guided bladder drainage, or nephrostomy, has been achieved in the presence of posterior urethral valves (Harrison et al), and in the presence of bilateral ureteropelvic junction stenosis (Vallancien et al). Blane et al have pointed out that preservation of renal function in a fetus with severe obstructive hydronephrosis may require very early intervention. Additional experience is obviously needed before definitive recommendations can be made regarding the efficacy and risk of these fetal procedures.

IMAGING OF THE NEONATE

Indications for evaluation of the neonatal kidneys range from abnormal urine findings, oliguria, or elevated blood urea nitrogen to a multitude of physical findings such as a single umbilical artery, malformed ears, abnormal external genitalia, exstrophy of the bladder, prune-belly syndrome, meningomyelocele, and other congenital abnormalities (Dunbar and Nogrady). The excretory urogram has traditionally been utilized for initial renal imaging. However, this imaging may prove suboptimal in the neonate. Limitations in the handling of intravenous contrast material are imposed by the relatively decreased glomerular filtration rate and concentrating power of the normal neonatal kidney. Thus, high dosages of contrast material, delayed imaging, and/or tomography may be required, particularly in the presence of impaired renal function. Consequently, ultrasonography is now widely utilized for initial delineation of the neonatal urinary tract. As underscored by Sumner et al, portable real-time scanning provides the means for examining fragile and severely compromised infants in the preferable environment of a temperature-controlled isolette (Fig. 9–6) and is a rapid and effective means of imaging which may obviate the need for more complex renal studies. The utility of either static or real-time imaging is perhaps best exemplified in the neonate presenting with a flank mass. In the great majority of instances, this is indicative of a renal abnormality. Distinguishing between intrarenal and extrarenal causes of a palpable mass is most often readily accomplished by ultra-

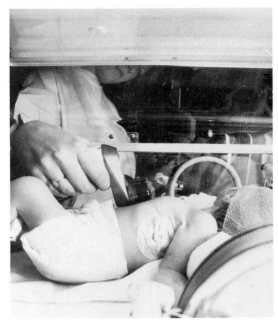

Figure 9–6. Real-time scanning in neonatal intensive care unit, performed through porthole of isolette.

sound. In either situation, the information provided by ultrasound will be extremely helpful in directing further investigation or treatment (Frank et al).

FLANK MASS IN THE NEONATE

Hydronephrosis

Nonobstructive pelvicalyceal dilatation can result in clinically apparent renal enlargement; however, obstructive uropathy is the most frequent etiology (Lebowitz and Griscom). The renal obstructions most commonly encountered are included below along with other abnormalities potentially responsible for an abdominal mass or masses in the neonate.

Ureteropelvic Junction (UPJ) Obstruction

The ultrasonic appearance of a severely obstructed renal pelvis is illustrated in Figure 9–7. A dilated ureter continuous with the distended renal pelvis characterizes ureterovesical junction obstruction, and can also be the result of vesicoureteral reflux. Ureteral dilatation distal to a UPJ obstruction can reflect the presence of coexistent vesicoureteral reflux (Lebowitz and Blickman) or a nonobstructed megaureter, as shown in Figure 9–8.

Multicystic Dysplastic Kidney

This represents the most common abdominal mass discovered during the first week of life. The characteristic appearance is that of a loculated cystic mass in which there is no identifiable renal pelvis (Bearman et al). As shown in Figure 9–9, the largest cyst is typically peripheral in location (Stuck et al).

Difficulty in differentiating a multicystic kidney from severe ureteropelvic junction obstruction can occur when the former is composed primarily of one large cyst. The reflection of renal function provided by radionuclide renal scanning can aid in this dis-

tinction (Harcke et al). As opposed to the hydronephrotic kidney, the multicystic dysplastic kidney is characteristically nonfunctional. Antegrade pyelography following percutaneous puncture of the fluid mass with ultrasonic guidance offers an alternate means of diagnostic confirmation.

Obstructed Duplex Kidney

The sonographic delineation of an upper-pole fluid mass (Fig. 9–10A), and an associated dilated ureter and ipsilateral intravesical fluid mass, indicative of a ureterocele (Fig. 9–10B), is diagnostic of this entity (Mascatello

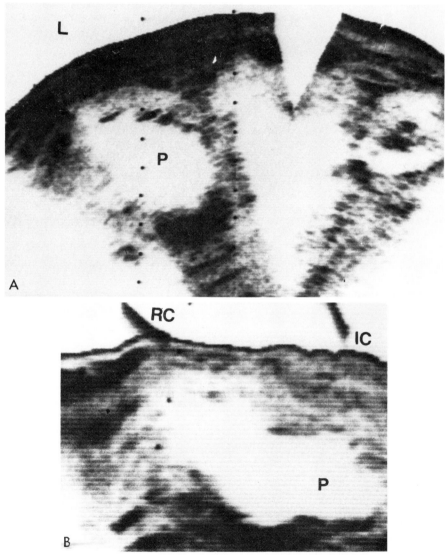

Figure 9–7. A, UPJ obstruction. Transverse prone sonogram demonstrates typical medial bowing of the dilated renal pelvis (P) of the left kidney. Right kidney appears normal. B, Longitudinally, dilated renal pelvis extends caudally. There was no evidence of ureteral dilatation. RC, base of rib cage; IC, posterior-superior iliac crest.

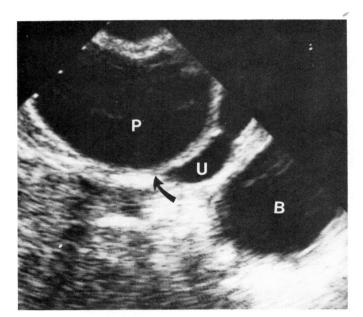

Figure 9–8. Coronal sonogram obtained from longitudinal real-time sector scan through the left mid-axillary line demonstrates point of UPJ obstruction (*arrow*), distal to which a dilated ureter (U) is seen. B, distended bladder; P, renal pelvis. Subsequent cystogram demonstrated no reflux; retrograde ureterogram confirmed a nonobstructed dilated ureter distal to the UPJ.

et al). A large ureterocele (Fig. 9–11) can also obstruct the ipsilateral lower renal duplication, as well as the contralateral kidney. The presence of upperpole hydroureteronephrosis without evidence of a ureterocele should suggest the possibility of extravesical termination of the obstructed ureter.

Posterior Urethral Valves

In this most common cause of bilateral hydroureteronephrosis in the male infant, the simultaneous delineation of both dilated ureters can be achieved by transverse scanning over the urine-distended bladder (Fig. 9–12). Confirmation of this abnormality is achieved by voiding cystourethrography. However, Gilsanz et al have described the associated sonographic findings of bladder wall thickening and a characteristic dilatation of the prostatic urethra (Fig. 9–13).

Renal Vein Thrombosis

This complication is prone to occur in the dehydrated or septic infant, and is also asso-

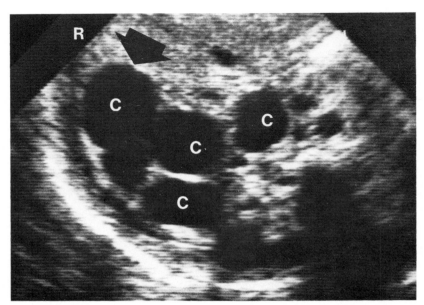

Figure 9–9. Multicystic dysplastic kidney seen on supine transverse sector sonogram of 6-day-old male. The largest of multiple cysts (C) is lateral (*arrow*).

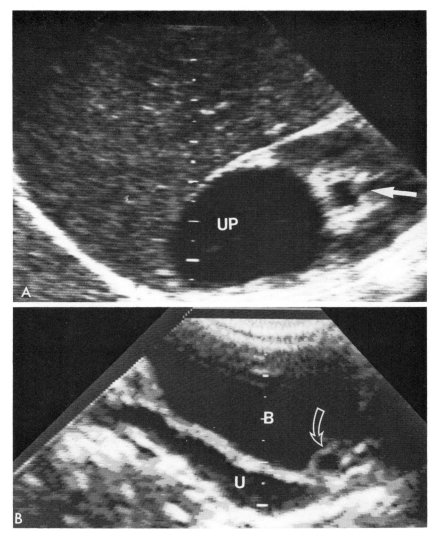

Figure 9 – 10. *A,* Etopic ureterocele. Longitudinal sector sonogram of supine infant girl reveals upper-pole fluid mass (UP) of right kidney. Mildly dilated pelvis of lower duplication is seen (*arrow*). *B,* Longitudinal supine sonogram displays distal dilated portion of the upper pole ureter (U). Small ureterocele (*arrow*) is seen within the urine-distended bladder (B).

Figure 9 – 11. Huge ureterocele (*arrow*) in left posterior bladder (B) seen on transverse sonogram, which resulted in hydrouretero-nephrosis of both elements of the duplicated left kidney, and of the right kidney.

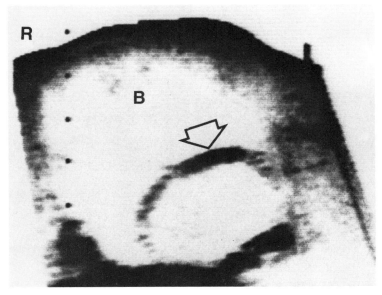

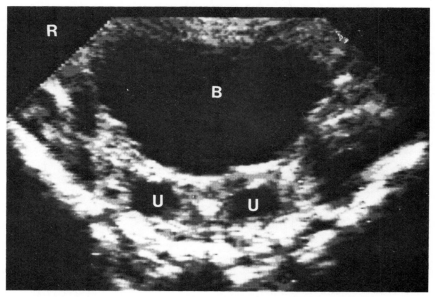

Figure 9–12. Posterior urethral valves. Dilated distal ureters (U) seen posterior to bladder (B) on transverse sector sonogram. Bilateral hydronephrosis was apparent on renal scans.

ciated with maternal diabetes. Ultrasonically, this disorder, which may be unilateral or bilateral, is typified by renal enlargement and a disordered internal echo pattern (Fig. 9–14). While the ultrasonic findings are not specific, this appearance in combination with hematuria, proteinuria, and a low platelet count indicating consumptive coagulopathy is virtually conclusive (Rosenberg et al).

Adrenal Hemorrhage

Unilateral or bilateral hemorrhage into the adrenal gland can occur as a result of a difficult delivery, fetal distress, asphyxia neona-

torum, or coagulation disorders. Clinical presentation includes a palpable mass, anemia, and jaundice that may be prolonged (Rose et al). As shown in Figure 9–14A, in the acute phase of hemorrhage, blood in the enlarged adrenal gland is essentially anechoic (Pery et al). The echogenicity that accompanies clot formation can render the adrenal mass indistinguishable from a neuroblastoma. However, unlike neuroblastoma, the hemorrhagic gland will subsequently decrease in size and echogenicity as a result of hemolysis of the blood clot (Coelho et al). Documentation of this sequential ultrasonic pattern (Fig. 9–15) may prevent unnecessary surgical exploration

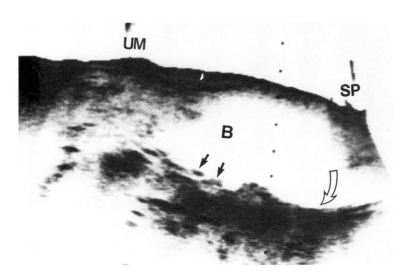

Figure 9–13. Longitudinal midline sonogram shows characteristic dilatation of prostatic urethra (curved arrow) in male infant with posterior urethral valves. Bladder (B) trabeculation is also noted (arrows). SP, symphysis pubis; UM, umbilicus.

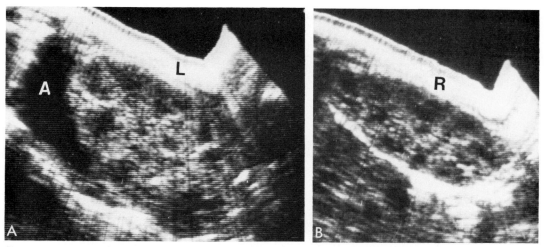

Figure 9–14. *A,* Renal vein thrombosis. Large left kidney is noted with disordered internal echo pattern in septic, dehydrated neonate. The presence of coexistent adrenal hemorrhage is indicated by suprarenal anechoic structure (A). *B,* Normal right kidney. (Courtesy of Dr. Carol Rumack, Health Sciences Center, University of Colorado, Denver, Colorado.)

Figure 9–15. *A,* Adrenal hemorrhage. Echogenic mass (*arrows*) is noted on longitudinal supine sonogram of 6-day-old jaundiced infant. The kidney (K) was displaced inferiorly, better seen on prone scans. *B,* Repeat scan 3 weeks later. The mass is now essentially anechoic and smaller (*arrows*), allowing return of kidney to more normal position. Suprarenal calcification was documented radiographically several weeks later.

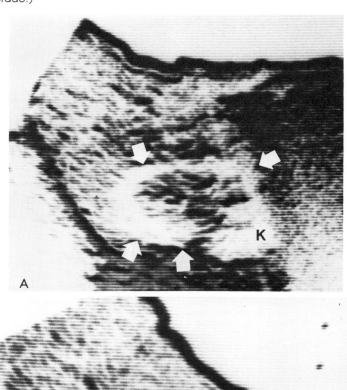

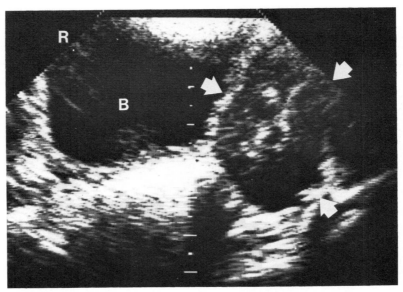

Figure 9 – 16. Transverse sector sonogram reveals a left pelvic kidney (*arrows*) adjacent to the bladder (B), accounting for the mass which was palpable in this 6-year-old girl.

(Mittelstaedt et al). Subsequent adrenal calcification can be recognized ultrasonically or radiographically.

OTHER DEVELOPMENTAL ABNORMALITIES

Renal Ectopia

Displacement of the kidney into the chest (Ramos et al) as well as pelvic ectopia can

be detected ultrasonically (Fig. 9 – 16). Fused crossed renal ectopia can be suspected when a unilateral elongated kidney is identified.

Horseshoe Kidney

The ultrasonic recognition of this anomaly requires delineation of the isthmus connecting the inferior pole of each kidney (Mindell and Kupic). The delineation may be facilitated when there is a morphologic abnormality of one or both kidneys (Fig. 9 – 17).

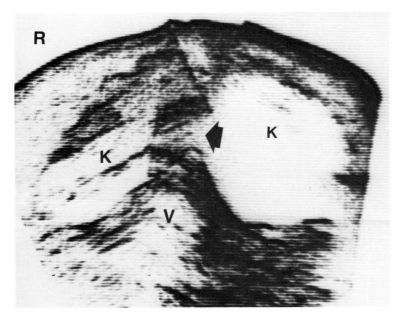

Figure 9 – 17. Supine transverse sonogram demonstrating isthmus (*arrow*) of horseshoe kidney. Note anterior position of both kidneys (K) relative to vertebra (V), and markedly hydronephrotic left kidney, the result of a UPJ obstruction.

RENAL NEOPLASMS

As stated by Markle and Potter, ultrasonic imaging is "one part of a multimodal evaluation to (1) confirm the organ of origin, and gross extent of the tumor, (2) identify large blood vessel involvement, (3) identify metastasis, and (4) define the status of the opposite kidney." The initial confirmation of a renal neoplasm is being more frequently achieved by ultrasonography, since there is a growing trend in the use of ultrasound for initial imaging of all pediatric patients presenting with an abdominal mass. Additionally, through the use of real-time scanning, immediate assessment for evidence of tumor extension to the vascular system can be achieved.

Mesoblastic Nephroma

This most common renal neoplasm of the neonate may be hyperechoic or hypoechoic (Fig. 9–18) or may produce a mixed echo pattern (Hartman et al). Benign congenital mesoblastic nephroma is thought to be part of a spectrum of mesenchymal renal neoplasms of infancy, including some that are malignant (Gonzalez-Crussi et al, 1981). These mass le-

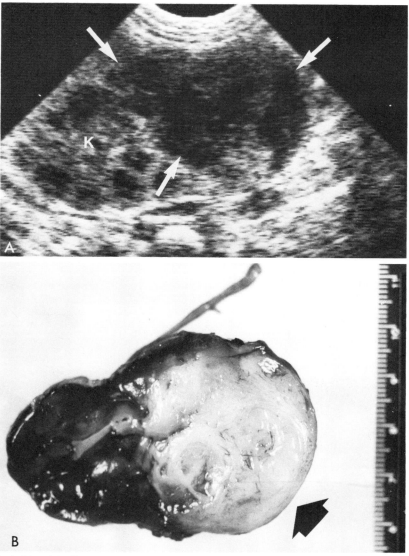

Figure 9–18. *A,* Mesoblastic nephroma. Supine longitudinal sector sonogram of 2-week-old boy reveals hypoechoic mass (*arrows*) in lower half of right kidney (K). *B,* Excised hemisected specimen showing tumor in lower pole (*arrow*). There was no histologic evidence of malignancy.

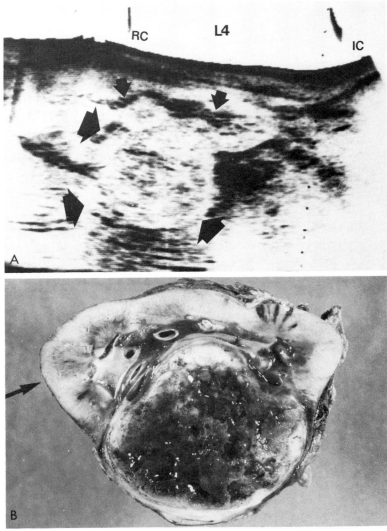

Figure 9–19. *A*, Wilms' tumor. Left longitudinal prone sonogram reveals echogenic mass (*large arrows*) extending from mid-anterior left kidney in 3-year-old girl. Note displacement of superior aspect of renal sinus echoes (*small arrows*). RC, base of rib cage. IC, posterior-superior iliac crest. *B*, Hemisected surgical specimen. Lower pole indicated (*arrow*).

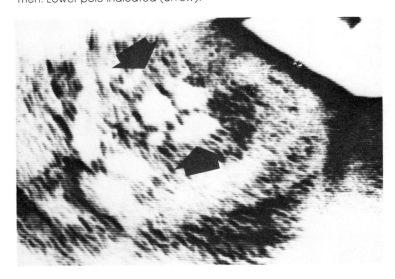

Figure 9–20. Wilms' tumor. Supine left longitudinal sonogram demonstrates multiple cystic compartments (*arrows*) within a large mass. No associated recognizable renal structure could be identified.

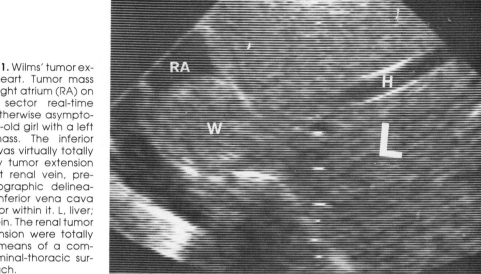

Figure 9–21. Wilms' tumor extension to heart. Tumor mass (W) seen in right atrium (RA) on longitudinal sector real-time scan in an otherwise asymptomatic 2-year-old girl with a left intrarenal mass. The inferior vena cava was virtually totally occluded by tumor extension from the left renal vein, precluding sonographic delineation of the inferior vena cava and the tumor within it. L, liver; H, hepatic vein. The renal tumor and its extension were totally excised by means of a combined abdominal-thoracic surgical approach.

sions are sonographically indistinguishable from Wilms' tumor. As with any suspect primary renal neoplasm, resection is indicated.

Wilms' Tumor

This represents the most common malignant abdominal tumor in children. One third of the cases are found in children under 1 year of age, and three fourths are found in children under 4 years of age (Markle and Potter). The tumor is usually large by the time of discovery, frequently presenting as a palpable mass. The renal origin of a predominantly exophytic Wilms' tumor may be difficult to establish (Jaffe et al). Teele has stressed the importance of carefully imaging the entire outline of the kidney (Fig. 9–19). When the tumor has largely replaced or displaced the kidney, specific ultrasonic documentation of its renal ori-

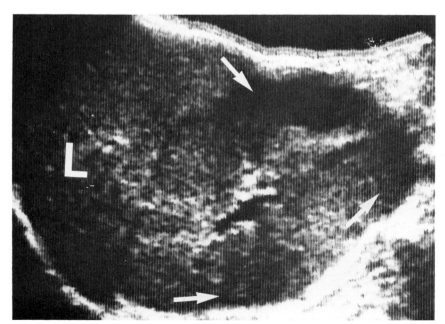

Figure 9–22. Nephroblastomatosis. Hypoechoic areas (*arrows*) seen longitudinally in enlarged lobulated right kidney. The size, shape, and echogenicity of the left kidney was similar in this 15-month-old girl. Multiple renal biopsies confirmed a superficial diffuse form of this abnormality. L, liver. (Courtesy of Dr. Lee H. Prewitt, Jr., Children's Health Center, Minneapolis, Minnesota.)

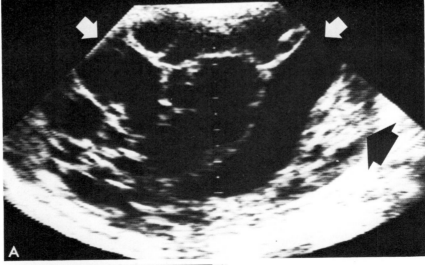

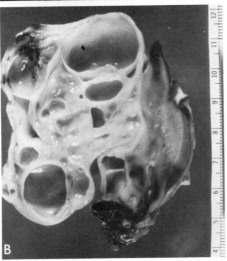

Figure 9–23. *A*, Cystic nephroma. Longitudinal supine sector sonogram of 8-month-old girl demonstrates a large right renal mass, predominantly composed of multiple fluid compartments (*light arrows*). A solid portion is noted inferiorly (*dark arrow*). *B*, Surgical specimen showing solid renal tissue.

gin may be virtually impossible. However, the depiction of multiple fluid compartments within the mass is highly suggestive of Wilms' tumor, since areas of cystic necrosis are a common feature of this neoplasm (Fig. 9–20). Conversely, neuroblastoma will most often appear entirely solid on the sonogram (Hartman and Sanders).

VASCULAR EXTENSION OF WILMS' TUMOR. Real-time scanning has greatly facilitated the detection of Wilms' tumor growth into the renal vein and inferior vena cava (Slovis et al, 1981) and into the heart (Shkolnik et al). Such tumor extension, even when reaching the right atrium, can be totally asymptomatic (Slovis et al, 1978). Therefore, whenever available, cardiovascular real-time imaging should be included in the work-up of patients in whom a renal tumor is apparent. Since the goal of surgery is total removal of the tumor, documentation of Wilms' tumor extensions can have significant bearing in determining the surgical approach (Fig. 9–21).

MONITORING THE PATIENT AT RISK. Ultrasonography is now widely accepted as the means for periodic renal monitoring of individuals who are at risk for the development of Wilms' tumor, such as patients with a previous Wilms' tumor, a family history of Wilms' tumor, or sporadic aniridia. Sonographic surveillance is similarly utilized for the detection of potential renal and extrarenal tumors in patients with the Beckwith-Wiedemann syndrome or syndromes associated with hemihypertrophy (Tolchin et al).

Nephroblastomatosis

This abnormality found in the kidneys of infants and children is characterized by the presence of persistent foci of immature renal blastema, which may be diffuse or multifocal. It can be found in up to one third of kidneys with Wilms' tumor, and also has an increased incidence in patients with the Beckwith-Wiedemann syndrome, syndromes associated with hemihypertrophy, or major chromosomal abnormalities (Franken et al). Nephroblastomatosis may result in renal enlargement and alteration in the renal parenchymal pattern (Fig. 9–22). The management and prognosis of nephroblastomatosis is uncertain. A decrease in renal size has been noted in some patients with nephromegaly who were treated with vincristine and actinomycin D. However, all patients with nephroblastomatosis, regardless of type, remain at risk for the development of Wilms' tumor (Franken et al).

Multilocular Cystic Nephroma

This uncommon renal neoplasm is characterized by well-circumscribed, noncommunicating, fluid-filled locules, which ultrasonically produce a whorled pattern (Madewell et al). An example of the ultrasonic and gross appearance of this tumor is demonstrated in Figure 9–23. Gonzalez-Crussi et al (1982) have noted a closer structural similarity of these lesions to nephroblastoma than to other known forms of cystic malformation, supporting the concept that nephrectomy is the treatment of choice.

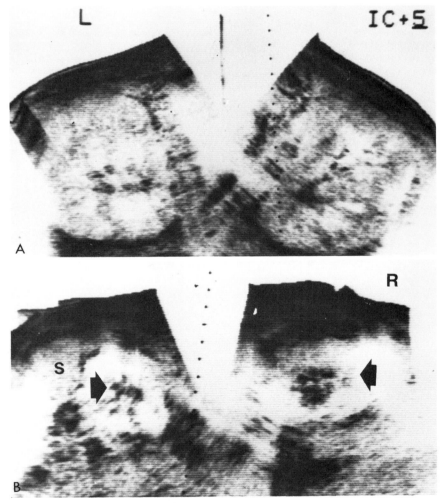

Figure 9–24. *A,* Renal leukemic infiltration. Transverse prone sonogram of 12-year-old boy with acute lymphoblastic leukemia reveals symmetrically enlarged kidneys with disordered internal echogenicity. *B,* Posttherapy sonogram reveals marked decrease in renal size, and normal appearance of renal sinus echoes bilaterally (*arrows*). S, spleen.

Leukemia and Lymphoma

Leukemic deposits or lymphomatous infiltration of the kidneys results in nephromegaly and distortion of the collecting systems. Lymphomatous infiltrate is typically hypoechoic in appearance. Leukemic infiltrate can be either hyperechoic or hypoechoic. Gore and Shkolnik noted that renal enlargement as an indicator of reactivated leukemia can precede bone marrow changes by up to 12 days. Ultrasonography provides the means for monitoring gross renal changes in response to therapy (Fig. 9 – 24).

CYSTIC ABNORMALITIES

Infantile Polycystic Kidney Disease

This abnormality has an autosomal recessive pattern of inheritance. Classically, infantile polycystic kidney disease presents with poorly functioning bilaterally enlarged kidneys. The "cysts" actually represent ectatic renal tubules, the walls of which produce intense echogenicity throughout the kidneys (Grossman et al). Owing to the marked echogenicity of the kidney, the renal sinus is often obscured. When mildly dilated, the pelvicalyceal systems can be identified (Fig. 9 – 25). Increased liver echogenicity in these patients signals the coexistence of hepatic fibrosis.

Tubular Ectasia and Hepatic Fibrosis

In the spectrum of cystic diseases affecting the kidneys and liver, the degree of renal tubular ectasia and renal symptomatology may be minimal. The clinical picture is dominated rather by the presence of hepatic fibrosis, and the subsequent development of portal hypertension and its complications. In such instances, the kidneys are enlarged but generally not to the degree of those in patients with infantile polycystic renal disease (Six et al). Dilated collecting tubules in the region of the renal pyramids can be seen on the excretory urogram, and ultrasonically they produce an intense echogenicity (Fig. 9 – 26).

Adult Polycystic Kidney Disease

This autosomal dominant abnormality can present in infants and children, but is much more frequently manifested in the adult, resulting in progressive diminution of renal function. Typically, well-defined cysts can be identified in the kidneys and liver (Fig. 9 – 27) and in the pancreas. Ultrasonography has been found more sensitive than excretory urography in documenting subclinical poly-

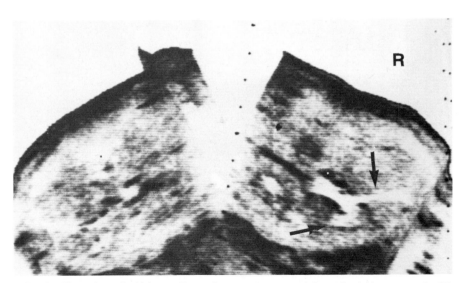

Figure 9 – 25. Infantile polycystic kidneys. Prone transverse scan of 4-week-old boy reveals diffuse accentuated echogenicity of markedly enlarged kidneys. Distortion of mildly ectatic collecting system of right kidney is seen (*arrows*).

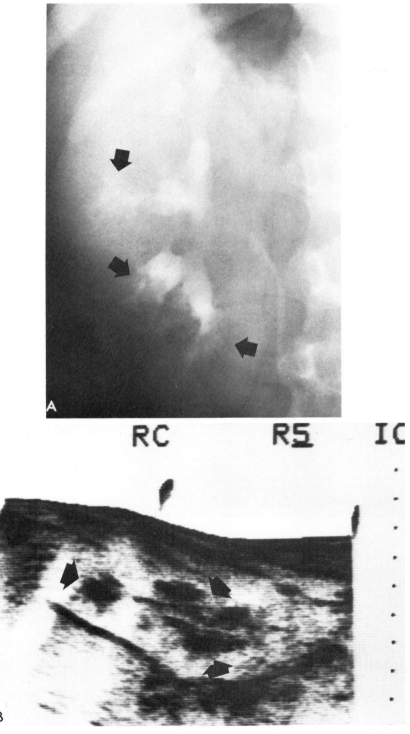

Figure 9–26. *A,* Tubular ectasia. Enlarged left kidney seen on excretory urogram revealed opacification of dilated tubules in region of medullary pyramids (*arrows*). Similar appearance was noted in smaller right kidney of this 4-year-old boy who presented with evidence of portal hypertension. Liver biopsy documented diagnosis of congenital hepatic fibrosis. *B,* Accentuated echogenicity as a result of dilated tubules in the medullary pyramids (*arrows*) as seen on prone longitudinal scan of right kidney. The left kidney displayed a similar appearance.

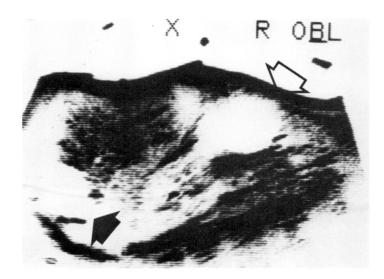

Figure 9–27. Adult polycystic renal disease. Oblique supine right-sided sonogram of 25-year-old woman reveals large cyst in lower pole of right kidney (*open arrow*) and cyst in right lobe of liver (*dark arrow*).

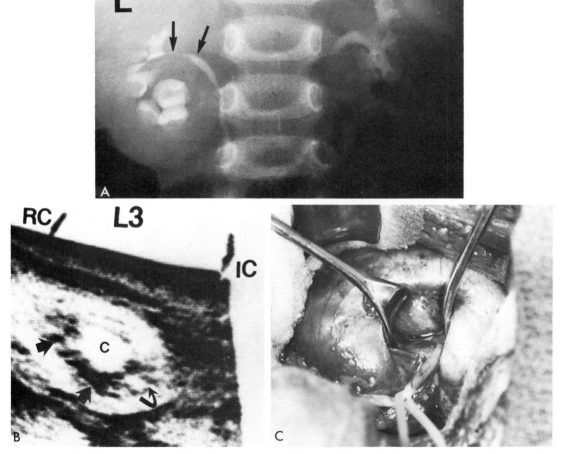

Figure 9–28. *A*, Parapelvic cyst. Excretory urogram of 3-year-old boy displayed in posteroanterior projection reveals pressure effect on left ureter (*arrows*). The renal pelvis is not seen. Mild ectasia of lower pole calyces is evident. *B*, Longitudinal prone sonogram of left kidney demonstrating anterior displacement of renal pelvic echoes (*solid arrows*) by adjacent cystic mass (C). Lower-pole calyectasis is demonstrated (*curved arrow*). RC, base of rib cage; IC, posterior-superior iliac crest. *C*, Intraoperative appearance of cyst. Excision undertaken because of clinical considerations.

cystic renal disease and has therefore been proposed for family screening studies (Lufkin et al).

Simple Cysts

These fluid masses are readily defined by ultrasound. In normotensive asymptomatic children, conservative management is sug-gested (Bartholomew et al) with or without cyst puncture (Kramer et al).

Parapelvic Cyst

This abnormality, rare in the pediatric age group, should not be mistaken for hydrone-phrosis (Cronan et al). As shown in Figure 9–28, a typical mass effect is noted on the

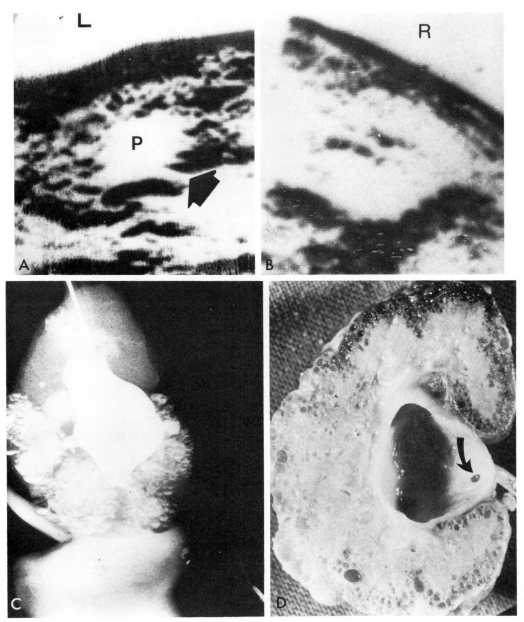

Figure 9–29. *A,* Transverse sonogram of prone 3-month-old girl in whom there was no evidence of left renal function documents presence of kidney with a dilated renal pelvis (P) and proximal ureter (*arrow*). The renal parenchymal echo pattern suggests multiple small cysts. *B,* Essentially normal-appearing right kidney. *C,* Contrast injection into excised left kidney reveals communication of obstructed pelvis with numerous ectatic collecting tubules. *D,* Cystic parenchyma and dilated pelvis seen in hemisected kidney. Orifice of ureter is seen (*arrow*); ureter was patent for 3 mm.

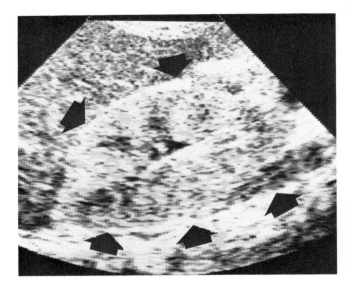

Figure 9–30. Congenital nephrotic syndrome. Large right kidney (*arrows*) of male neonate, as seen on longitudinal sonogram obtained in intensive care unit. Cortical echoes are stronger than those of adjacent liver. The left kidney was similar in size and echogenicity. A previous sibling with the identical abnormality is deceased.

excretory urogram, which ultrasonically is demonstrated as a cyst displacing the renal pelvis (Hidalgo et al).

Cystic Dysplasia

Varying degrees of cyst formation are known to occur as a result of severe obstructive uropathy (Fig. 9–29).

PARENCHYMAL ABNORMALITIES

Renal parenchymal disease occurring in the glomerulus or the interstitium results in recognizable, though nonspecific, changes in the internal echo pattern of the kidney. Cortical echogenicity becomes greater than that of normal liver parenchyma, with or without disruption of the normal recognizable corticomedullary junction (Fig. 9–30). The increased echogenicity has been attributed to the deposition of collagen, or to the acute phase of the parenchymal disease (LeQuesne). In comparing renal cortical echogenicity with the results of percutaneous renal biopsy in 25 patients with various forms of nephritis and nephrosis, Rosenfield and Siegel found no correlation between the nature and severity of glomerular disease and sonographic patterns. A correlation was noted, however, between the degree and severity of interstitial changes and the sonographic findings. Focal changes produced a minimal increase in cortical echogenicity, whereas the highest increases occurred in the presence of active interstitial infiltration. Hricak et al (1982a) noted a significant

positive correlation between cortical echogenicity and the severity of global sclerosis (Fig. 9–31), focal tubular atrophy, number of hyaline casts per glomerulus, and focal leukocyte infiltration. It is apparent that a clear distinction of different types of medical renal disease cannot be currently made on the basis of sonography alone. However, as stated by Hricak et al (1982a), "After the initial diagnosis has been made by biopsy, a good correlation between cortical echogenicity and the severity of histopathologic changes provides a promising noninvasive method of monitoring the progression of the renal disease."

NEPHROCALCINOSIS AND NEPHROLITHIASIS

Nephrocalcinosis with or without nephrolithiasis can occur as a result of renal tubular syndromes, enzyme disorders, hypercalcemic states, parenchymal renal disease, or vascular phenomena, and at times the cause may be unknown (Foley et al). Distal renal tubular acidosis and primary hyperoxaluria are the most common causes of nephrocalcinosis in the pediatric age group (Malek and Kelalis). Calcifications are intensely echogenic and are therefore very amenable to ultrasonic detection. The applications of ultrasonography in this regard can be categorized as follows:

1. Confirming a renal or extrarenal location of calculi identified radiographically. Macroscopic calculi produce classic acoustic shadowing (Figs. 9–32 and 9–33).
2. Screening patients who are predisposed to

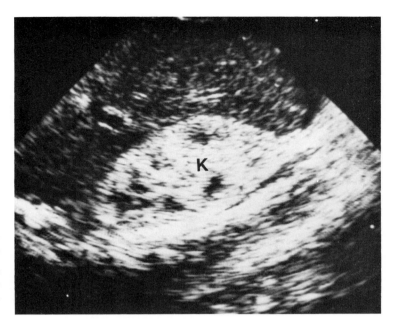

Figure 9–31. Biopsy-confirmed segmental sclerosis, resulting in intensely echogenic right kidney (K), as seen on longitudinal sonogram of 3-year-old boy with left-sided Wilms' tumor. (Courtesy of Dr. C. Keith Hayden, Jr., University of Texas Medical Branch, Galveston, Texas.)

nephrocalcinosis. Intensely echogenic foci without acoustic shadowing, corresponding to microscopic calcification, have been noted in an infant with hyperoxaluria (Brennan et al) and in infants with distal renal tubular acidosis (Fig. 9–34). These findings support the concept that acoustic shadowing requires macroscopic calcification (Glazer et al). Patients on long-term furosemide therapy are predisposed to the formation of renal calculi (Fig. 9–32) (Hufnagle et al).

3. Intraoperative localization of renal stones. Such definition can expedite the optimal surgical removal of renal calculi (Cook and Lytton). With the real-time scanning head encased in a sterile surgical glove or other appropriate container, scanning is preferably initiated prior to nephrotomy, with scanning performed directly on the surface

of the kidney, or through an intervening water bath. Ultrasonography has proved accurate in identifying stones 3 mm or greater in size (Marshall et al).

INFLAMMATORY DISEASE

Pyelonephritis

In the acute phase of pyelonephritis, ultrasonography can show swelling of the affected kidney, and diminished echogenicity of the parenchyma as a result of edema (Fig. 9–35). Reflux nephropathy is characterized by shrunken kidneys that demonstrate loss of renal parenchyma, retraction of one or more calyces, and increased echogenicity resulting from interstitial fibrosis (Kay et al). At times, mild dilatation of the pelvicalyceal system can be observed. A similar appearance may be

Figure 9–32. Supine left longitudinal sonogram confirms renal calculus (arrow) in collecting system of lower pole. Note characteristic anechoic acoustic shadow (S) deep to the calculus. This phenomenon is the result of the deficit of sound waves reaching the area deep to a strong reflector and absorber of sound such as a calcific mass. Sonography was performed in the neonatal intensive care unit on this infant with severe cardiopulmonary disease, whose treatment included administration of furosemide.

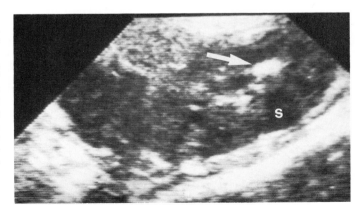

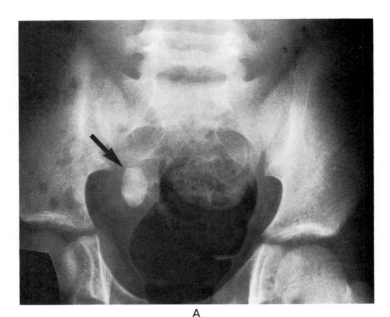

A

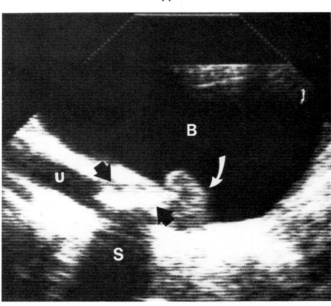

B

Figure 9–33. *A*, A large calculus (*arrow*) of unknown etiology, in right lower quadrant of 9-year-old male. Cystogram was unremarkable. Excretory urogram revealed delayed function of the hydronephrotic right kidney. *B*, Longitudinal sonogram confirms impaction of stone (*dark arrows*) at ureterovesical junction; the obstructed dilated distal ureter is noted. Marked right-sided hydronephrosis was also documented on renal scans. Inflammatory polyp (*curved arrow*), discovered during ultrasonic scanning, was also removed at surgery. B, bladder; U, ureter; S, acoustic shadow.

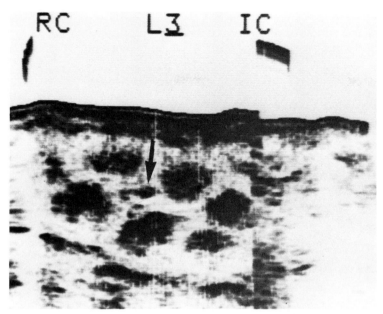

Figure 9–34. Medullary calcifications. Longitudinal prone sonogram of 6-week-old boy with clinical and laboratory evidence of distal renal tubular acidosis reveals densely echogenic pyramids of left kidney, virtually obscuring the renal pelvis (*arrow*). The right kidney demonstrated a similar appearance. Calcification was not apparent radiographically.

seen in virtually any chronic end-stage renal condition (Babcock).

Acute Focal Bacterial Nephritis (Acute Lobar Nephronia)

This abnormality is an acute localized renal infection resulting in a mass without liquefac-tion (Rosenfield et al, 1979). Retrograde infection with gram-negative bacteria secondary to vesicoureteral reflux is felt to play a major etiologic role (Siegel and Glasier). Lobar nephronia can simulate a mass lesion on the excretory urogram. Ultrasonically, a mass effect is noted, and unlike Wilms' tumor, it is most often less echogenic than the surround-

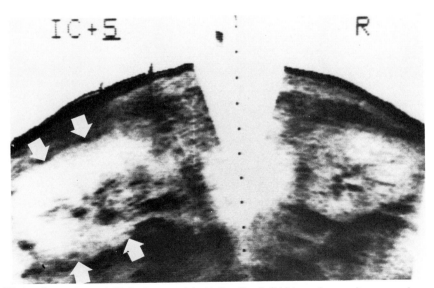

Figure 9–35. Acute pyelonephritis in 4-year-old girl. Swollen left kidney (*arrows*) seen on transverse prone sonogram. The edematous parenchyma is hypoechoic. Cortical-medullary distinction is obliterated.

ing renal tissue. A rapid change in this appearance typifies the response of this infectious process to antibiotic therapy (Fig. 9–36).

Renal Abscess

Ultrasonically, a renal abscess can present as a typical fluid mass with or without echo-

genic debris. An important aspect of ultrasonography is the ability to delineate an extrarenal extension of the process (Fig. 9–37).

Pyonephrosis

In the presence of an obstructed pelvicalyceal system, Coleman et al described persist-

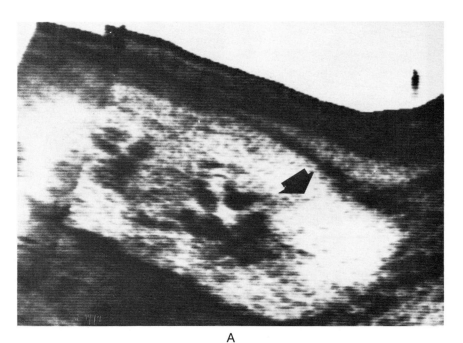

A

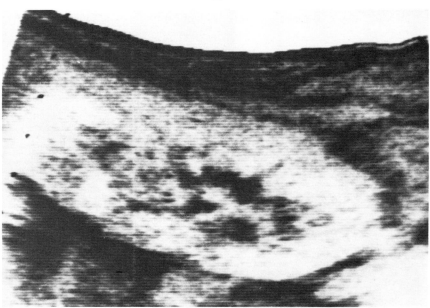

B

Figure 9–36. *A*, Lobar nephronia in 5-year-old girl. Hypoechoic area noted in lower pole of left kidney (*arrow*) on longitudinal prone sonogram. *B*, Sonogram after 7 days of antibiotic therapy reveals essentially normal appearance of lower pole.

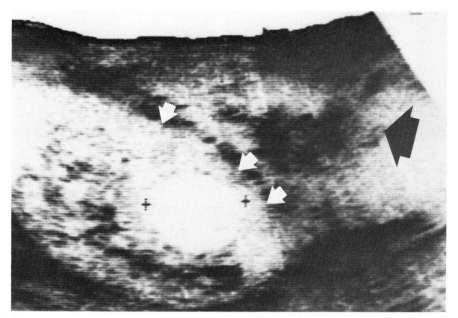

Figure 9–37. Renal abscess in lower pole of left kidney bracketed by electronic calipers (+), indicating a diameter of 3 cm. Extrarenal extension of the inflammatory processes is indicated by complex echogenic area (*dark arrow*) immediately adjacent to the posterior margin of the lower pole (*white arrows*), which is displaced anteriorly. The abscess and posterior extension were surgically confirmed and drained in this 2-year-old girl.

ent dependent echoes in the dilated pelvicalyceal system as one of the manifestations of pyonephrosis (Fig. 9–38). Additional findings noted in the presence of pyonephrosis included a fluid-debris level, echoes with acoustic shadowing as a consequence of gasforming pathogens, or low-level echoes completely filling the distended collecting system.

IMAGING FOLLOWING RENAL TRAUMA

The determination of renal function is paramount in the presence of suspected renal trauma. Thus, excretory urography, radionuclide imaging, or contrast-enhanced computed tomography should be the primary radiographic technique used. Ultrasonography

Figure 9–38. Pyonephrosis, surgically confirmed. Low-level echoes (*arrows*) in dependent portion of obstructed left renal pelvis of 6-year-old girl.

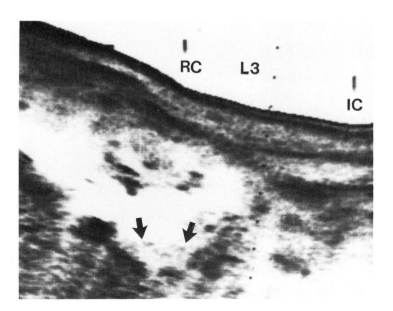

can often complement these studies, and is highly desirable when renal monitoring is indicated (Fig. 9 – 39).

POSTSURGICAL IMAGING

Following reconstructive renal surgery, ultrasonography can be quite useful in documenting changes in the degree of pelvicalyceal and/or ureteral dilatation. Fluid collections such as blood, lymph, or urine (Fig. 9 – 40) can be documented. Additionally, long-term postoperative sonographic follow-up can be used to document renal growth and rule out late obstruction.

Renal Transplant

Because of their superficial location in the lower abdomen and pelvis, renal transplants

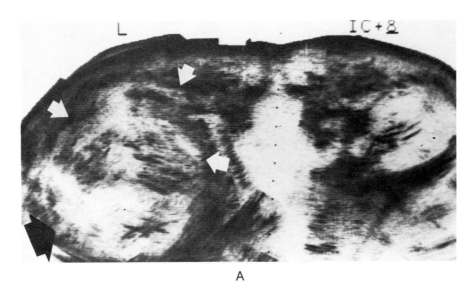

A

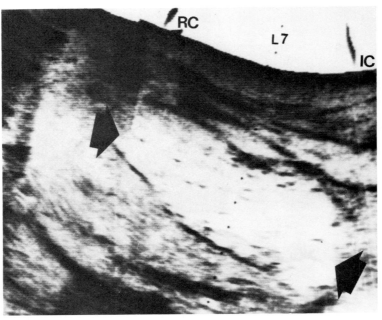

B

Figure 9 – 39. *A,* Subcapsular renal hematoma displaying heterogeneous echogenicity (*light arrows*), displacing left kidney (*dark arrow*) anteriorly, following left flank trauma to this 16-year-old boy. Renal function was not impaired. *B,* Hemolysis of clot, resulting in diminished echogenicity (*arrows*), is apparent on longitudinal sonogram performed 2 weeks later. The kidney remains displaced. Serial sonograms documented clot resorption and return of the left kidney to normal position.

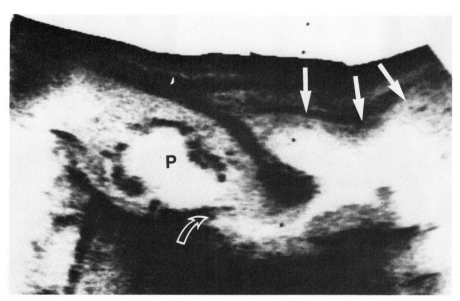

Figure 9–40. Post-pyeloplasty urinoma. Fluid mass (*solid arrows*) below left kidney, extending from the site (*open arrow*) of repair of the ureteropelvic junction obstruction in this 4-year-old boy. The lower pole of the kidney is displaced anteriorly by the fluid mass. P, renal pelvis.

are particularly well suited for ultrasonic imaging. Early and accurate diagnosis of renal transplant rejection is essential for the prompt initiation of appropriate therapy (Smith). Renal transplant rejection is manifested by an increase in renal size, accentuated cortical echogenicity, and increased prominence of the anechoic renal pyramids. Areas of infarction or necrosis may be reflected by large anechoic areas (Maklad et al). A decrease in the central sinus echogenicity has been noted

in relation to acute renal transplant rejection (Hricak et al, 1982b). While the role of ultrasonography in the detection of renal transplant rejection continues to evolve in relation to other imaging modalities and other diagnostic parameters (Firlit et al), its accuracy in detecting postoperative hydronephrosis (Fig. 9–41) and pararenal fluid collections (Fig. 9–42) is irrefutable. Such collections can mimic transplant rejection and may require surgical correction (Coyne et al).

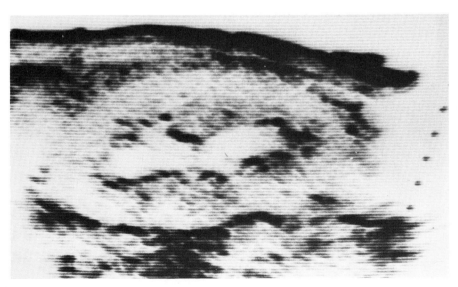

Figure 9–41. Moderately dilated pelvicalyceal system in renal transplant, seen on oblique supine sonogram of left lower quadrant in a 5-year-old patient.

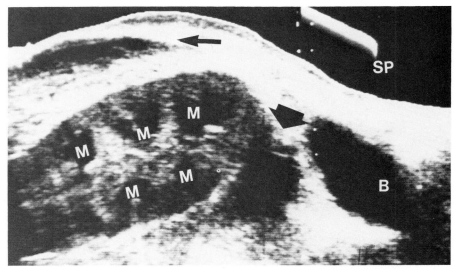

Figure 9–42. Longitudinal supine sonogram of 13-year-old girl reveals crescentic subcutaneous fluid collection immediately below site of surgical incision (*small arrow*). A larger rounded fluid collection (*large arrow*) is seen adjacent to lower pole of renal transplant. Findings suggesting renal rejection were supported by rather prominent medullary pyramids (M) and somewhat coarse cortical echogenicity of the transplant. The patient responded to conservative management. SP, symphysis pubis; B, bladder.

GUIDANCE FOR PERCUTANEOUS DIAGNOSTIC AND INTERVENTIONAL PROCEDURES

Accurate localization of the kidney and surrounding area can provide accurate guidance for percutaneous puncture procedures for both diagnosis and treatment. Accurate placement of probes or needles in association with articulated-arm scanning can be facilitated through the use of a slotted transducer (Fig. 9–43). Currently, needle guides are also available for use with real-time scanning transducers.

Ultrasonography is currently utilized for guiding diagnostic renal biopsy, including renal transplants (Spigos et al) and renal cyst

puncture. Needle penetration of the dilated renal pelvis for antegrade pyelography (Fig. 9–44), nephrostomy drainage (Babcock et al), and Whitaker tests can likewise be facilitated. Ultrasonic monitoring is likewise applicable for diagnostic aspiration and/or drainage of postrenal transplant accumulations (Silver et al) and more recently for inflammatory renal processes (Kuligowska et al).

THE BLADDER

The urine-distended bladder is ideally suited for ultrasonic imaging. Additionally, the distended bladder serves as an anatomic reference point and an optimal acoustic win-

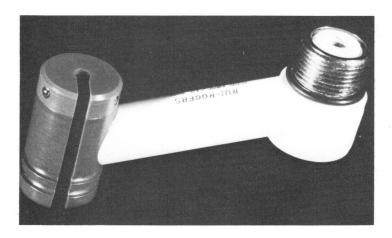

Figure 9–43. Slotted transducer for articulated-arm scanner, through which probe or needle can be passed after sonographic localization of desired plane. Following passage of instrument, transducer can be easily removed.

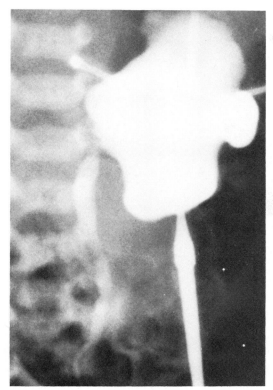

Figure 9–44. UPJ obstruction confirmed by antegrade pyelogram following sonographically guided puncture of renal pelvis.

dow through which sound can be transmitted to and from surrounding pelvic structures. Bladder displacement by an extrinsic mass is readily confirmed. The flow of fluid into an-

other fluid, as typified by the ureteral jet phenomenon and by vesicoureteral reflux, can be observed during real-time scanning.

The presence of a urachal cyst (Fig. 9–45) can be ultrasonically detected (Sanders et al). Bladder volume (McLean and Edell) as well as residual urine volume (Pedersen, Bartrum, et al) can be determined. Bladder wall thickening can be seen (Fig. 9–46) and diverticular outpouchings delineated (Fig. 9–47). Mass lesions arising from the posterior urethral or bladder wall and protruding into the bladder-filled lumen (Fig. 9–48) can be identified (Bree and Silver). Figure 9–49 demonstrates a fortuitous but valuable observation made during real-time scanning which was prompted by initial difficulty in catheterizing an infant in the intensive care unit.

GENITAL IMAGING

Uterus, Ovaries, and Vagina

Ultrasonography is being increasingly utilized for primary imaging of the young female presenting with lower abdominal pain, and is warranted when there is clinical suspicion or overt evidence of a pelvic mass. Pregnancy can be determined, and ovarian cysts (Fig. 9–50) as well as other adnexal masses are identifiable. Other indications for ultrasonic imaging of the female pelvis include primary and secondary amenorrhea, gonadal dysgenesis, precocious puberty, suspicion of pelvic

Figure 9–45. A superficial lower abdominal midline fluid mass (*large arrows*), delineated on longitudinal sonogram of 6-month-old girl with fluid drainage from the umbilicus (UM). Connection with bladder (B) was suggested (*small arrow*). A urachal cyst was surgically excised. SP, symphysis pubis.

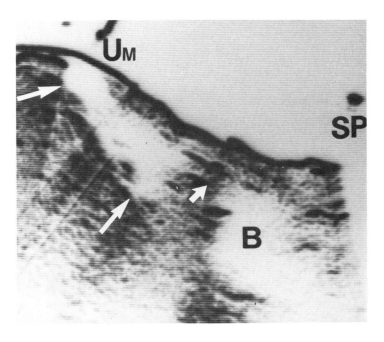

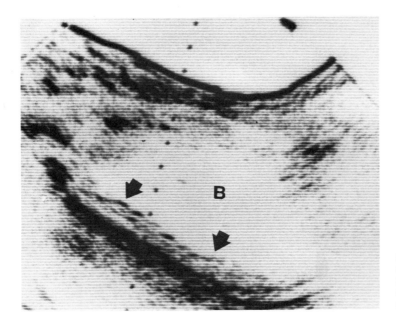

Figure 9–46. Thickened bladder (B) wall (*arrows*) seen on longitudinal midline scan of 8-year-old boy with cystitis. Edema of bladder wall was confirmed cystoscopically.

Figure 9–47. A bladder diverticulum (*arrow*) at left posterior aspect of bladder (B), as seen on transverse sector sonogram.

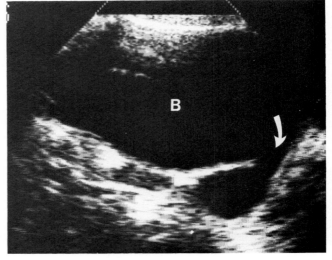

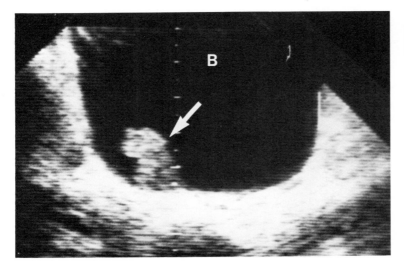

Figure 9–48. Myxomatous polyp later excised from right posterior bladder (B) wall of male infant.

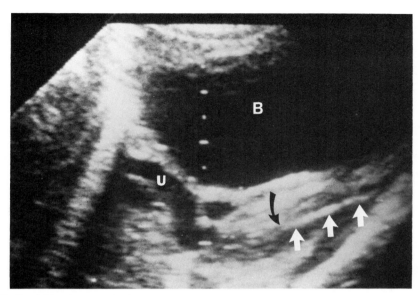

Figure 9–49. Real-time longitudinal scanning during catheterization of a male newborn with suspected posterior urethral valves demonstrated inadvertent passage of catheter (*white arrows*) into the dilated distal right ureter. Proximal tip of catheter is indicated (*dark arrow*) and dilated segment of proximal ureter (U) is seen. The catheter was subsequently repositioned appropriately in the distended bladder (B).

inflammatory disease, and abnormal vaginal discharge (Haller and Fellows). Masses originating in the vagina can be visualized, conceivably including dense foreign material.

Prostate Gland

Approximately 15 per cent of rhabdomyosarcomas in childhood originate in the bladder or prostate (Ravitch et al). Ultrasound can be used to assess the extent and consistency of the resultant mass (Fig. 9–51). Ultrasonography has been increasingly useful in the evaluation of the prostate gland in the adult.

Ambiguous Genitalia

Canty et al state: "The newborn with ambiguous genitalia must be regarded as a relative surgical emergency. . . . Parents should not be requested to take a newborn with ambiguous genitalia home before proper gender

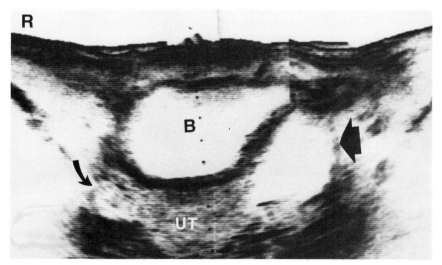

Figure 9–50. Large left ovarian cyst (*large arrow*) in 14-year-old girl with left lower quadrant pain. Uterus (UT), bladder (B), and normal right ovary (*curved arrow*) shown.

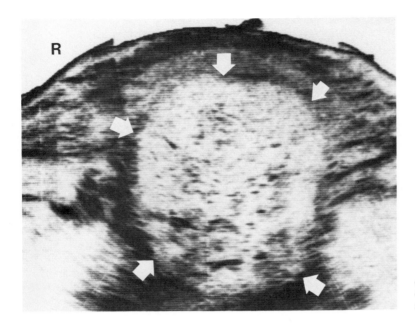

Figure 9–51. Prostatic rhabdomyosarcoma (*arrows*) as outlined on transverse pelvic sonogram of 4-year-old boy.

has been assigned and a carefully explained description given of specific plans for surgical reconstruction and endocrinological management." Ultrasonography provides a valuable addition to the multifaceted evaluation required in such infants (Shkolnik, 1980). The ovaries are generally not ultrasonically definable in the young infant, but the uterus can be consistently identified in the neonatal period. Such delineation in a newborn with abnormal external genitalia underscores the likelihood of a virilized female (Fig. 9–52) and further alerts the clinician to the risk of salt-losing adrenal hyperplasia (Lippe and Sample). Müllerian duct remnants may otherwise escape detection unless they become symptomatic (Fig. 9–53).

Scrotum

The diagnosis of scrotal disease is highly dependent on clinical history and physical examination. Palpation can be severely compromised in the presence of marked tenderness of the scrotum or scrotal contents. Ultrasonography provides an innocuous means of assessing the scrotal contents without much discomfort to the patient. Static ultrasonic examination of the testis was first described by Miskin and Bain in 1974. The development of real-time scanning as well as enhanced imaging provided by the development of high-frequency transducers has prompted an upsurge in the ultrasonic imaging of the scrotum and scrotal contents.

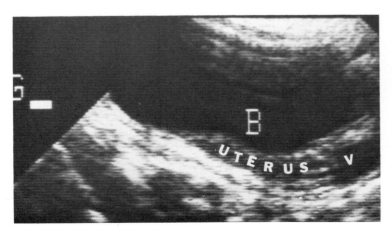

Figure 9–52. Virilizing adrenal hyperplasia. Infantile uterus is identified on longitudinal sonogram of neonate with ambiguous genitalia. Fluid-distended vagina (V) was the result of labial fusion. B, bladder.

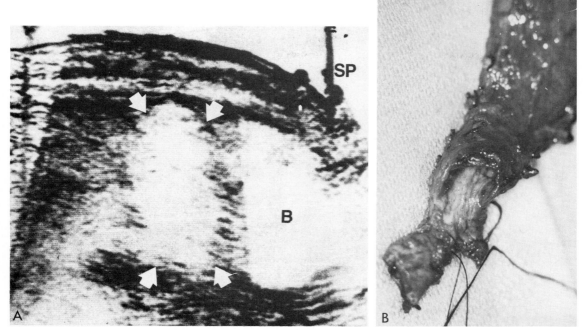

Figure 9–53. *A*, Supravesical fluid mass (*arrows*) identified on midline sonogram of 19-year-old male with dysuria. There was previous history of undescended testes, and multiple surgical repairs for severe hypospadias. SP, symphysis pubis; B, bladder. *B*, Müllerian duct remnant (''uterus masculinis'') which, at surgery, was fluid-filled. No adnexal structures were present.

Hydrocele

Hydrocele is common in the newborn and will resolve spontaneously in most instances as the processus vaginalis, connecting the peritoneum and scrotum, closes off. The diagnosis can be readily made by transillumination of the scrotum. In questionable cases, ultrasonography can provide verification of this condition. Additionally, testes that cannot be palpated well because of a massive hydrocele can be evaluated (Fig. 9–54).

Figure 9–54. Normal right testis (T) and epididymis (E) surrounded by large hydrocele (H) on sector sonogram obtained during real-time scanning of the scrotum in a 2-month-old boy.

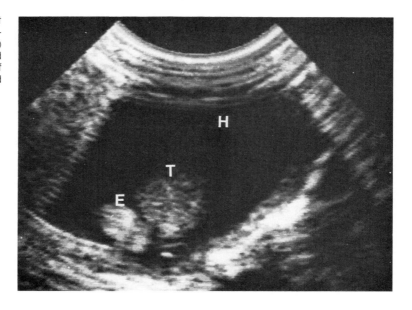

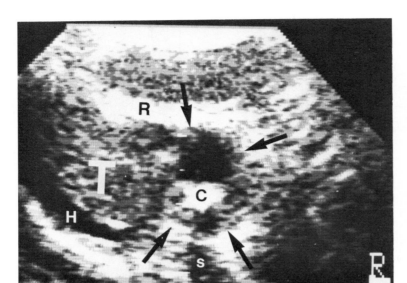

Figure 9–55. Palpable mass (*arrows*) at inferior aspect of right testicle, in 9-year-old boy with previous episode of local pain. Strongly echogenic structure (C) with acoustic shadowing (S) is identified in lower portion of otherwise predominantly fluid mass. Note reactive hydrocele (H) around the right testis (T). R, median raphe of scrotum. At surgery, the mass was found to be the result of torsion of a distal portion of the epididymis, resulting in a cystic mass which contained a calcification in area of earlier tissue necrosis.

Extratesticular Mass

The accuracy of static and real-time sonography in distinguishing between testicular and extratesticular masses has been stressed by numerous investigators (Sample et al; Richie et al; Carroll and Gross). An example of this application is presented in Figure 9–55.

Neoplasm

Testicular tumors may be hyperechoic or hypoechoic, or, as displayed in Figure 9–56, they may produce a combination of both patterns. In the leukemic patient in bone marrow remission, the ultrasonic definition of a focal or diffuse hypoechoic region in an enlarged

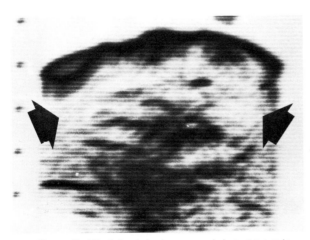

Figure 9–56. Articulated-arm scrotal sonogram in a 3-month-old infant defines irregular and accentuated echogenicity in an enlarged left testis (*arrows*) that proved to be a teratoma.

testicle has been documented as the first site of extramedullary relapse (Lupetin et al).

Torsion of the Spermatic Cord

This abnormality is usually accompanied by a history of sudden onset of scrotal pain. In the newborn, findings may be confined to swelling and redness of the scrotum (Hricak and Filly). Radionuclide imaging with technetium 99m pertechnetate is widely utilized as a primary diagnostic tool, and Doppler ultrasound may also be useful for determining the lack of blood flow to the affected testis (Pedersen, Holm, et al). Prompt surgery is of paramount importance if testicular necrosis is to be avoided. Ultrasonic changes following torsion occur rapidly and are characterized by an enlarged and hypoechoic testis. Torsion can be excluded when the ultrasonic appearance of the symptomatic testicle is normal in a patient whose symptoms have exceeded 6 hours in duration (Bird et al).

Inflammation

Orchitis in young boys is usually the result of trauma. It can also occur in later years as a complication of mumps, epididymitis, or systemic disorders. The involved testicle appears enlarged and hypoechoic. The inflamed epididymis also appears enlarged and either hypoechoic or hyperechoic (Fig. 9–57).

Cryptorchidism

In the great majority of instances, the undescended testis is located in the inguinal

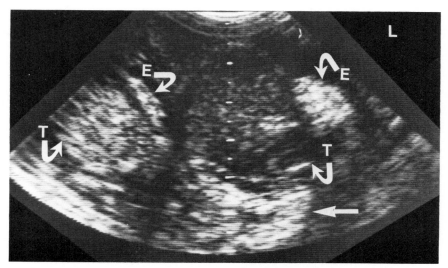

Figure 9-57. Orchitis and epididymitis in 13-year-old boy with parotitis and left-sided testicular and scrotal pain. Enlarged hypoechoic left testis (T) and prominent hyperechoic epididymis (E) seen during sector real-time scanning. Accentuated echogenicity (*straight arrow*) was the result of scrotal inflammation and enhanced sonic transmission through the edematous left testis.

canal, and may be palpable or identifiable sonographically (Madrazo). Some success, thus far limited, has been reported in the detection of intra-abdominal testes located on the surface of the iliac vessels (Wolverson et al).

Other Applications

The fluid nature of spermatoceles and varicoceles renders these abnormalities amenable to ultrasonic identification (Goodman and Haller). The diagnosis of scrotal hernia is most often achieved by clinical examination. Ultrasonographically, this abnormality is supported by identification of loops of bowel within the scrotum, continuous with a hernia sac in the inguinal region (Subramanyam et al).

Acknowledgment

I want to pay tribute to our outstanding ultrasound technologists, Suzanne Devine, R.T., R.D.M.S., and Maria Manolovic, R.T., R.D.M.S. I want to thank the many physicians at The Children's Memorial Hospital who have allowed us to help in the diagnostic evaluation and subsequent management of their patients, and Drs. Keith Hayden, Lee Prewitt, Carol Rumack, and Carlos Reynes for providing case material. I also want to express my gratitude to Diane Aljets and Debbie Krusen for their invaluable aid in the preparation of this manuscript.

BIBLIOGRAPHY

Babcock DS: Medical diseases of the urinary tract and adrenal glands. *In* Ultrasound in Pediatrics. Edited by JO Haller, A Shkolnik. New York, Churchill Livingstone, 1981, pp 113-134.

Babcock JR Jr, Shkolnik A, Cook WA: Ultrasound-guided percutaneous nephrostomy in the pediatric patient. J Urol 121:327, 1979.

Baker ML, Dalrymple GV: Biological effects of diagnostic ultrasound: a review. Radiology 126:479, 1978.

Bartholomew TH, Slovis TL, Kroovand RL, et al: The sonographic evaluation and management of simple renal cysts in children. J Urol 123:732, 1980.

Bartrum RJ Jr, Crow HC: Real-Time Ultrasound: A Manual for Physicians and Technical Personnel. Second ed. Philadelphia, WB Saunders Co., 1983.

Bearman SB, Hine PL, Sanders RC: Multicystic kidney: a sonographic pattern. Radiology 118:685, 1976.

Bird K, Rosenfield AT, Taylor KJW: Ultrasonography in testicular torsion. Radiology 147:527, 1983.

Blane CE, Koff SA, Bowerman RA, et al: Nonobstructive fetal hydronephrosis: sonographic recognition and therapeutic implications. Radiology 147:95, 1983.

Brandt TD, Neiman HL, Dragowski MJ, et al: Ultrasound assessment of normal renal dimensions. J Ultrasound Med 1:49, 1982.

Bree RL, Silver TM: Sonography of bladder and perivesical abnormalities. AJR 136:1101, 1981.

Brennan JN, Diwan RV, Makker SP, et al: Ultrasonic diagnosis of primary hyperoxaluria in infancy. Radiology 145:147, 148, 1982.

Canty TG, Leopold GR, Wolf DA: The female genital tract. *In* Ultrasonography of Pediatric Surgical Disorders. New York, Grune & Stratton, 1982, pp 1992-2009.

Carroll BA, Gross DM: High-frequency scrotal sonography. AJR 140:511, 1983.

Coelho JCU, Sigel B, Ryva JC, et al: B-mode sonography of blood clots. J Clin Ultrasound 10:323, 1982.

Coleman BG, Arger PH, Mulhern CB Jr: Pyelonephrosis: sonography in the diagnosis and management. AJR 137:939, 1981.

Conrad AR, Rao SAA: Ultrasound diagnosis of fetal hydrocele. Radiology 127:232, 1978.

Cook JH, Lytton B: Intraoperative ultrasound. In Diagnostic Imaging in Renal Disease. Edited by AT Rosenfield, MG Glickman, J Hodson. New York, Appleton-Century-Crofts, 1979, pp 249–255.

Cook JH, Rosenfield AT, Taylor KJW: Ultrasonic demonstration of intrarenal anatomy. AJR 129:831, 1977.

Coyne SS, Walsh JW, Tisnado J, et al: Surgically correctable renal transplant complications: an integrated clinical and radiologic approach. AJR 136:1113, 1981.

Cronan JJ, Amis ES, Yoder IC, et al: Peripelvic cysts: an imposter of sonographic hydronephrosis. J Ultrasound Med 1:229, 1982.

Dubbins PA, Kurtz AF, Wapner RJ, et al: Renal agenesis: spectrum of in utero findings. J Clin Ultrasound 9:189, 1981.

Dunbar JS, Nogrady B: Excretory urography in the first year of life. Radiol Clin North Am 10:367, 1972.

Firlit CF, Greenslade T, Bashoor R: The prognostic value of B₂ microglobulin in pediatric renal transplantation. Proc Dialysis Transplant Forum, 1978, pp 219–224.

Foley LC, Luisiri A, Graviss ER, et al: Nephrocalcinosis: sonographic detection in Cushing syndrome. AJR 139:610, 1982.

Frank JL, Potter BM, Shkolnik A: Neonatal urosonography. In Genitourinary Ultrasonography. Edited by AT Rosenfield. New York, Churchill Livingstone, 1979, pp 159–174.

Franken EA Jr, Yiu-Chiu V, Smith WL, et al: Nephroblastomatosis: clinicopathologic significance and imaging characteristics. AJR 138:950, 1982.

Friedberg JE, Mitnick JS, Davis DA: Antepartum ultrasonic detection of multicystic kidney. Radiology 131:198, 1979.

Gilsanz V, Miller JH, Reid BS: Ultrasonic characteristics of posterior urethral valves. Radiology 145:143, 1982.

Glazer GM, Callen PW, Filly RA: Medullary nephrocalcinosis: sonographic evaluation. AJR 138:55, 1982.

Gonzalez-Crussi F, Kidd JM, Hernandez RJ: Cystic nephroma: morphologic spectrum and implications. Urology 20:88, 1982.

Gonzalez-Crussi F, Sotelo-Avila C, Kidd JM: Mesenchymal renal tumors in infancy: a reappraisal. Human Pathology 12:78, 1981.

Goodman JD, Haller JO: The scrotum. In Ultrasound in Pediatrics. Edited by JO Haller, A Shkolnik. New York, Churchill Livingstone, 1981, pp 264–275.

Gore RM, Callen PW, Filly RA, et al: Prenatal percutaneous antegrade pyelography in posterior urethral valves: sonographic guidance. AJR 139:994, 1982.

Gore RM, Shkolnik A: Abdominal manifestations of pediatric leukemias: sonographic assessment. Radiology 143:207, 1982.

Grossman H, Rosenberg ER, Bowie JD, et al: Sonographic diagnosis of renal cystic diseases. AJR 140:81, 1983.

Habif DV Jr, Berdon WE, Yeh MN: Infantile polycystic kidney disease: in utero sonographic diagnosis. Radiology 142:475, 1982.

Hadlock FP, Deter RL, Carpenter R, et al: Sonography of fetal urinary tract anomalies. AJR 137:261, 1981.

Haller JO, Berdon WE, Friedman AP: Increased renal cortical echogenicity: a normal finding in neonates and infants. Radiology 142:173, 1982.

Haller JO, Fellows RA: The pelvis. In Ultrasound in Pediatrics. Edited by JO Haller, A Shkolnik. New York, Churchill Livingstone, 1981, pp 165–185.

Harcke HT, Williams JL, Popky GL, et al: Abdominal masses in the neonate: a multiple modality approach to diagnosis. RadioGraphics 2:69, 1982.

Harrison MR, Golbus MS, Filly RA, et al: Fetal surgery for congenital hydronephrosis. N Engl J Med 136:591, 1982.

Hartman DS, Lesar MSL, Madewell JE, et al: Mesoblastic nephroma: radiologic-pathologic correlation of 20 cases. AJR 136:69, 1981.

Hartman DS, Sanders RC: Wilms' tumor versus neuroblastoma: usefulness of ultrasound in differentiation. J Ultrasound Med 1:117, 1982.

Hidalgo H, Dunnick NR, Rosenberg ER, et al: Parapelvic cysts: appearance on CT and sonography. AJR 138:667, 1982.

Hricak H, Cruz, C, Romanski R, et al: Renal parenchymal disease: Sonographic histologic correlation. Radiology 144:141, 1982a.

Hricak H, Filly RA: Sonography of the scrotum. Invest Radiol 18:112, 1983.

Hricak H, Romanski RN, Eyler WR: The renal sinus during allograft rejection: sonographic and histopathologic findings. Radiology 142:693, 1982b.

Hufnagle KG, Khan SN, Penn D, et al: Renal calcifications: a complication of long-term furosemide therapy in preterm infants. Pediatrics 70:360, 1982.

Jaffe MH, White SJ, Silver TM, et al: Wilms' tumor: ultrasonic features, pathologic correlation, and diagnostic pitfalls. Radiology 140:147, 1981.

Jeanty P, Dramaix-Wilmet M, Elkhazen N, et al: Measurement of fetal kidney growth on ultrasound. Radiology 144:159, 1982.

Kay CJ, Rosenfield AT, Taylor KJW, et al: Ultrasonic characteristics of chronic atrophic pyelonephritis. AJR 132:47, 1979.

Kessler RM, Altman DH: Real-time sonographic detection of vesicoureteral reflux in children. AJR 138:1033, 1982.

Kramer SA, Hoffman AD, Aydin G, et al: Simple renal cysts in children. J Urol 128:1259, 1982.

Kremer RJ, Dobrinski W, Mikyska M, et al: Ultrasonic in vivo and in vitro studies on the nature of the ureteral jet phenomenon. Radiology 142:175, 1982.

Kremkau FW: Diagnostic Ultrasound. Physical Principles and Exercises. New York, Grune & Stratton, 1980.

Kuligowska E, Newman B, White SJ, et al: Interventional ultrasound in detection and treatment of renal inflammatory disease. Radiology 147:521, 1983.

Lawson TL, Foley WD, Berland LL, et al: Ultrasonic evaluation of fetal kidneys: analysis of normal size and frequency of visualization as related to stage of pregnancy. Radiology 138:153, 1981.

Lebowitz RL, Blickman JG: The coexistence of ureteropelvic junction obstruction and reflux. AJR 140:231, 1983.

Lebowitz RL, Griscom NT: Neonatal hydronephrosis: 146 cases. Radiol Clin North Am 15:49, 1977.

LeQuesne GW: Assessment of glomerulonephritis in children by ultrasound. In Ultrasound in Medicine. Vol. 4. Edited by D White, EA Lyons. New York, Plenum Press, 1978, pp 205–207.

Lippe BM, Sample WF: Pelvic ultrasonography in pediatric and adolescent endocrine disorders. J Pediatr 92:897, 1978.

Lufkin EG, Alfrey AC, Trucksess ME, et al: Polycystic kidney disease: earlier diagnosis and using ultrasound. Urology 4:5, 1974.

Lupetin AR, King W, Rich P, et al: Ultrasound diagnosis of testicular leukemia. Radiology 146:171, 1983.

Madewell JE, Goldman SM, Davis CJ, et al: Multilocular

cystic nephroma: a radiographic-pathologic correlation of 58 patients. Radiology 146:309, 1983.

Madrazo BL, Klugo RC, Parks JA, et al: Ultrasonographic demonstration of undescended testes. Radiology 133:181, 1979.

Maklad NF, Wright CH, Rosenthal SJ: Gray scale ultrasonic appearances of renal transplant rejection. Radiology 131:711, 1979.

Malek RS, Kelalis PP: Nephrocalcinosis in infancy and childhood. J Urol 114:441, 1975.

Markle BM, Potter BM: Surgical diseases of the urinary tract. In Ultrasound in Pediatrics. Edited by JO Haller, A Shkolnik. New York, Churchill Livingstone, 1981, pp 135–164.

Marshall FF, Smith NA, Murphy JB, et al: A comparison of ultrasonography and radiography in the localization of renal calculi: experimental and operative experience. J Urol 126:576, 1981.

Mascatello VJ, Smith EH, Carrera GF, et al: Ultrasonic evaluation of the obstructed duplex kidney. AJR 129:113, 1977.

McLean GK, Edell SL: Determination of bladder volumes by gray scale ultrasonography. Radiology 128:181, 1978.

Mindell HJ, Kupic EA: Horseshoe kidney: ultrasonic demonstration. AJR 129:526, 1977.

Miskin M, Bain J: B-mode ultrasonic examination of the testes. J Clin Ultrasound 2:307, 1974.

Mittelstaedt CA, Volberg FM, Merten DF, et al: The sonographic diagnosis of neonatal adrenal hemorrhage. Radiology 131:453, 1979.

Moskowitz PS, Carroll BA, McCoy JM: Ultrasonic renal volumetry in children: accuracy and simplicity of the method. Radiology 134:61, 1980.

Pedersen JF, Bartrum RJ, Grytter C: Residual urine determination by ultrasonic scanning. Am J Roentgenol Radium Ther Nucl Med 125:474, 1975.

Pederson JF, Holm HH, Hald T: Torsion of the testis diagnosed by ultrasound. J Urol 113:66, 1975.

Pery M, Kaftori JK, Bar-Maor JA: Sonography for diagnosis and follow-up of neonatal adrenal hemorrhage. J Clin Ultrasound 9:397, 1981.

Ramos AJ, Slovis TL, Reed JO: Intrathoracic kidney. Urology 13:14, 1979.

Ravitch MM, Welch KJ, Benson CD, et al: Pediatric Surgery. Third ed. Vol. 2. Chicago, Year Book Medical Publishers, 1979, p 317.

Richie JP, Birnholz J, Garnick MB: Ultrasonography as a diagnostic adjunct for the evaluation of masses in the scrotum. Surg Gynecol Obstet 154:694, 1982.

Rose J, Berdon WE, Sullivan T, et al: Prolonged jaundice as presenting sign of massive adrenal hemorrhage in newborn. Radiology 98:263, 1971.

Rose J, Goldberg BB: Basic Physics in Diagnostic Ultrasound. New York, John Wiley & Sons, 1979, p 49.

Rosenberg ER, Trought WS, Kirks DR, et al: Ultrasonic diagnosis of renal vein thrombosis in neonates. AJR 134:35, 1980.

Rosenfield AT, Glickman MG, Taylor KJW, et al: Acute focal bacterial nephritis (acute lobar nephronia). Radiology 132:553, 1979.

Rosenfield AT, Siegel NJ: Renal parenchymal disease: histopathologic-sonographic correlation. AJR 137:793, 1981.

Rumack CM, Johnson ML, Zunkel D: Antenatal diagnosis. In Ultrasound in Pediatrics. Edited by JO Haller, A Shkolnik, New York, Churchill Livingstone, 1981, pp 210–230.

Sabbagha RE, Shkolnik A: Ultrasound diagnosis of fetal abnormalities. Semin Perinatol 4:213, 1980.

Sample WF, Gottesman JE, Skinner DG, et al: Gray scale ultrasound of the scrotum. Radiology 127:225, 1978.

Sanders RC, Oh KS, Dorst JP: B-scan ultrasound: positive and negative contrast material evaluation of congenital urachal anomaly. Am J Roentgenol Radium Ther Nucl Med 120:448, 1974.

Scheible W, Leopold GR: High-resolution real-time ultrasonography of neonatal kidneys. J Ultrasound Med 1:133, 1982.

Shih WJ, Greenbaum LD, Baro C: In utero sonogram in prune belly syndrome. Urology 20:102, 1982.

Shkolnik A: B-mode ultrasound and the nonvisualizing kidney in pediatrics. AJR 128:121, 1977.

Shkolnik A: The role of ultrasound in pediatrics. Pediatr Ann 9:27, 1980.

Shkolnik A, Foley MJ, Riggs TW, et al: New application of real time ultrasound in pediatrics. RadioGraphics 2:422, 1982.

Siegel MJ, Glasier CM: Acute focal bacterial nephritis in children: significance of ureteral reflux. AJR 137:257, 1981.

Silver TM, Campbell D, Wicks JD, et al: Peritransplant fluid collections: ultrasound evaluation and clinical significance. Radiology 138:145, 1981.

Six R, Oliphant M, Grossman H: A spectrum of renal tubular ectasia and hepatic fibrosis. Radiology 117:117, 1975.

Slovis TL, Cushing B, Reilly BJ, et al: Wilms' tumor to the heart: clinical and radiographic evaluation. AJR 131:263, 1978.

Slovis TL, Perlmutter AD: Recent advances in pediatric urological ultrasound. J Urol 123:613, 1980.

Slovis TL, Philippart AI, Cushing B, et al: Evaluation of the inferior vena cava by sonography and venography in children with renal and hepatic tumors. Radiology 140:767, 1981.

Smith EH: Ultrasound in the evaluation of renal transplants. Postgrad Radiol 1:3, 1981.

Spigos D, Capek V, Jonasson O: Percutaneous biopsy of renal transplants using ultrasonographic guidance. J Urol 117:699, 1977.

Stuck KJ, Koff SA, Silver TM: Ultrasonic features of multicystic dysplastic kidney: expanded diagnostic criteria. Radiology 143:217, 1982.

Subramanyam BR, Balthazar EJ, Raghavendra BN, et al: Sonographic diagnosis of scrotal hernia. AJR 139:535, 1982.

Sumner TE, Phelps C, Crowe JE, et al: Neonatal abdominal real-time sonography. RadioGraphics 1:29, 1981.

Teele RL: Ultrasonography of the genitourinary tract in children. Radiol Clin North Am 15:109, 1977.

Tolchin D, Koenigsberg M, Santorineou M: Early detection of Wilms' tumor in a child with hemihypertrophy and ovarian cysts. Pediatrics 70:135, 1982.

Vallancien G, Dumez Y, Aubry MC, et al: Percutaneous nephrostomy in utero. Urology 20:647, 1982.

Waterhouse RK: The pediatric urologist's point of view. In Ultrasound in Pediatrics. Edited by JO Haller, A Shkolnik. New York, Churchill Livingstone, 1981, pp 10–12.

Whitaker J, Johnston GS, Lawson JD: Urinary outflow resistance estimation in children. Invest Urol 7:127, 1969.

Wladimiroff JW: Effect of furosemide on fetal urine production. Br J Obstet Gynaecol 82:221, 1975.

Wolverson MK, Houttuin E, Heiberg E, et al: Comparison of computed tomography with high-resolution real-time ultrasound in the localization of the impalpable undescended testis. Radiology 146:133, 1983.

10

CYSTOSCOPY

R. LAWRENCE KROOVAND

In 1877 Max Nitze, with the help of instrument maker Wilhelm Deicke, invented and demonstrated the first practical light cystoscope in Dresden, Germany. Since then, progress in both technical innovation and clinical application has made possible the remarkably high quality of present-day urologic endoscopy. Unfortunately, during this same time the indications for pediatric cystoscopy have remained so poorly defined that some urologists believe that no pediatric urologic evaluation is complete without cystoscopic examination, while others use cystoscopy only sparingly. This chapter details rational indications and contraindications for pediatric cystoscopy, describes the endoscopic instruments currently available and the design of a pediatric endoscopic suite, and discusses operative endoscopy.

INDICATIONS AND CONTRAINDICATIONS

The Controversy

Cystourethroscopy is an established essential tool for adult urologic investigation. However, in view of the current sophistication of uroradiographic techniques and the types of common pediatric urologic problems, the role of cystoscopy in the evaluation and management of pediatric urologic problems has become more limited. Of course, cystoscopic examination should always be done when required; however, in recommending cystoscopy for the pediatric patient, one must consider the sometimes questionable diagnostic and therapeutic benefit to the child. This must be balanced against the risk of anesthesia and the potential for urethral trauma.

Only three publications (Johnson et al; Walther and Kaplan; Dunn et al) have systematically reviewed and analyzed large series of cystoscopic examinations in children. Each study clarifies the indications for cystoscopic examination in childhood and indicates that the number of situations calling for cystoscopy is declining. The following section is intended to serve as an outline of the indications for diagnostic pediatric cystoscopy; operative endoscopy is discussed later in this chapter.

Indications for Cystoscopy

Prior to any endoscopic evaluation of the urinary tract in a child, voiding cystourethrography and excretory urography should be done. These studies will define the anatomic and functional status of the urinary tract and will also suggest specific abnormalities that can be evaluated at endoscopy. Cystoscopy in children may be unwise or dangerous in the presence of active infection or blood dyscrasia.

Urinary Tract Infection

The most common indication for cystoscopic examination in children has been urinary tract infection. Many urologists, including this author, feel that the child with an uncomplicated urinary tract infection who appears normal on x-rays (excretory urography and voiding cystourethrography) does not have pyelonephritis, and as such does not routinely require cystoscopy; results of cystoscopy in these children are almost always normal, or positive findings are incidental and do not alter treatment or eventual outcome. However, cystoscopy certainly should be part of the evaluation of persistent infections or of multiple recurrent urinary infections, especially where there are also symptoms of disturbed micturition. Children with such infections, usually girls over age 5 with a history of urge incontinence, frequently have cystitis follicularis (cystitis cystica) and require long-term antibiotic treatment (6 to 12 months or more) to control recurrent infection and to allow resolution of long-standing symptoms and inflammatory mucosal changes. Documentation of chronic cystitis cystica may improve parental compliance with recommended long-term medication programs, although this has not been proved.

Children with urinary infection and abnormal x-rays will be discussed in the section specific to the disease.

Voiding Dysfunction Without Urinary Infection

Children with voiding dysfunction (day wetting, frequency, urgency, or nocturnal enuresis) and without documented urinary infection usually have normal physical and neurologic examinations, normal urinalyses, and normal x-rays. Because cystoscopy here is generally normal or reveals only insignificant abnormalities and does not alter therapy or ultimate outcome, it seems generally unnecessary. Even in those children with voiding dysfunction and abnormal x-rays, cystoscopic examination may confirm or refute the x-ray findings, but these findings generally are incidental and do not explain the child's symptoms, unless the presence of trabeculation first makes the endoscopist think of the possibility of sphincter dyssynergia.

The value of urethral dilation in girls with urinary infections and/or voiding dysfunction remains controversial. Most pediatric urologists now believe that urethral manipulation (dilation or urethrotomy) has little or no effect on the recurrence rate of infection and only infrequently enhances resolution of symptoms. Routine urethral manipulation appears of little value in the treatment of children with urinary infections or voiding dysfunction (Kaplan et al).

Vesicoureteral Reflux

Because expression cystourethrography with the patient under general anesthesia may miss up to 50 per cent of known vesicoureteral reflux, its use for such purposes is to be discouraged (Timmons et al). Instillation of methylene blue during anesthesia to detect vesicoureteral reflux is similarly inaccurate.

The proper role for cystoscopy as part of the evaluation and treatment of children with vesicoureteral reflux remains controversial. For these children a decision to operate is most often based on several factors including the degree of reflux as judged from the cystogram, recurrent infection when under treatment, or noncompliance with antibacterial therapy; less absolute indications include renal scarring, failure of renal growth, and failure of reflux to resolve as expected.

Although cystoscopy at the time of initial evaluation may result in a recommendation for earlier ureteral reimplantation in some children, especially those with more severe grades of reflux (IV/V, V/V) and golf-hole orifices or large paraureteral diverticula, the majority of children with reflux and urinary infection can be safely managed by long-term prophylactic antibacterial coverage. With cessation of recurrent urinary infection, renal growth resumes, renal scarring does not progress, and the reflux may decrease in degree or completely resolve. Cystoscopy in children with reflux and infection appears to be of most value in assessing the prognosis of those with long-term persistent reflux by evaluating orifice configuration and measuring the length of the submucosal tunnel. A previously refluxing contralateral ureter may also be evaluated prior to ureteral reimplantation. Endoscopic evaluation can then generally be done at the time of the planned ureteral reimplantation.

Hematuria

Some have advocated routine cystoscopy for all children with hematuria. This appears unnecessary because the most common causes of microscopic hematuria in children are infection and glomerulonephritis, and reasons for gross hematuria not evident on x-ray studies, such as small bladder tumors, are extremely rare before puberty (Chan). All children with hematuria, gross or microscopic, should have an excretory urogram with a voiding film or a separate VCUG. When these studies are normal, cystoscopic evaluation invariably is normal and therefore unnecessary. As most significant bladder lesions in the pediatric age group are radiologically evident (Fig. 10–1), cystoscopy in this situation is indicated only to confirm the radiologic findings. Persistent hematuria occasionally leads to cystoscopic examination (usually in desperation). However, causal lesions are seldom discovered.

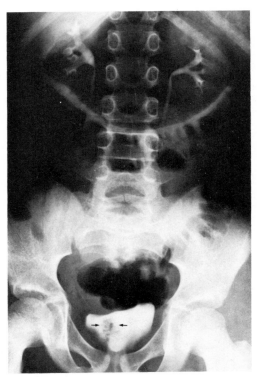

Figure 10-1. Inverted papilloma (*arrows*) in an 11-year-old girl with painless gross hematuria.

A prolonged course of intense chemotherapy (cyclophosphamide), particularly with concurrent radiotherapy to the pelvic region, may result in an atrophic cystitis causing profuse gross hematuria (Droller et al). Early cystoscopy in these children may confirm the diagnosis and alter the plan of chemotherapy.

In some boys anterior (bulbar) urethritis may produce characteristic terminal hematuria or blood spotting on the shorts, with or without dysuria but without pyuria, positive cultures, or abnormal x-rays. Cystoscopy may suggest anterior urethritis as a cause (Plate 10-1A) but is rarely indicated as the symptoms and signs are so pathognomonic. Further, cystoscopy in this condition has preceded stricture formation, giving rise to the thought that the additional trauma of urethroscopy may make stricture more likely (Kaplan and Brock).

Neoplasia

As noted, urothelial malignancy involving the upper or lower urinary tract is rare in the pediatric age group. When present, such lesions are usually visualized on x-ray studies (Fig. 10-1); cystoscopy is then confirmatory rather than diagnostic. Renal parenchymal tumors such as Wilms' tumor (more common) and renal cell carcinoma (uncommon) have such characteristic appearances on the urogram that endoscopic evaluation and retrograde ureteropyelography are seldom necessary. Rhabdomyosarcoma of the bladder and prostate is usually very characteristic in appearance on radiographic evaluation, and pretreatment endoscopy is then performed to judge the extent of the tumor and to obtain a specimen for biopsy.

Malignant or benign lesions arising in other organ systems, such as the retroperitoneum, the internal genital ducts, or the intestinal tract, and appearing to impinge upon the urinary tract sometimes may be best defined by cystoscopy with retrograde pyelography. The indications for endoscopic evaluation in this situation must be individualized.

Urinary Calculi and Foreign Bodies

Urinary calculi in children are relatively uncommon (Reiner et al). As in adults, they may pass or may be evaluated and manipulated by retrograde techniques. For those calculi that do not pass spontaneously, the criteria for endoscopic retrieval or open removal are the same as for adults. Unfortunately, the small size of the prepubertal male urethra places certain constraints on the size of instruments that can be used for endoscopic manipulation of ureteral or vesical calculi. In girls the urethra is more distensible and with gentle dilation permits passage of adult-size instruments, thus increasing the options for endoscopic stone manipulation. If the urethra will accommodate a 13 F or large sheath, a 4 F Pfister-Schwartz or 5 F Dormia stone retriever may facilitate ureteral calculus removal. Bladder calculi and foreign bodies often require open surgical removal.

Retrograde Ureteral Catheterization

With the increasing sophistication in uroradiographic techniques, radionuclide scans, and ultrasonography, the indications for retrograde ureteral catheterization have become relatively limited. Retrograde studies are only infrequently required to evaluate abnormalities of the upper urinary tract but may be useful whenever an obstructing process within the collecting system is incompletely visualized. A dilated megaureter that is in-

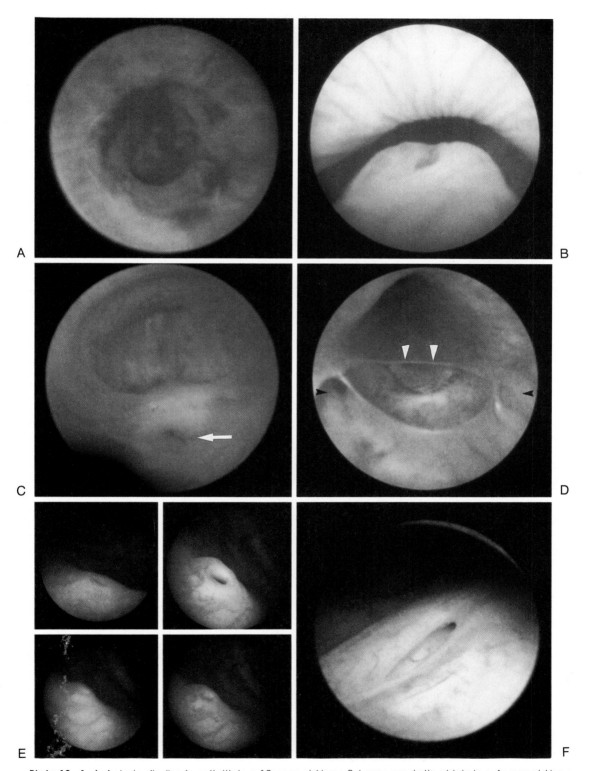

Plate 10–1. *A*, Anterior (bulbar) urethritis in a 10-year-old boy. *B*, Large prostatic utricle in a 4-year-old boy with penoscrotal hypospadias. *C*, Entrance of the vagina (*arrows*) into the urethra of a 3-year-old girl with congenital virilizing adrenogenital syndrome. *D*, Anomalous development of the Cowper's ducts with characteristic bulbar urethral diverticulum (*white arrows*); note the entrance of the Cowper's ducts into the urethra (*black arrows*). *E*, Cone- or volcano-shaped ureteral orifice. *F*, Stadium-shaped ureteral orifice.

completely visualized by intravenous urography or persistent ureterectasis that follows ureteral reimplantation or megaureter repair may be better defined by retrograde filling. In such instances fluoroscopy permits observation of ureteral peristalsis and drainage; manometric pressure perfusion recordings can be obtained if necessary.

In dealing with ureteropelvic junction obstruction, retrograde studies as a separate procedure are not necessary unless another ureteral abnormality that is not defined on the excretory urogram is suspected. A retrograde ureteropyelogram may be done at the time of the definitive operative procedure, thereby avoiding a separate induction of anesthesia and reducing the potential complications of iatrogenic infection.

The difficulties in obtaining adequate urine flow for split renal function studies through small caliber ureteral catheters, plus the ill-defined effect of general anesthesia on renal function in the anesthetized child, limit the success of this endeavor. Split cultures may be obtained after copious bladder washing; however, percutaneous nephrostomy is now preferred in cases of renal failure from severe upper urinary obstruction. When percutaneous drainage procedures fail, however, temporary retrograde catheterization of the ureter may still provide adequate drainage prior to definitive therapy.

Congenital Anomalies

Endoscopy can further define anatomic abnormalities associated with severe hypospadias, ambiguous genitalia, persistent urogenital sinus, and cloacal malformations that are not fully demonstrated uroradiographically. In boys with severe hypospadias a large utriculus masculinus not always visualized on voiding cystourethrography may be easily identified endoscopically (Plate 10–1B). Cystoscopy is not routinely performed in boys with hypospadias, however. The precise localization of the narrow entrance of the distal vagina into the urogenital sinus may be identified at the time of genital reconstruction or vaginoplasty in girls with virilizing adrenogenital syndrome (Plate 10–1C). When virilization is extreme, endoscopic insertion of a Fogarty balloon catheter through the tiny urethral connection into the vaginal cavity helps in identifying the vagina and may reduce the extent of perineal dissection required during repair.

ENDOSCOPIC INSTRUMENTS

During the past 80 years improvements in technique and instrumentation have made endoscopic evaluation of the lower urinary tract in infants and children a practical and safe procedure. Fiberoptic illumination and the Hopkins lens system now permit more reliable and intense illumination with increased perception and a clearer, less distorted visual field. One can visualize the lower urinary tract of infants and children accurately; transurethral manipulation and fulguration are easily accomplished. In addition, endoscopic photography and television recording are now routine at many centers.

The essentials of a pediatric cystoscopic set include interchangeable telescopes (direct vision and forward-oblique) and sheaths of assorted sizes to permit both observation (examination) and operative endoscopy. Several manufacturers (Storz,* ACMI,† Wolf,‡ Olympus§) produce pediatric endoscopic instruments. Most instruments are color coded and engraved for easy identification of French

* Karl Storz, Endoscopy-America, Inc., 10111 West Jefferson Boulevard, Culver City, CA 90230.
† American Cystoscope Makers, Division of American Hospital Supply Corporation, 300 Stillwater Avenue, Stamford, CT 06902.
‡ Richard Wolf Medical Instruments Corporation, 7046 Lundon Avenue, Rosemont, IL 60018.
§ Olympus Corporation of America, Medical Instrument Division, 4 Nevada Drive, New Hyde Park, NY 11042.

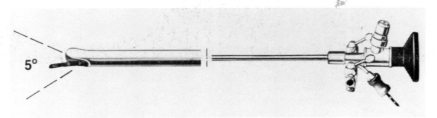

Figure 10–2. An 8 French infant cystoscope that will accommodate a 3 French ureteral catheter.

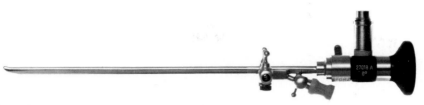

Figure 10–3. A 10 French sheath with interchangeable direct and forward-oblique lenses; the instrument will accommodate a 4 French ureteral catheter.

size and catheter capacity. The listed French sizes are approximate for sheaths with an oval cross section. Unfortunately, the true diameter of some of these instruments is sometimes greater than stated by the manufacturer; actual size should be verified by the prospective buyer. Because these instruments are very delicate and are readily damaged, they should be handled with utmost care and gentleness. The quality and availability of instrument repair is variable and should be considered by the prospective buyer, because even with appropriate use these instruments occasionally require repair.

Observation cystoscopes are available in 8 and 11 F sizes (Olympus, Storz, Wolf). Some have both observation (examination) and irrigating capability, while others permit observation only. I have not found either particularly useful because of the inability to fulgurate valves in small infants or to perform retrograde ureteropyelography. Storz and Wolf have an 8 F cystoscope with a side channel that will accommodate a 3 F ureteral catheter; this cystoscope is especially useful in small male infants for transurethral fulguration of valves (Fig. 10–2).

For larger infants and children instruments of 10 to 14 F sheath size are available; most will accommodate one or two ureteral catheters. Some have an integrated (not interchangeable) sheath and telescope, and the others have interchangeable direct vision and forward-oblique telescopes. Integrated instruments may add unnecessary expense in equipping a pediatric endoscopic unit and are therefore less desirable. However, such instruments may be more durable. For versatility, I find a 10 F sheath with interchangeable direction vision and forward-oblique telescopes the most useful (Fig. 10–3).

Pediatric resectoscopes in sizes from 9.5 to 14 F permit a wide variety of endoscopic surgery (Fig. 10–4). Most use an interchangeable direct-vision telescope and may also be used with a cold-knife blade for direct-vision internal urethrotomy for treatment of ureteral strictures (see Operative Endoscopy later in this chapter).

In addition, each manufacturer has available a variety of compatible accessories including operating bridges, grasping and foreign-body forceps, coagulating electrodes, urethrotomes, and teaching attachments. Space limitations prevent a detailed review of these instruments; the interested reader should consult the individual manufacturers' catalogues for additional information.

Light Sources

Fiberoptic light sources of infinitely variable intensity and flexible light-conducting systems are available from the various manu-

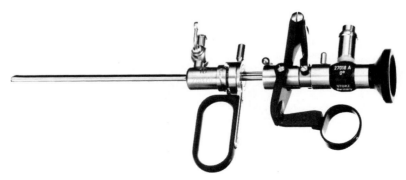

Figure 10–4. A 10 French pediatric resectoscope.

facturers. Storz has recently introduced a fluid light-conducting system that greatly reduces the slight yellow hue that the fiber bundle imparts to the visual field. Xenon light sources provide brighter illumination than standard light sources and are useful in performing endophotography. However, caution must be exercised to avoid thermal injury due to increased heat transfer.

Teaching Attachments

Improved illumination and better visualization afforded by modern lens systems have revolutionized teaching attachments. It is now possible for both the endoscopist and the observer to have sufficient illumination for good visualization. Both flexible and articulated attachments are available for teaching the student and house staff and for endophotography.

Retrograde Catheters

Sterile disposable whistle-tip, pigtail, and olive-tip ureteral catheters are available in 3 F and larger sizes. The smallest cone-tip ureteral catheter available is an 8 F tip on a 5 F stem and thus has limited application in pediatric patients.

Specialized ureteral catheters such as the double-J and Cook catheters are available in pediatric sizes and are appropriate for selected situations when longer-term ureteral intubation is necessary.

Irrigating Solutions

Either sterile water or saline, warmed to body temperature, may be used for endoscopic examinations. Because the risks of hemolysis or electrolyte disturbance from intravascular absorption or intraperitoneal perforation during endoscopic surgery are minimal in children, sterile water is appropriate for endoscopic surgery in infants and children.

Bougies and Sounds

Otis bougies à boule and female urethral sounds are familiar and commonly available instruments and require no additional comment. Because of the different curvature of the bulbar urethra and the rigidity of the urogenital diaphragm in the young male, infant male sounds must have a shape and tip that

conforms to the shorter curvature of the urethra in the young boy.

ENDOSCOPIC SUITE

Because urologic endoscopic procedures in children require some form of anesthesia, a fully equipped room within an operating or anesthesia suite is safest. Cystoscopic examination with the patient under local anesthesia is ill advised except possibly in older girls. Our cystoscopic table is hydraulically operated, including the movable table top. We have customized clamps to accommodate the smaller knee supports necessary for younger children (Fig. 10–5). An electrosurgical unit appropriately calibrated for pediatric endo-

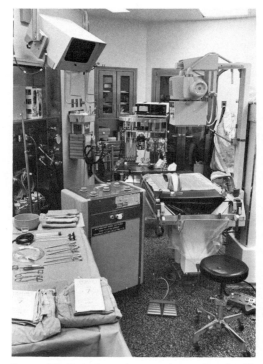

Figure 10–5. A view of our endoscopic suite. The power-operated table is as described. Custom clamps accommodate the smaller knee supports necessary for young children. Note the under table image-intensifier which includes a cine camera, variable collimator; the television monitor is conveniently located. The instrument storage cabinet, with side shelves elevated, serves as a surface for the sterile instrument table. A typical sterile setup is shown; less frequently used supplies are added as necessary. In actual use the electrosurgical unit and sterile table are positioned more conveniently for the endoscopist.

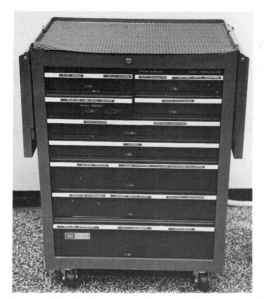

Figure 10-6. The author's portable instrument storage cabinet; the side shelves of this cabinet, when extended, serve as a surface for the sterile cystoscopic instrument table.

scopic surgery should be a permanent part of any pediatric endoscopic unit. For convenience we have a portable cabinet to organize and store our endoscopic equipment. The top of this cabinet expands to provide a larger surface for the sterile endoscopic supplies (Fig. 10-6).

The importance of the dynamic factors in evaluating certain urologic disorders in children cannot be overemphasized; accordingly, we have an image intensifier mounted on the cystoscopic table in our unit. The size of the x-ray field is easily and accurately controlled by a variable collimator that has separate vertical and lateral shutter adjustments as well as a swivel mount to rotate the axes of the field.

Videotape and 105 mm x-ray capability allow documentation of dynamic fluoroscopic studies for later review, or for conversion to 16 mm film or videotape for closed-circuit transmission to conferences. In addition, we have 35 mm photographic and television capabilities to record endoscopic findings.

CYSTOSCOPIC TECHNIQUES

Cystoscopic technique in the infant and child is similar to that in the adult and therefore will not be discussed in detail. However, certain precautions relevant to introducing the cystoscope into the urethra and a description of normal and abnormal ureterovesical anatomy will be reviewed.

Cystoscopy is done with the child in the lithotomy position, although in small infants and young girls an exaggerated frog-leg position is also acceptable. Appropriate surgical cleansing is done prior to cystoscopy, and sterile technique is maintained throughout the procedure. The surgeon should scrub preoperatively and wear a mask, surgical cap, and sterile gown and gloves.

Particular care is required to avoid urethral injury, and consistent gentleness is mandatory. When the sheath is being introduced, the obturator should generally be in place; the well-lubricated instrument must be guided, not pushed. Forcing a sheath through a tight urethra may result in subsequent urethral stricture.

Although there is a normal range of urethral caliber for each sex and age group, I generally use the largest caliber instrument appropriate for the examination that can be inserted without stretching the urethra. In the male child the range of urethral size is limited (Allen et al). The narrowest portion of the male urethra is the external meatus; meatotomy is frequently required before endoscopy. A simple crush meatotomy can be performed to permit easy passage of the instrument.

The elasticity and distensibility of the female urethra, even in neonates, allow greater flexibility in the choice of sheath size and operative endoscopic procedures that can be done in girls (Immergut and Wahman).

Generally the urethra of a male neonate will admit only an 8 or 10 F instrument, whereas the male urethra of mid childhood usually accommodates a 13 or 14 F sheath without difficulty. Available 8 F cystoscopes now permit not only observation but also limited endoscopic manipulation.

Occasionally the penile urethra is of insufficient size to permit passage of even the smallest infant cystoscope. In this situation a perineal urethrotomy can be done. Placing traction sutures in the urethral edges permits easy access to the larger caliber proximal bulbar urethra and allows the required endoscopic examination as well as manipulation for treatment of posterior urethral valves or for retrograde ureteropyelography. With the increased diagnostic yield of modern radiologic techniques, perineal urethrotomy solely

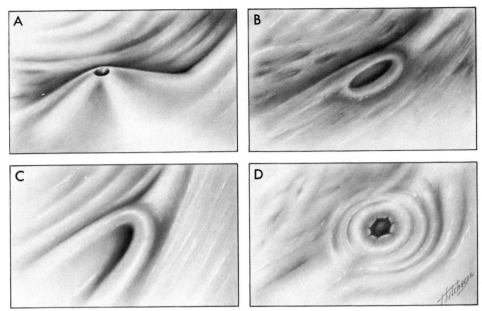

Figure 10-7. Appearances of ureteral orifice. Normal orifice (A). Stadium-type orifice (B), and horseshoe orifice (C) are variants of normal and generally do not reflux if a submucosal tunnel of adequate length is present. The "golf-hole" orifice (D) almost always refluxes; generally, no submucosal tunnel is present.

for cystoscopic observation now appears unwarranted.

We do not advocate routine dilation of the urethra prior to endoscopy, especially in the male child, as this may produce iatrogenic injury to the delicate urethral tissues. However, calibration with bougies allows one to employ instruments of appropriate size. Direct visual observation of the male urethra during passage of the instrument may be required to minimize urethral trauma and also to observe the entire urethra prior to any instrumentation and possible iatrogenic change.

In the female child the sheath and obturator may be introduced directly into the bladder and the telescope then inserted. Prior to formal examination of the bladder a urine specimen for urinalysis, culture, and sensitivity testing is usually obtained.

The normal prepubertal male urethra is pale pink and of uniform caliber except at the penoscrotal angle and at the urogenital diaphragm, where physiologic narrowing or sphincter spasm may be misinterpreted as a urethral stricture. In the deep bulbar urethra the entrances of Cowper's ducts are frequently visualized (Plate 10-1D). The normal longitudinal vasculature of the urethra becomes more prominent at the urogenital diaphragm and should not be misinterpreted as anterior (bulbar) urethritis or some other inflammatory process. Similarly, the verumontanum, prostatic urethra, and bladder neck are generally more vascular than the penile urethra.

The bladder neck in both sexes is usually supple and not prominent. In boys with posterior urethral valves or long-standing voiding dysfunction the bladder neck may be elevated and appear obstructive. Generally this proves not to be the case, and treatment of the bladder neck itself is seldom if ever necessary; these visual abnormalities generally resolve after relief of more distal outlet obstruction or voiding dysfunction.

The trigone is normally pale and smooth with ureteral orifices located symmetrically within one or two visual fields of the midline. The shape (cone, stadium, horseshoe, golf hole) (Fig. 10-7, Plates 10-1E and F and 10-2A and B) and position (Fig. 10-8) of the ureteral orifices should be recorded with the bladder empty and full. The visual appearance of the ureteral orifice varies, depending upon whether a direct-vision or forward-oblique telescope is used. The endoscopist should develop a routine best suited to his goals.

The normal ureteral orifice is cone- or volcano-shaped (Plate 10-1E) and located at the "A" position on the trigone. The orifice retains its appearance and does not migrate laterally with bladder filling. The stadium ori-

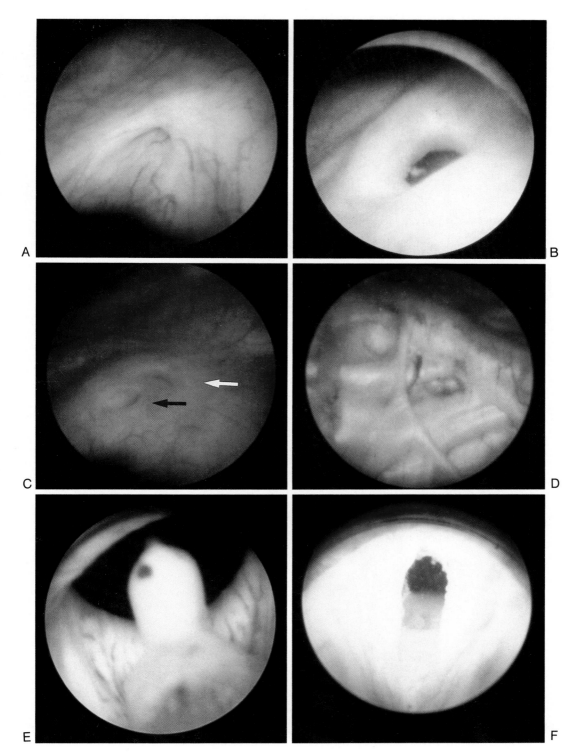

Plate 10–2. *A*, Horseshoe-shaped ureteral orifice; the orifice has lost its medial rim. *B*, Golf hole–shaped ureteral orifice; there is little or no submucosal ureteral tunnel. *C*, Duplicated ureteral orifices; the upper and more lateral orifice (*white arrow*) drains the lower renal segment; the lower and more medial orifice (*black arrow*) drains the upper renal segment. *D*, Bladder trabeculation in a boy with urinary outlet obstruction. *E*, A urethral polyp originating from the verumontanum in a boy with hematuria. *F*, Posterior urethral valves.

CHILDREN'S HOSPITAL OF MICHIGAN
CYSTOSCOPIC EXAMINATION

DATE
PATIENT NO.
PATIENT NAME
MEDICAL RECORD NO.
BIRTH DATE SEX
PHYSICIAN

HISTORY ____________________

PHYSICAL FINDINGS ____________________

IVP ____________________

CYSTOGRAM ____________________

URINALYSIS
BLADDER ________ (R)________ (L)________

URINE CULTURE
BLADDER ________ (R)________ (L)________

INSTRUMENT SIZE ________ LENS________ BLADDER RESIDUAL ________

URETHRA
MEATUS ________ LENGTH ________ MUCOSA ________

CALIBRATION FR. _____ DILATATION FR. _____ MEATOTOMY _____ URETHROTOMY _____ OTHER _____

BLADDER
BLADDER NECK ________TRIGONE________ CAPACITY ________

MUCOSA ________TRABECULATION ________

URETERAL ORIFICES

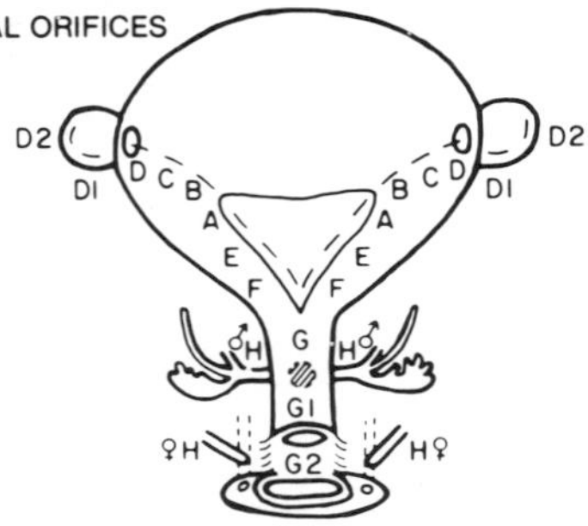

DO NOT WRITE IN THIS MARGIN

Rt. Orifice Posn (✓) Lt. Orifice Posn

H	G	F	E	D*	C	B	A	Shape	A	B	C	D	E	F	G	H
								Golf Hole								
								Horseshoe								
								Stadium								
								Normal								
								Size								
								Small(S) Med.(M) Large(L)								
								Patulous(P) NonPat(NP)								
								Submucosal Tunnel m.m.								

▒ If ureteric orifice is duplicated, describe U.O. corresponding with cranial renal segment in shaded part of appropriate column.

* Paraureteral Diverticulum R. Present ☐ Not Present ☐ L. Present ☐ Not Present ☐

If present, denote site of U.O. in relation to diverticulum as shown on diagram D, D1, D2 when possible in D column/s.

RETROGRADE STUDIES (R)________(L)________

PERISTALSIS (R)________(L)________

OTHER OBSERVATIONS & CONCLUSIONS ________

PLAN ________

SURGEON ________

FORM OR 3

White, MEDICAL RECORD — Canary, SURGEON — Pink, RESIDENT — Gold, DEPT.

Figure 10–8. Cystoscopy report. Endoscopic findings should be recorded on a cystoscopy record that becomes a permanent part of the patient record.

fice (Plate 10–1F) is more laterally positioned ("B" position) on the trigone, is oval in shape, and may migrate laterally with bladder filling. The horseshoe orifice (Plate 10–2A) has lost its medial rim and is usually in the "B" or "C" position on the trigone; lateral migration of the orifice commonly occurs with bladder filling. The golf-hole orifice (Plate 10–2B) has poor trigonal attachment and is usually found in the "D" position; there is little or no submucosal ureteral tunnel, giving this orifice its gaping golf-hole appearance.

The length of the submucosal ureteral tunnel can be estimated or measured using a ureteral catheter. The length of the submucosal ureteral tunnel and the position of the ureteral orifice when the bladder is fully distended are important guidelines in predicting spontaneous resolution of vesicoureteral reflux. The shape and position of the ureteral orifices, submucosal tunnel length, and observation for the presence of ureteral duplication (Plate 10–2C) or ectopia, trabeculation (Plate 10–2D), diverticulum, tumor, stone, foreign body, bleeding points (Plate 10–2E), or other abnormality and bladder capacity should be noted and recorded on a cystoscopy report that becomes a permanent part of the patient record (Fig. 10–8).

OPERATIVE ENDOSCOPY

Posterior Urethral Valves

Posterior urethral valves are usually diagnosed from a voiding cystourethrogram and represent an obstructing diaphragm distal to the verumontanum with an eccentric annulus (Plate 10–2F). Transurethral incision of the obstructing diaphragm (valves) can be done in the neonate and small infant through an 8 or 10 F cystoscope sheath or in the larger infant or young boy using a 13 or 14 F sheath or resectoscope with a direct-vision or forward-oblique telescope. When a cystoscope sheath is used, a 3 or 4 F ureteral catheter passed through the side channel may be converted into a satisfactory electrode using the catheter as the insulating sheath and advancing a wire stylet 1 to 2 mm beyond the end of the catheter to serve as a straight electrode; it may also be fashioned into a small hook. A flexible electrode or right-angle resectoscope electrode may also be used to incise the valve leaflets.

The electrosurgical unit should be calibrated before the valve leaflets are incised with the selected electrode. I use a cutting current to insure a clean incision. It is not necessary to remove the entire valve leaflet, which is most commonly quite thin. Simple incision in several places—posterolaterally on each side and distal to the verumontanum, taking care not to injure that structure—usually suffices and avoids accidental injury to the external sphincter. Residual obstruction can easily be dealt with at a later time.

After incision of the valve leaflets, contrast material may be instilled into the bladder and an expression cystourethrogram done to verify relief of the obstruction.

Anterior Urethral Valves and Urethral Diverticula

Anterior urethral valves and anterior urethral diverticula are rare causes of congenital urinary outlet obstruction. They appear to represent similar entities, fusion defects of the urethral floor. The distal edge of the diverticulum acts as an obstructing flap during voiding and obstructs micturition. Anterior valves with limited urethral undermining may be easily removed by transurethral incision or resection; larger diverticula require open repair.

Ureterocele

The role of transurethral management of ureteroceles is limited. Because transurethral incision or resection of an ectopic ureterocele usually trades obstruction for problematic reflux, most authors agree that ectopic ureteroceles in infants and children are best treated by open surgery. However, large ectopic ureteroceles associated with severe urinary sepsis may be treated on an emergency basis by transurethral incision with later planned reconstruction. During endoscopic evaluation of a child, an ectopic ureterocele may collapse during bladder filling or even evert through the ureteral hiatus and be mistaken for a bladder diverticulum (Plate 10–3A).

Simple ureteroceles are usually asymptomatic and are infrequently diagnosed in childhood. Occasionally they may be associated with significant obstruction or stone formation. Because incision of the ureteral wall with a loop electrode usually causes reflux, simple ureteroceles may be treated by careful medial incision of the stenotic meatus with a fine-tip flexible electrode or with endo-

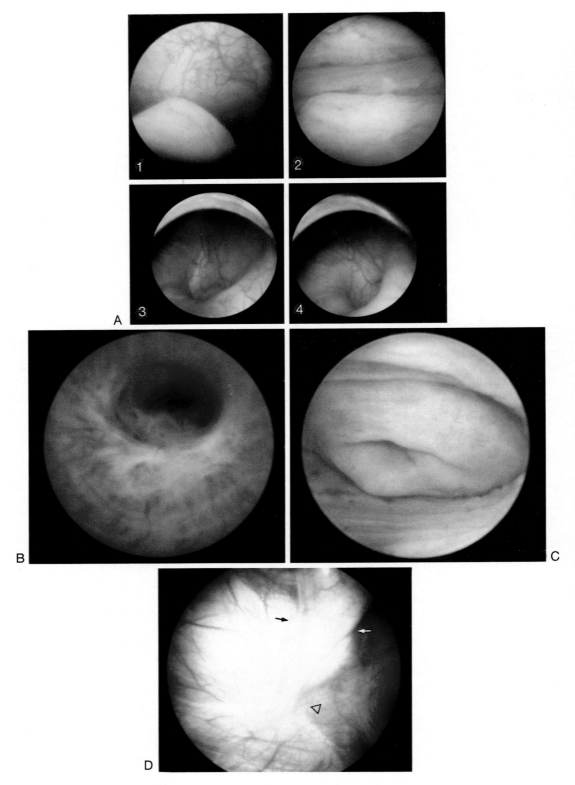

Plate 10–3. *A*, Ectopic ureterocele. The ureterocele bulges into the bladder (1), gradually flattens with increased bladder filling (2), and everts outside the bladder simulating a bladder diverticulum (3 and 4). *B*, Urethral stricture. *C*, Vaginoscopy; a normal prepubertal cervix. *D*, Laparoscopy; the lower pole of the testes and the gubernaculum (*black arrows*) at the internal ring (*open arrow*) in a boy with a nonpalpable undescended testicle. (Courtesy of M. Maizels and L. R. King.)

scopic scissors. Significant postincision reflux is unusual and may be treated later, electively, when it persists. Similarly, a stenotic ureteral meatus may be minimally incised to relieve any obstruction present.

Occasionally ureteral meatotomy is indicated for the treatment of ureteral obstruction following ureteral reimplantation if the obstruction appears to be the result of distal ureteral fibrosis or an excessively long intravesical tunnel; ureteral meatotomy may also be indicated if a stone is lodged in the distal ureter. When carefully done, ureteral meatotomy may relieve the obstruction or allow stone removal without causing reflux.

Bladder Neck Obstruction

Bladder neck obstruction and bladder neck hypertrophy are uncommon diagnoses in childhood; bladder neck hypertrophy is usually secondary to distal obstruction and will regress after relief of the obstruction. We have not had reason to perform transurethral surgery for either of these diagnoses. The possibility of retrograde ejaculation must be kept in mind as a potential complication after bladder neck resection (or incision) in males and vesicovaginal fistula after deep resection of the bladder neck in females.

Urinary Calculi

The indications and techniques for endoscopic manipulation of urinary calculi in children are similar to those for adults and are well elaborated in standard urologic texts. The small size of the male urethra in childhood limits endoscopic manipulation of urinary calculi. However, the distensibility of the urethra in little girls allows use of adult-sized instruments and more latitude in management. Endoscopic calculus manipulation should be done under fluoroscopic control.

Urethral Stricture and External Sphincter Spasm

Transurethral treatment of congenital or acquired urethral strictures (Plate 10–3B) can be done either by cold knife or by electroincision. The Otis urethrotome also may be used to incise strictures but is a blind instrument with a closed diameter of approximately 13 F and therefore not appropriate for infants and young children. The cold knife or Sachse urethrotome offers more versatility and allows direct-vision internal urethrotomy with inspection of the entire stricture and complete division of all scar under direct vision (Smith et al). Transcutaneous or transurethral injection of steroid into the stricture prior to incision may lessen postoperative reaction and therefore stricture recurrence.

Urinary outlet obstruction as a result of narrowing of the urethra at the urogenital diaphragm may be produced by external sphincter spasm in some forms of reflex neurogenic bladder and in children with myelodysplasia or prune-belly syndrome and may interfere with bladder emptying and contribute to urinary infection and/or upper tract deterioration. One form of treatment for such obstruction is anterior urethrotomy at the 12 o'clock position; cutting at other positions may cause excessive bleeding.

Complications of Pediatric Cystoscopy

The potential complications of pediatric cystoscopy may be avoided or minimized by using gentle technique and by keeping the procedure relatively brief. Adherence to meticulous sterile technique makes postinstrumentation urinary infection uncommon. Sepsis is more common after prolonged vigorous instrumentation or instrumentation of an anomalous or infected urinary tract with poor emptying characteristics. In such situations, maintenance of adequate postinstrumentation drainage is recommended to reduce the possibility of sepsis.

Mechanical injury to the urethra may occur with laceration, perforation, or false passage formation because of excessive trauma or from the use of a tightly fitting sheath. Because stricture of the male urethra may follow instrumentation, even months or years later, a difficult or complicated endoscopic examination requires careful long-term follow-up.

In infants and physically small boys even gently performed endoscopy may result in temporary postoperative urinary retention owing to dysuria or edema and may require brief catheterization.

Tearing of the bladder mucosa or rupture of the bladder may result from direct trauma from the cystoscope or may be caused by overdistention of the bladder. Perforation of the ureter or renal parenchyma may occur during forceful ureteral catheterization or endoscopic manipulation.

Deep resection of posterior urethral valves may result in incontinence or membranous urethral stricture. Transurethral resection of the female bladder neck or trigone is a procedure that may cause vesicovaginal fistula and can no longer be justified.

An infrequent but potentially serious complication of cystoscopy is hypothermia from the use of cold or room temperature irrigating solutions. Every effort should be made to utilize warm irrigating solutions and to carefully monitor body temperature during cystoscopy (Meyers and Oh).

OTHER ENDOSCOPIC PROCEDURES

Vaginoscopy

The indications for vaginoscopy include vaginal discharge, genital malformation, vaginal tumor, and vaginal cysts. Vaginoscopy done using a panendoscope with a direct-viewing telescope with the patient under general anesthesia provides a much clearer view of the vagina and cervix than can be obtained with a vaginal or nasal speculum. The juvenile vagina is narrow and relatively long; the cervix is small and pale and often hidden in the vaginal mucosal folds of the fornix, where it may be difficult to visualize (Plate 10–3C).

A snug panendoscope and high water pressure should be avoided, as retrograde passage of irrigating solution into the peritoneal cavity may cause peritonitis.

Nephroscopy

Nephroscopy is an important adjunct to open renal surgery. In pediatric urology it is useful to localize and manipulate intrarenal calculi and to identify the site of intrarenal bleeding. Pediatric nephroscopic techniques are analogous to those in the adult and therefore are not discussed further.

Laparoscopy

Laparoscopy using a pediatric laparoscope or panendoscope may allow identification of the nonpalpable undescended testis or an intraperitoneal anomaly such as an ovotestis, uterus, fallopian tube, or ovary. Identification of the internal spermatic vessels, vas deferens, or testicle (Plate 10–3D) may allow more appropriate operative exposure. When the spermatic vessels and vas deferens end blindly in a scarlike area, the child may be spared an operative exploration (Kaplan and Brock, King and Maizels).

Endophotography

The improved resolution and wide viewing angle afforded by the newer lens systems, along with improvements in light sources and light transmission, have markedly improved the quality of endoscopic photographs. Although the small lens system of pediatric telescopes limits the quality of endoscopic photographs in this age group, it is usually possible to document endoscopic findings with great accuracy.

Any good single-lens reflex camera may be utilized for endophotography, although a special adapter is necessary to secure the camera to the cystoscopic eyepiece. Storz, Wolf, and Olympus have excellent units with compatible light sources and flash generators.

Additionally, motion picture and television technology has advanced to the point that endoscopic procedures may now be recorded with amazing accuracy in both detail and color. Such photographs subsequently become valuable teaching aids.

BIBLIOGRAPHY

Allen JS, Summers JL, Wilkerson SE: Meatal calibration in newborn boys. J Urol 107:498, 1972.

Chan JCM: Hematuria and proteinuria in the pediatric patient. Diagnostic approach. Urology 11:205, 1978.

Droller MJ, Saral R, Santos G: Prevention of cyclophosphamide-induced hemorrhagic cystitis. Urology 20:256, 1982.

Dunn, M, Smith JB, Abrams PH: Endoscopic examination in children. Br J Urol 50:586, 1978.

Immergut MA, Wahman GE: The urethral caliber of female children with recurrent urinary tract infections. J Urol 99:189, 1968.

Johnson DK, Kroovand RL, Perlmutter AD: The changing role of cystoscopy in the pediatric patient. J Urol 123:232, 1980.

Kaplan GW, Sammons TA, King LR: A blind comparison of dilation, urethrotomy and medication alone in treatment of urinary tract infections in girls. J Urol 109:917, 1973.

King, LR, Maizels M: Personal communication.

Lowe, DH, Brock WA, Kaplan GW: Laparoscopy for localization of nonpalpable testes. J Urol 131:728, 1984.

Meyers MB, Oh TH: Prevention of hypothermia during cystoscopy in infants. Anesth Analg 55:592, 1976.

Reiner RJ, Kroovand RL, Perlmutter AD: Unusual aspects of urinary calculi in children. J Urol 121:480, 1979.

Smith PJB, Dunn M, Dounis A.: The early results of treatment of stricture of the male urethra using the Sachse optical urethrotome. Br J Urol 51:224, 1979.

Timmons JW, Watts FB, Perlmutter AD: A comparison of awake and anesthesia cystography. Birth Defects 13:363, 1977.

Walther PC, Kaplan GW: Cystoscopy in children: indications for its use in common urologic problems. J Urol 122:717, 1979.

11

GENITOURINARY INFECTIONS

Nonspecific Infections

A. BARRY BELMAN

Bacterial infections of the urinary tract in children are second in incidence only to bacterial infections of the respiratory tract. The importance of urinary tract infection, particularly in the very young, cannot be overstressed. Since it is unrealistic to advocate generalized screening of the urinary tract in all infants, infection is a major indication for investigating the possibility of anatomic abnormalities that have the potential for causing significant morbidity and renal damage.

DIAGNOSIS OF URINARY TRACT INFECTION

Urinary tract infection can be reliably diagnosed only on culture. Symptoms of dysuria, urgency, frequency, and enuresis are nonspecific and may be the result of vulvitis, urethritis, or nonurinary causes such as dehydration associated with a febrile illness. In 34 children with lower urinary symptoms alone, urine culture demonstrated significant bacilluria in only 18 per cent; 40 per cent of those with sterile urine had upper respiratory infection as compared with 21 per cent of the group with significant bacilluria (Dickinson). Heale et al found that of 378 children with urinary complaints, only 14.3 per cent had urinary infection. Thirty-three per cent with flank pain and dysuria and 31.5 per cent with the recent onset of wetting had urinary tract infection, while only 4.2 per cent with chronic nocturnal enuresis were infected. Of those without specific complaints 4.4 per cent had urinary tract infection (little different from those who were wet only at night).

Although urinalysis can be helpful in calling attention to those who might be infected,

the association of inflammatory cells in the urine is at best only 80 per cent reliable (Kass; Ginsburg and McCracken) and is oftentimes less reliable (Corman et al; Pryles and Eliot). Pyuria in the absence of urinary tract infection may be found in children following viral immunization (Hart and Cherry) and in association with gastroenteritis (Pryles and Lüders). The presumption of urinary tract infection based on history and result of urinalysis must be followed, then, by a positive urine culture to be definitive.

Specimen Collection

In the pre–toilet-trained group the urine specimen is initially obtained by applying a collection bag (U-Bag) to the perineum (Fig. 11–1). Although this method has been justifiably criticized as having a high rate of contamination, it is reliable when the culture is negative. Contamination is directly related to the length of time the collection device remains applied to the child. In a well-controlled office situation the reliability approaches 98 per cent (Randolph and Majors); however, if a specimen has not been obtained within 30 minutes of application, reliability begins to fall. This method has also been effectively carried out in a home screening program (Randolph et al, 1981). Removing the appliance and plating or refrigerating the urine immediately after the child voids is paramount. Having the parent apply the bag before leaving for the physician's office in an effort to shorten the wait is acceptable only when that culture is negative. Confirmation of all positive urine cultures collected by the external appliance technique is advisable prior to treatment. Invasive means (catheteri-

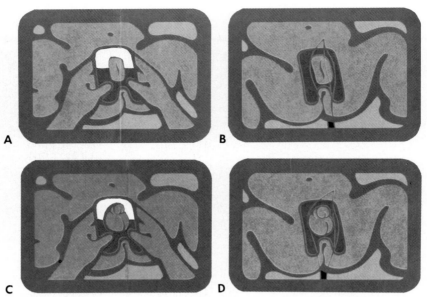

Figure 11-1. Application of Hollister U-Bag. *A*, In girls, stretch the perineum to separate skin folds and expose the vagina. When applying adhesive to the skin, be sure to start at the narrow bridge of skin separating the vagina from the anus. Work outward from this point. *B*, Press the adhesive firmly against the skin and avoid wrinkles. When the bottom part is in place, remove the paper from the upper portion of the adhesive. Work upward to complete application, pressing the adhesive all around the vagina. *C*, In boys, when pressing adhesive to the skin, be sure to start at the narrow bridge of skin between the anus and the base of the scrotum. Work outward from this point. Be sure the skin is dry before applying the collector. *D*, Continue to press the adhesive firmly against the skin, avoiding wrinkles. When the bottom part is in place, remove the paper from the upper portion of the adhesive patch. Work upward to complete application. (From Belman AB, Kaplan GW: Genitourinary Problems in Pediatrics. Philadelphia, WB Saunders Co., 1981.)

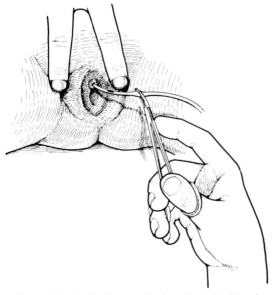

Figure 11-2. Sterile urethral catheterization for collection of a urine specimen for culture.

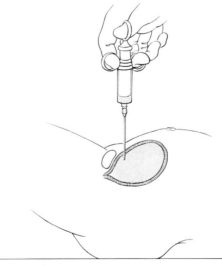

Figure 11-3. Suprapubic aspiration for collection of bladder urine with a full bladder. The needle is inserted 2 cm cephalad to the symphysis perpendicular to the axis of the child.

zation or suprapubic aspiration) should be employed when the clinical situation dictates the necessity for immediate treatment.

When a clean specimen is difficult or impossible to obtain or the institution of therapy is urgent, the urine should be collected by catheterization or direct bladder (suprapubic) aspiration (SPA). A feeding tube (7 to 10 F) is ideal for catheterization. The perineum is cleansed with soap and water or a mild antiseptic. Gloves are not necessary if a clean technique can be otherwise assured (Fig. 11–2). SPA has achieved great popularity in pediatric circles. This is most likely a response to the negative reputation urethral catheterization has gained through the years. Young children are particularly favorable candidates for SPA because of the abdominal location of their urinary bladders. However, the procedure cannot be expected to be successful when the bladder is empty. Therefore, a requirement for attempting aspiration is a palpable bladder. This requirement is the major drawback of SPA. If urine is not obtained initially, repeat attempts at aspiration should be delayed until such time as the bladder has filled.

SPA is performed after first cleaning the suprapubic area with an antiseptic solution. A 21 to 25 gauge needle is inserted perpendicular to the patient in the midline one fingerbreadth above the symphysis (Fig. 11–3). Although a local anesthetic can first be infiltrated, this appears not to be necessary and may actually cause more pain than a quick in-and-out aspiration. It is practical to apply a U-Bag to the perineum prior to cleansing the abdomen. Many times the child voids during preparation for aspiration, obviating the necessity for that procedure if the voided urine is immediately plated or refrigerated.

It has been stated that "any number of colonies" obtained by suprapubic bladder puncture are significant, but that "counts will generally exceed 5,000–10,000/ml of urine" (Kunin, 1979). Since the bladder is a reservoir and this method of collection depicts the number of bacteria in that reservoir, one should not anticipate colony counts significantly different from those properly collected by other means and then handled in a similar manner. Ginsburg and McCracken demonstrated greater than 100,000 colonies per ml in 96 per cent and 40,000 to 80,000 colonies in the remaining 4 per cent of 100 infants 5 days

to 8 months of age with bacilluria demonstrated on SPA. None had fewer than 40,000 colonies. Nelson and Peters had similar results. Colony counts from the bladder of less than 10,000 are suspect regardless of the manner in which that urine was collected.

Reported complications resulting from SPA are few, although transient hematuria is common. Pelvic hematomas requiring transfusion have been noted (Morrell et al). Additionally, a report of two cases of abdominal wall abscesses following aspiration of intestinal contents reinforces the conclusion that a palpable bladder is an absolute prerequisite (Polnay et al).

Culture Techniques

The bacteriology laboratories' calibrated loop culture techniques are being supplemented by less complicated and less expensive methods applicable to standard office use. *No matter the method of culture, the most significant determinant of the interpretive value of the findings on that culture is the time between collection of the specimen and inoculation into the culture medium.* If it is anticipated that inoculation is to be delayed for more than 10 minutes, the specimen should immediately be refrigerated or placed in an ice bath. Urine transported from the patient's home to the office or from the office to the laboratory should be kept in a cold environment.

In the past few years a number of commercial preparations have been introduced that have made office bacteriology both simple and economical. Means of both direct and indirect detection of bacteriuria exist (Craig et al). The popular indirect measurement employs the Griess test. Reagent paper is impregnated with sulfanilic acid and alpha-naphthylamine. Nitrite diazotizes the sulfanilic acid, which then reacts with the alpha-naphthylamine to form a red azo dye. Given adequate contact, bacteria convert nitrate, normally present in the urine, to nitrite. Thus, a positive colorimetric reaction implies the presence of bacteria in the bladder. However, a relatively long incubation period (4 hours) is required for conversion of nitrate to nitrite. For this reason, the first morning urine is really the only reliable specimen for this test. This study might serve as a means of home evaluation for patients being followed with chronic or recurrent cystitis (Kunin and De-Groot) but is probably not a reliable office

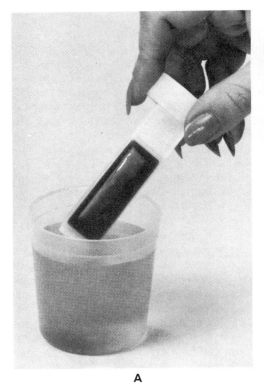

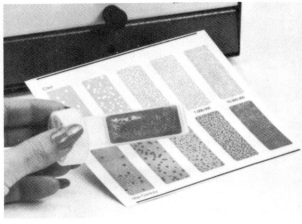

B

Figure 11-4. *A*, Inoculation of the dip slide in urine is demonstrated. *B*, Interpretation of the density of bacterial colonies on the dip slide. (From Schaeffer AJ: The office laboratory. Urol Clin North Am 7:29, 1980.)

A

screening test when used alone (Marr and Traisman).

The direct tests for bacteriuria involve urine culture. Two basic types are available. The first type of test employs a strip of filter paper impregnated with nitrite-sensitive dye and having two areas impregnated with culture media. One of these two media supports only the growth of gram-negative organisms, making it possible to delineate false positives based on gram-positive contaminants. A semi-quantitative colony count is achieved by comparison at 24 to 48 hours through a set of standards. This method correlates fairly accurately in the presence of infection (80 to 90 per cent) and has a low incidence of false negatives (Winter; Craig et al; Gillenwater et al, 1976).

The second type of test utilizes slides coated with culture media. Numerous methods are available and allow for subculturing if antibiotic sensitivities are indicated. A distinction can also be made between gram-negative and gram-positive organisms with the presence of a different medium on each side of the slide. The accuracy of the slide method is comparable to that of the dipstick method, again with few false-negative results. As in all culture techniques, accuracy depends on the rapidity

of inoculation and experience in interpretation (Fig. 11-4).

INCIDENCE

Neonates

The male:female ratio for bacteriuria in neonates is reversed from that seen in older children. The overall incidence of neonatal urinary tract infection has been recorded as 1.4 to 5 per 1,000 live births, with the male:female ratio ranging between 2.8:1 and 5.4:1 (Bergstrom et al; Drew and Acton). The explanation for this observation of a reversed sex ratio remains unclear, although it has been reliably documented and is even more apparent in low-birth-weight and premature neonates (Thrupp et al; Edelmann et al).

Newborn males have a higher incidence of sepsis than newborn females in approximately the same ratio as that for bacteriuria (Buetow et al). The source of the bacteria in urinary tract infections in this age group is thought to be primarily hematogenous and not ascending (Stamey). Nevertheless, 88 per cent of the infecting bacteria are *Escherichia coli* (Ginsburg and McCracken). Although the mature kidney prevents filtration of bacteria from blood into the urine, it would appear that in neonates, particularly in premature infants, circulating bacteria may indeed enter the urine by filtration. If this is true, it would explain both the high incidence of bacteriuria in neonates in the absence of obstructive urinary disease and the increased incidence of bacteriuria in males, who as a group are more susceptible to septicemia. The reason for this increased susceptibility is currently unknown.

School-Age Girls

At least 5 per cent of girls will acquire bacteriuria sometime during their school years (Kunin, 1970; Winberg et al, 1974; Randolph et al, 1975). The prevalence of bacteriuria as demonstrated by Kunin et al in their classic epidemiologic survey is 0.7 per cent in 5- to 9-year-old girls and 0.5 per cent in those 10 to 14 years of age. This trend toward decreasing incidence of bacteriuria with advancing age has been substantiated by others (Meadow et al; DeLuca et al). Additional data on the same population collected by Kunin (1970) reveal that infection will recur in 80 per cent of all white girls and 60 per cent of black girls within 5 years (Fig. 11–5). Fair et al also found that 80 per cent of their patients had recurrences following short-term treatment of a documented urinary tract infection. Belman, in the follow-up of a group of white girls on long-term prophylaxis for recurrent lower urinary tract infection and bladder changes of cystitis cystica (cystitis follicularis), also re-

Table 11–1. Sex Ratio of Urinary Tract Infections

	Females	Males
Neonate	0.4	1
1–6 mos.	1.5	1
6–12 mos.	4.0	1
1–3 yrs.	10.0	1
3–11 yrs.	9.0	1
11–16 yrs.	2.0	1

From Belman AB, Kaplan GW: Genitourinary Problems in Pediatrics. Philadelphia, WB Saunders Co., 1981. Modified from Winberg, J., Andersen, H. J., Bergström, L., et al.: Epidemiology of symptomatic urinary tract infection in childhood. Acta Paediatr. Scand. (Suppl.), 252:1, 1974.

ported an 80 per cent reinfection rate within 1 year following 6 to 12 months of continuous medication.

Boys

The incidence of symptomatic bacteriuria in boys other than neonates is extremely low. In the original survey by Kunin et al only 2 of 7,731 boys studied were found to have asymptomatic bacteriuria. The female : male ratio of children with urinary tract infections at various ages has been noted by Winberg et al (1974) (Table 11–1).

ETIOLOGY

Route of Entry

The route of bacterial entry into the urinary tract in all age groups other than the neonate is thought to be largely retrograde (urethral) in origin; the usual pathogens are fecal flora that contaminate the perineum. Stamey demonstrated that the organisms causing bladder infections in women can be found on perineal culture prior to bladder invasion. In contrast to adult females, in whom bacteria are virtually always found on the perineum, Stamey also noted that two thirds of randomly selected prepubertal girls did not have even a solitary gram-negative bacterium on the introitus on routine culture. Leadbetter and Slavin, and Bollgren and Winberg (1976b) reported that girls with recurrent infections also tend to have colonization of the introitus with the offending organism prior to infection, just as women do. The ensuing conclusion is that

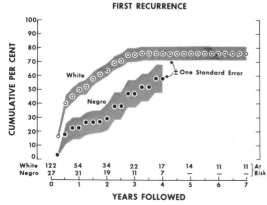

Figure 11–5. Recurrence of bacteriuria in girls following treatment of their first urinary tract infection. (From Kunin CM: The natural history of recurrent bacteriuria in schoolgirls. N Engl J Med 282:1443, 1970.)

the majority of normal girls and women have a degree of introital resistance (perineal defense mechanism) to pathogenic organisms. The mechanism of this resistance has not been elucidated. The susceptible group of females tend to allow perineal colonization with pathogenic organisms, presumably because of the absence of this defense mechanism.

Bollgren and Winberg (1976a) found massive aerobic periurethral bacterial flora in normal children of both sexes in the first few weeks of life. The numbers decrease during the first year of life, and the presence of periurethral pathogens becomes rare after 5 years.

The Urethra and Bladder

In addition to the as yet undetermined perineal defense mechanism described above, the urethra may also play a mechanical role preventing bladder contamination. Although particles instilled in the distal urethra in animals were noted in the urinary bladder after voiding (Corriere et al), none could be found in the bladder of girls based solely on spontaneous vulvourethral reflux (Ericsson et al).

Urethral caliber, chronically blamed as the pre-eminent factor influencing susceptibility to lower urinary tract infections in girls, probably plays little, if any, role. It has long been recognized that intrinsic urethral luminal size is not significantly different between those girls who become bacteriuric and those who are never infected (Graham et al; Immergut and Wahman). In fact, both studies demonstrated that urethral diameter was slightly larger in infected groups than in those never infected.

When bacteria find their way into the urinary tract, their elimination by frequent and complete bladder emptying plays a significant role in preventing infection. In a group of girls followed with asymptomatic bacteriuria (ABU), the incidence of recurrence related directly to bladder emptying. Average residual volumes in those with ABU was 23.7 ml, whereas normal controls had a mean residual volume of 1.1 ml. On follow-up, recurrences were present in 75 per cent of those with more than 5 ml of residual urine, while only 17 per cent of those with less than 5 ml of residual urine had recurrences (Lindberg, Bjure, et al).

After bacteria have found their way into the bladder, their adherence to the bladder wall appears to be inhibited by epithelial mucopolysaccharide (Parsons et al). The success of certain E. coli strains to resist washout relates to their pathogenicity; those most likely to cause clinical infections are those with the greatest ability to adhere to bladder epithelial cells (Svanborg Edén et al).

Immunology

Efforts have also been made to understand the mechanisms of immunologic response at the bladder level. Uehling and King recorded increased urinary IgA levels in children with chronic cystitis but were unable to appreciate any degree of resistance in this group. Indeed, it would appear that they fit into a relatively recalcitrant group despite (or because of) the apparently activated immune system. Clark et al were unable to find a circulating systemic antibody response to cystitis. However, Dubroff et al found a positive delayed phytohemagglutinin hypersensitivity response to cystitis equal to that of other acute infections. All this would appear to attest to the normalcy of the local and systemic immune mechanisms of children who develop urinary tract infection.

Efforts have been made to correlate immune mechanism abnormalities with upper urinary tract infection. There is no evidence demonstrating an abnormal response or immune deficit in this group either, except in infants under 2 months of age (Winberg et al, 1963).

There is no question, however, that the role immunology plays as it pertains to urinary tract infection has yet to be uncovered. Tamm-Horsfall glycoprotein antibodies are elevated following pyelonephritis and are highest in those individuals who also have vesicoureteral reflux. Yet, in the presence of renal scarring T-H antibodies are significantly depressed (Jodal and Fasth). The level of vaginal IgA in girls with a history of urinary tract infection is significantly lower as compared with those having nocturnal enuresis alone (Tuttle et al). Finally, 70 per cent of pyelonephritis is caused by only five different K capsular polysaccharide antigen E. coli types (Kaijser et al). The significance of these data awaits clinical correlation.

Heredity

As it becomes increasingly apparent that the primary underlying factor influencing susceptibility to urinary tract infection is perineal immunology, it is not surprising to discover that heredity plays a role. Kunin et al

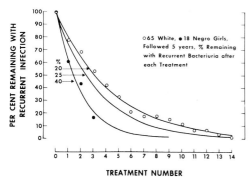

Figure 11–6. Theoretical rates of extraction of schoolgirls into remission after short courses of specific chemotherapy directed toward each episode of recurrence. Rates are presented for removal of 20, 25, and 40 per cent for each treatment. The observed percentage remaining in the population which required further treatment is superimposed on the theoretical projections for white and black girls followed for 5 years. (From Kunin CM: The natural history of recurrent bacteriuria in schoolgirls. N Engl J Med 282:1443, 1970.)

reported a 1.2 per cent bacteriuric prevalence rate in white girls versus a rate of 0.5 per cent in black girls in the same age group. In a retrospective review the number of black girls evaluated following urinary tract infection was one third that of white girls at an institution with equal numbers of black and white girls hospitalized (Askari and Belman). It is also evident that the rate of recurrent bacteriuria is racially dependent. Kunin (1970) reported an 80 per cent recurrence rate in white girls, while in black girls the rate was only 60 percent (Fig. 11–6). Additionally, it is becoming evident that daughters of mothers who had been bacteriuric in childhood have a higher incidence of UTI and female siblings tend also to have a higher incidence of bacteriuria (Gillenwater et al, 1979; Fennell et al, 1977).

Constipation

A definite correlation exists between constipation and the incidence of lower urinary tract infections. It is unclear if this correlation is based on increased bacterial contamination, mechanical voiding factors relating to a large mass of stool compressing the bladder outlet, or a relationship between infrequent voiding and constipation. Neumann et al found a marked improvement in recurrence rate of UTI with improvement in bowel habits. An important part in obtaining the patient's history is a careful documentation of the frequency of bowel movements. Additionally, symptoms ranging from severe urinary frequency to overflow incontinence can result from a fecal impaction. Rectal examination as a routine part of the physical examination should be considered in this group of patients.

Irritation

Local urethral factors have been implicated as playing a causative role in UTI. Bubble bath and pinworms are two most commonly indicted; however, objective data supporting irritation as an underlying cause of infection is lacking. It is important to recognize that the symptoms caused by introital or urethral irritation may in fact mimic those of infection (Demetriou et al). The differentiation is made primarily by urine culture.

MICROBIOLOGY

Bacterial Infections

Approximately 80 per cent of urinary tract infections are caused by E. coli. The majority of the remainder are due to Proteus, Klebsiella, Enterobacter, and Pseudomonas. Identification of these organisms by standard culture techniques is routine and available in all laboratories and many office practices.

The pathogenicity of different organisms appears to vary and may account for the presence of renal involvement in some cases and not in others. A high correlation exists between pyelonephritis and specific types of E. coli. Seventy per cent of pyelonephritis can be accounted for by E. coli types K1, 2, 3, 12, and 13 (K capsular polysaccharide antigen) (Kaijser et al) (Fig. 11–7). Eight specific O antigen types were found to cause 80 per cent of pyelonephritis in a report published by Lindberg et al (1975). Interestingly, these types accounted for slightly less than 60 per cent of the E. coli causing cystitis and only 31 per cent of those involved in asymptomatic bacteriuria. It may be that an asymptomatic patient infected with a less virulent bacterial form is better left untreated to avoid the risk of reinfection with a more pathogenic type.

Occasionally organisms not usually considered as urinary pathogens are isolated from the urinary tract. Hermansson et al reported 15 of 525 children in whom coagulase-negative staphylococci were identified as a cause

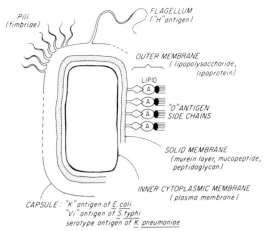

Pili (timbriae)

FLAGELLUM ("H" antigen)

OUTER MEMBRANE (lipopolysaccharide, lipoprotein)

LIPID

"O" ANTIGEN SIDE CHAINS

SOLID MEMBRANE (murein layer, mucopeptide, peptidoglycan)

INNER CYTOPLASMIC MEMBRANE (plasma membrane)

CAPSULE: "K" antigen of E. coli "Vi" antigen of S. typhi serotype antigen of K. pneumoniae

Figure 11–7. Schematic presentation of the antigenic structure of gram-negative enteric bacteria. (From Young LS, Martin WJ, Meyer RD, et al: Gram-negative rod bacteremia: microbiologic, immunologic, and therapeutic considerations. Ann Int Med 86:456, 1977.)

of symptomatic urinary tract infections in children. Although rare in young children, these organisms represented 41 per cent of those isolated in the 11 to 15 year age group. Maskell also reported coagulase-negative staphylococci (micrococcus 3) as the most common organism in sexually active females. He found it difficult to grow these bacteria on standard culture media. In older boys both staphylococci and streptococci are not infrequently found as infecting organisms.

Urinary infections have been attributed to *Hemophilus influenzae* type B (Granoff and Roskes). *H. influenzae* epididymo-orchitis in infant males probably secondary to hematogenous spread has also been recently recognized (Thomas et al). Anaerobic bacteria including *Fusobacterium nucleatum, Bacteroides fragilis* and *melaninogenicus, Peptococcus asaccharolyticus* and *Bifidobacterium adolescentis* have been reported as urinary pathogens and may account for 1 to 2 per cent of all urinary infections (Segura et al; Brook; Ribot et al). Immune deficient individuals appear to be the most susceptible. Anaerobic bacteria, *H. influenzae*, and coagulase-negative staphylococci are poorly grown on standard culture media. Special techniques become necessary when the clinical situation suggests the possibility of urinary infections caused by any of these agents.

Viral Cystitis

The clinical picture of severe urinary frequency, urgency, incontinence, and gross hematuria with clots in the face of a negative routine urine culture suggests acute viral cystitis. Adenoviruses 11 and 21 are the most common offending organisms (Mufson et al, 1973). The bladder changes that result can be quite impressive and may mimic the picture of bladder sarcoma (Fig. 11–8A). However, the symptom complex is acute and quite typical,

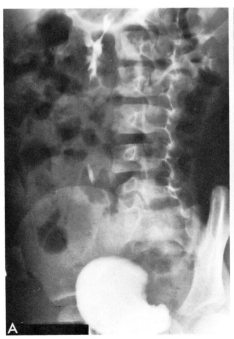

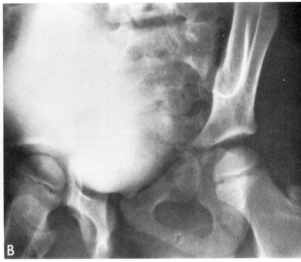

Figure 11–8. A, Excretory urogram in a girl with acute viral hemorrhagic cystitis demonstrating filling defect on posterior wall of bladder. B, Cystogram phase of excretory urogram 2 weeks following acute viral hemorrhagic cystitis. Filling defect in bladder has resolved.

Table 11-2. Prominent Symptoms in Neonatal* Nonobstructive UTI (N = 75)

Symptom	Per Cent
Weight loss†	76
Fever	49
Cyanosis or gray color	40
Distended abdomen	16
CNS symptoms (purulent meningitis not included)	23
Generalized convulsions	7
Purulent meningitis	8
Jaundice (conjugated bilirubin increased)	7
Other	16

From Harrison JH, Gittes RF, Perlmutter AD, et al: Campbell's Urology. Fourth ed. Vol. 1. Philadelphia, WB Saunders Co., 1978.

* Zero to 30 days old.

† Registered for only 46 patients falling ill on days 0 to 10. Weight loss was not explained by vomiting, diarrhea, or refusal to eat.

and both hematuria and x-ray changes resolve within 2 to 3 weeks (Fig. 11-8B). Cystoscopy is not recommended in this group unless a mass is felt on bimanual rectal exam or the bladder lesion does not resolve in that period of time. Since this is not an ascending infection, one can presume that no anatomic urinary tract abnormalities underlie viral cystitis, and evaluation is not recommended if

the diagnosis is confirmed (Mufson et al, 1971).

CLINICAL PRESENTATION AND LOCALIZATION

As one would anticipate, the classic symptoms and signs of UTI do not present themselves in the very young. Instead, nonspecific symptoms such as irritability, poor feeding, failure to gain weight, vomiting, and diarrhea may be the only suggestions of an underlying problem (Table 11-2). Fever is often absent in this group. As the child reaches the toddler age, more classic symptoms present themselves, with fever as the most common. A screening urine culture is required whenever a nonverbal, non-toilet-trained child presents with unexplained fever.

As the child becomes verbal and toilet training can be anticipated, urinary tract pathology is more readily recognizable. Through the years the peak time of diagnosis of urinary tract infection has been at age 3 years. It is obvious, however, that infection occurs more frequently in younger children but is often missed, although fever is a frequent concomitant in this group (Fig. 11-9). Urgency, frequency, enuresis, and dysuria are the common presenting symptoms in older children. Failure to become toilet trained at the proper

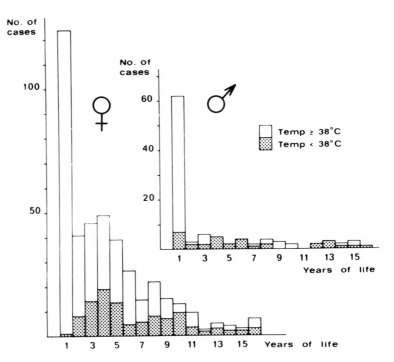

Figure 11-9. Apparently primary onset of urinary tract infection in 419 girls and 104 boys between 2 months and 16 years of age (neonates zero to 30 days old excluded.) The proportion of nonfebrile infections was very small during the first year of life but increased with age. Fifty-four male and 21 female neonatal infections were not included. (From Winberg J, Andersen HJ, Bergström T, et al: Epidemiology of symptomatic urinary tract infection in childhood. Acta Pediatr Scand (Suppl 252):1, 1974.)

age is frequently a sign of unrecognized chronic lower urinary tract infection.

Pyelonephritis

Febrile urinary tract infections suggest renal involvement and the presence of vesicoureteral reflux (Govan and Palmer). Reliable laboratory attempts at objectively localizing the site of infection have not met with great success. The presence of antibody-coated bacteria in the urine, a means of differentiating renal involvement, was reported as moderately successful by Pylkkänen. Antibody-coated bacteria were noted in 76 per cent of those who had symptomatic pyelonephritis for *more* than 1 week. Generally, however, this test has not been found to be reliable in children.

Elevated C-reactive protein levels (greater than or equal to 30 μg/ml) correlated well with the diagnosis of pyelonephritis as determined by clinical findings (temperature greater than 38.4° C and constitutional complaints) (Wientzen et al; Jodal et al). Lorentz and Reznick noted elevation of urinary LDH isoenzymes in 14 of 15 with positive upper tract cultures and found that LDH levels correlated as anticipated in 14 of 14 with lower urinary tract infection. Absolute confirmation of upper versus lower tract infection can be determined by direct thin-needle aspiration of renal pelvic urine under ultrasonic guidance, the bladder washout test (Fairley et al), or split urine cultures collected by ureteral catheterization (Table 11–3).

Pyelonephritis in childhood in the absence of obstruction is almost always a consequence of bacterial infection plus vesicoureteral as well as pyelotubular reflux (Ransley and Risdon, 1978). Renal damage and scarring appear to occur almost exclusively in children under 5 years of age and most frequently in children under 1 year. New scarring in older children and adults is exceedingly rare (Hodson and Wilson).

This potential for severe renal scarring in infants reinforces the necessity for early recognition. Welch et al reported scars developing in 41 per cent of neonates with bacteriuria and septicemia. Although lower rates of scarring have been reported in other studies, the incidence of reflux in neonates with bacteriuria has been reported to be close to 50 per cent by virtually all observers. The recurrent infection rate within the first year was reported as 25 per cent by Bergstrom et al. A single episode of pyelonephritis in infancy can lead to significant renal damage (Fig. 11–10). Ransley and Risdon (1980) suggest that the portions of the kidney at risk are those susceptible to pyelotubular backflow.

Progressive renal scarring is probably the result of repeated episodes of infection (Filly et al). In nonobstructed systems bacteria cannot be isolated from the kidney after an adequate course of antibiotic therapy, suggesting that a chronic or indolent form of bacterial pyelonephritis does not exist. However, an ongoing antigen-antibody reaction may be set up leading to progressive damage in some (Intorp et al). This may be the underlying explanation for the extremes of reflux nephropathy presenting in late adolescence and early adulthood with renal insufficiency and severe hypertension (Lloyd-Still and Cottom; Stickler et al). This has also been referred to as pyelonephritis lenta (MacGregor), and its presence demonstrates the importance of discovering reflux early and preventing further episodes of infection.

FOCAL BACTERIAL NEPHRITIS. An unusual form of pyelonephritis termed "focal bacterial nephritis" or acute lobar nephronia has occasionally been recognized presenting as a renal mass. Reflux is present in the majority of these cases, and its diagnosis may be confused with abscess or tumor. Localized parenchymal density is reduced, and on sonography the renal substance is ill defined with areas of liquefaction (Siegel and Glasier; Rosenfield et al).

RENAL ABSCESS. Renal abscesses are another rare form of renal infection that, in the past, were generally not thought to be caused by ascending infection. *Staphylococcus aureus* has historically been the offending organism, and in most cases a peripheral cutaneous site of origin could be localized. Lebowitz et al applied four etiologic categories to this problem: (1) a minor remote bacterial focus in a child who is otherwise well; (2) a

Table 11–3. Split Cultures

Culture Site	Colony Count
Bladder	100,000 *Enterococcus*, group D
Bladder wash	15,000 *Enterococcus*, group D
Left renal pelvis	25,000 *Enterococcus*, group D
Right renal pelvis	80,000 *Enterococcus*, group D

Example of split cultures that localize urinary tract infection in both kidneys as well as the bladder, thus proving the presence of upper tract infection. (From Belman AB, Kaplan GW: Genitourinary Problems in Pediatrics. Philadelphia, WB Saunders Co., 1981.)

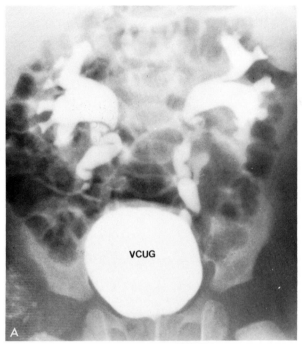

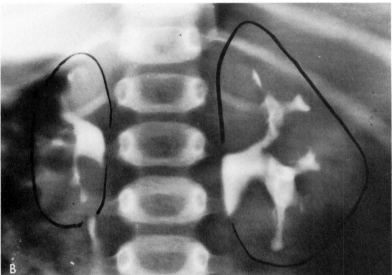

Figure 11–10. *A,* Cystogram in a 6-month-old boy with a single febrile urinary tract infection. The kidneys appear of equal size. *B,* Excretory urogram 2 years later demonstrating a small right kidney. This picture is typical of the potential effects of bacterial pyelonephritis associated with reflux in infancy. (From Belman AB, Kaplan GW: Genitourinary Problems in Pediatrics. Philadelphia, WB Saunders Co., 1981.)

structural urinary abnormality; (3) another organ defect; (4) a defective host response due to systemic illness. One can predict that a gram-positive organism will be present in group 1, and a gram-negative organism in group 2. However, the organisms in groups 3 and 4 are not predictable. Cases have recently been reported in children in which gram-neg-

ative organisms in the presence of vesicoureteral reflux are most common (Timmons and Perlmutter; Rote et al). It may be that these are more accurately examples of focal bacterial nephritis rather than classic renal cortical abscesses.

XANTHOGRANULOMATOUS PYELONEPHRITIS. Xanthogranulomatous pyelonephritis is rare in children; 15 cases have been reported to date in the English-language literature (Bagley et al). Two types appear to exist: focal involvement more commonly occurring in girls (9 of 9), whereas 5 of 6 boys had diffuse involvement. All those kidneys with diffuse xanthogranulomatous pyelonephritis were nonfunctioning and renal or ureteral calculi were present. No calculi have been reported in those with focal involvement. Yazaki et al added 8 cases from the Japanese literature. All were diffusely involved with no associated functioning renal tissue. Of the 8 affected Japanese children, 7 were male.

Cystitis

Lower urinary tract symptoms alone in the absence of fever suggest cystitis without reflux and renal involvement. Only 6 per cent of 46 patients with urinary tract infections but no demonstrated reflux had systemic complaints, whereas 80 per cent of 55 children with infections and reflux had a history of fever and abdominal pain and were toxic (Govan and Palmer). Although the recurrence rate of lower urinary tract infections is high, most cases can be considered little more than a nuisance, and recurrences will tend to disappear by adolescence. However, slightly less than 10 per cent of girls susceptible to urinary infection will go on to have recurrences virtually at the completion of each course of antibiotic therapy. Symptoms of severe urgency, frequency, and urinary incontinence accompanied by bladder spasms become con-

stant. Squatting in response to these spasms is common in this group (Fig. 11–11). Endoscopically, multiple raised "cysts" are seen in the area of the bladder neck and trigone. Histologically, submucosal lymphoid follicles are present (Fig. 11–12). Clinically, this entity has been termed cystitis cystica, although the histologic appearance suggests it would be more accurately referred to as cystitis follicularis. The presence of these follicles suggests an immunologic response to chronic infection (Uehling and King).

Asymptomatic Bacteriuria

The presence of unrecognized bacteriuria in 0.5 to 1.6 per cent of school girls at any one time (Kunin et al; Emans et al) suggests that in many girls urinary bacteria do not present a health hazard. In a review of 116 girls with asymptomatic bacteriuria Lindberg et al (1978) found that 21 per cent had reflux, 10 per cent had reduction of renal parenchymal size, and 30 per cent had previous urinary tract infections. Follow-up by the Cardiff-Oxford Bacteriuria Study Group revealed that those children who presented initially with a radiographically normal urinary tract remained normal in spite of persistent infections. Only those children who had previous renal scarring developed new scars or had progression of scarring, and all of these children had vesicoureteral reflux. Nevertheless, all children, even those with progressive scarring, continued to grow normally and had normal blood pressure at the end of 4 years of follow-up.

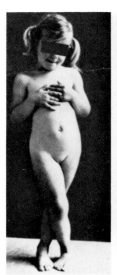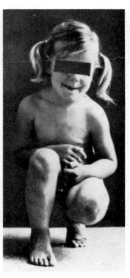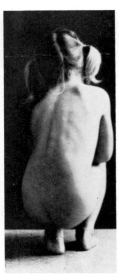

Figure 11–11. Typical posturing of child with the *urge syndrome*, characterized by an unpredictable urge to void, often associated with urge incontinence. To avoid wetting, the child assumes a posture that provides for external urethral compression, usually by squatting onto one heel until the urgency disappears. The urge incontinence is often associated with diurnal or nocturnal enuresis and may be associated with infection in some cases, although for many children the syndrome appears to be an abnormality of micturition. (From DeJonge GA: The urge syndrome. *In* Bladder Control and Enuresis. Edited by I Kolvin, RC MacKeith, SR Meadow. London, W. Heinemann Medical Books, Ltd., 1973.)

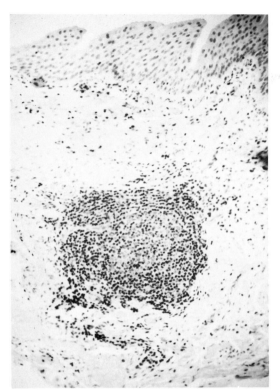

Figure 11-12. "Cystitis cystica." Submucosal lymphoid follicle (cystitis follicularis) is typical of the histologic changes seen in children with long-standing cystitis. (From Belman AB, Kaplan GW: Genitourinary Problems in Pediatrics. Philadelphia, WB Saunders Co., 1981.)

EVALUATION

The evidence strongly supports the necessity for radiographic evaluation after the first urinary tract infection in all boys and white girls. Recurrence can be anticipated in 80 per cent, and one third will have reflux. Reflux has been reported in over half of children under 3 years of age who have UTI (Monahan and Resnick). Additionally, how can one be sure that the presenting infection is indeed the "first infection"? In a carefully controlled health environment (Sweden) 4.5 per cent of 440 girls with their "first" UTI already had established renal scarring. Seventeen per cent of 41 with a known second infection had scars (Winberg et al, 1975).

The necessity for evaluating black girls raises additional questions. It is apparent that both the prevalence and recurrence of urinary infections are less in this group (Kunin et al). Additionally, there is strong evidence that vesicoureteral reflux is also significantly reduced (Askari and Belman). Evaluation in black girls might well be reserved for infants and those with febrile urinary tract infections.

Evaluation includes a preliminary radiograph (plain film) followed by a dynamic cystogram with a urethrogram in all males. The spine should be carefully inspected and attention paid to the amount of stool in the colon. Visualization of the urethra in females is helpful only in those rare individuals with refluxing ectopic ureters. The radiographic configuration of the female urethra otherwise adds nothing to the evaluation (Lyon). The most common abnormality found is vesicoureteral reflux. For this reason one might consider screening the urinary tract with an isotope cystogram in girls, since urethral visualization is unimportant. In males, however, visualization of the urethra is needed to rule out urethral obstruction.

A post-void film is helpful to demonstrate if the bladder empties. Failure to empty the bladder completely may have no significance, however, in a child facing an anxiety-provoking radiographic study. Filled bladder capacity should also be noted. An especially large bladder suggests a history of infrequent voiding. This is often found in conjunction with large amounts of stool in the colon. Visualization of the upper tract is classically obtained by excretory urogram. On the other hand, renal sonography is an alternative method of screening for renal number, size, and position. Obstruction is readily recognizable sonographically. Radioisotope renography is also a means of evaluating the upper urinary tract; early flow studies and computerization add the potential for an objective baseline assessment of renal function. Additionally, in children under 3 to 4 months of age, renal visualization can be difficult to obtain by excretory urography because of poor concentrating ability and excessive bowel gas (Fig. 11-13).

The timing of radiographic evaluation has been a topic of recent interest. It has been suggested that studies should be delayed 4 to 6 weeks following the acute inflammatory episode to avoid demonstrating transient low grade vesicoureteral reflux. Grade I/V reflux in the absence of scarring or a febrile infection may have no clinical relevance. On the other hand, the absence of reflux in a child with a febrile UTI suggests transient intrarenal reflux at the time of the acute episode, and serious consideration should be given long-term antibiotic prophylaxis.

Regardless of when studies are performed, it is recommended that patients with febrile

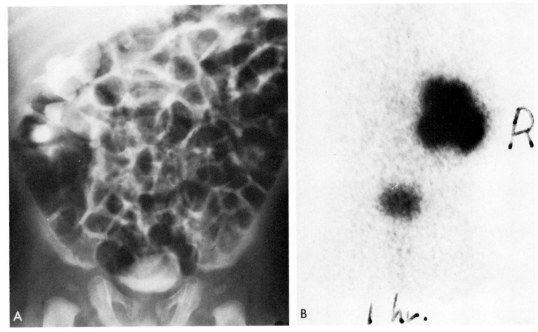

Figure 11–13. *A,* Excretory urogram in newborn with right flank mass. Hydronephrotic system is visible on the right. Excessive bowel gas obscured adequate interpretation on the left. *B,* Delayed renal scan in the same patient (posterior view). Hydronephrosis secondary to ureteropelvic junction obstruction is evident. No isotope is present on the left to indicate renal presence or function on that side. Imagine the consequences if one had thought that a collecting system was present on the left and removal of the right hydronephrotic kidney had been elected. (From Belman AB, Kaplan GW: Genitourinary Problems in Pediatrics. Philadelphia, WB Saunders Co., 1981.)

UTI be maintained on prophylaxis until that time and that children requiring hospitalization at least be screened for obstruction prior to discharge. Trimethoprim-sulfamethoxazole or nitrofurantoin is the drug of choice for prophylaxis prior to radiographic evaluation and is started as soon as the initial medication is discontinued.

Cystoscopy no longer plays a diagnostic role in the evaluation of the urinary tract in children with UTI. No additional information can be acquired in those who have a normal urinary tract demonstrated by an adequate radiographic study (Johnson et al). Although prognosis may be predicted in those with cystitis cystica (cystitis follicularis) or vesicoureteral reflux, an unexpected finding at cystoscopy cannot be anticipated.

More sophisticated studies including computed tomography, arteriography, or gallium scanning are rarely necessary in children with urinary tract infection. Nonetheless, to establish the correct diagnosis of renal cortical abscess, focal bacterial nephritis, or xanthogranulomatous pyelonephritis, these studies may occasionally be required (Fig. 11–14).

TREATMENT

Acute Infection

The initial treatment should, ideally, be based on in vitro antibiotic sensitivities. Frequently treatment is initiated before these results are available. As a general rule, success can be anticipated with the tried-and-true urinary "antiseptics" for the first infection. Sulfa, nitrofurantoin, or nalidixic acid can be used as the initial drug in the nonfebrile child with her "first" urinary tract infection. Unfortunately, ampicillin and amoxicillin are used commonly by primary health care physicians. High intestinal levels result in rapid development of resistant enteric organisms, which then become the infecting bacteria. This limits the effectiveness of these synthetic penicillins as first-line urinary tract agents.

The child with suspected pyelonephritis requires a greater degree of assurance of immediate therapeutic success since the degree of scarring and renal damage resulting from an infection can be influenced by the rapidity of effective therapy (Ransley and Risdon, 1980).

Oral medication can be initiated in those who are not septic or vomiting. Trimethoprim-sulfamethoxazole is not used frequently by the pediatric practitioner and can be anticipated to be effective. Additionally, bowel flora returns to normal within 1 month of discontinuation of this combination antibacterial agent (Grüneberg, et al).

Cephalosporins are rarely used by pediatricians and are a good choice for initial therapy in the febrile child who does not require parenteral therapy. Treatment can be changed to less expensive agents when the antibiotic sensitivities become known.

The toxic child or infant under 1 year old with suspected pyelonephritis is a candidate for immediate parenteral therapy. After appropriate cultures (blood, urine, and cerebrospinal fluid) have been obtained, combination therapy including an aminoglycoside and synthetic penicillin are initiated.

Prophylaxis

Long-term *continuous* prophylaxis is recommended in those children under 7 to 8 years of age with vesicoureteral reflux and those with frequent recurrences (greater than four per year) or endoscopically demonstrated cystitis cystica (cystitis follicularis). The effectiveness and safety of trimethoprim-sulfamethoxazole and nitrofurantoin have been proved (Smellie and Grüneberg). Pure sulfamethoxazole is less effective than either of these, and synthetic penicillins are poor pro-

phylactic agents and should not be used beyond the usual 10 day course. Methenamine requires a highly acid environment and at least 2 hours for sufficient formaldehyde to be liberated for bactericidal activity. Therefore, this group can be anticipated to be effective only in the presence of urinary stasis.

Prophylaxis prevents infection but cannot be expected to reduce the recurrence rate of urinary infection after therapy has been discontinued (Fennell et al, 1980). In those with cystitis cystica (cystitis follicularis), 80 per cent had recurrences within 1 year after 6 to 12 months of continuous prophylaxis (Belman).

Short-Course Therapy

Recently single-dose or short-course antimicrobial therapy has come into vogue in the treatment of uncomplicated adult female urinary tract infections. Studies using a short-acting sulfa, nitrofurantoin, trimethoprim-sulfamethoxazole, or amoxicillin all demonstrate a satisfactory immediate response to both single doses and a 3-day mini-course in children with *uncomplicated* lower urinary tract infections (Shapiro and Wald; Pitt et al; Lohr et al; Kallenius and Winberg). Long-term recurrence rates were not appreciably different between those having single-dose or short-course therapy and those treated for 7 to 10 days, although those treated with a single dose or short-term course tended to have recurrences more rapidly than those treated for 10 days.

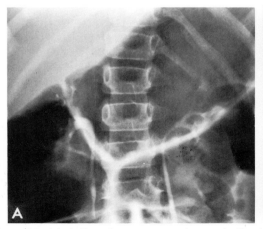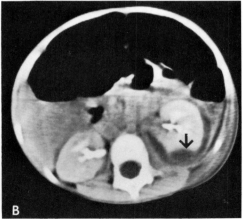

Figure 11–14. *A*, Excretory urogram demonstrating lateral deviation of left upper collecting system in a child with flank pain and fever. *B*, Computed tomographic cut revealing a filling defect in the upper pole of the left kidney confirming the diagnosis of renal parenchymal abscess.

Antibacterial Agents

SULFONAMIDES. Sulfonamides act by competitively blocking the conversion of para-aminobenzoic acid to folic acid (Feingold). About 75 per cent of the oral dose is absorbed. Free sulfonamide is excreted by filtration and tubular secretion. Although high tissue levels are not achieved, excellent urine levels result. Sulfonamides are most effective against *E. coli* but also may be effective against other gram-negative and gram-positive organisms. Sensitivity testing for this class of drugs is not particularly useful when the disk method is employed.

Sulfonamides are well tolerated by children, are inexpensive, and have few side effects. They affect the gastrointestinal flora when used for long-term prophylaxis but are effective agents for short-term acute therapy of uncomplicated infections. They displace protein-bound bilirubin and hence in the neonate have the potential to interfere with bilirubin excretion and cause jaundice. Once the infant has passed through the period of "physiologic jaundice" these agents can be utilized safely. Some patients are allergic to sulfa, but fortunately most reactions are of a minor cutaneous nature such as urticaria. There have been some problems with major hypersensitivity reactions such as the Stevens-Johnson syndrome, but these are rare. The most widely used agent is sulfisoxazole employed in a dose of 150 mg/kg of body weight per day, given acutely in four to six divided doses orally (Vaughan and McKay).

NITROFURANTOIN. Nitrofurantoin is quite useful in the treatment of simple cystitis and is also a very effective agent for long term low dose prophylaxis. It is thought to interfere with early stages of the bacterial Krebs cycle (AMA Drug Evaluations). It is well absorbed from the gastrointestinal tract and has minimal effect on bowel flora. Tissue levels are low because it is excreted almost entirely in the urine by glomerular filtration. Urinary levels tend to be quite high. Urinary alkalinization increases urine levels, whereas acidification increases tissue levels. It works well against most *E. coli* and enterococci but is not particularly effective against *Klebsiella, Proteus,* or *Pseudomonas.*

Nausea and vomiting are frequent troublesome side effects in children; however, these can be minimized by administering the agent immediately following a meal or by utilizing nitrofurantoin macrocrystals supplied in capsule form. For the small child the contents of the capsule can be emptied and administered dry on bread or in potatoes or applesauce.

In neonates nitrofurantoin has the potential to cause a hemolytic anemia due to glutathione instability. Consequently it should not be used in this age group. Additionally, the drug is ineffective in patients with significant renal impairment. Other side effects are rare but do include peripheral neuropathy and pulmonary infiltrates. The usual dose is 6 mg/kg/day given orally in three to four divided doses (Vaughan and McKay, 1975).

TRIMETHOPRIM - SULFAMETHOXAZOLE. The trimethoprim-sulfamethoxazole combination is useful both in the management of simple cystitis and for long-term antibacterial prophylaxis. This combination has a diminished effect on bowel flora and has the advantage of entering vaginal secretions in the adult female (Stamey et al). This latter characteristic appears to be of particular utility in its effectiveness as a prophylactic agent. Trimethoprim interferes with dihydrofolic acid reductase, while sulfa blocks the conversion of para-aminobenzoic acid to dihydrofolic acid. The combination is effective against many gram-negative as well as gram-positive organisms. It is well absorbed, attains high levels in both serum and urine, and is well tolerated by children. Neutropenia and thrombocytopenia are not uncommon with its use. The significance of these changes, however, is unknown (Asmar et al).

The combination is available as a suspension containing 40 mg of trimethoprim and 200 mg of sulfamethoxazole per 5 ml. The dose employed is 10 mg of trimethoprim and 50 mg of sulfamethoxazole per kg of body weight per day in two divided doses (Howard and Howard).

NALIDIXIC ACID. Nalidixic acid is an antibacterial agent that produces good urinary levels and is effective against gram-negative organisms. It is especially effective against *Proteus.* Previous negative reports regarding the effectiveness of this agent can probably be accounted for by inadequate dosage (Stamey and Bragonzi, 1976). Nalidixic acid is well absorbed from the gastrointestinal tract and is readily tolerated by children. It is rapidly inactivated by the liver. It is thought to interfere with DNA synthesis. The development of pseudotumor cerebri has been reported as a complication of its use in children (Anderson et al). Nalidixic acid is available in both tablet and suspension form and the recommended dose is 50 mg/kg/day in two to four divided doses (Vaughan and McKay).

METHENAMINE MANDELATE AND METHENAMINE HIPPURATE. These agents are readily absorbed from the intestinal tract and remain inactive until they are excreted by the kidney and concentrated in the urine. Methenamine in an acid urine is converted to the bactericidal agent formaldehyde; however, this conversion takes a minimum of 2 hours to achieve adequate bactericidal levels. Mandelic and hippuric acids are urinary acidifiers that have some additional inherent but weak antibacterial agent. Efficacy of methenamine may be enhanced further by supplementary urinary acidification, such as with ascorbic acid. Both can cause dysuria when administered in high doses, and methenamine mandelate has on rare occasions produced hemorrhagic cystisis (Ross and Conway). The recommended dose for these agents is 40 to 50 mg/kg per day given orally in two to three divided doses (Vaughan and McKay, 1975).

PENICILLIN. The penicillins as a class are probably the most widely used antibiotics. All act by blocking mucopeptide synthesis in the cell walls so that the bacterium is unprotected from its high internal osmotic pressure (Goodman and Gilman, 1970). This effect occurs only in growing cells, however. These agents should not be administered to patients with a known history of penicillin allergy.

Penicillin G. Extremely high urine levels can be achieved with penicillin G in patients with normal renal function, and under those circumstances this drug may be very effective against both E. coli and Proteus. Its major toxic effect is allergy manifested by rash or anaphylaxis.

Ampicillin. Ampicillin is the most widely used penicillin in the treatment of urinary tract infections. It is not well absorbed from the gastrointestinal tract; therefore, high fecal levels do occur and diarrhea is common. High serum and urine concentrations are achievable. The usual dose is 50 to 200 mg/kg/day given every 6 to 8 hours. It can be administered either orally or intravenously (Vaughan and McKay, 1975).

Amoxicillin. Amoxicillin is a derivative of ampicillin that is absorbed more readily and therefore produces less diarrhea. It is administered orally in a dose of 20 to 40 mg/kg/day every 6 to 8 hours (Vaughan and McKay, 1975).

Carbenicillin. Carbenicillin is an agent that is especially useful in the treatment of Pseudomonas and indole-positive Proteus. It is available as tablets and as a parenteral solution. When it is used parenterally for urinary tract infection in children, the usual dose is 50 to 200 mg/kg/24 hours given every 4 to 6 hours (Vaughan and McKay, 1975). The oral form is not predictably effective in children.

CEPHALOSPORINS. Cephalosporins are usually effective against most of the gram-negative and gram-positive pathogens. Excretion is by both glomerular filtration and tubular secretion. Although there can be some cross reactivity in patients who are allergic to penicillin in general, these agents can be cautiously administered to patients with penicillin allergy. Cephalexin is well absorbed from the gastrointestinal tract and can be given orally in a dose of 25 to 100 mg/kg/day. Parenteral forms include cefazolin, cephalothin, and cephapirin (Vaughan and McKay, 1975).

AMINOGLYCOSIDES. The aminoglycosides are well tolerated by children and are of special utility in the treatment of complicated gram-negative urinary tract infections. They interfere with protein synthesis by binding proteins of the bacterial ribosomes.

Gentamicin. Gentamicin is probably the most widely used of the aminoglycosides in children and is especially effective against Pseudomonas. The usual pediatric dose is 5 to 7.5 mg/kg/day parenterally in two or three divided doses depending upon age. It achieves high tissue concentration and can be ototoxic particularly to the vestibular cells. Nephrotoxicity also occurs in 3 to 6 per cent of patients and should be watched for by checking serum creatinine periodically during the course of therapy. Nephrotoxicity occurs particularly frequently when gentamicin is given in combination with cephalosporins. Both ototoxicity and nephrotoxicity are usually transient.

Tobramycin. A newer aminoglycoside, tobramycin has the advantage of particular efficacy against Pseudomonas. It is said to be less nephrotoxic than gentamicin (Kurnin).

TETRACYCLINES. *Tetracyclines should not be used in children under 8 years of age because they stain the permanent teeth.* The need for tetracycline is extremely unusual in modern-day pediatrics.

Treatment in Renal Failure

The dynamics of antibiotic detoxification and excretion are usually deranged in the child with renal failure. Antibacterial doses need to be adjusted in such patients to avoid adverse reactions. Certain drugs—those dependent on renal function for efficacy — are useless in these patients. The frequency of administration of those drugs that are effective in the face of renal failure, rather than their dosages, should be modified based on the degree of renal insufficiency.

Specific Therapy

In addition to appropriate antimicrobial therapy, other factors must be taken into consideration in patient management. *Voiding frequency* and control of *constipation* are the two most common variables that are readily changeable and may be the most important in effecting changes in susceptibility to infection. Establishing a voiding schedule in small children is extremely difficult and often provokes conflict in the parent-child relationship. The physician can interject his or her influence by explaining the treatment goal to the child and requesting that a regular voiding pattern be instituted and maintained. The child should be told that she will be reminded by her parents to void regularly and that she should follow this request even if she does not feel the urge to void at this time. Constipation often requires an intensive therapeutic approach. In the most severe cases enemas given for several days may initially be necessary to disrupt a high fecal impaction and relax an overstretched colon. Increased intake of fiber and fluid and regular toilet habits must then be instituted. In most cases these are long-term requirements, and failure to continue this regimen generally results in recurrence of both constipation and urinary tract infection.

The most severe voiding problems in the otherwise normal child are associated with non-neuropathic voiding dyssynergia. Recognition and differentiation of this entity from neuropathic disease is mandatory. Treatment is described in Chapter 13.

Urinary stasis for any other reason needs to be addressed if infection cannot be otherwise controlled with antibiotic prophylaxis. Causes may include severe reflux with secondary poor bladder emptying (megacystis-megaureter syndrome), dilatation in the absence of obstruction, bladder diverticula, or residual ureteral stumps. Since otherwise unexplained urinary infection is so common, it is incumbent upon the physician to document the influence of any of these entities on infection prior to recommending surgical correction; for example, a culture may be obtained by needle aspiration of a dilated, nonobstructed upper collecting system to ascertain its involvement prior to surgical revision.

Treatment of *asymptomatic bacteriuria* appears not to be necessary if the urinary tract is otherwise normal, although a slight risk of pyelonephritis does exist (Lindberg et al, 1978). Spontaneous resolution or nonrecurrence after a course of therapy can be anticipated as voiding habits improve. If nontreatment is elected, one might consider a course of short-term antibiotic therapy periodically, particularly if there is historical evidence that a change in voiding pattern has been established. Those with either vesicoureteral reflux or renal scarring are best maintained on antibacterial prophylaxis.

Those children with *lower urinary symptoms* or evidence of cystitis cystica (cystitis follicularis) should be maintained on *continuous* prophylaxis. Medication is not discontinued for urine culture. When breakthrough infection occurs, the offending organism will be resistant to the current agent and the culture media will not be sterilized by the excreted drugs. Even discontinuing medication for 2 to 3 days for culture in these exquisitely sensitive children may result in reinfection with a resistant organism. A minimum of a 6 to 12 month block of therapy is used for prophylaxis with treatment discontinued at the end of each of these periods. Medication is reinstituted for an additional 12 months if infection recurs within 3 months of discontinuation. This cycle is continued until such time as there are no further recurrences. Children with vesicoureteral reflux are maintained on prophylaxis until the decision is made to correct the reflux or discontinue prophylaxis. Prophylaxis should be maintained until the child is at least 8 years old.

Prophylactic doses are generally less than those used to treat acute infection. Smellie and Grüneberg effectively used 10 mg of sulfamethoxazole plus 2 mg of trimethoprim per kg per day, or nitrofurantoin 1 to 2 mg/kg/day in one to two doses. My practice is to administer half to one third of the therapeutic dose twice daily. Requesting a twice-daily dose schedule has a pragmatic advantage: if one dose is missed, the child still receives some medication each day. However, in a highly compulsive family, a single nighttime dosage schedule is usually effective. Harding et al reported successful prevention of recurrent infection in preadolescent girls with low-dose trimethoprim-sulfamethoxazole administered only three times per week.

Pyelonephritis is treated with a 10 day course of appropriate bactericidal medication. A urine culture is obtained at completion and prophylaxis instituted until evaluation of the urinary tract is completed and a course of treatment planned.

The classic treatment of *renal abscesses* has included surgical drainage in addition to appropriate systemic antibiotic therapy. Recently, however, with improved diagnostic techniques and the ability to obtain a culture percutaneously under ultrasonic control, the necessity for surgery may be less absolute (Pederson et al). Ten days of parenteral treatment followed by an additional 2 weeks of appropriate oral therapy was successful in seven patients reported by Schiff et al. (1977). A sterile abscess cavity was secondarily drained in one. Nevertheless, surgical drainage and nephrectomy remain the most common treatments (Rote et al; Timmons and Perlmutter).

The role the female urethra plays in urinary tract infections has been one of the most controversial subjects in pediatric urology. The "mechanical school" has long advocated that urinary tract infection is the result of voiding problems secondary to urethral obstruction, resistance, or turbulence. As Graham et al and Immergut and Wahman demonstrated years ago, the urethral caliber of girls with infection is slightly larger than those of age-matched controls. Nevertheless, the practice of urethral dilation, meatotomy, and urethrotomy has continued to have its extreme advocates.

Hendry et al and Van Gool and Tanagho found that the incidence of recurrence of urinary infection was not affected by urethral dilation. Nevertheless, both reports concluded that a dysfunctioning voiding cycle can be disrupted by overstretching the urethra but that the same results can probably be achieved with control of infection using antibacterials, and institution of a regular voiding schedule aided by anticholinergic therapy. Govan et al reported no decreased recurrence rate in a group of girls followed 3 years before and after urethral dilation, and Kaplan et al found no difference between controls and a group subjected to dilation that were each on antibacterial prophylaxis for 3 months. Forbes et al found no change in either voiding patterns or recurrent infection rates in those girls subjected to urethral meatotomy alone. The radiographic appearance of the urethra was altered, however.

The most difficult data to interpret are those regarding urethrotomy. Kaplan et al found no difference in rate of recurrence of urinary tract infection between groups subjected to urethral dilation, urethrotomy, or medication alone. Immergut and Gilbert reported success in a group of 57 girls having urethrotomy. Only one third became reinfected, but the follow-up was limited to 6 months. Halverstadt and Leadbetter found a 10 per cent recurrence rate in those given 3 months of prophylaxis after urethrotomy and a 40 per cent recurrence rate in those given only 2 weeks of prophylaxis compared with a 70 per cent recurrence rate when medication was stopped in those on prophylaxis alone. The follow-up period in this group was 6 to 18 months. In a report of a 2 year follow-up of the same group, Vermillion et al reported an 18 per cent recurrence rate in the group on prophylaxis for 3 months following urethrotomy versus 67 per cent for controls. Nevertheless, Leadbetter and Slavin in a paper on perineal defenses suggested that anatomic abnormalities did not appear to play the most significant role as a cause for urinary infection in children. This appears to be confirmed by a prospective study carried out by Busch et al in which no significant difference in the incidence of urinary infections could be found in a group of girls and women before and after urethrotomy.

Therefore, it would appear that urethral manipulation in girls is rarely, if ever, necessary. In the absence of significant anatomic abnormalities that require further diagnostic evaluation, the role cystoscopy, urethral calibration, dilation, meatotomy, and urethrotomy play in the current practice of pediatric urology is minimal.

BIBLIOGRAPHY

American Medical Association: AMA Drug Evaluations. Chicago, AMA, 1971.

Anderson EE, Anderson B Jr, Nashold BS: Childhood complications of nalidixic acid. JAMA 216:1023, 1971.

Askari A, Belman AB: Vesicoureteral reflux in black girls. J Urol 127:747, 1982.

Asmar BI, Maqbool S, Dajani AS: Hematologic abnormalities after oral trimethoprim-sulfamethoxazole therapy in children. Am J Dis Child 135:1100, 1981.

Bagley FH, Stewart AM, Jones PF: Diffuse xanthogranulomatous pyelonephritis in children: an unrecognized variant. J Urol 118:434, 1977.

Belman AB: Clinical significance of cystitis cystica in girls: results of a prospective study. J Urol 119:661, 1978.

Bergstrom T: Sex differences in childhood urinary tract infection. Arch Dis Child 47:227, 1972.

Bergstrom T, Larson K, Lincoln K, et al. Studies of urinary

tract infections in infancy and childhood. J Pediatr 80:858, 1972.

Bollgren I, Winberg J: The periurethral aerobic bacterial flora in healthy boys and girls. Acta Paediatr Scand 65:74, 1976a.

Bollgren I, Winberg J: The periurethral aerobic flora in girls highly susceptible to urinary infections. Acta Paediatr Scand 65:81, 1976b.

Brook, I: Urinary tract infections caused by anaerobic bacteria in children. Urology 16:596, 1980.

Buetow KC, Klein SW, Lane RB: Septicemia in premature infants. Am J Dis Child 110:29, 1965.

Busch R, Huland H, Kollermann MW et al: Does internal urethrotomy influence susceptibility to recurrent urinary tract infection? Urology 20:134, 1982.

Cardiff-Oxford Bacteriuria Study Group: Sequelae of covert bacteriuria in school children. Lancet 1:889, 1978.

Clark H, Ronald AR, Turck M: Serum antibody response in renal versus bladder bacteriuria. J Infect Dis 123:539, 1971.

Corman LI, Foshee WS, Kotchmar GS: Simplified urinary microscopy to detect significant bacteriuria. Pediatrics 70:133, 1982.

Corriere JN Jr, McClure JM III, Lipschultz LI: Contamination of bladder urine by urethral particles during voiding: urethrovesical reflux. J Urol 107:399, 1972.

Craig WA, Kunin CM, DeGroot J: Evaluation of new urinary screening devices. Appl Microbiol 26:196, 1975.

DeLuca FG, Fisher JH, Swenson O: Review of current urinary tract infections in infancy and early childhood. N Engl J Med 268:75, 1963.

Demetriou E, Emans SJ, Masland RP Jr: Dysuria in adolescent girls: urinary tract infection or vaginitis? Pediatrics 70:299, 1982.

Dickinson JA: Incidence and outcome of symptomatic urinary tract infection. Br Med J 1:1330, 1979.

Drew JH, Acton CM: Radiological findings in newborn infants with urinary infection. Arch Dis Child 51:628, 1976.

Dubroff LM, Duckett JW, Corriere JN Jr: Phytohemagglutinin lymphocyte stimulation in children with recurrent urinary tract infections. Urology 5:744, 1975.

Edelmann CM Jr, Ogwo JE, Fine BP, et al: The prevalence of bacteriuria in full-term and premature newborn infants. J Pediatr 82:125, 1973.

Emans SJ, Grace E, Masland RP Jr: Asymptomatic bacteriuria in adolescent girls. Pediatrics 64:433, 1979.

Ericsson NO, Van Hedenberg C, Teger-Nilsson AC: Vulvourethral reflux: a fiction? J Urol 110:606, 1973.

Fair WR, Govan DE, Friedland GW, et al: Urinary tract infections in children. West J Med 121:366, 1972.

Fairley KF, Bond AG, Brown RB, et al: Simple test to determine the site of urinary tract infection. Lancet 2:427, 1967.

Feingold DS: Antimicrobial chemotherapeutic agents: the nature of their action and selective toxicity. N Engl J Med 269:900, 1963.

Fennell RS, Luengnaruemitchai M, Iraveni A, et al: Urinary tract infections in children: effect of short course antibiotic therapy on recurrence rate in children with previous infections. Clin Pediatr 19:121, 1980.

Fennell RS, Wilson SG, Garin EH et al: Bacteriuria in families of girls with recurrent bacteriuria. Clin Pediatr 16:1132, 1977.

Filly R, Friedland GW, Govan DE, et al: Development of progression of clubbing and scarring in children with recurrent urinary tract infections. Radiology 113:145, 1974.

Forbes PA, Drummond KN, Nogrady MB: Meatotomy in girls with meatal stenosis and urinary tract infection. J Pediatr 75:937, 1969.

Gillenwater JY, Gleason CH, Lohr JA, et al: Home urine cultures by the dipstick method: results in 289 children. Pediatrics 58:508, 1976.

Gillenwater JY, Harrison RB, Kunin CM: Natural history of bacteriuria in schoolgirls. N Engl J Med 301:396, 1979.

Ginsburg CM, McCracken GH: Urinary tract infections in young infants. Pediatrics 69:409, 1982.

Goodman LS, Gilman A: The Pharmacological Basis of Therapeutics. Fourth ed. New York, Macmillan Co., 1970.

Govan DE, Fair WR, Friedland GW, et al: Management of children with UTI. Urology 6:275, 1975.

Govan DE, Palmer JM: Urinary tract infection in children: the influence of successful antireflux operations in morbidity from infection. Pediatrics 44:677, 1969.

Graham JB, King LR, Kropp KA, et al: The significance of distal urethral narrowing in young girls. J Urol 97:1045, 1967.

Granoff DM, Roskes S: Urinary tract infection due to Hemophilus influenzae type B. J Pediatr 84:414, 1974.

Grüneberg RN, Smellie JM, Leakey A, et al: Long term low dose cotrimoxazole in prophylaxis of childhood urinary tract infection: bacteriologic aspects. Br Med J 2:206, 1976.

Halverstadt DB, Leadbetter GW Jr: Internal urethrotomy and recurrent urinary tract infection in children: results in the management of infection. J Urol 100:297, 1968.

Harding GKM, Buckwold FJ, Marrie TJ, et al: Prophylaxis of recurrent urinary tract infection in female patients. JAMA 242:1975, 1979.

Hart AF, Cherry JD: Cytology of the urine in children after poliovirus vaccine. N Engl J Med 272:174, 1965.

Heale WF, Weldone DP, Hewstone AS: Reflux nephropathy: presentation of urinary infection in children. Med J Aust 1:1138, 1973.

Hendry WF, Stanton SL, Williams DI: Recurrent urinary tract infections in girls: effects of urethral dilatation. Br J Urol 45:72, 1973.

Hermansson G, Bollgren I, Bergström T, et al: Coagulase negative staphylococci as a cause of symptomatic urinary infections in children. J Pediatr 84:807, 1974.

Hodson CJ, Wilson S: Natural history of chronic pyelonephritis scarring. Br Med J 2:191, 1965.

Howard JB, Howard JE: Trimethoprim-sulfamethoxazole vs sulfamethoxazole for acute urinary tract infections in children. Am J Dis Child 132:1085, 1978.

Immergut MA, Gilbert EC: Internal urethrotomy in recurring urinary infections in girls. J Urol 109:126, 1973.

Immergut MA, Wahman GE: The urethral caliber of female children with urinary tract infection. J Urol 99:189, 1968.

Intorp HW, Kloke O, Losse H: Autoimmune concomitants of chronic pyelonephritis. In Urinary Tract Infection. Vol. IV. Pyelonephritis. Edited by H Losse, AW Asscher, AE Lison. New York, Thieme Stratton Inc., 1980.

Jodal U, Fasth A: Diagnostic implications of immunological responses to urinary tract infection. In Urinary Tract Infection. Vol. IV. Pyelonephritis. Edited by H Losse, AW Asscher, AE Lison. New York, Thieme Stratton Inc., 1980.

Jodal U, Lindberg U, Lincoln K: Level diagnosis of symptomatic urinary tract infections in childhood. Acta Paediatr Scand 64:201, 1975.

Johnson DK, Kroovand RL, Perlmutter AD: The changing role of cystoscopy in the pediatric patient. J Urol 123:232, 1980.

Kaijser B, Hanson LA, Jodal U, et al: Frequency of *E. coli* K antigens in urinary tract infections in children. Lancet 1:663, 1977.

Kallenius G, Winberg J: Urinary tract infections treated with single dose of short-acting sulphonamide. Br Med J 1:1175, 1979.

Kaplan GW, Sammons TA, King LR: A blind comparison of dilation, urethrotomy and medication alone in the treatment of urinary infections in girls. J Urol 109:917, 1973.

Kass EH: Asymptomatic infections of the urinary tract. Trans Assoc Amer Phys 69:56, 1956.

Kunin CM: The natural history of recurrent bacteriuria in schoolgirls. N Engl J Med 282:1443, 1970.

Kunin CM: Detection, Prevention and Management of Urinary Tract Infections. Third ed. Philadelphia, Lea & Febiger, 1979.

Kunin CM, DeGroot JE: Sensitivity of a nitrate indicator strip method in detecting bacteriuria in preschool girls. Pediatrics 60:244, 1977.

Kunin CM, Deutscher R, Paquin A Jr: Urinary tract infection in schoolchildren: an epidemiologic, clinical and laboratory study. Medicine 4:91, 1964.

Kurnin GD: Clinical nephrotoxicity of tobramycin and gentamicin: a prospective study. JAMA 244:1808, 1980.

Leadbetter G Jr, Slavin S: Pediatric urinary tract infection: significance of vaginal bacteria. Urology 3:581, 1974.

Lebowitz RL, Fellows KE, Colodny AH: Renal parenchymal infections in children. Radiol Clin North Am 15:37, 1977.

Lindberg U, Bjure J, Haugstvedt S, et al: Asymptomatic bacteriuria in schoolgirls. III. Relation between residual urine volume and recurrence. Acta Paediatr Scand 64:437, 1975.

Lindberg U, Claessen I, Hanson L, et al: Asymptomatic bacteriuria in schoolgirls. J Pediatr 92:194, 1978.

Lindberg U, Hanson LA, Lidin-Janson G, et al: Asymptomatic bacteriuria in schoolgirls. II. Differences in *E. coli* causing asymptomatic and symptomatic bacteriuria. Acta Paediatr Scand 64:432, 1975.

Lloyd-Still J, Cottom D: Severe hypertension in childhood. Arch Dis Child 42:34, 1967.

Lohr JA, Nunley DH, Howards SS, et al: Prevention of recurrent urinary tract infections in girls. Pediatrics 59:562, 1977.

Lorentz WB, Resnick MI: Comparison of urinary lactic dehydrogenase with antibody coated bacteria in the urinary sediment as a means of localizing the site of urinary tract infection. Pediatrics 64:672, 1979.

Lyon RP: Distal urethral stenosis. *In* Reviews in Paediatric Urology. Edited by JH Johnston, WE Goodwin. Amsterdam, Excerpta Medica, 1974.

MacGregor M: Pyelonephritis lenta. Consideration of childhood urinary tract infection as the forerunner of renal insufficiency in later life. Arch Dis Child 45:159, 1970.

Marr TJ, Traisman HS: Detection of bacteriuria in pediatric outpatients. Am J Dis Child 129:940, 1975.

Maskell R: Importance of coagulase-negative staphylococci as pathogens in the urinary tract. Lancet 1:1155, 1974.

Meadow SR, White RHR, Johnston NM: Prevalence of symptomless urinary tract disease in Birmingham school children. I. Pyuria and bacteriuria. Br Med J 3:81, 1969.

Monahan M, Resnick JS: Urinary tract infections in girls: age of onset and urinary tract abnormalities. Pediatrics 62:237, 1978.

Morrell RE, Duritz G, Oltorf C: Suprapubic aspiration associated with hematuria. Pediatrics 69:455, 1982.

Mufson MA, Belshe RB, Horrigan TJ, et al: Cause of acute hemorrhagic cystitis in children. Am J Dis Child 126:605, 1973.

Mufson MA, Zollar LM, Mankad VN, et al: Adenovirus infection in acute hemorrhage cystitis. Am J Dis Child 121:281, 1971.

Nelson JD, Peters PC: Suprapubic aspiration of urine in premature and term infants. Pediatrics 36:132, 1965.

Neumann PZ, de Domenico IJ, Nogrady MB: Constipation and urinary infection. Pediatrics 52:241, 1973.

Parsons CL, Greenspan C, Moore SW, et al: Role of surface mucin in primary antibacterial defense of bladder. Urology 9:48, 1977.

Pederson JF, Hancke S, Kristensen JK: Renal carbuncle: antibiotic therapy governed on ultrasonically guided aspiration. J Urol 109:777, 1973.

Pitt WR, Dyer SA, McNee JL, et al: Single dose trimethoprim sulfamethoxazole treatment of symptomatic urinary tract infection. Arch Dis Child 57:229, 1982.

Polnay L, Fraser AM, Lewis JM: Complications of suprapubic bladder aspiration. Arch Dis Child 50:80, 1975.

Pryles CV, Eliot CR: Pyuria and bacteriuria in infants and children: the value of pyuria as a diagnostic criterion of urinary tract infections. Am J Dis Child 110:628, 1965.

Pryles CV, Lüders D: Bacteriology found in infants and children with gastroenteritis. Pediatrics 28:877, 1961.

Pylkkänen J: Antibody-coated bacteria in the urine of infants and children with their first two urinary tract infections. Acta Paedr Scand 67:275, 1978.

Randolph MF, Hodson J, Woods S, et al: Home screening for urinary tract infections in infants. Am J Dis Child 135:122, 1981.

Randolph MF, Majors F: Office screening for bacteriuria in early infancy: collection of a suitable urine specimen. J Pediatr 76:934, 1970.

Randolph MF, Morris KE; Office screening for bacteriuria in infants: collection of the voided specimen by the parent at home. J Pediatr 82:888, 1973.

Randolph MF, Morris KE, Gould EB: The first urinary tract infection in the female infant. J Pediatr 86:342, 1975.

Ransley PG, Risdon RA: Reflux and renal scarring. Br J Radiol (Suppl) 14, 1978.

Ransley PG, Risdon RA: Reflux nephropathy: the effects of antibiotic treatment on the development of pyelonephritis scar. *In* Urinary Tract Infection. Vol. IV. Pyelonephritis. Edited by H Losse, AW Asscher, AE Lison. New York, Thieme Stratton Inc., 1980.

Ribot S, Gal K, Goldblat M, et al: The role of anaerobic bacteria in the pathogenesis of urinary tract infections. J Urol 126:852, 1981.

Rosenfield AT, Glickman MG, Taylor KJW, et al: Acute focal bacterial nephritis. Radiology 132:553, 1979.

Ross RR Jr, Conway GF: Hemorrhagic cystitis following accidental overdose of methenamine mandelate. Am J Dis Child 119:86, 1970.

Rote AR, Bauer SB, Retik AB: Renal abscess in children. J Urol 119:254, 1978.

Schiff M Jr, Glickman M, Weiss RM, et al: Antibiotic treatment of renal carbuncle. Ann Intern Med 8:305, 1977.

Segura JW, Kelalis PP, Martin WJ, et al: Anaerobic bacteria in the urinary tract. Mayo Clin Proc 47:30, 1972.

Shapiro ED, Wald EF: Single dose amoxicillin treatment of UTI. J Pediatr 99:989, 1981.

Siegel MJ, Glasier CM: Acute focal bacterial nephritis in children: significance of ureteral reflux. AJR 137:257, 1981.

Smellie JM, Grüneberg RN: The treatment of childhood urinary tract infection with special reference to the use of trimethoprim and talampicillin for prophylaxis. *In* Urinary Tract Infection. Vol. IV. Pyelonephritis. Edited by H Losse, AW Asscher, AE Lison. New York, Thieme Stratton Inc., 1980.

Stamey TA: Urinary infections in infancy and childhood. *In* Urinary Infections. Baltimore, Williams and Wilkins, 1972.

Stamey TA, Bragonzi J: Resistance to nalidixic acid: a misconception due to underdosage. JAMA *236*:1857, 1976.

Stamey TA, Condy M, Mihara G: Prophylactic efficacy of nitrofurantoin macrocrystals and trimethoprim-sulfamethoxazole in urinary infections: biologic effects on the vaginal and rectal flora. N Engl J Med *296*:780, 1977.

Stickler GB, Kelalis PP, Burke EC, et al: Primary interstitial nephritis with reflux: a cause of hypertension. Am J Dis Child *122*:144, 1971.

Svanborg Edén C, Ericksson B, Hanson LA, et al: Adhesions to normal human uroepithelial cells of *E. coli* from children with various forms of urinary tract infection. J Pediatr *93*:398, 1978.

Tanagho EA, Miller ER, Lyon RF, et al: Spastic striated external sphincter and urinary tract infection in girls. Br J Urol *43*:69, 1971.

Thomas D, Simpson K, Ostojic H, et al: Bacteremic epididymo-orchitis due to *Hemophilus influenzae* type B. J Urol *126*:832, 1981.

Thrupp LD, Hodgman JE, Karelitz M, et al: Transurethral reflux during cleansing procedure for clean-voided urine specimen in low birth weight infants. J Pediatr *82*:1057, 1973.

Timmons JW, Perlmutter AD: Renal abscess: a changing concept. J Urol *115*:299, 1976.

Tuttle JP Jr, Sarvas H, Koistinen J: The role of vaginal immunoglobulin A in girls with recurrent urinary tract infections. J Urol *120*:742, 1978.

Uehling D, King LR: Secretory immunoglobulin A excretion in cystitis cystica. Urology *1*:305, 1973.

Uehling DT, Steihm ER: Elevated urinary secretory IgA in children with urinary tract infection. Pediatrics *47*:40, 1971.

Van Gool J, Tanagho EA: External sphincter activity and recurrent urinary infection in girls. Urology *10*:348, 1977.

Vaughn VC III, McKay RJ: Nelson Textbook of Pediatrics. Tenth ed. Philadelphia, WB Saunders Co., 1975.

Vermillion CD, Halverstadt DB, Leadbetter GW: Internal urethrotomy and recurrent urinary tract infection in female children. II. Long-term results in the management of infection. J Urol *106*:154, 1971.

Welch TR, Nogrady MB, Outerbridge EW: Roentgenologic sequelae of neonatal septicemia and urinary tract infection. Am J Roentgenol Radium Ther Nucl Med *118*:28, 1973.

Wientzen RL, McCracken GH Jr, Patruska ML, et al: Localization and therapy of urinary tract infections of childhood. Pediatrics *63*:467, 1979.

Winberg J, Andersen HJ, Bergström T, et al: Epidemiology of symptomatic urinary tract infection in childhood. Acta Paediatr Scand (Suppl) *252*:1, 1974.

Winberg J, Andersen HJ, Hanson LA, et al: Studies of urinary tract infections in infancy and childhood. Br Med J *2*:524, 1963.

Winberg J, Bergström T, Jacobsson B: Morbidity, age and sex distribution, recurrences and renal scarring in symptomatic urinary tract infection in childhood. Kidney Int *8*:S101, 1975.

Winter CC: Rapid miniaturized test for bacteriuria: Microstix and Bacturcult and urine tests. J Urol *114*:755, 1975.

Yazaki T, Ishikawa S, Ogawa Y, et al: Xanthogranulomatous pyelonephritis in childhood: case report and review of English and Japanese literature. J Urol *127*:80, 1982.

Specific Infections

STEPHEN A. KRAMER

TUBERCULOSIS

The advent of effective antituberculosis agents has made genitourinary tuberculosis an uncommon occurrence in the Western world. In 1979, 27,669 cases were reported in the United States. Approximately 10 per cent of these were in children and adolescents. The infection rate in children living in the United States whose parents were born in this country ranges between 1 and 2 cases per 10,000 per year. No new clinical cases of genitourinary tuberculosis have been seen at the Babies Hospital, Columbia Presbyterian Medical Center, since 1966. We have seen no new cases of genitourinary tuberculosis in children at the Mayo Clinic since 1956.

Tuberculosis in children occurs most often in lower socioeconomic groups. Black children and other minorities have higher tuberculosis case rates than Caucasian children. Transmission of tuberculous infection from mother to infant via the placenta or amniotic fluid has been reported in 130 to 200 patients (Smith and Marquis).

PATHOGENESIS. *Mycobacterium tubercu-*

losis, the tubercle bacillus, is a slow-growing, acid-fast organism, which is usually acquired through inhalation of respiratory droplets from an infected person. Renal tuberculosis is always preceded by a focus of infection in some other organ system, usually pulmonary (Robbins and Cotran). The tubercle bacilli gain access to the kidneys via hematogenous dissemination, and therefore renal infection must be considered bilateral in nature.

PATHOLOGY. Genitourinary tuberculosis occurs in 4 to 9 per cent of patients with tuberculosis (Cinman; Cos and Cockett). Renal tuberculosis is a late and uncommon complication of pulmonary disease, which rarely occurs less than 4 to 5 years after primary infection. Predisposing conditions such as malnutrition, diabetes mellitus, and chronic corticosteroid administration play a significant role in the development of genitourinary tuberculosis. The tuberculous bacillary emboli are deposited initially in the glomerular and cortical arterioles and cause small tubercles to develop. These tubercles undergo necrosis, with eventual caseation and cavitation of sloughed material into the calyceal walls at the papillary tips. These lesions may extend throughout the renal parenchyma and cause total destruction of the renal pyramids. Rupture of the bacilli into the calyx and collecting system results in dissemination of disease to other calyces, renal pelvis, ureter, and bladder.

Progression of disease results in fibrosis and may lead to stenosis at the calyceal neck, infundibulum, ureteropelvic junction, mid ureter, and ureterovesical junction. Ureteral fibrosis results in straightening and shortening of the ureter and ultimately produces the classic gaping golf-hole ureteral orifice with vesicoureteral reflux. Alternatively, ureteral stricture may produce hydroureteronephrosis and ultimately a nonfunctioning "autonephrectomized" kidney (Murphy et al).

Involvement of the bladder by tubercle bacilli causes ulceration and bleeding with destruction of the vesical mucosa. In the later stages of the disease, progressive fibrosis produces vesical contraction and scarring, which may lead to vesicoureteral reflux or ureterovesical junction obstruction.

Tuberculosis of the genital tract is uncommon in both sexes before puberty. In males, involvement of the genital tract usually occurs either hematogenously or through retrograde passage of infected urine through the posterior urethra in the prostatic ducts. Tubercu-

lous epididymitis or epididymo-orchitis can occur in early childhood and may be the initial method of presentation. In females with genital tuberculosis, the fallopian tubes are involved in approximately 90 per cent of cases, the endometrium in 50 per cent, the ovaries in 20 to 30 per cent, and the cervix in 2 to 4 per cent (Smith and Marquis).

SYMPTOMS. The majority of young children with genitourinary tuberculosis have no symptoms during the initial infection (Ehrlich and Lattimer). The lag time between pulmonary infection and the clinical onset of renal tuberculosis explains why most patients are adolescents at the time of initial presentation. Symptoms of frequency, dysuria, hematuria, and pyuria occur late in the course of disease, when the lesions ulcerate through the calyces and renal pelvis, and tubercle bacilli are disseminated to the bladder. Some children may present with systemic symptoms of generalized malaise, fatigue, low-grade persistent fever, or night sweats. Genitourinary tuberculosis must be suspected in patients with chronic or recurrent urinary tract infections who do not respond to standard antibiotic therapy. Furthermore, children with sterile pyuria, patients with draining sinuses, and those with a history of tuberculosis elsewhere in the body or in the family should be suspected of having genitourinary involvement.

DIAGNOSIS. Microscopic hematuria and pyuria are usually present. Routine urine culture is often negative; however, 15 to 20 per cent of patients with tuberculous bacilluria may have coexistent bacterial infection. The diagnosis of genitourinary tuberculosis is suggested by the demonstration of acid-fast bacilli in the stained urinary sediment and is confirmed by culture, usually guinea pig inoculation. Collection of fresh morning urine specimens appears to be just as accurate as 24-hour urinary concentrates in providing the diagnosis (Kenney et al). The acid-fast tubercle bacilli are discharged intermittently, and therefore at least three separate specimens should be collected for study. Tetracycline and sulfa medications have mild bacteriostatic effects on tuberculosis cultures, and these drugs should be discontinued before urine collection (Lattimer et al). Skin tests for tuberculosis (PPD) are usually positive except in cases of overwhelming infection. The erythrocyte sedimentation rate may be elevated, and anemia may be seen in advanced disease.

Plain films of the abdomen may reveal punctate calcification overlying the renal parenchyma (Hartman et al). Approximately 10 per cent of patients with renal tuberculosis have calculi. The earliest radiographic findings on the excretory urogram may be minimal calyceal dilatation or erosion of the papillary tip. As the infection proceeds, there is increased destruction of the calyces (Fig. 11–15). With advanced disease, there may be cavitation and cicatricial deformity of the collecting system, which may progress to pyonephrosis and nonfunction (Fig. 11–16). On the other hand, the urogram is within normal limits in as many as 33 per cent of children, and thus a normal excretory urogram does not rule out active genitourinary tuberculosis (Lattimer and Wechsler). In patients with hydroureteronephrosis or nonfunctioning renal units, ureteral catheterization may be helpful for selective urinary collection, and retrograde pyelography may be necessary to provide accurate delineation of pyelocalyceal architecture.

Cystoscopic examination reveals only minimal inflammatory changes in the early stages of disease. With coalescence of the tubercles, there may be areas of white or yellow raised nodules with a halo of hyperemia. With advanced localized disease, bladder capacity may become markedly diminished, with fixed and incompetent ureteral orifices, mucosal ulceration, and diffuse cystitis.

TREATMENT. The advent of effective antituberculosis chemotherapy has obviated surgical intervention in virtually all patients (Cinman; Cos and Cockett). Furthermore, Lattimer and Wechsler have stated that it is

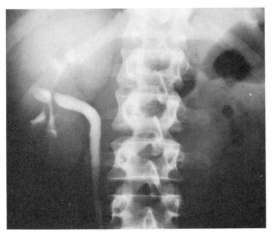

Figure 11–15. Excretory urogram in a 19-year-old male demonstrates extensive papillary necrosis involving upper pole of right kidney from renal tuberculosis.

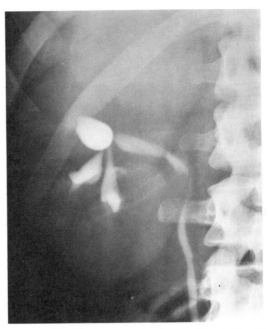

Figure 11–16. Same patient as in Figure 11–15, showing cicatricial deformity of collecting system with amputation of upper pole infundibulum.

most often possible to arrest all cases of genitourinary tuberculosis, regardless of the extent of disease, by persistent reapplication of new drug combinations in patients who have a relapse.

Antituberculosis drugs inhibit multiplication of tubercle bacilli and arrest the course of disease progression. A variety of antituberculosis agents are currently available, as discussed in the following paragraphs (Glassroth et al; Smith and Marquis; American Academy of Pediatrics). The efficacy of combination chemotherapy over single drug administration has been well documented (Lattimer and Wechsler). Furthermore, analysis of long-term patient follow-up has demonstrated that oral therapy is as effective as parenteral drug administration.

Isoniazid. The dosage of isoniazid (INH) is 10 to 30 mg/kg per day, up to 300 mg daily, given in one dose. The drug is the most effective of the antituberculosis agents available and remains the keystone of all therapeutic regimens. Isoniazid is metabolized in the liver and is excreted primarily through the kidney. It is available in both liquid form (50 mg/5 ml) and in tablets, which may be dissolved in fruit juice or water; this makes drug administration easier in infants and young children. Peripheral neuritis is the most common side effect and is probably caused by inhibition of pyridoxine metabolism. Neurotoxic side effects have not been reported in children less than 11 years old, and thus pyridoxine supplementation is not recommended unless nutrition is inadequate. Hepatotoxicity, which is seen often in older patients, rarely occurs in children.

Rifampin. The dosage of rifampin is 10 to 20 mg/kg per day, up to 600 mg daily. Rifampin, one of the newest antituberculosis agents, is extremely effective and virtually nontoxic for childhood administration. Rare cases of minor hepatic and renal dysfunction have been reported. This drug is indicated for the initial treatment of genitourinary tuberculosis and for cases requiring re-treatment. Rifampin is excreted in the bile and urine and may cause orange discoloration of urine, tears, and sweat.

Ethambutol. The dosage of ethambutol is 15 to 20 mg/kg per day, up to 1,500 mg daily, divided into two to three doses. This is an extremely effective antituberculosis drug, which has replaced para-aminosalicylic acid in most adults. It is rapidly absorbed and excreted in the urine. Optic neuritis is a major toxic effect of ethambutol, and monthly visual examinations are required. This drug is not recommended for use in small children who are not able to cooperate in examination of visual acuity and color vision.

Streptomycin. The dosage of streptomycin is 20 mg/kg per day intramuscularly, up to 1,000 mg daily. Although streptomycin is still a useful drug for the treatment of genitourinary tuberculosis, the risk of eighth nerve damage prohibits use of this medication for longer than a 4-week period.

Para-aminosalicylic acid (PAS). The dosage of PAS is 200 mg/kg per day, up to 12 g daily. PAS is an effective bactericidal drug for the treatment of renal tuberculosis when used in combination with other antituberculosis medications. However, PAS is not effective when used alone. Major side effects are gastrointestinal problems, including nausea, vomiting, diarrhea, and anorexia. It is best to give PAS after meals and in the form of sodium and potassium PAS to reduce gastrointestinal irritability.

Other Drugs. Ethionamide, cycloserine, kanamycin, pyrazinamide, and capreomycin may be useful in treating drug-resistant cases of genitourinary tuberculosis.

Specific Therapy for Genitourinary Tuberculosis. The accepted treatment for genitourinary tuberculosis is triple-drug chemotherapy administered daily for a period of 2 years (Wechsler and Lattimer). Recently, short-course chemotherapy (9-month treatment regimen) has been advocated in an attempt to (1) increase patient compliance, (2) reduce the cost of medication, (3) lower drug toxicity, and (4) produce an equally successful regimen when compared with the standard therapy (Fox; Gow). At this time, only limited data are available on short-course chemotherapy in children, and the American Academy of Pediatrics does not recommend this treatment regimen for childhood genitourinary tuberculosis. The recommended treatment for children with genitourinary tuberculosis is isoniazid, ethambutol, and rifampin for a period of 2 years (Wechsler).

The majority of relapses occur within the first 2 years; however, late recurrence is not uncommon, and therefore meticulous and long-term follow-up is mandatory. Routine urinalyses to check for pyuria and urine cultures for acid-fast bacilli are recommended every 2 months during treatment. The urine from patients with renal tuberculosis is highly infectious, and therefore children should be isolated for weeks or months until their urine becomes sterile. Excretory urography and voiding cystourethrography are done every 6 months during treatment and then yearly thereafter for 10 years to rule out urothelial strictures or renal parenchymal disease.

Although aggressive surgical therapy in patients with genitourinary tuberculosis has been recommended (Flechner and Gow; Wong and Lau), the results of chemotherapy are so impressive that surgical intervention should be limited to exceptional cases such as ureteral stricture (Murphy et al), ureterovesical junction reconstruction, or augmentation cytoplasty in children with small contracted bladders (Zinman and Libertino).

FUNGAL DISEASES

Fungal infestation should be considered in the differential diagnosis of children with inflammatory disease of the genitourinary tract. Opportunistic fungal infections in adults and children have increased significantly in recent years. These fungal infections occur most often in patients with obstructive uropathy and in patients with impaired host resistance due to causes such as extensive burns, blood dyscrasias, collagen vascular disease, and long-term steroid therapy. Glycosuria provides a favorable environment for mycotic growth, and patients with diabetes mellitus, in particular, are at increased risk for fungal involvement of the genitourinary tract.

Candidiasis

Candida albicans and, more rarely, *C. tropicalis* are yeast forms that may exist as commensals in the mouth, intestinal tract, vagina, and skin of normal persons. *Candida* is the most common of the opportunistic mycoses, and systemic disease occurs almost exclusively in patients with impaired host resistance. *Candida* may also be recoverable in the urine of persons with asymptomatic infection, usually as a result of overgrowth after broad-spectrum antibiotic therapy.

PATHOGENESIS AND PATHOLOGY. Conditions that predispose to candidemia include contamination of intravenous catheters, long-term antibiotic therapy, steroid administration, immunosuppressive agents, cytotoxic drug therapy, blood dyscrasias, burns, and open surgical wounds (MacMillan et al; Stone et al). In patients with gram-negative bacteremia, antibiotic therapy appears to be one of the most important predisposing factors in the development of subsequent candidemia (Stone et al).

Primary candidiasis of the genitourinary tract may involve the kidneys, ureters, and bladder. Candiduria may lead to the formation of fungus balls in the collecting system with obstruction, pyelonephritis, or perinephric abscess formation. Up to 88 per cent of patients with disseminated candidiasis have microorganisms demonstrable within the renal parenchyma.

SYMPTOMS. Patients with renal candidiasis may present with fever, chills, flank pain, renal colic, or urosepsis. Pyelonephritis and ureteral obstruction due to fungus ball infestation have been reported (Schönebeck et al; Kozinn et al, 1976). Anuria in infants can result from bilateral renal pelvic fungus balls (Eckstein et al; Khan). In patients with localized candidal cystitis, urinary urgency, frequency, and dysuria are typical findings.

DIAGNOSIS. Schönebeck stated that any number of *Candida* cultured from a midstream urine collection in the male or from a catheterized specimen in the female is significant for *Candida* infection. Recent evidence suggests that colony counts greater than 15,000 per ml obtained by midstream clean catch or a single urethral catheterization are evidence of renal *Candida* infection (Wise et al, 1976; Kozinn et al, 1978). Conversely, colony counts of more than 100,000 per ml in patients with indwelling urethral catheters appear to have no relationship to upper tract candidal infection.

Criteria for determining significant candidal infection should be based on clinical data, urinary findings, and serum precipitin titers. The presence of agglutinating antibodies and serum precipitins, as detected by agar gel diffusion techniques, provides an accurate index of parenchymal or invasive candidal infection (Wise et al, 1972; Dolan and Stried; Everett et al). In a series of patients with systemic candidiasis, Kozinn et al (1976) reported true-positive precipitin reactions in 65 of 69 patients (94 per cent). Interestingly, fewer than 50 per cent of patients with systemic candidiasis have positive blood cultures.

The excretory urogram may suggest papillary necrosis, tuberculosis, calculous disease, or neoplasm. A fungus ball may appear as a filling defect in the collecting system and cause obstructive uropathy or nonvisualization of the kidney. Cystoscopic examination reveals diffuse cystitis with purulent material distributed over the mucosal surface.

TREATMENT. Candiduria that occurs in healthy patients after long-term broad-spectrum antibiotic therapy should clear after use of the antibiotic has been stopped. Localized infections of the kidney or bladder may be controlled and eradicated by irrigation with a solution of 5 per cent amphotericin B (Fungizone) in sterile water via a nephrostomy tube or three-way bladder catheter (Wise et al, 1973, 1982). Infants with renal fungus balls may require emergency pyelotomy and insertion of nephrostomy tubes for irrigation. Continuous irrigation with a slow-drip infusion can be maintained for several days without systemic toxic effects. Alkalinization of the urine to a pH of 7.5 with oral sodium bicarbonate is recommended.

The treatment of choice for systemic candidiasis is amphotericin B, a nephrotoxic, fungistatic agent that must be given intravenously. Amphotericin B must be administered in 5 per cent dextrose in water. Initially, a test dose of 0.1 mg/kg up to a total dose of 1 mg is given over a period of 3 to 4 hours with careful monitoring of temperature, respirations, and blood pressure. The drug should be increased gradually in daily increments of 0.25 mg/kg over a 4-day period, until a total dose of 1 mg/kg is achieved. Peak serum levels should be twice the mean inhibitory concentration for the infectious organism, and trough levels should be approximately equal to the mean inhibitory concentration for the fungus. Toxic side effects include fever, nausea and vomiting, generalized malaise, and phlebitis. Decreased renal function is not uncommon, and thus careful and prolonged determinations of serum creatinine are required. The duration of therapy is dependent upon the extent of the infection, but intravenous drug administration is usually required for several weeks to eradicate disseminated disease.

Flucytosine (Ancobon) is a much less toxic agent than amphotericin B and is very effective in the treatment of systemic candidiasis (Wheeler et al; Wise et al., 1974). The drug is administered orally and is excreted primarily unchanged in the urine. The dose is 150 mg/kg per day given orally at 6-hour intervals. Adverse side effects are infrequent; however, thrombocytopenia, leukopenia, rash, hepatic dysfunction, and diarrhea may occur, especially in patients with diminished renal function.

Miconazole, a relatively new intravenous antifungal agent, lacks hepatic and renal toxicity. The use of miconazole in the treatment of genitourinary candidiasis in a newborn has been reported (Noe and Tonkin). There is limited experience with this drug in the clinical setting, however, and amphotericin B and flucytosine remain the initial drugs of choice in children with *Candida* sepsis (Wise).

Ketoconazole is a new oral antimycotic agent that has been shown to be effective for both superficial and deep fungal infections (Graybill et al). It is well absorbed orally and appears to have minimal toxicity (Borgers et al). The efficacy of this agent in the treatment of pediatric systemic fungal infections will depend on future clinical trials.

Aspergillosis

Aspergillosis is the second most common fungal infection in patients with hematologic malignancies (Hinson et al). Aspergillosis species are prevalent worldwide and grow on decaying vegetation, in damp hay or straw, and in the soil (Young et al).

PATHOGENESIS AND PATHOLOGY. The disease is caused by inhalation of fungal spores. The organism is occasionally introduced through an operative wound, via trauma, or from a foreign body such as an intravenous or urinary catheter. Three separate patterns of disease have been described: (1) disseminated hematogenous spread with multiple organ involvement (Young et al), (2) involvement limited to the renal pelvis or parenchyma (Comings et al; Warshawsky et al; Eisenberg et al), and (3) panurothelial disease involving the urethra, bladder, ureters, and kidneys (Flechner and McAninch). Renal infection is characterized by vascular invasion, focal microabscess formation, and, occasionally, papillary necrosis.

SYMPTOMS. Microscopic hematuria and pyuria are often present in patients with aspergillosis. Obstructive uropathy from a fungus ball or "aspergilloma" in the renal pelvis may be the initial method of presentation (Comings et al; Young et al; Melchior et al; Eisenberg et al).

DIAGNOSIS. The fungi may be identified as branched septate hyphae on potassium hydroxide preparations of infected material. Results of urine cultures are variable, and multiple cultures are often required to identify the organism. Serum precipitins are useful in certain forms of aspergillosis; however, approximately 40 per cent of patients with pulmonary tuberculosis may have elevation of these antibodies (Weinstein and Farkas). Skin tests are usually positive but are nondiagnostic. Definitive diagnosis of invasive aspergillosis is established by tissue biopsy or by identification of sloughed tissue and fungus balls per urethra. Excretory urographic findings are nonspecific and may demonstrate filling defects in the renal pelvis secondary to fungus ball infestation.

TREATMENT. Invasive aspergillosis is usually a rapidly fatal disease, and treatment is generally unsuccessful. Amphotericin B is the most potent and reliable drug available. Flucytosine is inactive against aspergillosis (Bennett). In patients with fungus balls in the kidney, upper tract irrigation through a nephrostomy tube may be indicated (Warshawsky et al). Alternatively, Flechner and McAninch reported successful upper tract irrigation through ureteral catheters by the use of a solution of sterile water with 15 mg of amphotericin B and one ampule of neomycin and polymyxin B administered at 100 ml per hour.

Actinomycosis

Actinomycosis bovis is an anaerobic fungus with worldwide distribution. The organism is normally present in the mouth and throat and may also be found elsewhere in the gastrointestinal tract. Although rare, actinomycotic infection in infants and children has been reported (Kretschmer and Hibbs; Drake and Holt).

PATHOGENESIS AND PATHOLOGY. Actinomycosis is a chronic, progressive suppurative disease characterized by multiple abscesses and draining sinuses (Berardi). Progression of disease is associated with pronounced fibrosis and development of spontaneous fistulas. Three major varieties of clinical disease are cervicofacial, thoracic, and abdominal. Genitourinary involvement by actinomycosis has been well documented (Deshmukh and Kropp; Crosse et al; Grierson and Zelas; Isaacson and Jennings). Renal involvement usually occurs as a result of hematogenous dissemination or of direct extension from a pulmonary or gastrointestinal lesion (Robbins and Scott).

SYMPTOMS. Patients with actinomycosis of the kidney may present with a painful flank mass or urosepsis secondary to a perinephric abscess. The bladder may become involved secondarily from direct extension of infection in the appendix, colon, or fallopian tube. Patients with vesical involvement may present with dysuria, urgency, and frequency.

DIAGNOSIS. The demonstration of "sulfur granules" in pus establishes the diagnosis of actinomycosis. A Gram stain reveals a dense reticulum of filaments which stains violet and projects around the periphery of the granule. Specimens must be cultured anaerobically on selective media. Although there have been no serodiagnostic techniques available for the diagnosis of actinomycosis, the recent use of fluorescent antibody reagents has been promising (Holmberg et al).

Excretory urography may demonstrate calyceal erosion and simulate genitourinary tuberculosis. The urogram may also show a mass lesion simulating a parenchymal abscess or neoplasm (Fig. 11–17).

TREATMENT. The drug of choice for actinomycosis is penicillin in dosages of 300,000 units per kg per day up to 20 million units over 3 months (Eastridge et al). Tetracycline, erythromycin, lincomycin, chloramphenicol, and clindamycin have been employed with successful results (Rose and Rytel; Fass et al). In unresponsive cases and in patients with extensive renal parenchymal destruction, surgical drainage and occasionally nephrectomy may be required.

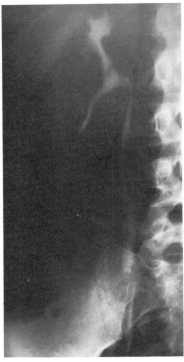

Figure 11–17. Right retrograde pyelogram demonstrates calyceal splaying and mass lesion suggesting renal tumor in a patient with actinomycosis. (From Hunt VC, Mayo C: Actinomycosis of the kidney. Ann Surg 93:501–505, 1932. By permission of JB Lippincott Company.)

Blastomycosis

Blastomyces dermatitidis, the etiologic agent of North American blastomycosis, is a dimorphic fungus found in the soil. Endemic sites of disease in the United States include Ohio, the Mississippi and Missouri River valleys, and the area along the western shores of Lake Michigan (Furcolow et al).

PATHOGENESIS. Infection from blastomycosis usually occurs from inhalation of the fungus, which produces a primary pulmonary focus. Dissemination of the fungus may occur to any organ of the body through hematogenous or lymphogenous routes. Genitourinary involvement occurs in approximately 20 to 30 per cent of cases (Denton et al), and childhood involvement has been documented (Gill and Gerald; Eickenberg et al; Yogev and Davis).

SYMPTOMS. Blastomycosis should be considered in the differential diagnosis of any granulomatous or suppurative disease of the genitourinary tract. The fungus has a predilection for males; no female patients with genitourinary involvement were documented in a series of 51 patients recorded by Eickenberg et al. Blastomycosis may involve the kidney, prostate, epididymis, and testes (Furcolow et al; Schwarz and Salfelder; Macher; Bergner et al). Symptoms vary with the organ involved; however, dysuria, urgency, frequency, hematuria, and epididymo-orchitis have been frequent modes of presentation.

DIAGNOSIS. Potassium hydroxide preparations of urine demonstrate the thick-walled, single-budding yeast forms of blastomycosis. Definitive diagnosis is substantiated only by culture or by histologic examination of tissue specimens. Complement fixation, immuno-diffusion antibody, and skin sensitivity testing are not sensitive diagnostic aids.

TREATMENT. Amphotericin B is the drug of choice for genitourinary blastomycosis. Surgical excision of localized lesions may be indicated, particularly in cases of epididymo-orchitis.

Cryptococcosis

Cryptococcosis is an infectious disease caused by a spherical fungus, *Cryptococcus neoformans.* Cryptococcosis occurs most often in debilitated patients, especially those with Hodgkin's disease.

PATHOGENESIS. Infection with *C. neoformans* may be acquired by inhalation of infected particles during exposure to pigeon excreta (Wittner). The primary site of disease is pulmonary; however, hematogenous dissemination of the fungus often occurs, and renal involvement is well documented (Randall et al; Lewis and Rabinovich). In a review of autopsy cases of disseminated cryptococcal infection, Salyer and Salyer found that 20 of 39 patients (51 per cent) had involvement of the kidneys. Cryptococcal involvement of the prostate has been documented both at autopsy (Cohen and Kaufmann; Bowman and Ritchey; Salyer and Salyer) and as a cause of lower urinary tract obstruction (Huynh and Reyes; O'Connor et al; Tillotson and Lerner).

SYMPTOMS. Microscopic hematuria and pyuria occur in the majority of patients with genitourinary cryptococcosis. In patients with diffuse granulomatous involvement of the kidneys, pyelonephritis may be the initial method of presentation.

DIAGNOSIS. The encapsulated yeasts may be demonstrated in urine, pus, or India ink preparations of cerebrospinal fluid. Pre-

cise diagnosis, however, depends on identification of the organism by culture techniques. In patients with disseminated cryptococcosis, urine and blood cultures have usually been positive. The latex agglutination test for cryptococcal antigen is highly specific and may have both diagnostic and prognostic value (Gordon and Vedder).

TREATMENT. The drug of choice for disseminated cryptococcosis is amphotericin B.

Coccidioidomycosis

Coccidioidomycosis is an infection caused by a dimorphic fungus, *Coccidioides immitis.* Endemic areas are confined to the Western Hemisphere. In the United States, these areas include the Southwest, encompassing western Texas, New Mexico, Arizona, and California (Granoff and Libke).

PATHOGENESIS AND PATHOLOGY. Genitourinary involvement is common with disseminated disease. In an autopsy series of patients with disseminated coccidioidomycosis, renal involvement was recorded in 30 of 50 cases (60 per cent) (Conner et al). Fungal involvement of the kidney appears confined to the cortex as small miliary granulomas or microabscesses. Genital involvement with bilateral epididymitis may be the initial method of presentation (Cheng).

DIAGNOSIS. In disseminated disease, microscopic examination of exudates or biopsy specimens is diagnostic if typical spherules are visualized. Skin tests are helpful and become positive 1 to 3 weeks after exposure to the fungus. Definitive identification requires animal inoculation or special culture techniques. Serologic studies are useful and include serum precipitins and latex agglutination (Drutz and Catanzaro; Weinstein and Farkas). Immunodiffusion and counterimmunoelectrophoresis are alternative methods for the detection of specific coccidioidal antibodies (Aguilar-Torres et al).

The radiographic findings of advanced renal coccidioidomycosis may mimic those of tuberculosis and demonstrate infundibular stenosis, blunted or sloughed calyces, and calcified granulomas.

TREATMENT. Amphotericin B is the drug of choice for disseminated disease. Miconazole has been used successfully in a number of patients (Stevens et al). Ketoconazole is a new, orally active antifungal agent that is presently undergoing clinical trials (Granoff and Libke).

Mucormycosis

Mucormycosis is a ubiquitous saprophyte and opportunistic pathogen that may cause rapidly fatal disease in patients with impaired host resistance (Baker; Meyer et al).

PATHOGENESIS. Mucormycosis develops subsequent to ingestion of fungal elements from decaying food and vegetation. The organism has a predilection for growth in the walls of blood vessels and may lead to arterial thrombosis and infarction.

SYMPTOMS. Most cases of mucormycosis occur in patients with diabetes mellitus and ketoacidosis. Renal abscesses may occur alone (Prout and Goddard; Langston et al) or in conjunction with disseminated disease (Dansky et al). Hematuria has been reported in most patients with genitourinary involvement; obstructive uropathy may be the initial method of presentation.

DIAGNOSIS. The diagnosis of mucormycosis requires organ identification by culture techniques. There are no good serologic tests available.

TREATMENT. Amphotericin B is the drug of choice for disseminated mucormycosis. Partial or total nephrectomy may be indicated in selected cases with extensive renal parenchymal involvement.

PARASITIC INFECTIONS

Schistosomiasis

Urinary schistosomiasis, or bilharziasis, is a vascular, parasitic infectious disease caused by the blood fluke *Schistosoma haematobium.* It is estimated that between 200 and 300 million people in Africa, Asia, South America, and the Caribbean area are infected by schistosoma (Hanash and Bissada). The disease is endemic in Egypt. Rare cases are seen in the United States and always originate from an endemic area.

PATHOGENESIS. The life cycle of *S. haematobium* begins when a person with schistosomiasis urinates and discharges the parasite's egg into the stagnant water of a lake or river. During warm hours of the day the egg swells, ruptures, and liberates a miracidium. The miracidium swims toward and penetrates a specific species of fresh-water snail. After penetration, the miracidium matures into a sporozoite. These sporozoites bud and produce thousands of cercariae, which are liberated into the water. The cercariae penetrate

the skin or mucous membranes of a human host. After cutaneous penetration, the cercariae become schistosomula, enter the venous and lymphatic systems, and are carried to the right side of the heart. They then migrate to the portal circulation, where copulation between males and females occurs. The male carries the female to the pelvic venules, where the eggs are deposited. These eggs (ova) pass through the vessels and are either buried in the bladder wall or excreted with the urine and thereby complete the life cycle (von Lichtenberg and Lehman).

PATHOLOGY. The basic response to schistosome eggs is a pronounced eosinophilic infiltrate, with the formation of granulomas or "pseudotubercles" around the ova. With advanced disease, collagen formation occurs, with scarring of the bladder wall, deposition of calcareous material, and calcification sclerosis.

Urothelial changes occur in all stages of disease and include mucosal hyperplasia, squamous metaplasia, and epithelial dysplasia. Involvement of the trigone may lead to fibrosis of the bladder neck and cause vesical outlet obstruction. Outlet obstruction with stasis of infected urine predisposes to the formation of bladder calculi in older patients. In children, however, urinary bilharziasis does not appear to play a role in the cause of vesical calculi (Kambal). In patients with long-standing disease, chronic vesical irritation may predispose the bladder to squamous cell carcinoma.

In the ureter, tissue reaction to the ova may result in ureteritis cystica, ureteritis calcinosa, or stricture formation. Vesicoureteral reflux is a result of fibrosis and lateral displacement of the intramural ureter and is seen in up to 50 per cent of patients (Hanna).

The kidneys are involved infrequently with bilharzial infection; however, it has been suggested that glomerulonephritis may result from an immune-complex reaction (Hanash and Bissada).

SYMPTOMS. Humans become infected with *Schistosoma* after coming into contact with contaminated water through drinking, swimming, bathing, or washing clothes. Children of any age are at risk for infection. Acute schistosomiasis occurs between 3 and 9 weeks after infection and coincides with the deposition of eggs in the bladder wall. Terminal hematuria and dysuria are classic findings. Occasionally, bleeding becomes so extensive as to result in anemia. In patients with bladder ulceration, symptoms include urinary urgency, frequency, and severe suprapubic pain.

In the later stages of disease (inactive phase of infection), fibrosis and contracture of the bladder and ureter have the potential to produce obstructive uropathy. The disease process is insidious, and massive hydroureteronephrosis or renal nonfunction may occur before the onset of clinical symptoms.

DIAGNOSIS. The diagnosis of schistosomiasis is established by the presence of terminal-spined eggs in the urine. A 24-hour urine collection with microscopic examination of the sediment is recommended. In the absence of eggs from multiple urine specimens, bladder biopsies or rectal biopsies provide a satisfactory method of obtaining the diagnosis (von Lichtenberg and Lehman). Intradermal skin tests and serologic techniques including fluorescent antibody, latex flocculation, complement fixation, and precipitin tests have been described (Kagan). Positive tests indicate prior exposure to schistosome infection, but these studies do not identify the present status of disease and therefore may remain positive in the absence of eggs or living worms.

Peripheral blood examination usually demonstrates eosinophilia. With chronic worm infestation, the patient may be anemic as a result of destruction of erythrocytes by the blood fluke or as a consequence of chronic disease and uremia.

RADIOGRAPHIC AND CYSTOSCOPIC EVALUATION. A plain film of the abdomen may reveal calcification within the urinary tract or in other organs (Hanna). Egg-shell calcification over the bladder in an appropriate clinical setting is likely to indicate chronic urinary schistosomiasis (Fig. 11–18). Excretory urography may demonstrate ureteral strictures, hydronephrosis, or filling defects in the bladder and ureter secondary to polypoid lesions. In chronic disease, vesicoureteral reflux can occur.

Endoscopic evaluation with or without transurethral bladder biopsies may yield characteristic findings. In patients with active lesions, the bilharzial tubercles predominate over the trigone and posterior bladder wall as granular, white or yellow lesions with a halo or hyperemia (Hanash et al). Overdistention of the bladder results in bleeding and is reminiscent of interstitial cystitis or hemorrhagic cystitis. Coalescence of these tubercles may form a bilharzioma, which is a multinodular, hypervascular lesion usually attached by a narrow pedicle. In patients with chronic disease, fibrosis and calcification of the tubercles

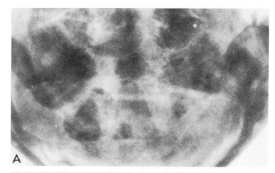

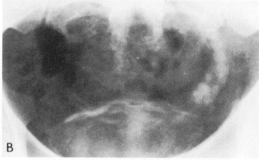

Figure 11–18. *A,* Plain film shows curvilinear calcification of the bladder and both distal ureters. *B,* There are numerous calculi in the left ureter. (From Hanash KA, Bissada NK, Lewall DB, et al: Genito-urinary schistosomiasis (bilharziasis). Part 2: Clinical, parasitologic, immunologic, and radiologic diagnosis. King Faisal Specialist Hosp Med J 1:119–130, 1981. By permission of the King Faisal Specialist Hospital and Research Centre.)

in the submucosa form dull, granular "sandy patches" that resemble grains of sand under water.

TREATMENT. Although various chemotherapeutic agents are available for the treatment of urinary schistosomiasis, all drugs are potentially dangerous and difficult to use. Historically, antimony-containing compounds—for example, sodium or potassium antimonyltartrate (tartar emetic)—formed the basis of medical treatment. These drugs must be given intravenously or intramuscularly and are accompanied by frequent side effects, including nausea, vomiting, peripheral neuritis, joint pains, and diarrhea. Tartar emetic is cardiotoxic and has been associated with ventricular irritability and Adams-Stokes syndrome.

The drugs available for use in the United States can be obtained only from the Parasitic Disease Drug Service, Centers for Disease Control. The most widely used drug for the treatment of urinary schistosomiasis is niridazole (Ambilhar), which is given orally, 25 mg/kg daily divided into two doses, for a period of 5 to 7 days (Sullivan). The patient usually must be hospitalized during therapy with niridazole because of frequent side effects such as headache, dizziness, nausea, vomiting, diarrhea, and cramping abdominal pain. Patients with hepatic, psychiatric, or central nervous system disease or seizure disorders should not receive this drug.

Metrifonate is an effective alternative to niridazole for the treatment of *S. haematobium* infections. The drug is an inexpensive, orally administered agent, which is currently being evaluated in several endemic areas in Africa. The dosage for children is 10 mg/kg administered every other week for three doses (American Academy of Pediatrics).

Patients should be evaluated monthly to ascertain that no living eggs are being passed. The presence of living ova indicates either failure of treatment or reinfection. Dead eggs may be recovered for long periods after therapy and are not necessarily an indication for re-treatment.

Surgical intervention in schistosomiasis should be reserved until the effects of medical management can be assessed. Not infrequently, however, genitourinary schistosomiasis may cause fibrosis and contracture of the bladder, requiring augmentation cystoplasty. Bilharzial strictures of the ureter can produce obstructive uropathy, with damage to the upper tracts, recurrent urinary tract infections, and renal calculi. The lower ureter is involved in approximately two thirds of cases and often requires surgical reconstruction at the ureterovesical junction. Extensive fibrosis of the ureteral wall and vesical mucosa usually precludes ureteroneocystostomy by a submucosal tunnel technique. Partial flap ureteroneocystostomy has produced improved or stabilized upper tracts radiographically in 83 per cent of patients (Bazeed et al). It is noteworthy that vesicoureteral reflux developed in 30 per cent of the patients postoperatively. In patients requiring surgery, it is important that the urine be sterilized preoperatively and that chemotherapy be continued postoperatively to prevent reinfection.

Echinococcosis

Echinococcosis, or hydatid cyst disease, is an infestation caused by the dog tapeworm *Echinococcus granulosus.* The major endemic sites of echinococcosis occur in sheep-raising areas such as Argentina, Australia, Spain, and Greece.

PATHOGENESIS. The adult tapeworm inhabits the intestinal tracts of dogs. The dogs become infected by swallowing the parasite scolex, which is encysted in the liver or lungs of sheep. Worm eggs from the dog are then excreted in the feces and may be ingested by sheep, cattle, pigs, and occasionally humans. After human ingestion, larval eggs pass through the intestinal wall and are disseminated throughout the body. Hydatid cysts have been found in virtually all human organs (Hunter et al). In man, the liver is the primary organ affected. *Echinococcus* gains access to the kidney in approximately 3 per cent of the cases, usually from rupture of hepatic cysts into the peritoneal cavity with subsequent retroperitoneal penetration (Musacchio and Mitchell; Silber and Moyad).

SYMPTOMS. Auldist and Myers reported 114 cases of hydatid cyst disease in children. Children of any age may be affected; however, the disease occurs infrequently in patients less than 5 years of age. Echinococcosis in children has been reported in the kidneys (Sharma et al; Gharbi et al; Gajjar and Sinclair-Smith; Shulman and Morales), in the bladder (Fuloria et al), and as a cause of bilateral hydronephrosis (Keramidas et al). Echinococcosis has been implicated as a cause of eosinophilic cystitis (Hansman and Brown).

The growth of the hydatid cyst occurs slowly over a number of years, and the size of the cyst can be extremely large at the time of initial presentation. Hydatid cyst of the kidney usually presents as a painful flank mass, and microscopic hematuria is often present. Rupture of the cyst into the renal pelvis causes acute flank pain and passage of scolices or daughter cysts with hematuria, with or without urinary obstruction (Gilsanz et al).

DIAGNOSIS. A history of contact with sheep dogs in an endemic area is most helpful in diagnosing echinococcosis. The findings of scolices and hooklets in the urine is pathognomonic for echinococcosis. Eosinophilia is present in approximately one third of affected children (Apt and Knierim). A positive Casoni skin sensitivity test is useful, and positive reactions have been reported in approximately 90 per cent of patients at 24 hours (Hunter et al). Serologic methods are particularly important in the diagnosis of echinococcal infections. The indirect hemagglutination test is the most specific of these techniques and is

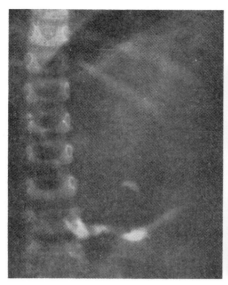
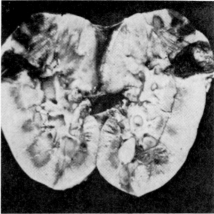

Figure 11–19. *A,* Left retrograde pyelogram in a 7-year-old girl demonstrates a large renal mass with distortion of the upper and middle calyces. *B,* Right nephrectomy specimen from a 17-year-old male shows hydatid cyst involving upper calyces. (From Shawket TN, Al-Waidh M: Hydatid cysts of the kidney: simulating similar kidney lesions. Br J Urol *46:*371–376, 1974. By permission of the British Association of Urological Surgeons.)

available through the Centers for Disease Control.

Plain films of the abdomen reveal spherical cysts with peripheral calcification overlying the kidneys. Excretory urography demonstrates a calcified renal mass lesion, with or without calyceal distortion, which mimics a renal abscess or neoplasm (Fig. 11–19). Nephrotomography and selective renal arteriography are useful in clarifying the diagnosis (Baltaxe and Fleming).

TREATMENT. Surgical intervention may be required in some patients with hydatid cyst disease. Nephrectomy remains the mainstay of treatment of hydatid disease of the kidney. Meticulous care is necessary to prevent spillage of the cyst contents, a complication that can produce systemic anaphylactoid symptoms. Excision of the cyst wall is often difficult because of an inadequate plane of cleavage between the renal parenchyma and the fibrous cyst capsule. Marsupialization of the cyst wall or partial nephrectomy may result in spillage of infective scolices and, in turn, increased morbidity. The hydatid fluid should be aspirated and replaced with one of several chemical scolicidal agents before the cyst cavity is opened; hydrogen peroxide, sodium hypochloride, glycerin, and formalin are useful agents. Meymerian et al have recommended a solution of hydrogen peroxide, 0.1 per cent,

and cetrimide, 0.005 per cent, as an effective and less toxic agent than formalin. In patients with systemic echinococcosis, mebendazole appears to be an effective antihelminthic agent (Nabizadeh et al).

Chlamydial Infection

Chlamydia trachomatis is an obligate intracellular parasite that may be responsible for 50 per cent of cases of nongonococcal urethritis and up to 66 per cent of cases of pelvic inflammatory disease in women (Rettig and Nelson). *Chlamydia* has only rarely been isolated from the genital tracts of prepubertal children. Rettig and Nelson were able to recover *C. trachomatis* from boys with coexistent or previous anogenital gonorrhea.

SYMPTOMS. Chlamydial infection in males typically presents as urethritis, epididymitis, or Reiter's syndrome and may be a rare cause of prostatitis (Smith et al.; Berger et al). The most common symptom is a clear, mucoid urethral discharge with or without urinary urgency and frequency. In females, acute inflammatory changes in the vagina or cervix lead to mucopurulent cervicitis, endometritis, or salpingitis. Conversely, asymptomatic carriage of *Chlamydia* in the endocervix may occur in the absence of urogenital symptoms.

DIAGNOSIS. *Chlamydia* should be suspected in patients who have persistent urethral or vaginal discharge and a history of anogenital gonorrhea. The organism may be visualized in smears with the use of the immunofluorescent antibody typing test or Giemsa stain. Definitive diagnosis is established through isolation of the organism by inoculation into selected cell culture lines.

TREATMENT. Sulfonamides, erythromycin, and tetracycline, administered for 10 days to 2 weeks, are effective agents for the treatment of *Chlamydia* infection (Oriel et al). (Tetracycline should not be administered in children less than 8 years of age.) Cephalosporins have not proved effective in vitro against *Chlamydia* (Ridgway and Oriel). In prepubertal female patients with persistent asymptomatic genitourinary colonization with *Chlamydia*, Rettig and Nelson recommend treatment to prevent possible adverse side effects of prolonged genital carriage. Persistence or recurrence of disease after treatment is not uncommon, and repeat cultures and prolonged antibiotic therapy may be required.

OTHER DISORDERS

Pinworm Infestation

Pinworm is caused by the nematode *Enterobius vermicularis*. The disease is distributed worldwide and occurs commonly in families.

PATHOGENESIS. The adult worm lives in the large intestine of the human. The gravid female migrates to the rectum, deposits her eggs on the perianal skin and perineum at night, and then dies. Autoinfection and infection of other persons continues as long as adult gravid females deposit eggs on the perianal skin.

SYMPTOMS. Pinworm infection causes pruritus ani and occasionally pruritus vulvae. *Enterobius* has been implicated as a factor in secondary enuresis and also in acute and chronic urinary tract infection (Mayers and Purvis; Sachdev and Howards). In a study of female children, Kropp et al demonstrated that 22 per cent of patients with documented urinary tract infections had pinworm infestation, compared with only 5 per cent of the control population. While the relationship between female urinary tract infections and the presence of introital enteric organisms is well recognized, the association between pinworms and positive introital cultures is also noteworthy. Kropp et al found that the incidence of pinworms recovered from the perineum of females was higher in girls with enteric organisms present on a swab of the introitus than in those with negative introital cultures.

DIAGNOSIS. *Enterobius* is recovered by application of Scotch tape to the perianal skin to pick up any eggs. The tape is then applied to a glass slide and examined under low-power magnification (Graham). Specimens should be obtained early in the morning before washing of the genitalia.

TREATMENT. The drugs of choice for enterobiasis are pyrantel pamoate, given orally, 100 mg twice daily for 3 days, or mebendazole, as a single 100-mg dose, which is repeated in 2 weeks. Neither drug is recommended for children less than 2 years of age. These medications should be administered to all family members (Hoekenga).

Trichomoniasis

Trichomonas vaginalis, a flagellate protozoan, often affects the genitourinary tract and may cause significant urologic complications.

PATHOGENESIS. Vaginal trichomoniasis in the newborn may result from nonsexual transmission via infected mothers to the fetus at the time of delivery (Al-Salihi et al; Postlethwaite; Krieger). In adolescents, the majority of cases are acquired through sexual intercourse.

SYMPTOMS. Approximately 25 per cent of females with culture-proven *Trichomonas* infection have no symptoms (Rein). Conversely, *Trichomonas* may be responsible for abacterial cystitis or may occur concomitantly with recurrent bacterial urinary tract infections. Symptoms of urgency, frequency, pruritus, and vaginal discharge are typically present (Fouts and Kraus).

In males, *T. vaginalis* infection is usually asymptomatic; however, this organism has been implicated as an infrequent cause of nonspecific urethritis, prostatitis, epididymitis, balanoposthitis, and urethral stricture disease, and it may result in infertility (Meares; Krieger).

DIAGNOSIS. The diagnosis of *T. vaginalis* infection is made by direct microscopic examination of a wet-mount specimen or by growth of the trichomonads in a selective culture medium. Recovery of *T. vaginalis* requires meticulous culture techniques under anaerobic conditions with optimal incubation at 37° C

(Rothenberg et al). Serologic techniques remain research tools at this time. The association between *Trichomonas* and gonorrhea is well documented, and patients treated for gonorrhea who have persistent urinary symptoms or culture-proven reinfection should be investigated for trichomoniasis.

TREATMENT. The drug of choice for *T. vaginalis* infection is metronidazole (Flagyl), which is effective in 90 to 95 per cent of patients (Perl and Ragazzoni). Side effects include vertigo, nausea, and headaches. The dosage recommended by the Bureau of Venereal Disease Control is 250 mg orally three times a day for 7 days, or 2 g orally as a single dose. In females with neonatal vaginitis, Postlethwaite recommends 50 mg three times a day for 10 days.

Ureaplasma *Infection*

Ureaplasma urealyticum is a common inhabitant of male and female genital tracts after puberty. Colonization is primarily the result of sexual contact (McCormack et al, 1973a, 1973b). Infants become colonized with *U. urealyticum* during passage through the birth canal of an infected mother (Klein et al). In prepubertal children, *Ureaplasma* has been recovered infrequently from the urine or external genitalia (Foy et al).

Ureaplasma has been implicated in approximately 20 to 30 per cent of patients with nongonococcal urethritis (McCormack et al, 1973a; Taylor-Robinson and McCormack). Microscopic examination of the urethral discharge is essential to rule out gonorrhea. Definitive diagnosis is established by culture techniques.

The treatment of choice is tetracycline, 40 mg/kg over 24 hours in four divided doses for 10 days (Holmes et al; Handsfield). Erythromycin is the preferred antimicrobial agent in children less than 9 years of age. In adolescent patients, sexual partners should be treated as well.

Cyclophosphamide Cystitis

Cyclophosphamide (Cytoxan) is an effective and widely utilized antineoplastic agent in children. A major side effect of this drug is hematuria, which has been reported in 2 to 40 per cent of patients (Lawrence et al; Texter et al). Although acute hemorrhagic cystitis is usually reversible, extensive chronic bleeding may lead to irreversible changes of vesical fibrosis and contracture. The long-term complications of cyclophosphamide appear to be related to the duration of therapy and the total dose of drug administration.

PATHOGENESIS. The cyclophosphamide molecule itself does not appear to be responsible for damage to the bladder mucosa (Philips et al). Cyclophosphamide is converted by the liver into an active, toxic metabolite, acrolein, which is excreted through the kidneys and produces cell damage by local contact with the urothelium. The bladder is the organ most susceptible to damage because the surface contact with urine is longest here. However, the entire uroepithelial surface may be affected, and lesions of the renal pelvis and ureter have been reported.

SYMPTOMS. Hemorrhagic cystitis can occur after oral or intravenous cyclophosphamide administration. Bleeding may develop soon after intravenous drug injection but more commonly occurs several weeks to months after therapy (Liedberg et al). The initial onset of symptoms may be delayed for several years after cyclophosphamide therapy (Kende et al). There appears to be additive toxicity between radiation therapy and cyclophosphamide administration. Children with extensive disease present with urinary urgency, frequency, suprapubic pain, and passage of blood clots. Profuse bleeding has been reported and may be life threatening.

DIAGNOSIS. Cystoscopic examination demonstrates diffuse erythematous changes with patchy mucosal sloughing and necrosis. Slow oozing of blood is demonstrable from most areas of the bladder. Bladder biopsy demonstrates nonspecific inflammatory changes with edema in the mucosa and submucosa.

TREATMENT. In an experimental model (Tolley) and in the clinical setting (Primack), *N*-acetylcysteine has been shown to be of value in protecting the bladder from developing hemorrhagic cystitis without impairing the therapeutic efficacy of cyclophosphamide. This agent contains sulfhydryl groups that may bind and inactivate active sites within the toxic metabolites of cyclophosphamide. The recommended dose ratio of *N*-acetylcysteine to cyclophosphamide is 1:1 weight per weight given within 2 hours of drug administration. *N*-acetylcysteine does not appear to speed resolution of the inflammatory changes if given after a course of cyclophosphamide therapy.

Erlich et al recently reported success in preventing cyclophosphamide cystitis by administering sodium 2-mercaptoethane sulfonate. This drug prevents the formation of acrolein.

Hemorrhagic cystitis can be prevented by promoting overhydration and frequent micturition during therapy. An indwelling urethral catheter can be justified in patients in whom frequent voiding is not possible.

Adequate hydration and maintenance of vigorous diuresis are recommended in patients with extensive hemorrhagic cystitis (Droller et al). Attempts at bladder fulguration usually prove ineffective because of the diffuse nature of the vesical involvement. In extensive bleeding, a variety of treatment regimens have included instillation of formalin (Shrom et al), phenol (Duckett et al), or silver nitrate (Kumar et al); intravenous vasopressin administration (Pyeritz et al); bilateral hypogastric artery ligation; and cystectomy with urinary diversion. Rabinovitch has reported success with suprapubic cystostomy and continuous bladder irrigation for evacuation of clots.

Eosinophilic Cystitis

Eosinophilic cystitis is an uncommon inflammatory disease of the bladder which is characterized by irritative urinary symptoms, hematuria, and suprapubic pain. This entity has been reported in all age groups (Champion and Ackles; Goldstein; Nkposong and Attah; Hellstrom et al; Tauscher and Shaw). There is often a personal or family history of allergy (Rubin and Pincus).

PATHOGENESIS AND PATHOLOGY. No causative agent has been definitively identified, although food allergens, medications, bladder injury, and parasites have been suggested as the cause of the disease. Others have postulated an antigen–immune-complex reaction in the bladder that stimulates eosinophilic infiltration (Hellstrom et al; Littleton et al).

SYMPTOMS. Dysuria, urgency, frequency, and hematuria are usually present, and symptoms last for 1 to 3 weeks. Gross hematuria has been reported (Nkposong and Attah). Physical examination may reveal suprapubic tenderness with or without a palpable pelvic mass.

DIAGNOSIS. The differential diagnosis includes bacterial cystitis, interstitial cystitis, parasitic infection of the bladder, and vesical neoplasia. Peripheral eosinophilia is a routine finding in children with eosinophilic cystitis. Results of urinalysis are nonspecific; most patients have microscopic pyuria and hematuria. Urine culture is negative. Excretory urographic findings range from normal to the demonstration of filling defects in the bladder (Farber and Vawter). Bilateral hydroureteronephrosis may result (Nkposong and Attah). Cystoscopic findings reveal inflammatory mucosal changes with polypoid lesions and thickening of the bladder wall. Bladder biopsies demonstrate intense eosinophilic infiltration of the bladder mucosa and musculature.

TREATMENT. Steroids, antihistamines, cytotoxic drugs, radiotherapy, and long-term antibiotics have all been advocated in the treatment of eosinophilic cystitis. Each of these has had limited success. Powell et al have recommended that these patients be evaluated by an allergist to rule out a specific allergen as the cause of the disease. In rare cases of advanced disease, extirpative surgery may be necessary (Sidh et al).

Chronic Granulomatous Disease

Chronic granulomatous disease of infancy is a hereditary disorder of leukocyte metabolism that is associated with chronic and recurrent bacterial infections. The disease is transmitted as a sex-linked disorder in males and as an autosomal recessive disease in females (Young and Middleton).

PATHOGENESIS. In patients with chronic granulomatous disease, the leukocytes have ineffective bactericidal and fungicidal activity (Rodey et al; Lehrer). One of the normal mechanisms of bacterial destruction involves halogenation of the bacterial cell wall and requires hydrogen peroxide and peroxidase (Klebanoff and White). In children with chronic granulomatous disease, granulocytes are capable of normal ingestion of bacteria; however, hydrogen peroxide production is impaired. Thus, these leukocytes are unable to destroy bacteria that do not produce their own hydrogen peroxide, such as *Staphylococcus aureus* and gram-negative enteric organisms (Holmes et al; Elgefors et al). These defective granulocytes also produce inadequate amounts of superoxide, an agent that has significant bactericidal activity (Curnutte et al).

SYMPTOMS. This disease should be suspected in children who have an increased propensity to infection. The most frequent sites of involvement include the skin, lymphatics, respiratory tract, gastrointestinal system, liver, spleen, and bone. Urologic involvement has been reported and may be manifest as xanthogranulomatous pyelonephritis (Johansen et al) or cystitis (Young and Middleton).

DIAGNOSIS. The laboratory diagnosis of chronic granulomatous disease is established by the nitroblue tetrazolium dye test (Baehner and Nathan). Ninety per cent of normal leukocytes reduce nitroblue tetrazolium during phagocytosis of latex particles. However, in children with chronic granulomatous disease, only 10 per cent of the leukocytes are capable of reducing nitroblue tetrazolium. Definitive diagnosis of the disease depends on the demonstration of impaired intracellular bactericidal activity.

TREATMENT. Continuous and long-term prophylactic antibiotic therapy appears indicated in these children (Philippart et al). The frequency and severity of bacterial infections appear to be reduced in children undergoing long-term sulfonamide therapy (Johnston et al).

BIBLIOGRAPHY

TUBERCULOSIS

American Academy of Pediatrics: Report of the Committee on Infectious Diseases. Nineteenth ed. Evanston, Ill., American Academy of Pediatrics, 1982.

Cinman AC: Genitourinary tuberculosis. Urology 20:353, 1982.

Cos LR, Cockett ATK: Genitourinary tuberculosis revisited. Urology 20:111, 1982.

Ehrlich RM, Lattimer JK: Urogenital tuberculosis in children. J Urol 105:461, 1971.

Flechner SM, Gow JG: Role of nephrectomy in the treatment of non-functioning or very poorly functioning unilateral tuberculous kidney. J Urol 123:822, 1980.

Fox W: The chemotherapy of pulmonary tuberculosis: a review. Chest 76(Suppl):785, 1979.

Glassroth J, Robins AG, Snider DE: Letter to the editor. N Engl J Med 303:940, 1980.

Gow JG: Genitourinary tuberculosis: a 7-year review. Br J Urol 51:239, 1979.

Hartman GW, Segura JW, Hattery RR: Infectious diseases of the genitourinary tract. In Emmett's Clinical Urography: An Atlas and Textbook of Roentgenologic Diagnosis. Vol 2. Fourth ed. Edited by DM Witten, GH Myers Jr, DC Utz. Philadelphia, WB Saunders Co., 1977, pp 898–918.

Kenney M, Loechel AB, Lovelock FJ: Urine cultures in tuberculosis. Am Rev Respir Dis 82:564, 1960.

Lattimer JK, Vasquez G, Wechsler H: New drugs for treatment of genitourinary tuberculosis: a comparison of efficacy. J Urol 83:493, 1960.

Lattimer JK, Wechsler M: Genitourinary tuberculosis. In Campbell's Urology. Vol 1. Fourth ed. Edited by JH Harrison, RF Gittes, AD Perlmutter, et al. Philadelphia, WB Saunders Co., 1978, pp 557–575.

Murphy DM, Fallon B, Lane V, et al: Tuberculous stricture of ureter. Urology 20:382, 1982.

Robbins SL, Cotran RS: Pathologic Basis of Disease. Second ed. Philadelphia, WB Saunders Co., 1979, pp 396–404.

Smith MHD, Marquis JR: Tuberculosis and other mycobacterial infections. In Textbook of Pediatric Infectious Diseases. Vol 1. Edited by RD Feigin, JD Cherry. Philadelphia, WB Saunders Co., 1981, pp 1016–1060.

Wechsler H: Update on chemotherapy of renal tuberculosis. J Urol 124:319, 1980.

Wechsler H, Lattimer JK: An evaluation of the current therapeutic regimen for renal tuberculosis. J Urol 113:760, 1975.

Wong SH, Lau WY: The surgical management of non-functioning tuberculous kidneys. J Urol 124:187, 1980.

Zinman L, Libertino JA: Antirefluxing ileocecal conduit. Urol Clin North Am 7:503, June 1980.

CANDIDIASIS

Borgers M, Van Den Bossche H, DeBrabander M: The mechanism of action of the new antimycotic, ketoconazole. Am J Med Suppl 74:2, 1983.

Dolan CT, Stried RP: Serologic diagnosis of yeast infections. Am J Clin Pathol 59:49, 1973.

Eckstein C, Koss EJ, Koff SA: Anuria in a newborn secondary to bilateral ureteropelvic fungus balls. J Urol 127:109, 1982.

Everett ED, LaForce FM, Eickhoff TC: Serologic studies in suspected visceral candidiasis. Arch Intern Med 135:1075, 1975.

Graybill GR, Galgiani GN, Jorgensen JH, et al: Ketoconazole therapy for fungal urinary tract infections. J Urol 129:68, 1983.

Khan MY: Anuria from Candida pyelonephritis and obstructing fungal balls. Urology 21:421, 1983.

Kozinn PJ, Galen RS, Taschdjian CL, et al: The precipitin test in systemic candidiasis. JAMA 235:628, 1976.

Kozinn PJ, Taschdjian CL, Goldberg PK, et al: Advances in the diagnosis of renal candidiasis. J Urol 119:184, 1978.

MacMillan BG, Law EJ, Holder IA: Experience with Candida infections in the burn patient. Arch Surg 104:509, 1972.

Noe HN, Tonkin ILD: Renal candidiasis in the neonate. J Urol 127:517, 1982.

Schönebeck J: Studies on Candida infection of the urinary tract and on the antimycotic drug 5-fluorocytosine. Scand J Urol Nephrol [Suppl] 11:1, 1972.

Schönebeck J, Andersson L, Lingårdh G, et al: Ureteric obstruction caused by yeast-like fungi. Scand J Urol Nephrol 4:171, 1970.

Stone HH, Kolb LD, Currie CA, et al: Candida sepsis: pathogenesis and principles of treatment. Ann Surg 179:697, 1974.

Wheeler JG, Boyle R, Abramson J: Candida tropicalis pyelonephritis successfully treated with 5-fluorocytosine and surgery. J Pediatr 102:627, 1983.

Wise GJ: Letter to the editor. J Urol 128:828, 1982.

Wise GJ, Goldberg P, Kozinn PJ: Genitourinary candidiasis: diagnosis and treatment. J Urol 116:778, 1976.

Wise GJ, Kozinn PJ, Goldberg P: Amphotericin B as a urologic irrigant in the management of noninvasive candiduria. J Urol 128:82, 1982.

Wise GJ, Ray B, Kozinn PJ: The serodiagnosis of significant genitourinary candidiasis. J Urol 107:1043, 1972.

Wise GJ, Wainstein S, Goldberg P, et al: Candidal cystitis: management by continuous bladder irrigation with amphotericin B. JAMA 224:1636, 1973.

Wise GJ, Wainstein S, Goldberg P, et al: Flucytosine in urinary *Candida* infections. Urology 3:708, 1974.

ASPERGILLOSIS

Bennett JE: Chemotherapy of systemic mycoses (second of two parts). N Engl J Med 290:320, 1974.

Comings DE, Turbow BA, Callahan DH, et al: Obstructing *Aspergillus* cast of the renal pelvis: report of a case in a patient having diabetes mellitus and Addison's disease. Arch Intern Med 110:255, 1962.

Eisenberg RL, Hedgcock MW, Shanser JD: *Aspergillus* mycetoma of the renal pelvis associated with uretero-pelvic junction obstruction. J Urol 118:466, 1977.

Flechner SM, McAninch JW: Aspergillosis of the urinary tract: ascending route of infection and evolving patterns of disease. J Urol 125:598, 1981.

Hinson KFW, Moon AJ, Plummer NS: Broncho-pulmonary aspergillosis: a review and a report of eight new cases. Thorax 7:317, 1952.

Melchior J, Mebust WK, Valk WL: Ureteral colic from a fungus ball: unusual presentation of systemic aspergillosis. J Urol 108:698, 1972.

Warshawsky AB, Keiller D, Gittes RF: Bilateral renal aspergillosis. J Urol 113:8, 1975.

Weinstein AJ, Farkas S: Serologic tests in infectious diseases: clinical utility and interpretation. Med Clin North Am 62:1099, September 1978.

Young RC, Bennett JE, Vogel CL, et al: Aspergillosis: the spectrum of the disease in 98 patients. Medicine (Baltimore) 49:147, 1970.

ACTINOMYCOSIS

Berardi RS: Abdominal actinomycosis. Surg Gynecol Obstet 149:257, 1979.

Crosse JEW, Soderdahl DW, Schamber DT: Renal actinomycosis. Urology 7:309, 1976.

Deshmukh AS, Kropp KA: Spontaneous vesicocutaneous fistula caused by actinomycosis: case report. J Urol 112:192, 1974.

Drake DP, Holt RJ: Childhood actinomycosis: report of 3 recent cases. Arch Dis Child 51:979, 1976.

Eastridge CE, Prather JR, Hughes FA Jr, et al: Actinomycosis: a 24 year experience. South Med J 65:839, 1972.

Fass RJ, Scholand JF, Hodges GR, et al: Clindamycin in the treatment of serious anaerobic infections. Ann Intern Med 78:853, 1973.

Grierson JM, Zelas P: Actinomycosis involving urachal remnants. Med J Aust 1:849, 1977.

Holmberg K, Nord C-E, Wadström T: Serological studies of *Actinomyces israelii* by crossed immunoelectrophoresis: taxonomic and diagnostic applications. Infect Immunol 12:398, 1975.

Isaacson P, Jennings M: Bilateral ureteric obstruction in a patient with ileocaecal Crohn's disease complicated by actinomycosis. Br J Urol 49:410, 1977.

Kretschmer HL, Hibbs WG: Actinomycosis of the kidney in infancy and childhood. J Urol 36:123, 1936.

Robbins TS, Scott SA: Actinomycosis: the disease and its treatment. Drug Intell Clin Pharm 15:99, 1981.

Rose HD, Rytel MW: Actinomycosis treated with clindamycin (letter to the editor). JAMA 221:1052, 1972.

BLASTOMYCOSIS

Bergner DM, Kraus SD, Duck GB, et al: Systemic blastomycosis presenting with acute prostatic abscess. J Urol 126:132, 1981.

Denton JF, McDonough ES, Ajello L, et al: Isolation of *Blastomyces dermatitidis* from soil. Science 133:1126, 1961.

Eickenberg H-U, Amin M, Lich R Jr: Blastomycosis of the genitourinary tract. J Urol 113:650, 1975.

Furcolow ML, Chick EW, Busey JF, et al: Prevalence and incidence studies of human and canine blastomycosis. I. Cases in the United States, 1885–1968. Am Rev Respir Dis 102:60, 1970.

Gill JA, Gerald B: Blastomycosis in childhood. Radiology 91:965, 1968.

Macher A: Histoplasmosis and blastomycosis. Med Clin North Am 64:447, 1980.

Schwarz J, Salfelder K: Blastomycosis: a review of 152 cases. Curr Top Pathol 65:165, 1977.

Yogev R, Davis AT: Blastomycosis in children: a review of the literature. Mycopathologia 68:139, 1979.

CRYPTOCOCCOSIS

Bowman HE, Ritchey JO: Cryptococcosis (torulosis) involving the brain, adrenal and prostate. J Urol 71:373, 1954.

Cohen JR, Kaufmann W: Systemic cryptococcosis: a report of a case with review of the literature. Am J Clin Pathol 22:1069, 1952.

Gordon MA, Vedder DK: Serologic tests in diagnosis and prognosis of cryptococcosis. JAMA 197:961, 1966.

Huynh MT, Reyes CV: Prostatic cryptococcosis. Urology 20:622, 1982.

Lewis JL, Rabinovich S: The wide spectrum of cryptococcal infections. Am J Med 53:315, 1972.

O'Connor FJ, Foushee JHS Jr, Cox CE: Prostatic cryptococcosis: a case report. J Urol 94:160, 1965.

Randall RE Jr, Stacy WK, Toone EC, et al: Cryptococcal pyelonephritis. N Engl J Med 279:60, 1968.

Salyer WR, Salyer DC: Involvement of the kidney and prostate in cryptococcosis. J Urol 109:695, 1973.

Tillotson JR, Lerner AM: Prostatism in an eighteen-year-old boy due to infection with *Cryptococcus neoformans*. N Engl J Med 273:1150, 1965.

Wittner M: Cryptococcosis. *In* Textbook of Pediatric Infectious Diseases. Vol 2. Edited by RD Feigin, JD Cherry. Philadelphia, WB Saunders Company., 1981, pp 1505–1509.

COCCIDIOIDOMYCOSIS

Aguilar-Torres FG, Jackson LJ, Ferstenfeld JE, et al: Counterimmunoelectrophoresis in the detection of antibodies against *Coccidioides immitis*. Ann Intern Med 85:740, 1976.

Cheng SF: Bilateral coccidioidal epididimitis. Urology 3:362, 1974.

Conner WT, Drach GW, Bucher WC Jr: Genitourinary aspects of disseminated coccidioidomycosis. J Urol 113:82, 1975.

Drutz DJ, Catanzaro A: Coccidioidomycosis. Part I. Am Rev Respir Dis 117:559, 1978.

Granoff DM, Libke RD: Coccidioidomycosis in children. *In* Textbook of Pediatric Infectious Diseases. Vol 2. Edited by RD Feigin, JD Cherry. Philadelphia, WB Saunders Co., 1981, pp 1488–1500.

Stevens DA, Levine HB, Deresinski SC: Miconazole in coccidioidomycosis. II. Therapeutic and pharmacologic studies in man. Am J Med 60:191, 1976.

Weinstein AJ, Farkas S: Serologic tests in infectious diseases: clinical utility and interpretation. Med Clin North Am 62:1099, 1978.

MUCORMYCOSIS

Baker RD: Resectable mycotic lesions and acutely fatal mycoses. JAMA 150:1579, 1952.

Dansky AS, Lynne CM, Politano VA: Disseminated mucormycosis with renal involvement. J Urol 119:275, 1978.

Langston C, Roberts DA, Porter GA, et al: Renal phycomycosis. J Urol 109:941, 1973.

Meyer RD, Rosen P, Armstrong D: Phycomycosis complicating leukemia and lymphoma. Ann Intern Med 77:871, 1972.

Prout GR Jr, Goddard AR: Renal mucormycosis: survival after nephrectomy and amphotericin B therapy. N Engl J Med 263:1246, 1960.

SCHISTOSOMIASIS

American Academy of Pediatrics: Schistosomiasis: Report of the Committee on Infectious Diseases. Nineteenth ed. Evanston, Ill., American Academy of Pediatrics, 1982, pp 180–182.

Bazeed MA, Ashamalla A, Abd-Alrazek A-A, et al: Partial flap ureteroneocytostomy for bilharzial strictures of the lower ureter. Urology 20:237, 1982.

Hanash KA, Bissada NK: Genito-urinary schistosomiasis (bilharziasis). Part 1. King Faisal Specialist Hosp Med J 1:59, 1982.

Hanash KA, Bissada NK, Lewall DB, et al: Genito-urinary schistosomiasis (bilharziasis). Part 3. Endoscopic and pathologic diagnosis. King Faisal Specialist Hosp Med J 2:31, 1982.

Hanna AAZ: Genitourinary bilharziasis (schistosomiasis). In Emmett's Clinical Urography. Vol 2. Fourth ed. Edited by DM Witten, GH Myers Jr, DC Utz. Philadelphia, WB Saunders Co., 1977, pp 921–939.

Kagan IG: Current status of serologic testing for parasitic diseases. Hosp Pract 9:157, 1974.

Kambal A: The relation of urinary bilharziasis to vesical stones in children. Br J Urol 53:315, 1981.

Sullivan TJ: Schistosomiasis. In Textbook of Pediatric Infectious Diseases. Vol 2. Edited by RD Feigin, JD Cherry. Philadelphia, WB Saunders Co., 1981, pp 1625–1633.

von Lichtenberg F, Lehman JS: Parasitic diseases of the genitourinary system. In Campbell's Urology. Vol 1. Fourth ed. Edited by JH Harrison, RF Gittes, AD Perlmutter, et al. Philadelphia, WB Saunders Co., 1978, pp 598–615.

ECHINOCOCCOSIS

Apt W, Knierim F: An evaluation of diagnostic tests for hydatid disease. Am J Trop Med Hyg 19:943, 1970.

Auldist AW, Myers NA: Hydatid disease in children. Aust NZ J Surg 44:402, 1974.

Baltaxe HA, Fleming RJ: The angiographic appearance of hydatid disease. Radiology 97:599, 1970.

Fuloria HK, Jaiswal MSD, Singh RV: Primary hydatid cyst of bladder. Br J Urol 47:192, 1975.

Gajjar PD, Sinclair-Smith CC: Renal echinococcosis in children: a report of 2 cases. S Afr Med J 54:984, 1978.

Gharbi HA, Ben Cheikh M, Hamza R, et al: Les localisations rares de l'hydatidose chez l'enfant. (Rare sites of hydatid disease in children.) Ann Radiol (Paris) 20:151, 1977.

Gilsanz V, Lozano F, Jimenez J: Renal hydatid cysts: communicating with collecting system. AJR 135:357, 1980.

Hansman DJ, Brown JM: Eosinophilic cystitis: a case associated with possible hydatid infection. Med J Aust 2:563, 1974.

Hunter GW III, Swartzwelder JC, Clyde DF: Tropical Medicine. Fifth ed. Philadelphia, WB Saunders Co., 1976, pp 609–615.

Keramidas DC, Doulas N, Fotis G, et al: Bilateral hydronephrosis and hydroureter due to hydatid cyst in the pouch of Douglas. J Pediatr Surg 15:345, 1980.

Meymerian E, Luttermoser GW, Frayha GJ, et al: Host-parasite relationships in echinococcosis: X. Laboratory evaluation of chemical scolicides as adjuncts to hydatid surgery. Ann Surg 158:211, 1963.

Musacchio F, Mitchell N: Primary renal echinococcosis: a case report. Am J Trop Med Hyg 15:168, 1966.

Nabizadeh I, Morehouse HT, Freed SZ: Hydatid disease of kidney. Urology 22:176, 1983.

Sharma RS, Tiwari DS, Tiwari R: Hydatid cyst of the kidney. Indian J Pediatr 43:211, 1976.

Shulman Y, Morales P: Case profile: renal echinococcosis. Urology 20:452, 1982.

Silber SJ, Moyad RA: Renal echinococcus. J Urol 108:669, 1972.

CHLAMYDIAL INFECTION

Berger RE, Alexander ER, Monda GD, et al: Chlamydia trachomatis as a cause of acute 'idiopathic' epididymitis. N Engl J Med 298:301, 1978.

Oriel JD, Ridgway GL, Tchamouroff S: Comparison of erythromycin stearate and oxytetracycline in the treatment of non-gonococcal urethritis: their efficacy against Chlamydia trachomatis. Scott Med J 22:375, 1977.

Rettig PJ, Nelson JD: Genital tract infection with Chlamydia trachomatis in prepubertal children. J Pediatr 99:206, 1981.

Ridgway GL, Oriel JD: Activity of antimicrobials against Chlamydia trachomatis in vitro (letter to the editor). J Antimicrob Chemother 5:483, 1979.

Smith TF, Weed LA, Segura JW, et al: Isolation of Chlamydia from patients with urethritis. Mayo Clin Proc 50:105, 1975.

PINWORM INFESTATION

Graham CF: A device for the diagnosis of Enterobius infection. Am J Trop Med 21:159, 1941.

Hoekenga MT: Intestinal parasites. In Current Therapy 1976. Edited by HF Conn. Philadelphia, WB Saunders Co., 1976, pp 49–52.

Kropp KA, Cichocki GA, Bansal NK: Enterobius vermicularis (pinworms), introital bacteriology and recurrent urinary tract infection in children. J Urol 120:480, 1978.

Mayers CP, Purvis RJ: Manifestations of pinworms. Can Med Assoc J 103:489, 1970.

Sachdev YV, Howards SS: Enterobius vermicularis infestation and secondary enuresis. J Urol 113:143, 1975.

TRICHOMONIASIS

Al-Salihi FL, Curran JP, Wang J-S: Neonatal Trichomonas vaginalis: report of three cases and review of the literature. Pediatrics 53:196, 1974.

Fouts AC, Kraus SJ: Trichomonas vaginalis: reevaluation of its clinical presentation and laboratory diagnosis. J Infect Dis 141:137, 1980.

Krieger JN: Urologic aspects of trichomoniasis. Invest Urol 18:414, 1981.

Meares EM Jr: Prostatitis syndromes: new perspectives about old woes. J Urol 123:141, 1980.

Perl G, Ragazzoni H: Further studies in treatment of female and male trichomoniasis with metronidazole. Obstet Gynecol 22:376, 1963.

Postlethwaite RJ: Trichomonas vaginitis and Escherichia coli urinary infection in a newborn infant. Clin Pediatr (Phila) 14:866, 1975.

Rein MF: Trichomonas vaginalis. In Principles and Practice of Infectious Diseases. Vol 2. Edited by GL Mandell,

RG Douglas Jr, JE Bennett. New York, John Wiley & Sons, 1979, pp 2147–2150.

Rothenberg RB, Simon R, Chipperfield E, et al: Efficacy of selected diagnostic tests for sexually transmitted diseases. JAMA 235:49, 1976.

UREAPLASMA *INFECTION*

Foy H, Kenny G, Bor E, et al: Prevalence of *Mycoplasma hominis* and *Ureaplasma urealyticum* (T strains) in urine of adolescents. J Clin Microbiol 2:226, 1975.

Handsfield HH: Gonorrhea and nongonococcal urethritis: recent advances. Med Clin North Am 62:925, 1978.

Holmes KK, Johnson DW, Floyd TM: Studies of venereal disease. III. Double-blind comparison of tetracycline hydrochloride and placebo in treatment of nongonococcal urethritis. JAMA 202:474, 1967.

Klein JO, Buckland D, Finland M: Colonization of newborn infants by mycoplasmas. N Engl J Med 280:1025, 1969.

McCormack WM, Braun P, Lee Y-H, et al: The genital mycoplasmas. N Engl J Med 288:78, 1973a.

McCormack WM, Lee Y-H, Zinner SH: Sexual experience and urethral colonization with genital mycoplasmas: a study in normal men. Ann Intern Med 78:696, 1973b.

Taylor-Robinson D, McCormack WM: The genital mycoplasmas. N Engl J Med 302:1003, 1063, 1980.

CYCLOPHOSPHAMIDE CYSTITIS

Droller MJ, Saral R, Santos G: Prevention of cyclophosphamide-induced hemorrhagic cystitis. Urology 20:256, 1982.

Duckett JW Jr, Peters PC, Donaldson MH: Severe cyclophosphamide hemorrhagic cystitis controlled with phenol. J Pediatr Surg 8:55, 1973.

Erlich RM, Freidman A, Goldsobel A, et al: Prevention of cyclophosphamide cystitis with sodium 2-mercaptoethane sulfonate—an experimental and clinical investigation. Presented at the meeting of the American Academy of Pediatrics, Section of Urology, San Francisco, October 22–27, 1983.

Kende G, Wajsman Z, Thomas PRM, et al: Chronic hematuria and localized bladder damage following combined cyclophosphamide and local radiotherapy. J Surg Oncol 12:169, 1979.

Kumar APM, Wrenn EL Jr, Jayalakshmamma B, et al: Silver nitrate irrigation to control bladder hemorrhage in children receiving cancer therapy. J Urol 116:85, 1976.

Lawrence HJ, Simone J, Aur RJA: Cyclophosphamide-induced hemorrhagic cystitis in children with leukemia. Cancer 36:1572, 1975.

Liedberg C-F, Rausing A, Langeland P: Cyclophosphamide hemorrhagic cystitis. Scand J Urol Nephrol 4:183, 1970.

Philips FS, Sternberg SS, Cronin AP, et al: Cyclophosphamide and urinary bladder toxicity. Cancer Res 21:1577, 1961.

Primack A: Amelioration of cyclophosphamide-induced cystitis. J Natl Cancer Inst 47:223, 1971.

Pyeritz RE, Droller MJ, Bender WL, et al: An approach to the control of massive hemorrhage in cyclophosphamide-induced cystitis by intravenous vasopressin: a case report. J Urol 120:253, 1978.

Rabinovitch HH: Simple innocuous treatment of massive cyclophosphamide hemorrhagic cystitis. Urology 13:610, 1979.

Shrom SH, Donaldson MH, Duckett JW Jr, et al: Formalin treatment for intractable hemorrhagic cystitis: a review of the literature with 16 additional cases. Cancer 38:1785, 1976.

Texter JH Jr, Koontz WW Jr, McWilliams NB: Hemorrhagic cystitis as a complication of the management of pediatric neoplasms. Urol Surv 29:47, 1979.

Tolley DA: The effect of *N*-acetyl cysteine on cyclophosphamide cystitis. Br J Urol 49:659, 1977.

EOSINOPHILIC CYSTITIS

Champion RH, Ackles RC: Eosinophilic cystitis. J Urol 96:729, 1966.

Farber S, Vawter GF: Clinical pathological conference. J Pediatr 62:941, 1963.

Goldstein M: Eosinophilic cystitis. J Urol 106:854, 1971.

Hellstrom HR, Davis BK, Shonnard JW: Eosinophilic cystitis: a study of 16 cases. Am J Clin Pathol 72:777, 1979.

Littleton RH, Farah RN, Cerny JC: Eosinophilic cystitis: an uncommon form of cystitis. J Urol 127:132, 1982.

Nkposong EO, Attah EB: Eosinophilic cystitis. Eur Urol 4:274, 1978.

Powell NB, Powell EB, Thomas OC, et al: Allergy of the lower urinary tract. J Urol 107:631, 1972.

Rubin L, Pincus MB: Eosinophilic cystitis: the relationship of allergy in the urinary tract to eosinophilic cystitis and the pathophysiology of eosinophilia. J Urol 112:457, 1974.

Sidh SM, Smith SP, Silber SB, et al: Eosinophilic cystitis: advanced disease requiring surgical intervention. Urology 15:23, 1980.

Tauscher JW, Shaw DC: Eosinophilic cystitis. Clin Pediatr (Phila) 20:741, 1981.

CHRONIC GRANULOMATOUS DISEASE

Baehner RL, Nathan DG: Quantitative nitroblue tetrazolium test in chronic granulomatous disease. N Engl J Med 278:971, 1968.

Curnutte JT, Kipnes RS, Babior BM: Defect in pyridine nucleotide dependent superoxide production by a particulate fraction from the granulocytes of patients with chronic granulomatous disease. N Engl J Med 293:628, 1975.

Elgefors B, Olling S, Peterson H: Chronic granulomatous disease in three siblings. Scand J Infect Dis 10:79, 1978.

Holmes B, Page AR, Good RA: Studies of the metabolic activity of leukocytes from patients with a genetic abnormality of phagocytic function. J Clin Invest 46:1422, 1967.

Johansen KS, Borregaard N, Koch C, et al: Chronic granulomatous disease presenting as xanthogranulomatous pyelonephritis in late childhood. J Pediatr 100:98, 1982.

Johnston RB Jr, Wilfert CM, Buckley RH, et al: Enhanced bactericidal activity of phagocytes from patients with chronic granulomatous disease in the presence of sulphisoxazole. Lancet 1:824, 1975.

Klebanoff SJ, White LR: Iodination defect in the leukocytes of a patient with chronic granulomatous disease of childhood. N Engl J Med 280:460, 1969.

Lehrer RI: Measurement of candidacidal activity of specific leukocyte types in mixed cell populations. II. Normal and chronic granulomatous disease eosinophils. Infect Immun 3:800, 1971.

Philippart AI, Colodny AH, Baehner RL: Continuous antibiotic therapy in chronic granulomatous disease: preliminary communication. Pediatrics 50:923, 1972.

Rodey GE, Park BH, Windhorst DB, et al: Defective bactericidal activity of monocytes in fatal granulomatous disease. Blood 33:813, 1969.

Young AK, Middleton RG: Urologic manifestations of chronic granulomatous disease of infancy. J Urol 123:119, 1980.

Genital Infections
STEPHEN A. KRAMER

URETHRITIS

Gonococcal Urethritis

Gonorrhea is the most common reportable communicable disease in the United States today (Clark). Infection with *Neisseria gonorrhoeae* occurs most commonly in sexually active teenagers and young adults, but prepubertal involvement is not uncommon (Meek et al; Farrell et al).

PATHOGENESIS. The incubation period of *N. gonorrhoeae* is 2 to 8 days. Urethral infection in males is localized in the glands of Littre. Rectal carriage may occur in the absence of urethral colonization. Transmission of gonorrhea to prepubertal children may occur via nonsexual contact in social settings in which the parents are infected (Shore and Winkelstein). Conversely, Branch and Paxton noted a history of sexual exposure in 43 of 45 children, either from molestation from relatives or from voluntary sexual contact in older children.

SYMPTOMS. In adolescent males, gonorrhea is typically associated with dysuria and a profuse, yellow urethral discharge. Occasionally, asymptomatic pyuria may be the initial method of presentation. In younger children, penile swelling and the inability to void may be presenting complaints (Meek et al). Barrett-Connor reported a 23-month-old boy whose presenting symptom was an abscess on the glans penis.

DIAGNOSIS. Specimens should be obtained by stripping the urethra or by gently inserting a swab into the distal urethra. Demonstration of ovoid, gram-negative diplococci on staining is presumptive evidence of gonorrhea. Cultures must be obtained and should be plated and incubated immediately in a modified Thayer-Martin medium (Kellogg et al). Chocolate agar should also be used because an occasional strain of gonococcus is susceptible to the vancomycin present in modified Thayer-Martin medium. Serologic tests for syphilis should be performed on all patients with urethral discharge.

TREATMENT. In males with urethritis, the Centers for Disease Control recommend 75,000 to 100,000 units of aqueous procaine penicillin G per kilogram intramuscularly (Meek et al). Recent data have demonstrated that amoxicillin, 50 mg/kg orally to a maximum dose of 3.5 g, is as effective as penicillin G (Nelson et al). Each of these treatment regimens should be preceded by the administration of oral probenecid, 25 mg/kg, to a maximum dose of 1 g. In patients who are allergic to penicillin, alternate therapies for children more than 8 years of age include oral tetracycline, 25 mg/kg, as an initial dose, followed by 40 to 60 mg/kg per day for 7 days (Karney et al). In children less than 8 years of age, spectinomycin, 40 mg/kg in a single intramuscular dose, is recommended. Repeat urethral cultures should be taken approximately 1 week after completion of therapy to identify patients infected with penicillinase-producing organisms (Kellogg et al). It is important that infected contacts with gonorrhea be similarly treated with the dosage regimen described above.

Nongonococcal Urethritis

Nongonococcal urethritis, or nonspecific urethritis, is currently the most common sexually transmitted disease in males (Felman and Nikitas). Nongonococcal urethritis is quite common in the sexually active adolescent male but is rare in children.

PATHOGENESIS. *Chlamydia* and *Ureaplasma* have both been implicated as causative organisms in at least 50 to 60 per cent of cases of nonspecific urethritis (Smith et al). In the remaining 30 to 40 per cent of patients who have neither *Chlamydia* nor *Ureaplasma* isolated from the urethra, *Trichomonas vaginalis*, yeasts, or viruses may be the etiologic agents responsible for the urethritis.

SYMPTOMS. The onset of symptoms is usually more gradual in patients with nongonococcal urethritis than in those with gonococcal urethritis. Virtually all patients with gonorrhea have a urethral discharge with or without dysuria. Conversely, Jacobs and Kraus reported that only 38 per cent of patients with nongonococcal urethritis have both dysuria and urethral discharge. Whereas the urethral discharge in patients with gonococcal urethritis is characteristically purulent, the discharge in nongonococcal urethritis is clear, thin, and watery.

DIAGNOSIS. Nonspecific urethritis should be suspected in patients with a clear mucoid urethral discharge, persistent urethral discharge after treatment for gonococcal urethritis, or a history of anogenital gonorrhea. Examination of the first 10 to 15 ml of an early-morning voided urine demonstrates increased polymorphonuclear leukocytes and establishes the diagnosis of urethritis. It is imperative to rule out gonococcal urethritis by staining for gram-negative diplococci and obtaining Thayer-Martin cultures.

TREATMENT. Sulfonamides, erythromycin, and tetracycline, administered for 10 days to 2 weeks, are all effective agents for the treatment of chlamydial urethritis (Oriel et al). The drug of choice for *T. vaginalis* is metronidazole (Flagyl). Tetracycline and erythromycin are both effective agents for the treatment of *Ureaplasma* (see the preceding article in this chapter).

HERPES SIMPLEX INFECTION

Herpes simplex is an infectious venereal disease caused by Herpesvirus hominis that is the most common cause of vesiculoulcerative lesions of the genitalia in males and females.

PATHOGENESIS. The virus is transmitted via sexual intercourse, oral–genital contacts, or oral–anal contacts. Newborns may acquire infection during passage through a virus-infected birth canal (Nahmias et al, 1967 and 1970). The incubation period for herpes is 3 to 14 days for primary infections and 12 to 24 hours for repeat infections.

SYMPTOMS. In adolescent males, herpetic infections present as painful, clear vesicles on the shaft of the penis, scrotum, or thigh. These vesicles eventually coalesce and form pustules with ulceration. Herpesvirus has been implicated as a cause of urethritis.

In female infants and children, contact of the external genitalia with contaminated hands or by sexual abuse may be responsible for vulvovaginitis. In adolescent females, herpetic ulcers may develop at the introitus, within the vagina, or on the cervix. Symptoms of dysuria may be a clue to the diagnosis of herpetic cystitis (Person et al).

The vesiculoulcerative lesions heal spontaneously within 7 to 14 days. The disease is characterized by latency and repeated recurrent localized lesions, which may remain asymptomatic for long periods of time.

DIAGNOSIS. The diagnosis of herpes simplex is established by the clinical appearance of the vesicular lesions and the associated history of recurrences or exposure to disease. Herpes simplex virus can be grown in vitro in a variety of tissue cultures, with recovery of the virus in approximately 1 week. Serologic tests are available in some centers. Cytologic techniques involve scraping cells from the base of vesicular lesions and observing multinucleate giant cells and nuclear inclusion bodies.

Concurrent infection with *Treponema pallidum* is not uncommon, and therefore vesicular lesions on the genitalia should be tested by dark-field examination and patients should be followed serologically until recovery is complete (Fiumara et al).

TREATMENT. There is no effective treatment for herpes simplex virus infection. Topical therapy has proved ineffective and there is no immunologic vaccine available at this time. Idoxuridine (IDU) has been used to treat superficial keratitis, but it does not reduce the rate of recurrent disease. Photodynamic inactivation by means of tricyclic dyes—for example, neutral red—has been disappointing and furthermore may enhance the oncogenic potential of the virus.

SYPHILIS

Syphilis is caused by infection with the anaerobic spirochete *Treponema pallidum*. The overall rate of infectious syphilis in the United States has increased significantly since 1958 and parallels the increase in other venereal diseases (Wilfert and Gutman). In children, syphilis occurs much less often than gonorrhea.

PATHOGENESIS. *T. pallidum* has the ability to invade the intact mucous membrane or open wounds. Sexual contact is the most common method of disease transmission; however, other sites of inoculation include the lips, oral cavity, and abraded areas of skin. After tissue invasion, the organisms multiply and are disseminated by perivascular lymphatics to the systemic circulation (Robbins and Cotran).

Congenital syphilis may result from transplacental infection of the developing fetus or by contact with a primary syphilitic lesion during passage through the birth canal (Taber and Huber). Between 70 and 100 per cent of all pregnant women with untreated syphilis may transmit infection to the fetus. Congenital syphilis may be responsible for up to 25 per cent fetal mortality in utero and an additional 25 to 30 per cent mortality in the perinatal period (Wilfert and Gutman).

SYMPTOMS. Approximately 3 to 4 weeks after contact, the patient experiences an inflammatory response to infection at the site of inoculation. The chancre of primary syphilis is characteristically a single, nonpainful, nontender, firm lesion, which occurs most commonly on the penis in males and the vagina or cervix in females. Other sites of involvement include the lips, mouth, face, and abraded areas of skin.

Two to 10 weeks after the primary lesions, the patient may experience secondary disease manifested by maculopapular skin and mucous membrane lesions, fever, pharyngitis, generalized lymphadenopathy, headache, and flat moist lesions around the anus or vagina (condylomata lata). These secondary lesions of the skin and mucous membrane are highly infectious.

Tertiary syphilis develops years after secondary disease and may be characterized by gumma formation and also by neurologic and cardiovascular involvement.

DIAGNOSIS. The primary penile lesions of syphilis must be differentiated from chancroid, lymphogranuloma venereum, granuloma inguinale, herpes, and gangrenous balanitis (see below). The diagnosis is made by direct visualization of the pathogenic spirochetes on dark-field examination of the serous fluid from a syphilitic ulcer. Serologic methods for syphilis include both nontreponemal antigen tests and treponemal antigen tests. Nontreponemal studies identify nonspecific antitreponemal antibodies and include complement fixation and flocculation tests (VDRL). These studies demonstrate rising and falling antibody titers, which correlate well with adequacy of treatment.

Treponemal tests identify specific antitreponemal antibodies and include *T. pallidum* immobilization, fluorescent antibody, and hemagglutination tests. The *T. pallidum* immobilization test is based on the capacity of reaginic antibody and complement to immobilize living and motile treponemes. The fluorescent treponemal antibody absorption test is used for confirmation of positive nontreponemal tests.

TREATMENT. Penicillin remains the drug of choice for syphilis. For primary disease, the Centers for Disease Control recommend treatment with either a single intramuscular injection of benzathine penicillin G in a dosage of 2.4 million units intramuscularly or aqueous procaine penicillin G, 600,000 units daily for 8 days. In patients with penicillin allergies, erythromycin and tetracycline are alternative regimens.

Early treatment affords a high cure rate with excellent prognosis and minimal relapse. Patients should be followed with VDRL determinations every 3 months for a minimum of 1 year. Re-treatment is indicated in patients with persistently high serologic titers or in cases of decreasing titers that subsequently become elevated. Family members should be examined for syphilis, and case reports should be forwarded to local public health officials.

PROSTATITIS

Bacterial prostatitis is extremely rare in prepubertal children. Mann reported three neonates with prostatic abscesses, each associated with *Staphylococcus aureus*. Children may present with vesical irritative symptoms, urinary retention, or urethral discharge. Physical examination may reveal a cystic prostatic or seminal vesicle swelling that is exquisitely tender to palpation. The majority of patients with symptoms of prostatitis have negative urine cultures. In cases in which specific organisms are isolated, gram-negative bacteria and *Ureaplasma urealyticum* are usually identified. *Trichomonas vaginalis* infection of the prostate has been reported. There have also been rare cases of fungal prostatic infection, which is usually secondary to generalized systemic disease (Meares).

TREATMENT. The rare case of acute prostatitis in children and adolescents responds well to the initiation of appropriate antimicrobial therapy. Supportive treatment such as bed rest, hydration, antipyretics, and analgesics is recommended. Urethral instrumentation and prostatic massage should be avoided in the acute phase of the disease.

EPIDIDYMITIS

Acute epididymitis is rare in prepubertal boys; most childhood cases occur in adolescents (Doolittle et al; Amar and Chabra). In a

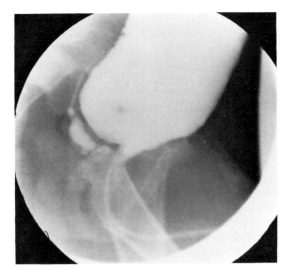

Figure 11–20. Voiding cystourethrogram. Contrast medium is demonstrated in left seminal vesicle and left vas deferens.

retrospective analysis of 136 patients with acute epididymitis, Barker and Raper reported no patients less than 14 years of age.

PATHOGENESIS. Infection in the epididymis may result from distal urethral obstruction, ectopic ureter draining into the seminal vesicle or vas deferens, or instrumentation, or it may be idiopathic in nature (Coran and Perlmutter; Waldman et al). Although infection with bacteria or viral organisms has been implicated as a cause of epididymitis, most cases are not associated with urinary tract infection (Hodgson and Hasan). Thus, it appears that sterile urine in the epididymis may be sufficient to incite an inflammatory response and clinical symptoms. Epididymal infection usually occurs via abnormal retrograde passage of urine from the prostatic ducts through the vas deferens (Kiviat et al) (Fig. 11–20). Hematogenous spread from an acute staphylococcal infection can occur subsequent to pneumonia, peritonitis, or other systemic infections. Epididymal involvement may also occur as a result of direct extension from a pre-existing orchitis.

SYMPTOMS. Patients with epididymitis have an enlarged and exquisitely tender epididymis and vas deferens. Scrotal edema, pain, and tenderness are early features of the disease. A reactive hydrocele usually develops with disease progression as a result of inflammatory changes in the tunica vaginalis.

DIAGNOSIS. Prepubertal boys with suspected epididymitis should have an excretory urogram to rule out the presence of an ectopic ureter. The differential diagnosis of epididymitis in children should always include testicular torsion, torsion of a testicular or epididymal appendage, and idiopathic scrotal edema. The onset of pain is usually more insidious in children with epididymitis than in those with testicular torsion. The physical examination in children with epididymitis usually reveals erythema and edema of the scrotum. Epididymal tenderness with or without urethral discharge is usually, but not invariably, present. The presence of a horizontal testicular lie or testicular retraction is characteristic of torsion of the testis. Prehn's sign is often unreliable in distinguishing epididymitis from testicular torsion. Urinalysis most often demonstrates pyuria with or without bacteriuria. However, results of urinalysis are abnormal in approximately 10 per cent of patients with testicular torsion (Ransler and Allen). Leukocytosis (> 10,000 leukocytes per high-power field) occurs in 30 to 50 per cent of children with epididymitis, testicular torsion, and torsion of a testicular appendage and, therefore, is not a helpful discriminator among these entities (Levy et al; Ransler and Allen). The Doppler ultrasonic stethoscope and radionuclide testicular scanning have been utilized to differentiate epididymitis from testicular torsion. Our experience and that of others (Brereton; Ransler and Allen) has been that the Doppler flowmeter is associated with false-negative results. Similarly, although nuclear scrotal scanning has proved to be a highly accurate diagnostic tool in large series of children with acute scrotum (Levy et al; Valvo et al), this method of investigation is not universally available or reliable. It must be remembered that epididymitis is extremely rare in children, and the safe and sure method of resolving the diagnosis of an acute scrotum requires scrotal exploration (Kelalis and Stickler).

TREATMENT. The treatment of acute epididymitis involves administration of broad-spectrum antibiotics (usually on an empiric basis), scrotal support with elevation, bed rest, and application of ice packs to the affected area. Injection of the spermatic cord with 1 to 2 ml of lidocaine hydrochloride may be used to alleviate severe pain (Smith).

ORCHITIS

Acute infection involving solely the testis is a relatively rare occurrence in boys (Kaplan and King). Malkin et al reported a case of bacterial orchitis in a newborn due to hematogenous spread of *Escherichia coli*.

PATHOGENESIS. In the majority of cases, orchitis develops as a result of extension of inflammation in the epididymis with the production of epididymo-orchitis. Less often, orchitis may develop by hematogenous or lymphogenous dissemination. Gram-negative coliforms, streptococci, or staphylococci account for most of the cases of bacterial orchitis. Mumps orchitis, which may occur in up to 20 per cent of adults with the virus, is exceedingly rare before puberty.

SYMPTOMS. Acute pyogenic orchitis presents as a swollen, tender, and sometimes fluctuant testis. The scrotal skin is erythematous and edematous, and there is usually an associated hydrocele due to inflammation of the tunica vaginalis. Pain may radiate to the inguinal canal and may be associated with nausea and vomiting. The differential diagnosis of acute orchitis includes acute epididymitis, torsion of the testicle or testicular appendages, and strangulated inguinal hernia.

TREATMENT. Broad-spectrum antibiotics are recommended pending the results of urine cultures. Supportive therapy includes bed rest, scrotal elevation, and hot or cold compresses for symptomatic relief. Aspiration of the associated symptomatic hydrocele may afford considerable relief of pain in selected patients.

VULVOVAGINITIS

Most female babies have a rather profuse, thick vaginal discharge during the newborn period as a consequence of prenatal stimulation by maternal hormones. This is a limited and physiologic condition, which does not require therapy. Similarly, copious vaginal secretion associated with swelling of the vulvar and vaginal tissues may occur at the time of puberty, as a result of the normal increase in estrogen stimulation. Vaginal discharge may result from an ectopic ureter that inserts into the vagina, and therefore excretory urography is recommended.

PATHOGENESIS. In premenarchial females, vulvovaginitis occurs most commonly between 2 and 7 years of age. Vulvovaginitis in this age group may be due to specific infections from bacteria, fungi, *Trichomonas, Mycoplasma, Chlamydia,* parasites, or viruses (Heller et al; Rein). Vulvovaginitis may be nonspecific in origin or may be related to chemical or allergic agents or foreign bodies in the vagina. In adolescent females, vulvovaginitis is usually the result of sexual promiscuity.

SPECIFIC VULVOVAGINITIS. Gonococcal vulvovaginitis in prepubertal girls may result from sexual abuse or from nonsexual contact with freshly infected material on clothing or towels (Burry; Tunnessen and Jastremski). Rarely, gonococcal vaginitis may be acquired during passage of the newborn through an infected birth canal (Stark and Glode). In prepubertal females, the endocervical glands are not well developed and do not harbor the gonococcus. Thus, prepubertal gonorrhea is limited to the vagina. The majority of adolescent females have no symptoms; however, an occasional patient may present with endometritis and salpingitis.

The child with gonococcal vulvovaginitis may complain of vulvar discomfort, dysuria, frequency, and pain on walking. The vulvar tissues are edematous and hyperemic and are covered by a profuse, thick, yellowish discharge that exudes from the vagina. The diagnosis is established by smears and cultures of urethral, vaginal, and rectal swabs. Endocervical cultures are not recommended in prepubertal females. Penicillin is the treatment of choice (see Gonococcal Urethritis).

T. vaginalis may cause vulvovaginal infection in infants and children. The disease may be acquired during passage of the newborn through an infected birth canal. Symptoms include vulvar pruritus, and physical examination reveals a grayish-white frothy vaginal discharge. The diagnosis is established by finding numerous leukocytes and trichomonads in saline wet-mount vaginal preparations. The treatment for trichomonal vaginitis is metronidazole, 125 mg three times daily for 10 days.

Mycotic infections, particularly those due to *Candida albicans,* may produce vulvovaginitis in infants and children. In most instances, the child will have received antibiotic therapy before the onset of genital symptoms. Children usually have vulvar pruritus. Physical examination reveals diffuse vulvar hyperemia with whitish plaques on the vaginal wall and minimal vaginal discharge. The diagnosis is established by finding leukocytes and mycelia in potassium hydroxide preparations and confirmed by identifying *C. albicans* in culture. The treatment for mycotic vulvovaginitis is miconazole or clotrimazole, 100 mg intravaginally daily for 7 days. Alternatively, 1 ml of 0.5 per cent aqueous solution of gentian violet may be injected intravaginally with a sterile eye dropper each night for 10 days (Huffman).

NONSPECIFIC VULVOVAGINITIS. Nonspecific vulvovaginitis may result from pinworm infestation, foreign bodies, anaerobic bacteria such as *Bacteroides* and *Peptococcus* species, *Gardnerella* infection, or upper respiratory infections. There is usually a moderate vaginal discharge, which is whitish-gray in appearance. Microscopic examination of the discharge demonstrates few leukocytes, and there are epithelial cells coated with small bacteria (clue cells). Vaginal smears and cultures are mandatory to rule out *Neisseria gonorrhoeae* and other specific infections. Therapy is based on good perineal hygiene, including proper cleansing after defecation.

GANGRENOUS BALANOPOSTHITIS

Inflammation of the glans penis and foreskin occurs commonly in infants and appears to be related to chronic irritation from wet or soiled diapers and from poor genital hygiene. Mild cases usually respond to local cleansing.

Gangrenous balanoposthitis is a result of an anaerobic fusospirochetal infection of the glans penis. The lesion begins as an ulcer in the region of the corona, beneath a tight and unclean prepuce. Spread of the ulcer produces a foul, profuse discharge with secondary edema of the glans. Gangrenous change may occur in both the glans and the shaft of the penis.

DIAGNOSIS. The diagnosis of gangrenous balanoposthitis is made by clinical appearance and by demonstration of spirochetes and fusiform bacilli in stained smears of the discharge. Dark-field examination is necessary to rule out infection with *Treponema pallidum*. It is important to remember that hair wrapped around the coronal sulcus may produce gangrenous balanoposthitis.

TREATMENT. Penicillin is the drug of choice. Hydrogen peroxide soaks are helpful in reversing the anaerobic process. A dorsal slit may be necessary in the acute stage of the disease; circumcision is recommended electively after resolution of edema.

LYMPHOGRANULOMA VENEREUM

Lymphogranuloma venereum is an infectious venereal disease caused by a specific type of chlamydial bacterium. The disease is characterized by granulomatous ulceration, abscess formation, and fibrosis of the inguinal, perineal, and rectal lymphatics (Abrams). There have been several reports of lymphogranuloma venereum in children (Levy; Weinstock and Keesal; Banov).

PATHOGENESIS AND PATHOLOGY. Acquisition of lymphogranuloma venereum in childhood occurs as a result of genital contact and may be transmitted by handling towels or clothes that contain drainage from an ulcerated lesion. In adolescents, the disease is transmitted by sexual intercourse.

The initial form of childhood presentation is painful and tender inguinal adenitis with subsequent abscess formation and draining sinuses. Extension of disease into the deep pelvic tissue may result in rectal and colonic strictures and also elephantiasis of the external genitalia.

DIAGNOSIS. Lymphogranuloma venereum should be suspected in persons with acutely painful inguinal lymphadenopathy or with an ulcerative or granulomatous lesion on the vulva or perineum. Definitive diagnosis is established by a positive intradermal skin test (Frei test) with the use of antigens from killed organisms. Serum complement fixation is highly accurate in the detection of initial infections and can be used to follow the course of the disease (Holder and Duncan). Biopsy of involved tissues is indicated to confirm the diagnosis. Patients with lymphogranuloma venereum should be evaluated for concurrent syphilitic infection and for other granulomatous and ulcerative genital diseases.

TREATMENT. Tetracycline, administered four times daily for 3 weeks, is the treatment of choice. Sulfonamides are also effective. The discharge from ulcerated lesions is infectious, and thus appropriate precautions should be taken to prevent transmission of disease.

GRANULOMA INGUINALE

Granuloma inguinale is a chronic venereal infection of the genital skin and subcutaneous tissues of the perineum (Davis; Lal and Nicholas). The etiologic agent is the encapsulated gram-negative bacillus *Calymmatobacterium granulomatis*. This disease occurs most commonly in the tropics and is relatively unusual in the United States.

PATHOGENESIS AND PATHOLOGY. Granuloma inguinale is sexually transmitted;

however, children may become infected by coming in contact with contaminated clothing or towels. The initial lesion is a reddish nodule on the penis, groin, vulva, or perineum that develops into a soft mass of granulation tissue (Douglas). A purulent discharge is common, and ulceration occurs with progressive disease. The ulcerative process may extend into the urethra and anus and cause extensive scarring and elephantiasis.

DIAGNOSIS. The diagnosis of granuloma inguinale is established by identification of Donovan bodies in smears of the affected tissue. Biopsy of the granulation tissue is helpful in confirming the diagnosis. The differential diagnosis includes other venereal diseases, and thus dark-field examination and serologic studies for syphilis, smears, biopsies, complement fixation, and skin sensitivity testing are indicated.

TREATMENT. Tetracycline administered four times daily for a 2-week period is the treatment of choice. Alternative drugs include chloramphenicol and gentamicin.

CHANCROID

Chancroid is an acute ulcerative disease of the external genitalia that occurs infrequently in children (Willcox). The causative agent is the gram-negative bacillus *Hemophilus ducreyi.*

PATHOGENESIS AND PATHOLOGY. Chancroid is transmitted by physical contact, most often via sexual intercourse. The incubation period is 1 to 5 days. The initial lesion is a single painful erythematous ulcer on the corona of the glans in males and on the labia minora or vulva in females. The ulcer multiplies by autoinoculation and forms an erosive lesion with purulent exudate. Inguinal lymphadenitis (buboes) occurs in approximately half the cases. With advanced disease, the inguinal nodes may abscess and produce draining sinuses.

DIAGNOSIS. The diagnosis of chancroid is made by identification of *H. ducreyi* in smears (Gram's or Wright's stain) or cultures and by the histologic appearance of biopsied tissue. Intradermal skin tests with bacillary antigen become positive in 1 to 4 weeks in approximately 75 per cent of patients. Urethral smears and cultures for gonococcus, dark-field examination for spirochetes, and serologic tests for syphilis are indicated to rule out other venereal infections.

TREATMENT. Chancroidal infection should respond to a 10-day course of sulfonamides. Fluctuant inguinal abscesses should be aspirated rather than drained openly. Discharge from these buboes is highly infectious, and therefore appropriate precautionary measures should be taken to prevent transmission of disease.

BIBLIOGRAPHY

GONOCOCCAL URETHRITIS

Barrett-Connor E: Gonorrhea and the pediatrician. Am J Dis Child 125:233, 1973.
Branch G, Paxton R: A study of gonococcal infections among infants and children. Public Health Rep 80:347, 1965.
Clark DO: Gonorrhea: changing concepts in diagnosis and management. Clin Obstet Gynecol 16:3, 1973.
Farrell MK, Billmire ME, Shamroy JA, et al: Prepubertal gonorrhea: a multidisciplinary approach. Pediatrics 67:151, 1981.
Karney WW, Pedersen AHB, Nelson M, et al: Spectinomycin versus tetracycline for the treatment of gonorrhea. N Engl J Med 296:889, 1977.
Kellogg DS Jr, Holmes KK, Hill GA: Laboratory diagnosis of gonorrhea. Cumitech 4:1, 1976.
Meek JM, Askari A, Belman AB: Prepubertal gonorrhea. J Urol 122:532, 1979.
Nelson JD, Mohs E, Dajani AS, et al: Gonorrhea in preschool- and school-aged children: report of the Prepubertal Gonorrhea Cooperative Study Group. JAMA 236:1359, 1976.
Shore WB, Winkelstein JA: Nonvenereal transmission of gonococcal infections to children. J Pediatr 79:661, 1971.

NONGONOCOCCAL URETHRITIS

Felman YM, Nikitas JA: Nongonococcal urethritis: a clinical review. JAMA 245:381, 1981.
Jacobs NF Jr, Kraus SJ: Gonococcal and nongonococcal urethritis in men: clinical and laboratory differentiation. Ann Intern Med 82:7, 1975.
Oriel JD, Ridgway GL, Tchamouroff S: Comparison of erythromycin stearate and oxytetracycline in the treatment of non-gonococcal urethritis: their efficacy against *Chlamydia trachomatis.* Scott Med J 22:375, 1977.
Smith TF, Weed LA, Segura JW, et al: Isolation of *Chlamydia* from patients with urethritis. Mayo Clin Proc 50:105, 1975.

HERPES SIMPLEX INFECTION

Fiumara NJ, Schmidt-Ulrick B, Comite H: Primary herpes simplex and primary syphilis: a description of seven cases. Sex Transm Dis 7:130, 1980.
Nahmias AJ, Alford CA, Korones SB: Infection of the newborn with *Herpesvirus hominis.* Adv Pediatr 17:185, 1970.
Nahmias AJ, Josey WE, Naib ZM: Neonatal herpes simplex infection: role of genital infection in mother as the source of virus in the newborn. JAMA 199:164, 1967.
Person DA, Kaufman RH, Gardner HL, et al: Herpesvirus type 2 in genitourinary tract infections. Am J Obstet Gynecol 116:993, 1973.

SYPHILIS

Robbins SL, Cotran RS: Pathologic Basis of Disease. Second edition. Philadelphia, WB Saunders Co., 1979, pp 406–410.

Taber LH, Huber TW: Congenital syphilis. Prog Clin Biol Res 3:183, 1975.

Wilfert C, Gutman L: Syphilis. *In* Textbook of Pediatric Infectious Diseases. Vol 1. Edited by RD Feigin, JD Cherry. Philadelphia, WB Saunders Co., 1981, pp 388–400.

PROSTATITIS

Mann S: Prostatic abscess in the newborn. Arch Dis Child 35:396, 1960.

Meares EM Jr: Prostatitis: a review. Urol Clin North Am 2:3, Feb. 1975.

EPIDIDYMITIS

Amar AD, Chabra K: Epididymitis in prepuberal boys: presenting manifestation of vesicoureteral reflux. JAMA 207:2397, 1969.

Barker K, Raper FP: Torsion of the testis. Br J Urol 36:35, 1964.

Brereton RJ: Limitations of the Doppler flow meter in the diagnosis of the "acute scrotum" in boys. Br J Urol 53:380, 1981.

Coran AG, Perlmutter AD: Mumps epididymitis without orchitis. N Engl J Med 272:735, 1965.

Doolittle KH, Smith JP, Saylor ML: Epididymitis in the prepuberal boy. J Urol 96:364, 1966.

Hodgson NB, Hasan S: Unusual cause of acute scrotal swelling. Society for Pediatric Urology Newsletter, April 9, 1980, p. 17.

Kelalis PP, Stickler GB: The painful scrotum: torsion versus epididymo-orchitis. Clin Pediatr (Phila) 15:220, 1976.

Kiviat MD, Shurtleff D, Ansell JS: Urinary reflux via the vas deferens: unusual cause of epididymitis in infancy. J Pediatr 80:476, 1972.

Levy OM, Gittelman MC, Strashun AM, et al: Diagnosis of acute testicular torsion using radionuclide scanning. J Urol 129:975, 1983.

Ransler CW, Allen TD: Torsion of the spermatic cord. Urol Clin North Am 9:245, 1982.

Smith DR: Treatment of epididymitis by infiltration of spermatic cord with procaine hydrochloride. J Urol 46:74, 1941.

Valvo JR, Caldamone AA, O'Mara R, et al: Nuclear imaging in the pediatric acute scrotum (abstract). Am J Dis Child 136:831, 1982.

Waldman LS, Kosloske AM, Parsons DW: Acute epididymo-orchitis as the presenting manifestation of *Hemophilus influenzae* septicemia. J Pediatr 90:87, 1977.

ORCHITIS

Kaplan GW, King LR: Acute scrotal swelling in children. J Urol 104:219, 1970.

Malkin RB, Joshi VV, Koontz WW Jr: Bacterial orchitis, abscess and sepsis in a newborn: a case report. J Urol 112:530, 1974.

VULVOVAGINITIS

Burry VF: Gonococcal vulvovaginitis and possible peritonitis in prepubertal girls. Am J Dis Child 121:536, 1971.

Heller RH, Joseph JM, Davis HJ: Vulvovaginitis in the premenarcheal child. J Pediatr 74:370, 1969.

Huffman JW: Gynecologic infections in childhood and adolescence. *In* Textbook of Pediatric Infectious Diseases, Vol 1. Edited by RD Feigin, JD Cherry. Philadelphia, WB Saunders Co., 1981, pp 407–415.

Rein MF: Current therapy of vulvovaginitis. Sex Transm Dis 8:316, 1981.

Stark AR, Glode MP: Gonococcal vaginitis in a neonate. J Pediatr 94:298, 1979.

Tunnessen WW Jr, Jastremski M: Prepubescent gonococcal vulvovaginitis. Clin Pediatr (Phila) 13:675, 1974.

LYMPHOGRANULOMA VENEREUM

Abrams AJ: Lymphogranuloma venereum. JAMA 205:199, 1968.

Banov L Jr: Rectal lesions of lymphogranuloma venereum in childhood: review of the literature and report of a case in a ten-year-old boy with rectal stricture. Am J Dis Child 83:660, 1952.

Holder WR, Duncan WC: Lymphogranuloma venereum. Clin Obstet Gynecol 15:1004, 1972.

Levy H: Lymphogranuloma venereum in childhood: review of the literature with report of a case. Arch Pediatr 57:441, 1940.

Weinstock HL, Keesal S: Lymphogranuloma venereum: report of a case in a child. Urol Cutan Rev 50:520, 1946.

GRANULOMA INGUINALE

Davis CM: Granuloma inguinale: a clinical, histological, and ultrastructural study. JAMA 211:632, 1970.

Douglas CP: Lymphogranuloma venereum and granuloma inguinale of the vulva. J Obstet Gynaecol Br Commonw 69:871, 1962.

Lal S, Nicholas C: Epidemiological and clinical features in 165 cases of granuloma inguinale. Br J Vener Dis 46:461, 1970.

CHANCROID

Willcox RR: Chancroid (soft sore). Recent Adv Sex Transm Dis No. 1, 1975, pp 185–187.

12
URODYNAMIC EVALUATION AND NEUROMUSCULAR DYSFUNCTION

STUART B. BAUER

PHYSIOLOGY OF MICTURITION

The lower urinary tract has two primary functions with regard to the transport of urine: adequate storage capacity and efficient emptying capability. These functions are governed by a complex physiologic process that involves several centers within the brain, various levels along the spinal cord, the intrinsic properties of the smooth muscles of the bladder and posterior urethra, and the striated muscle portion of the external urethral sphincter. These components work in a coordinated manner to maintain proper functioning of the lower urinary tract.

At the present time not all the neurologic pathways that control micturition have been elucidated by laboratory studies; nor is there a precise knowledge of the exact anatomic arrangement of the muscles composing the lower urinary tract. Enough information is available, however, to provide a reasonably accurate description of the mechanics of the vesicourethral unit.

The fundus of the bladder is composed of three layers of smooth muscle which crisscross one another, producing a powerful supporting wall (Woodburne). Many of the muscle bundles then interdigitate around the bladder neck and extend down the posterior urethra toward the external sphincter region (Tanagho and Smith, 1966; Woodburne) (Fig. 12-1). Their net effect is to act as a sphincter mechanism in this region, even though they

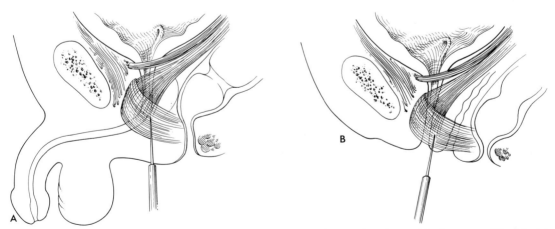

Figure 12-1. The detrusor is not oriented in a circular fashion to create a true sphincter around the bladder neck. Rather, muscle bundles interdigitate between one another and extend down the posterior urethra towards the external sphincter region as described by Woodburne. Note the position of an EMG electrode in the external sphincter muscle in both males (A) and females (B).

are not oriented in a circular fashion. A second area in the posterior urethra at the level of the pelvic diaphragm contains an arrangement of both smooth and skeletal muscles, creating another sphincter mechanism (Bradley et al; Hutch; Hutch and Rambo; Tanagho and Smith, 1968). The anatomy of these muscle groups is not clearly defined, and controversy still exists regarding their make-up and exact orientation (Donker et al; McNeal).

Lower urinary tract function is under the control of the somatic and autonomic nervous systems. The latter is composed of the sympathetic and parasympathetic nervous systems (Bradley et al; Bors and Comarr; Kuru; Nyberg-Hansen) (Fig. 12–2). Sympathetic nervous system control is derived from neurons that originate in the thoracolumbar region of the spinal cord at T10 to L1 and lead to synapses in the sympathetic chain. Postganglionic nerve fibers from this chain reach the bladder via the hypogastric plexus to supply primarily the fundus, bladder neck, and posterior urethral areas of the vesicourethral unit. The parasympathetic nervous system arises from the sacral area of the spinal cord at the level of S2 to S4. Preganglionic neurons from this level of the cord course through the pelvic

nerve plexus to ganglia at or near the muscular wall of the bladder or posterior urethra, where they synapse with postganglionic nerve fibers that primarily supply the fundus of the bladder. Somatic nerves from the sacral cord also course through the pelvic plexus and the pudendal nerve to the external sphincter region, where they innervate the skeletal muscle component of the external urethral sphincter.

Although the trigone and portions of the posterior urethra appear to be anatomically and embryologically separate, these areas behave similarly both neuroanatomically and neuropharmacologically (El-Badawi and Schenk, 1968, 1971, 1974). The sympathetic nervous system stimulates both alpha and beta receptor sites in the smooth muscle, the net effect being related to the predominant receptor found in the area (Fig. 12–3). Alpha adrenergic receptor sites are located primarily in the trigone, bladder neck, and proximal portion of the posterior urethra. The beta adrenergic receptor sites are located predominantly in the fundus of the bladder.

The primary neurohumoral transmitter for sympathetic postganglionic innervation is norepinephrine (Koelle). When this agent

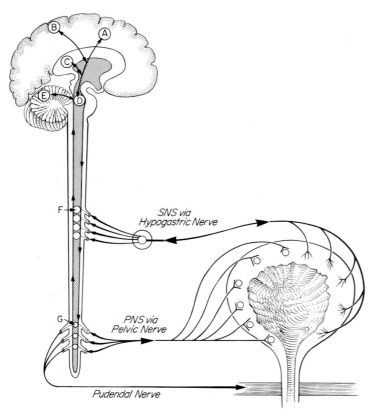

Figure 12–2. The frontal (A) and parietal (B) lobes of the cerebral cortex, the cingulate gyrus (C), the hypothalamus (D), the cerebellum (E), the sympathetic nervous system (F) from T10 to L1, the parasympathetic nervous system (G) from S2 to S4, and the pudendal nerve to the external sphincter all interact in a coordinated way to achieve proper and efficient function of the lower urinary tract.

SNS via Hypogastric Nerve

PNS via Pelvic Nerve

Pudendal Nerve

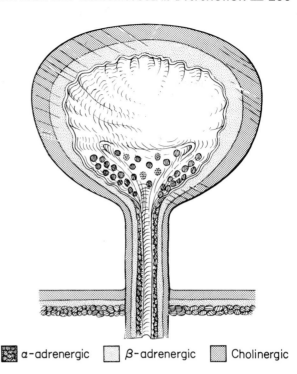

Figure 12-3. Distribution of alpha and beta sympathetic and parasympathetic (cholinergic) receptor sites in the vesicourethral unit.

▨ α-adrenergic   ☐ β-adrenergic   ▦ Cholinergic

reacts with alpha adrenergic receptors in the bladder neck and posterior urethra, a muscular contraction occurs, increasing the resistance in these areas. When norepinephrine is released to the beta adrenergic receptors in the fundus of the bladder, relaxation of the muscle occurs. This produces accommodation and allows the bladder to enlarge without significantly increasing the tension within its wall. Thus, the sympathetic nervous system exerts an important regulatory influence on bladder function during the filling phase of the micturition cycle by facilitating the storage of urine (Edvardsen, 1968a; Khanna) (Fig. 12-4).

The primary neurohumoral transmitter of the parasympathetic nervous system is acetylcholine. The receptor sites for this agent are located throughout the fundus of the bladder and to a lesser extent in the posterior urethra (El-Badawi and Schenk, 1968; Raezer et al) (Fig. 12-3). A bladder contraction is initiated when the pelvic nerves are stimulated, causing a release of acetylcholine by the postganglionic nerve cells, which in turn produces a detrusor contraction (Gyermek) (Fig. 12-4). It is postulated that at the same time a reflexic inhibition of the sympathetic nervous system occurs, causing a reduction in the release of norepinephrine (DeGroat and Saum; DeGroat and Theobold). This diminishes the alpha

adrenergic effect on the trigone, bladder neck, and posterior urethra, resulting in a relaxation of the muscles in this area. In addition, the beta receptor site stimulation in the fundus of the bladder ceases, further enhancing the contractile force generated by the parasympathetic discharge. The net effect is a sustained contraction of the bladder until all the urine is expelled (Fig. 12-4).

Just before a bladder contraction is about to begin, impulses traveling along the pudendal nerve act to relax both the smooth and skeletal muscle components of the external urethral sphincter area (Barrington; Kuru) (Fig. 12-5). This minimizes the resistance to flow through the urethra and improves emptying efficiency. The two phases of lower urinary tract function, namely storage and evacuation, have been labeled the sympathetic and parasympathetic phases, depending on which system is predominantly affecting the vesicourethral unit (Khanna) (Fig. 12-4).

Central nervous system control over lower urinary tract function is less well understood. Most of the information has been derived from physiologic experiments in animals, usually the cat, with few studies having been performed in man. The following summary is an extrapolation of that data.

From the sacral spinal micturition center, afferent and efferent pathways connect to the

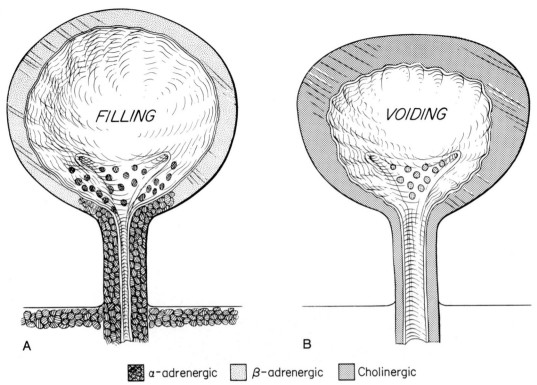

A   B

▨ α-adrenergic   ▢ β-adrenergic   ▢ Cholinergic

Figure 12–4. *A,* During filling of the bladder, stimulation of alpha sympathetic receptor sites increases muscle tone in the bladder neck and posterior urethra, and beta receptors decrease tone in the fundus. This allows adequate bladder volume at low filling pressures and increases outflow resistance to prevent leakage. *B,* During voiding, stimulation of sympathetic receptors diminishes while stimulation of cholinergic receptors increases. In addition, stimulation of somatic nerves to the external sphincter muscle ceases. This produces a sustained contraction of the detrusor with lowering of urethral resistance.

lower brain stem. Kuru has described two ascending spinal cord tracts — the pelvic sensory (in the dorsal funiculus) and the sacrobulbar (in the lateral funiculus) — and three descending tracts: (1) a lateral reticulospinal tract, which when stimulated facilitates bladder contractility; (2) a ventral reticulospinal tract, which inhibits the detrusor from contracting; and (3) a medial reticulospinal tract, which causes the external spincter to contract.

There is still considerable disagreement over the exact location and number of these

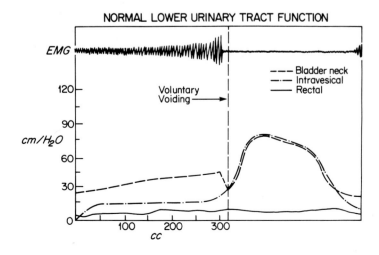

Figure 12–5. The interaction of intravesical, intraurethral, and rectal pressures, and electromyographic activity of the external urethral sphincter during a micturition cycle is shown here.

pathways and their total effect on micturition (Nathan; Ruch).

These tracts terminate in the brain stem, where, it has been postulated, three centers may exist: a facilitatory center in the anterior pons, an inhibitory center in the midbrain, and a second facilitatory center in the posterior hypothalmus (Ruch) (Fig. 12–2). The net effect is inhibitory. In addition, this area, also called the pontine center, regulates the external sphincter to act in a coordinated manner during voluntary voiding (Fig. 12–2).

The cerebral cortex plays the final role in the micturition cycle (Fig. 12–2). The areas most extensively involved with control over voiding are located in the supramedial portion of the middle of the frontal lobe, the anterior portion of the cingulate gyrus, and the genu of the corpus callosum (Bradley et al; Nathan; Raezer et al). Here too, the net effect is inhibitory, but whether or not each locality stimulates or inhibits micturition is unknown (Kuru; Ruch; Tang; Yeates, 1974). Rather, the effect is determined by the destructive or irritative nature of the particular disease process affecting the individual area.

Thus, micturition can be looked upon as a triple circuit affair (Barrington; Bradley et al; DeGroat; Kuru) (Fig. 12–2). Distention of the bladder results in impulses being sent along afferent pathways via the pelvic nerve to the sacral spinal cord. Internuncial neurons in the cord allow stimulation of parasympathetic, sympathetic (at the thoracolumbar level), and somatic efferent fibers that travel to the detrusor, bladder neck mechanism, and external urethral sphincter area, respectively (loop 1). Other intraspinal pathways carry messages to and from the sacral and thoracolumbar areas and the brain stem (loop 2). Frontal and parietal lobe communications to the brain stem, the third limb of the circuit, act to facilitate or inhibit these efferent spinal cord pathways. Brain stem inhibition facilitates urine storage by stimulating sympathetic efferent nerves to the bladder neck and fundus of the bladder and somatic efferents to the striated muscle component of the external sphincter. Complete transection of the spinal cord above the sacral reflex center leads to a loss of central control and an uncoordinated spinal reflex. This results in an unsustained detrusor contraction, a failure of the bladder neck and/or external sphincter area muscles to relax, and produces inefficient emptying of the bladder.

Although a paucity of experimental data exists, it is conjectured that these pathways are present and intact (although not completely myelinated) in the newborn and coordinated activity between detrusor and sphincter muscles is present when bladder emptying takes place (Allen and Bright). During the first 2 years of life, bladder capacity enlarges slowly as the brain stem inhibitory center acts to control micturition (MacKeith et al; Muellner; Yeates, 1973a). Maturation of the frontal and parietal lobes also progresses, first with an awareness of bladder fullness, then with the ability to inhibit voiding, and finally with the ability to facilitate voiding (Yeates, 1973b). As discussed in Chapter 13, the age at which this awareness and the eventual ability both to inhibit and to facilitate micturition develop is variable. Sexual as well as cultural and familial factors appear to be involved. Girls seem to gain control earlier than boys, and bowel control is apparently learned before urinary control (Bellman).

URODYNAMIC ASSESSMENT

Urodynamic tests are methods used to evaluate the function of the lower urinary tract. Every attempt to reproduce the natural act of voiding is exercised when studying this organ system in children with suspected dysfunction (Blaivas et al, 1977b). Unfortunately, urodynamics is an invasive procedure employing multi-channel or suprapubic catheters, rectal pressure balloons, and needle or surface electrodes to determine specific areas of dysfunction (Bauer, 1979; Blaivas et al, 1977a; Diokno et al). There are also inherent difficulties with present day urodynamic techniques, and unfortunately there are no reliable indirect methods to assess bladder and sphincter function accurately. These problems are compounded further in children because of their small size, shorter attention span, and decreased tolerance to discomfort and the dynamic process of maturation, which is occurring at a variable rate in each individual child. Thus, children with overt or suspected lower urinary tract dysfunction must be systematically evaluated to determine, first, the appropriateness of urodynamic testing, and second, whether the results will assist in therapy.

All children with overt neuropathic bladder dysfunction should have a urinalysis and urine culture, a serum creatinine test, a partial or complete urodynamic assessment, and an excretory urogram (or renal sonogram) to de-

Table 12–1. Evaluation of Children with Neurogenic Bladder Dysfunction

---

History
Bowel and bladder habits

Pattern of incontinence

Birth and development

Physical Examination
Spine

Lower extremities
    Reflexes
    Muscle mass
    Gait
    Perineal sensation/tone/reflexes

Laboratory
Urine analysis/culture

Urine specific gravity

Serum creatinine

X-Rays
Excretory urogram (or renal sonogram)

Voiding cystourethrogram

Spine

Urodynamics
Flow rate

Residual urine

Cystometrogram

External urethral sphincter EMG

Static and voiding urethral pressure profile

---

termine the status and drainage of the upper urinary tract (Table 12–1). The studies should be done soon after an injury occurs or, in the case of congenital lesions, within the early postnatal period. A voiding cystourethrogram is needed if (1) there is an abnormality on the excretory urogram, (2) the child has uncoordinated detrusor–external sphincter function on the urodynamic study (because this group is at high risk for bladder decompensation and/or upper urinary tract deterioration), or (3) urinary infection is present (Bauer, in press). The voiding cystogram documents the presence of reflux, the characteristics of the bladder wall, the appearance of the bladder neck and posterior urethra during both filling and voiding, the presence of functional urethral obstruction, and the emptying characteristics of the bladder. These findings, however, must be correlated with the measurements taken during urodynamic assessment.

Of paramount importance in the workup of children with neuropathic bladder dysfunction are the history and physical examination. The child's voiding habits prior to any injury

and the current pattern of bladder emptying should be delineated. It is imperative to note whether the child voids voluntarily, spontaneously, or only with the Credé maneuver. Does the child have periods of dryness between voiding, or is there constant urinary leakage? Is the incontinence characterized by urgency and an inability to get to the bathroom on time? Does the urine flow with a good stream or only dribble during emptying? Does leakage occur with crying or laughing? Has the child had urinary infection? How much urine is produced each day? What is the pattern of bowel function? A careful assessment is made of perianal and perineal sensation, anal sphincter tone, and the presence of bulbocavernosus and anocutaneous reflexes. The bulbocavernosus reflex is elicited by placing one's finger just at or slightly inside the external anal sphincter and briskly squeezing the glans or compressing the clitoris. If the reflex is present, the external anal sphincter should contract. The anocutaneous reflex is elicited by scratching the pigmented skin directly adjacent to the anal opening, which results in a contraction of the perianal muscle. In children with suspected neurogenic bladder dysfunction, complete evaluation of the back, including looking for agenesis of the sacrum or a cutaneous manifestation of an underlying occult spinal dysraphism, is an important diagnostic aid (Bauer, 1983; Mandell et al). Examination of the lower extremities, comparing muscle mass and strength of each leg, eliciting deep tendon reflexes, and observing gait, may provide clues to the presence of an occult spinal dysraphism affecting not only the sacral but the lumbar cord as well.

Technique of Urodynamic Studies

A very small dose of intramuscular meperidine, 1 mg/kg, is administered to children over the age of 1 year to reduce both discomfort and anxiety while maintaining their cooperation and responsiveness (Evans et al). Older children are instructed not to empty their bladders for 2 to 3 hours prior to the scheduled appointment. This allows the examiner to see the child first with a full bladder and to observe the presence of stress incontinence and the pattern of voiding. If the child has voluntary control, a urinary flow rate is obtained using a DISA uroflow meter,* which

---

* DISA Electronics, Franklin Lakes, NJ 07417.

records not only the characteristics of the urinary flow, but also the peak and mean flow and the volume. For those children who have no control, either a reflex bladder contraction is attempted or Credé voiding is used to empty the bladder and to allow an estimate of residual urine.

Next, a balloon catheter is inserted into the rectum to monitor intra-abdominal pressure. Artifacts of movement or straining, which may be confused with contractions of the bladder when one monitors only intravesical pressure, can then be eliminated (Bates et al).

Next, the child is catheterized with either a specially designed triple lumen 7 or 11 F urodynamic catheter.* In newborn males, a 5 F feeding tube may be substituted if necessary because of size restrictions in the urethra. On occasion, a hypotonic bladder will not empty completely even after a catheter has been inserted, and a Credé maneuver or aspiration of the contents of the bladder via the catheter may be necessary to measure the residual urine volume accurately (Bauer, 1983).

Urethral pressure profilometry measures the passive resistance of a particular point within the urethra to stretching (Gleason et al, 1974). Many factors contribute to this resistance, such as the elastic properties of the urethra and the tone of both the smooth and skeletal muscles that make up the urethral wall (Abrams; Evans et al) (Fig. 12–6). The tension generated by both muscle groups changes continuously throughout the micturition cycle. Urethral pressure recordings will be affected also by any neurologic lesion and the degree of denervation it produces. Finally, the actual measurements may change based on several variables, including size of catheter, number and total area of side openings on the catheter, rate of catheter withdrawal, type and rate of medium instilled, and position of the patient (Meunier and Mollard; Tanagho; Yalla et al, 1977). The variability of these latter factors has prompted several investigators to use a transducer-mounted catheter, which, because of its stiffness, must be used with caution in boys (Yalla et al, 1976) (Table 12–2).

Thus, the static urethral pressure profile is merely a measure of the passive resistance of the posterior urethra under a very specific set of circumstances. When the profile is recorded while the bladder is empty, it does not reflect the degree of resistance to flow during void-

* Bard Urological Division, Murray Hill, NJ 07974.

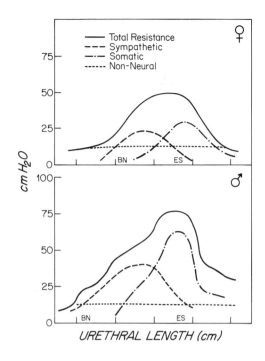

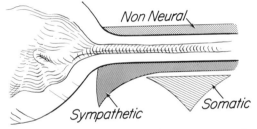

Figure 12-6. A schematic of the components of urethral wall tension according to their geographic distribution and effect along the urethra in males and females. BN, bladder neck. ES, external sphincter.

ing. A recording of urethral wall tension during voiding, by whatever means, is the only accurate measurement of urethral wall tension during emptying. Any attempt to extrapolate data from one condition to another during the micturition cycle will lead only to false

Table 12-2. Variables in Urethral Pressure Profilometry

Neurologic lesion
Bladder volume
Bladder contractions
Catheter size
Number and size of side holes
Rate of catheter withdrawal
Infusion medium and rate of instillation

impressions and assumptions, and improper treatment.

Urethral pressure profile measurements are made via the profile channel on the triple lumen catheter using saline infused at a rate of 2 ml per minute. The catheter is withdrawn at 0.5 cm per second with the child supine. Profile measurement is combined with fluoroscopic imaging to pinpoint accurately the various points of resistance along the urethra. It is performed with the bladder empty and repeated during filling and during emptying of the bladder either when the detrusor actually contracts or when the bladder is evacuated with a Credé maneuver. The second channel monitors bladder pressure continuously throughout the urethral pressure studies to detect uninhibited contractions. A comparison is made between the pressures within the bladder and the urethra during voiding to determine if outlet obstruction is present (Fig. 12–5). During voiding, pressures in the bladder and urethra should be equal. These pressures should be between 50 and 80 cm H_2O in girls and between 60 and 90 cm H_2O in boys (Gierup et al; Gierup and Ericsson) (Fig. 12–5). If a pressure differential is noted between the intravesical and intraurethral measurements, then outlet obstruction exists at the bladder neck; if both the bladder and urethral pressures are elevated, and the peak flow rate is less than 20 ml per second, an obstruction may be present at or beyond the external sphincter region.

Cystometry has long been a tool for measuring bladder function. The development of cystometers using carbon dioxide as an infusion medium has greatly facilitated our ability to evaluate the bladder (Merrill et al). This method allows for rapid filling and for studies that can easily be repeated with the patient in the supine, sitting, and standing positions. However, it has been shown convincingly that CO_2 cystometry does not give results similar to water cystometry, especially during voiding (Gleason et al, 1977). However, CO_2, being a gas, exhibits the common properties of all gases. For instance, when a pressure is applied, its volume contracts. Therefore, it is difficult to measure a detrusor contraction accurately with CO_2 because a damping effect is produced from the diminishing space of the gas.

The triple lumen catheter allows for bladder filling through one port while intravesical pressure is measured through another. The bladder can be filled rapidly or slowly depending on whether one is looking for uninhibited contractions or determining its actual capacity (Turner-Warwick).

Saline, warmed to body temperature, is infused. Filling is performed with the child supine and again when the child is upright. The patient is asked to cough during the filling phase in an attempt to elicit an uninhibited contraction (Mayo). At capacity, the child is asked to inhibit voiding as long as he or she can. When voiding actually begins, the child is again asked to stop urinating to determine how strongly he or she can block the micturition reflex. During emptying, voiding pressures are recorded continuously in the bladder and urethra to determine if there is any increased resistance to flow. If the patient has neither voluntary nor reflex bladder contractions, then a Credé or Valsalva maneuver is added to help achieve emptying of the bladder.

Placement of a suprapubic catheter to perform cystometry and assess voiding dynamics is not routinely undertaken even in children with neurogenic bladder dysfunction (Table 12–3). Most evaluations are made via the triple lumen urethral catheter. Only children who repeatedly fail to empty their bladder, have urethral pathology suggestive of outflow obstruction, require bladder cycling and lower urinary tract evaluation prior to urinary undiversion, or have had previous studies that failed to produce reliable data will undergo anesthesia with placement of a double lumen suprapubic catheter. Urodynamic studies are performed several days after placement of the catheter, when dysuria has subsided.

Currently, there is no single totally satisfactory or universally accepted method for assessing the degree of functional impairment of the striated muscle component of the external urethral sphincter during the micturition cycle. Various approaches have included perineal surface electrodes (Maizels and Firlit), blindly placed wire electrodes (Scott et al), surface catheter electrodes (Bradley et al, 1974a), anal plugs (Bradley et al, 1974b), and standard EMG needle electrodes (Blaivas et al,

Table 12–3. Indications for Urodynamic Study via Suprapubic Cystoscopy

Inability to empty
Outflow obstruction
Bladder cycling prior to undiversion
Previous unreliable data
Need cystoscopy for other reasons

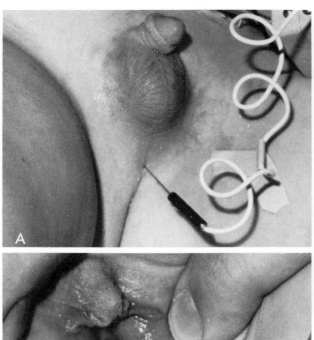

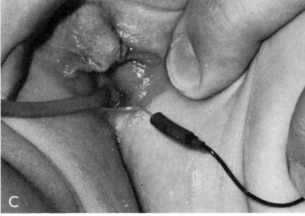

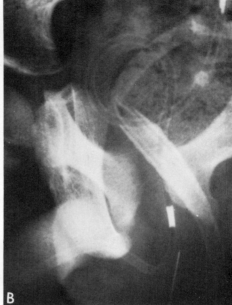

Figure 12–7. *A*, Placement of the EMG electrode in the male perineum. *B*, The position of the electrode is checked fluoroscopically. Note: Two radiopaque markers in the catheter allow the position of pressure recording openings to be determined. *C*, The EMG electrode in the female is inserted paraurethrally and advanced until the external sphincter muscle is reached (shown by injury potential).

1977a). The preferential and most accurate method, and the one used in our urodynamics facility, employs a standard concentric EMG needle electrode positioned in the periurethral striated muscle component of the external urethral sphincter under fluoroscopic and oscilloscopic control monitored by an EMG amplifier with audio output (TECA TE4 Electromyograph).* In boys, the external sphincter is pinpointed by inserting a finger in the rectum. The electrode is passed through the midline perineal skin and advanced toward the apex of the prostate at the level of the pelvic floor (Figs. 12–1*A* and 12–7*A* and *B*). In girls, the needle is inserted adjacent to the urethral meatus and advanced parallel to the lumen until the striated muscle component of the external urethral sphincter is reached (Figs. 12–1*B* and 12–7*C*). An anesthetic is sprayed on the skin prior to insertion of the needle.

When the electrode is in the muscle, characteristic motor unit action potentials are seen on the oscilloscope and heard from the audio output channel. Permanent recordings can be made on light-sensitive photographic paper using an electron beam display. Artifacts that are not readily discernible on a graphic recorder with a heat stylus pen can be easily detected and eliminated by observing the oscilloscopic screen, listening to the audio channel, and studying the recordings made on the photographic paper (Bauer, 1983; Blaivas, 1979). This method allows for accurate assessment of the degree of denervation involving the striated muscle component of the external urethral sphincter. Evidence of both acute and chronic denervation involving the sacral cord is easily discernible. Repositioning the needle allows the investigator to determine variations in the degree of denervation on one side of the external sphincter versus the other.

The electromyographic activity of the

---

* TECA Corp., Pleasantville, NY 10570.

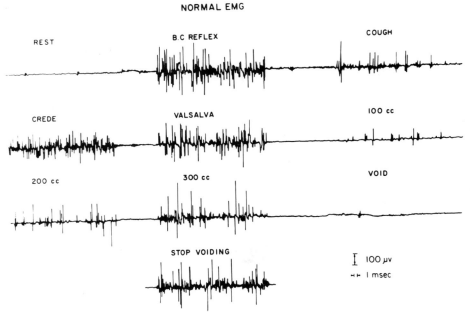

Figure 12-8. Normal external urethral sphincter electromyogram. Minimal activity is noted with the bladder empty. A complete interference pattern is seen with the bulbocavernosus reflex, cough, and Credé and Valsalva maneuvers. A gradual increase in electrical activity occurs with bladder filling. Voiding results in complete electrical silence. A command to stop voiding results in a complete interference pattern and a cessation of the urinary stream several seconds later.

striated muscle component of the external urethral sphincter is monitored in response to bulbocavernosus and anocutaneous reflexes, Credé and Valsalva maneuvers, voluntary control, and filling and emptying of the bladder (Fig. 12-8). The integrity of the sacral cord reflex arc can thus be determined (Blaivas et al, 1977a).

CLASSIFICATION OF NEUROPATHIC BLADDER

The classification of neuropathic bladder dysfunction used in this chapter is that which is being adopted by the Urology Section of the American Academy of Pediatrics in conjunction with the Urodynamic Society's classification.

Under normal conditions, all portions of the lower urinary tract (detrusor, bladder neck, and external sphincter mechanism) function as a coordinated unit for adequate storage and efficient evacuation of urine. When a neurourologic lesion exists, these components usually fail to act in unison. A classification has been adopted based on dysfunction of a specific area of the vesicourethral unit rather than specific etiology (Table 12-4).

Improper storage may be related to an alteration in detrusor function or an inadequate urethral closure mechanism. The bladder may have increased tone secondary to loss of elasticity of the muscle, overactivity from excessive or unopposed sympathetic discharges, or hyperreflexia due to a central nervous system lesion above the sacral cord that prevents the normal inhibitory centers from influencing the sacral reflex arc. Incontinence may occur with any one of these conditions despite a normal level of resistance in the bladder neck and urethra. Alternatively, incontinence may occur when the bladder neck and external sphincter areas do not provide adequate resistance during filling of the bladder or do not generate a reciprocal increase in outflow resistance as abdominal pressure is raised. An injury to the spinal cord or nerve roots affecting the sympathetic, parasympathetic, or sacral somatic nervous systems may alter both bladder neck and urethral tone. Periodic relaxation of the external urethral sphincter during filling of the bladder, the result of loss of central nervous system inhibition, may also lead to urinary incontinence.

Incomplete evacuation of the bladder may be due to a hypoactive or an areflexic detrusor muscle. Central nervous system lesions af-

Table 12–4. Functional Classification of Vesicourethral Dysfunction

Storage
Detrusor Tone
Normal

Increased
    Nonelastic
    Overactive
    Hyperreflexic

Decreased

Urethral Closing Mechanism
Incompetent
    Bladder neck
    External sphincter

Nonreciprocal

Periodic hypoactivity

Evacuation
Detrusor Contraction
Normoactive

Underactive
    Areflexic (nonreactive)
    Hypoactive (unsustained)

Urethral Closing Mechanism
Nonsynchronous
    Bladder neck
    External sphincter

fecting the parasympathetic efferents may be responsible. However, nonsynchronous relaxation of the bladder neck or external sphincter area mechanisms (dyssynergia) resulting from a lesion in the central nervous system above the sacral cord—e.g., the pontine center or the cerebral cortex—can produce a similar effect. Myogenic failure occurs as the detrusor muscle hypertrophies and then decompensates owing to persistent outflow resistance. Eventually this may produce an overflow type of incontinence.

In general, medical treatment of neuropathic bladder dysfunction is based on the functional impairment produced by the specific neurourologic defect (Table 12–5). Inadequate storage capacity may be enhanced by lowering detrusor tone or abolishing uninhibited contractions with anticholinergic medication, such as oxybutynin, pantheline, or propantheline. These drugs block cholinergic receptor sites in the detrusor muscle, diminishing its tone and suppressing involuntary contractions of the bladder. Other drugs, for example, flavoxate, act directly on the smooth muscle cells and lower detrusor tone without affecting contractility. Failure of drug therapy to increase bladder capacity and lower detrusor tone results in the need for subtotal cystectomy and augmentation cystoplasty to enhance bladder storage capability. This procedure is satisfactory so long as outflow resistance is normal or increased.

If inadequate urethral resistance is the primary reason for impaired storage of urine, the bladder neck mechanism or the external sphincter area, or both, may be responsible. Alpha sympathomimetic agents, such as ephedrine sulfate and phenylpropanolamine, stimulate receptors in the bladder neck area to enhance the tone of these muscles in this area. There are no drugs commercially available that will increase the tone of denervated skeletal muscle in the external sphincter region.

Incomplete emptying of the bladder may also be due to an areflexic bladder, unsustained detrusor contractions, or uncoordinated activity at the bladder neck or external sphincter area. Emptying may be facilitated by cholinergic drugs, such as bethanechol chloride or alpha sympatholytic agents, or

Table 12–5. Drug Therapy for Neuropathic Bladder Dysfunction

Type	Minimum	Maximum
Cholinergic		
Bethanechol	0.7 mg/kg TID	0.8 mg/kg QID
Anticholinergic		
Propantheline	0.5 mg/kg BID	0.5 mg/kg QID
Oxybutynin	0.2 mg/kg BID	0.2 mg/kg QID
Sympathomimetic		
Phenylpropanolamine	2.5 mg/kg BID	2.5 mg/kg TID
Ephedrine	0.5 mg/kg BID	1.0 mg/kg TID
Sympatholytic		
Phenoxybenzamine	0.3 mg/kg BID	0.5 mg/kg TID
Smooth muscle relaxant		
Flavoxate	3.0 mg/kg BID	3.0 mg/kg TID
Other		
Imipramine	0.7 mg/kg BID	0.8 mg/kg TID

skeletal muscle relaxants. Although conflicting reports have been published regarding the efficacy of bethanechol, it does seem to improve emptying of the bladder in most instances. It should be administered with alpha sympatholytic agents because bethanechol also increases urethral resistance at the bladder neck. Alpha sympatholytic agents, such as phenoxybenzamine or regitine, act primarily in the bladder neck area, whereas diazepam and baclofen diminish skeletal muscle tone at the external sphincter region to lower outlet resistance to voiding.

Most neurologic conditions affecting vesicourethral function in children, including myelomeningocele, lipomeningocele, sacral agenesis, and occult lesions, are congenital neurospinal dysraphisms (Table 12 – 6). Cerebral palsy is an acquired nonprogressive form of dysfunction occurring in the perinatal period as a consequence of cerebral anoxia from a variety of conditions. Other traumatic causes of spinal cord or cerebral dysfunction resulting in neuropathic bladder are rare and will not be dealt with in any detail in this chapter. Indications for evaluation, however, are proposed for each specific type of dysfunction.

Children without obvious neurologic disease may have a voiding abnormality on a functional or maturational basis. Most children gain urinary control before age 5. Persistent day and night incontinence with no prolonged period of dryness or the recurrence of wetting lasting into puberty are indications for urodynamic evaluation in neurologically normal children. Although an overwhelming number have normal findings, a significant percentage may have a dysfunctional voiding state. The types of abnormalities will be discussed separately along with individual approaches to therapy.

Table 12 – 6. Etiologic Classification of Vesicourethral Dysfunction

Neuropathic
Spinal Cord
Congenital
    Neurospinal dysraphism
    Other anatomic
Acquired
    Trauma
    Tumor
    Infection
    Vascular
    Miscellaneous
Supraspinal Cord
Anatomic/congenital
Trauma
Tumor
Infection
Vascular
Degenerative
Miscellaneous
Temporary
Peripheral
Trauma
Tumor
Degenerative
Guillain-Barré syndrome

Nonneuropathic
Anatomic
Myopathic
Psychologic
Endocrinologic
Toxic

MYELOMENINGOCELE

Myelomeningocele is the single most common cause of neuropathic bladder dysfunction in children. The incidence is one per thousand live births in North America but is higher in Wales and Ireland. Worldwide, the incidence is decreasing (Stein et al). Prenatal detection may further reduce the number of children being born with this condition (Hobbins et al).

Management of the child with myelomeningocele must be individualized. Not only the level of the vertebral bony defect (Ericsson et al) but also the degree of involvement of the spinal cord, the peripheral nerve roots, and the brain and brain stem (due to the Arnold-Chiari malformation) will vary (Stark; Fry et al). There may be differences in the neurologic deficit on opposite sides of the spinal cord, even at the same level (Bauer et al, 1977). It has been shown clearly that the level of the bony defect is not a good indicator of the type of nerve dysfunction affecting the lower urinary tract (Bauer et al, 1977; Ericsson et al).

At one time, urodynamic studies were performed in these children only after simple attempts at achieving continence were unsuccessful, usually during school-age years. This obviously necessitated waiting a number of years after the appearance of the initial lesion to evaluate bladder and sphincter function. Oftentimes the urodynamic findings did not correlate well with the x-ray appearance of

Table 12–7. Reasons for Urodynamic Evaluation in Newborns with Myelodysplasia

Provides baseline value of the neurourologic status of the lower urinary tract

Identifies babies at risk for urinary tract deterioration

Permits detection of progressive denervation on subsequent studies

Determines appropriateness and effectiveness of Credé voiding

Aids in counseling parents regarding future sexual function

the lower urinary tract (Ericsson et al). Thus, it seemed more appropriate to perform urodynamic studies in the newborn period, as soon as possible after the back was closed and the cerebrospinal fluid shunted (if necessary).

Studies at this time (1) determine the neurologic status of the lower urinary tract so that subsequent studies may detect signs of progressive denervation, and (2) identify babies at risk for urinary tract deterioration in the first year or two of life (Table 12–7). High bladder filling and voiding pressures, especially in the face of an incoordinated external urethal sphincter, are ominous signs suggesting that either bladder decompensation or upper urinary tract deterioration will occur (McGuire et al; Van Gool et al) (Fig. 12–9A). Seventy-two per cent of newborns with myelodysplasia in our series who had these findings subsequently developed urinary tract changes that required intervention (Bauer et al, in press). Finally, such studies aid in counseling parents regarding future sexual and reproductive function.

At the present time, a urinalysis, urine culture, serum creatinine measurement, excretory urogram, urodynamic assessment, and a measurement of residual urine volume are obtained in the newborn period. Based on the urodynamic findings, the newborns are divided into three groups: those with detrusor–external urethral sphincter incoordination (dyssynergia); those with detrusor–external urethral sphincter coordination (synergia); and those with no bioelectric activity or complete neurologic lesions.

The children with dyssynergia have a voiding cystourethrogram to ascertain the presence of vesicoureteral reflux. Follow-up studies include periodic determinations of residual urine volume, an excretory urogram or renal sonogram, and a voiding cystourethrogram or radionuclide cystogram, semiannually until age 2 to detect vesicoureteral reflux, hydroureteronephrosis, or increasing residual urine volume (Fig. 12–9B and C). A urodynamic study is repeated yearly to determine if there is progressive denervation of the external urethral sphincter.

Children with synergic sphincter activity are not at risk for urinary tract deterioration unless their neurologic picture changes and dyssynergia occurs. These babies are followed with an excretory urogram or renal sonogram and urodynamic study yearly as long as their studies reveal coordinated sphincter activity. In our series 22 per cent of these children converted to dyssynergia and subsequently all in this latter group developed bladder decompensation.

Babies with a complete neurologic lesion need only a yearly renal sonogram and a periodic check of residual urine volume. The lower urinary tract acts as a conduit without causing obstruction to urine flow. These children are at low risk for deterioration (6 per cent in our series) unless they have an increase in residual urine volume or urodynamic studies reveal elevated urethral pressure from denervation fibrosis of the skeletal muscle component of the external urethral sphincter (Bauer et al, 1977).

If a child has an abnormal excretory urogram or a urinary tract infection, a voiding cystogram is obtained, or repeated, to look for vesicoureteral reflux. Residual urine volume is then checked every 3 months. Credé voiding is contraindicated in children with intact sacral reflex function, since these children will have a reflexic increase in external urethral sphincter electromyographic activity during a Credé maneuver (Fig. 12–10). This will result in increased urethral resistance and high "voiding" pressures.

Intervention to improve upper or lower urinary tract drainage is undertaken at the first sign of hydroureteronephrosis, bladder enlargement, or vesicoureteral reflux. As a result of the findings on urodynamic assessment in newborns in our series and in older children by others (Van Gool et al; McGuire et al) and the high degree of predictability for urinary tract deterioration, we have proposed early intervention in children with detrusor–external sphincter incoordination and outflow obstruction (Bauer et al, in press). Intermittent catheterization may be started in girls as young as 2 months of age or in boys over the age of 1 year, as long as the social situation permits. Younger boys and some girls may

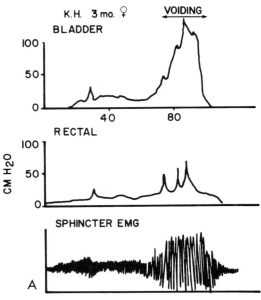

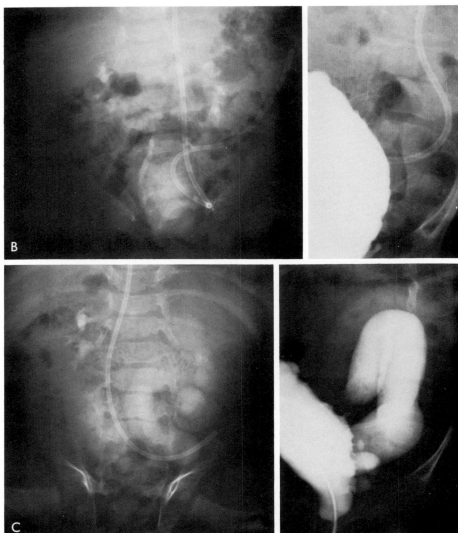

Figure 12–9. *A,* An urodynamic study in a 3-month-old girl with myelodysplasia demonstrates high voiding pressures and bladder–external urethral sphincter dyssynergia. *B,* Her initial excretory urogram and voiding cystogram were normal. *C,* At 6 months of age she had a urinary tract infection. A repeat excretory urogram revealed severe left hydroureteronephrosis, and the voiding cystogram demonstrated massive left-sided reflux.

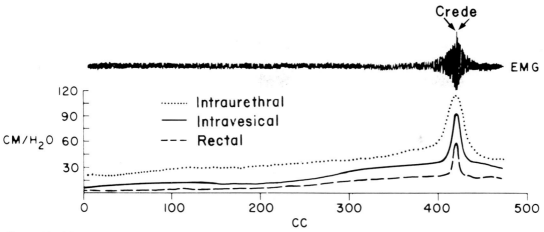

Figure 12–10. In children with a reactive external urethral sphincter, a Credé manuever produces a reflexic increase in external urethral sphincter EMG activity with a concomitant rise in urethral resistance. This results in high-pressure voiding.

require cutaneous vesicostomy for a variable period of time until they are old enough to be started on intermittent catheterization. This preserves the bladder neck and urethral sphincter mechanisms and bladder contractility. Urethral dilatation and external sphincterotomy are no longer performed because they may destroy the only level of resistance in the urethra that can act as a continence mechanism.

Urodynamic studies in babies with moderate to severe degrees of reflux will determine the presence of elevated filling or voiding pressures, factors that may contribute to the severity of the reflux. Anticholinergic drugs and frequent intermittent catheterization to empty the bladder may be necessary to lower filling and voiding pressures and to help minimize the reflux (Kass et al; Bauer et al, 1982). When a reactive external urethral sphincter is found, the Credé maneuver is contraindicated because the high voiding pressure generated by the reflexic sphincter activity in response to the Credé maneuver may be transmitted to the kidneys via the reflux.

The indications for antireflux surgery in children with myelodysplasia (or other types of neuropathic bladder dysfunction) are not very different from those in children with normal bladder function. They are recurrent urinary infection while the child is on adequate antibacterial therapy and appropriate intermittent catheterization techniques; the development or progression of pyelonephritic scarring; persistent hydroureteronephrosis despite effective emptying of the bladder; severe reflux with a definitive anatomic abnor-

mality at the ureterovesical junction; and planned implantation of an artificial urinary sphincter (Bauer et al, 1982). Trabeculation of the bladder is not a contraindication. However, a cross trigonal procedure is preferred over the Politano-Leadbetter reimplant because the trigone is usually less trabeculated than the fundus and the chance of postoperative obstruction is minimized with the former technique. Bilateral surgery is not recommended for unilateral disease because reflux does not commonly develop on the nonoperated side. Of paramount importance postoperatively is effective emptying of the bladder. Prior to the advent of clean intermittent catheterization, the success rate of ureteral reimplantation in patients with neuropathic bladder dysfunction was less than 50 per cent. Jeffs et al, and later Kass et al, demonstrated that by combining ureteral reimplantation with intermittent catheterization, a success rate equal to that for children with normal bladder function could be achieved.

Urodynamic testing is performed in older children only after the initial attempts at achieving continence are unsuccessful (Bauer et al, 1977). If a child is incontinent on intermittent catheterization or despite regular use of the Credé maneuver, this may be due to elevated bladder filling pressure, uninhibited detrusor contractions, low urethral resistance, or excessive urine volume. Except for the last condition, the specific etiology can be determined only by urodynamic testing. Appropriate therapy with anticholinergic drugs, such as oxybutynin and propantheline, to lower detrusor tone and contractility, and/or alpha sympathomimetic agents, such as phenylpropanolamine and ephedrine, to raise urethral resistance, may be necessary to improve continence between emptyings (Raezer et al, 1977). The urine volume may be measured easily each time the child is catheterized. If fluid intake is excessive, it can be curtailed.

Reconstructive surgery may be needed if the child fails to achieve continence with drug therapy and intermittent catheterization. Augmentation cystoplasty is suitable for the patient with either a poorly compliant bladder with high filling pressure or an uninhibited detrusor that does not respond to drug therapy. Conversely, if drug therapy fails to raise urethral resistance sufficiently to maintain continence, surgery to improve bladder neck resistance may be required. Several alternatives are possible, and urodynamic studies will determine which procedure is most appropriate. Bladder neck reconstruction is undertaken if the vesical neck is patulous and has minimal or no resistance, the external urethral sphincter muscle is innervated sufficiently to provide some resistance and is responsive to increases in intra-abdominal pressure (i.e., Credé or Valsalva maneuver), and the bladder has adequate volume so that it will not be compromised when a portion is used to create a new bladder neck. If the bladder is not large enough, then augmentation cystoplasty should be combined with bladder neck reconstruction and urethral lengthening.

The implantation of an artificial urinary sphincter is indicated in those children with complete or nearly complete neurologic lesions involving the external urethral sphincter who have had either an exhaustive trial of drug therapy with intermittent catheterization or previous bladder neck reconstruction yet are still incontinent. These children should have absent or controllable uninhibited detrusion contractions and a highly compliant bladder.

If bladder outlet resistance is very low, it may be difficult to assess detrusor tone during cystometry. Bladder filling pressure may be falsely low due to the escape of fluid around the catheter. If a balloon catheter is used to occlude the vesical neck, simulating an artificial sphincter, compliance may be measured more accurately during filling to determine if the child is a candidate for the device (Woodside and McGuire).

If the bladder has a low compliance or cannot accommodate at least 6 to 8 oz of urine, augmentation cystoplasty is needed to keep the filling pressure low enough to allow the upper urinary tracts to drain freely into the bladder and to maintain continence for an acceptable period of time. Bladder flap urethroplasty in girls, advocated at one time as a preliminary procedure for achieving total emptying, is not recommended now because intermittent catheterization may be used in conjunction with placement of an artificial sphincter if residual urine volume is high postoperatively.

Urinary diversion is rarely if ever performed today in children with neurogenic bladder dysfunction. Ileal conduit diversion, once considered a panacea for reflux, hydronephrosis, or urinary incontinence has been shown to open a Pandora's box of new clinical problems. Pyelonephritis and renal scarring, renal calculi, ileal strictures, and stomal stenoses are common long-term complications (Shapiro et al). The indications for urinary diversion are very specific and include a urethra that cannot be catheterized because of anatomic reasons or mental or physical handicaps, a bladder that cannot be salvaged even with an augmentation procedure, persistent hydroureteronephrosis despite exhaustive surgical and mechanical measures to improve urinary drainage, and intractable incontinence. Once the necessity for a diversion procedure is established, the choice between a nonrefluxing sigmoid colon or ileocecal conduit is determined by the size of the ureters, for it is difficult to create an effective antireflux tunnel in the wall of the sigmoid if the ureters are dilated. Ureterosigmoidostomy or other types of internal diversion are not an option in children with myelodyplasia because fecal incontinence is such a prominent feature.

Many children with previously diverted urinary tracts should be considered for possible undiversion. Diversion would not be performed in many of these individuals if they were seen for the first time today rather than 10 to 15 years ago.

The evaluation process includes tests of serum creatinine and creatinine clearance; an excretory urogram, loopogram, cystogram, and retrograde ureterograms (in the absence of reflux) to determine distal ureteral length and the feasibility of using the lower ureters to bridge the gap between ureteral segments. Suprapubic cycling of the bladder may be tried to see if it will re-expand to sufficient size and to determine whether the patient requires intermittent catheterization to empty the bladder (Perlmutter). If necessary, intermittent catheterization is begun during this period of cycling to test the child's ability to perform self-catheterization and to see if this provides continence. Once it has been determined that the child cannot void voluntarily nor be dry on intermittent catheterization, a urodynamic study is useful in deciding appropriate drug therapy or alternatives for achieving continence, either at the time of, or preferably prior to, the undiversion procedure (Bauer et al, 1980). Psychologic testing is of major importance in many adolescents. It is imperative that such children become continent after reconstitution of the urinary tract.

LIPOMENINGOCELE AND OTHER OCCULT DYSRAPHISMS

A lipoma or lipomeningocele is the second most common congenital spinal anomaly. It produces a neurologic deficit that is as variable as myelomeningocele. The extent of denervation is not determined so much by size but rather by the extent of fatty tumor infiltration into the spinal cord and surrounding nerve roots (Dubrowitz et al; James and Lassman). Other dysraphic states include: diastematomyelia, neurenteric cyst or sinus, aberrant sacral roots, fibrous traction on the conus medullaris, or a tight filum terminale. These conditions also produce variable patterns of denervation. The exact lesion affecting the spinal cord and nerve roots cannot always be determined by performing a cursory neurologic examination of the lower extremities (Mandell et al). These lesions produce abnormalities varying from no loss of nerve function to extensive lower motor neuron denervation and/or upper motor neuron dysfunction.

Urodynamic studies performed preoperatively for either a lipomeningocele or an occult spinal dysraphism will determine the true extent of nerve dysfunction involving the sacral cord and guide the neurosurgeon in his approach to excising the fatty tumor or the occult lesion. Such studies may be repeated 6 to 12 weeks postoperatively to see if further denervation, stabilization, or improvement has occurred as a result of the surgery. Subsequent testing may be necessary to determine if there is progressive loss of function as the child continues to grow.

Despite the presence of minor degrees of denervation, a period of observation may be necessary in children who have not yet been toilet trained to see if they will develop control of urination before deciding whether or not they have significant neurogenic bladder dysfunction. Urodynamic studies need not be repeated until such children are old enough to be continent, but are not.

Most lipomeningoceles, because of their size, are discovered and repaired within the first year or two of life. Other occult lesions are not generally discovered until the children are older. Urinary incontinence or infection, gait abnormalities, disparity in lower extremity size or strength, and cutaneous lesions overlying the spine are signs of an occult dysraphic condition (Anderson; James and Lassman; Mandell et al). An excretory urogram, a renal sonogram or renal scan, and a voiding cystourethrogram (particularly if the urine has been infected) are necessary in all symptomatic children. Long-term follow-up is needed only if the child is prepubertal at the time the lesion is discovered. Progressive denervation may occur during the pubertal growth spurt as a result of tethering and increased traction on the lower spinal cord.

SACRAL AGENESIS

Agenesis of the sacrum is a rare congenital anomaly that involves absence of part or all of two or more sacral vertebrae (Fig. 12–11). This can affect lumbar vertebrae as well, in which case the condition is related to the caudal regression syndrome, which includes other anomalies of the urinary and gastrointestinal tracts.

Most children with sacral agenesis are discovered during the neonatal examination. Some children escape detection until they are referred for evaluation of daytime and nighttime incontinence and/or fecal incontinence (Braren and Jones; White and Klauber; Thompson et al). All children with incontinence should have their lower back inspected and the sacral spine palpated. In sacral agenesis the gluteal cleft is usually absent and the buttocks are flattened. Any suspicion should be confirmed by anteroposterior and lateral x-ray views of the lower spine. One per cent of diabetic mothers have offspring with sacral agenesis, and 16 per cent of children with this anomaly have mothers with insulin-dependent diabetes. Thus, a family history of diabetes should be ascertained in all children with suspected sacral agenesis (Passarge and Lenz; Guzman et al). Sacral agenesis is sometimes found in conjunction with other abnormalities, such as with imperforate anus or as a part of the VATER syndrome.

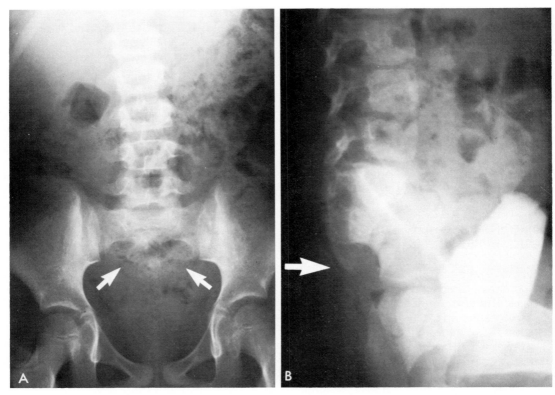

Figure 12–11. The diagnosis of partial or complete sacral agenesis is best confirmed by an AP (*A*) and lateral (*B*) film of the spine.

Neurourologic testing reveals that the degree of nerve root loss is variable and cannot be predicted from the number of affected vertebral bodies (Koff and DeRidder). In a recent review of 16 patients with sacral agenesis (Guzman et al), 9 children had detrusor contractions and 7 had an areflexic bladder. The type of bladder function could not be predicted by the level of affected vertebrae (Fig. 12–12). Of the 9 with bladder contractions, 3 had normal sphincter activity and voluntary

control with no apparent neurologic deficit, and 6 had exaggerated sacral reflexes without voluntary control (upper motor neuron type dysfunction). Of the 7 patients with an areflexic bladder, 4 had complete lower motor lesions with no electrical activity in the sphincter muscle. Again, the type of lesion, upper versus lower motor neuron, could not be predicted by the number of affected vertebrae. Seventy-five per cent of the children had completely normal sensation in the skin

COMPARISON OF TYPE OF BLADDER FUNCTION
TO HEIGHT OF ABSENT VERTEBRAE

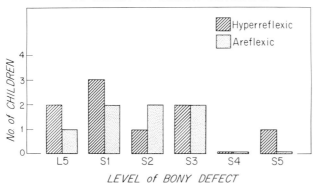

Figure 12–12. Bladder function cannot be correlated with any one level of affected vertebrae.

innervated by the sacral dermatomes. Thus, sensory afferents do not appear to be affected as commonly as motor efferents.

Therefore, it again becomes apparent that urodynamic studies are necessary to define accurately the level of denervation involving the vesicourethral unit. Studies should be coupled with either an excretory urogram or a renal sonogram and a voiding cystogram to determine the presence of reflux and the competency of the bladder neck and urethra. As a result of these tests, appropriate treatment plans can be formulated as outlined above.

CEREBRAL PALSY

Cerebral palsy is the result of a nonprogressive injury to the brain in the perinatal period that produces neuromuscular disability and/or specific symptom complexes of cerebral dysfunction. Its incidence is approximately 1.5 per thousand births and it is usually due to a perinatal infection or a period of hypoxia or anoxia to the central nervous system. It is most commonly seen in babies who are premature, but it may be discovered following neonatal seizures, infections, or intracranial hemorrhage. Affected children have delayed gross motor development, abnormal motor performance, altered muscle tone, abnormal posture, and exaggerated reflexes. Although five types of dysfunction have been identified, spastic diplegia is the most common, accounting for nearly two thirds of the cases. The other types are termed athetoid, ataxic, rigid, and mixed.

Most children with cerebral palsy develop total urinary control. Urinary incontinence is a feature in some, but the exact incidence has never been determined. A number of these children have such a severe degree of mental retardation that they are not trainable. The majority, however, have sufficient intelligence to learn basic social protocol. Many do achieve control over urination, albeit at a somewhat later age than normal children. Therefore, urodynamic evaluation is reserved for those children who appear trainable but who have not achieved total urinary continence by late childhood or early puberty.

In a recent review of this subject, urodynamic testing was performed in 16 children with cerebral palsy who fit the above criteria (Khoshbin et al). Twelve of them, or 75 per cent, had upper motor neuron type neuro-

pathic bladder dysfunction; that is, exaggerated sacral reflexes and uninhibited bladder contractions despite voluntary control and normal sphincter electromyographic activity. Half of these children demonstrated detrusor sphincter incoordination during their involuntary voiding.

The remaining 4 of the original 16 children had evidence of both upper and lower motor neuron dysfunction with bladder areflexia and/or external sphincter denervation as judged by electromyographic criteria. In this latter group spinal cord injury must have occurred at the same time as the cerebral insult. Thus, lower motor neuron dysfunction can develop in addition to the suspected upper motor neuron type dysfunction in children with cerebral palsy. Once the exact type of neuropathic bladder dysfunction is defined by urodynamic evaluation, a specific treatment program can be initiated to achieve continence. A renal sonogram, or an excretory urogram and a voiding cystourethrogram (only if the child has had urinary infection, or an inability to empty the bladder) are obtained.

DETRUSOR HYPERREFLEXIA

Urinary continence is achieved in most children between the ages of 2 and 5, with daytime control attained before nighttime dryness. Many children have persistent daytime symptoms of frequency, urgency, or urge or sudden incontinence in addition to enuresis (Firlit et al). Some may outgrow their nighttime wetting but have nocturia one or more times. During the day they urinate frequently, and unless they can use a bathroom immediately, incontinence will result. Despite this, these children can void normally and on command. Often there is a history of delayed training in other family members, and one or both parents may have been bedwetters until their teenage years (Bauer et al). The adults have compensated for their symptoms by voiding frequently during the day and awakening one or more times at night.

No evidence of outlet obstruction is found on voiding cystourethrography, and the upper urinary tract has normal drainage. A neurologic examination may reveal mild hyperreflexia of the lower extremities, but usually no abnormalities are found. The child's birth, developmental milestones, fine motor coordination, and learning abilities are normal also.

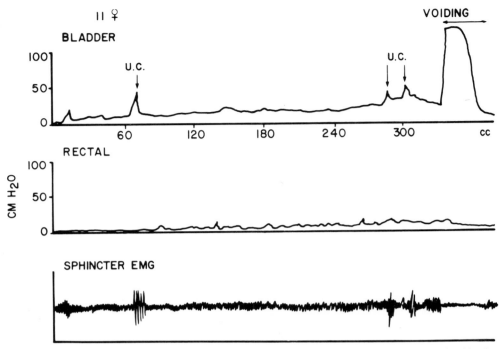

Figure 12 – 13. Uninhibited contractions (U.C.) of the bladder are associated with a rise in electrical activity of the external urethral sphincter. During voluntary voiding a coordinated vesicourethral unit exists.

Urodynamic evaluation reveals uninhibited contractions of the bladder during filling, which the child may or may not abolish by increasing the activity of the external urethral sphincter (Fig. 12 – 13). At capacity, a normal detrusor contraction takes place with sustained relaxation of the sphincter, which results in complete emptying of the bladder. The uninhibited contractions are thought to account for the wetting.

It is postulated that the infant has no ability to abolish a bladder contraction. Sometime between the first and second years of life the child develops the ability to inhibit voiding, first by tightening the external urethral sphincter and then by suppressing the detrusor contraction. Eventually this becomes an automatic response on a subconcious level. In children with no apparent or overt neuropathy, detrusor hyperreflexia has been linked to delayed maturation of the reticulospinal pathways and/or the inhibitory centers in the midbrain and cerebral cortex. Thus, total central nervous system control of the vesicourethral unit may be lacking (MacKeith et al; Muellner; Yeates). Torrens and Collins found a similar urodynamic profile in a significant number of adults with enuresis and/or day-

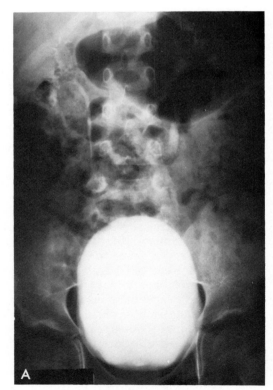

Figure 12 – 14. An excretory urogram in a girl who urinates infrequently demonstrates a large-capacity bladder with a normal upper urinary tract.

Illustration continued on opposite page.

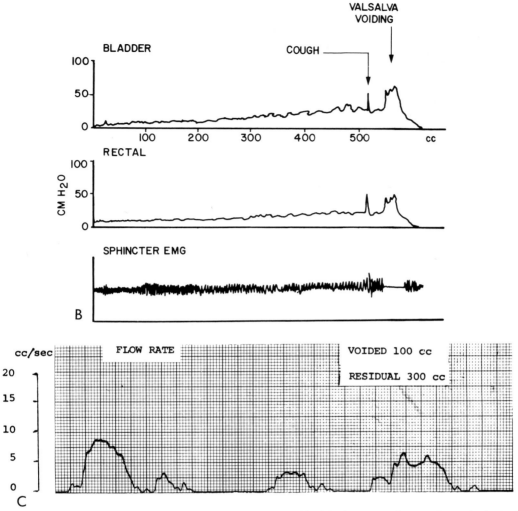

Figure 12-14 *Continued. B*, A large-capacity, low-pressure bladder is seen on her urodynamic study. She emptied entirely by straining, with no apparent detrusor contraction even though she relaxed her external sphincter. *C*, A urinary flow rate reveals an intermittent voiding pattern consistent with the clinical, radiologic, and urodynamic pictures.

time symptoms. Although parents of children with this pattern of urinary frequency and/or incontinence have not been studied, there may be a familial cause of delay in maturation that results in late control of bladder function.

Anticholinergic medication (oxybutynin, propantheline, and imipramine) have been effective in controlling the detrusor hyperreflexia (Bauer et al; Kass et al; Firlit et al).

THE INFREQUENT VOIDER

Most children void three to five times per day and defecate daily or every other day.

Some children, mostly girls, urinate only twice a day, once in the morning and once at night. These children have usually exhibited normal voiding patterns as infants, but after toilet training learned to avoid micturition for long periods of time (DeLuca et al). Some develop a fear of contamination in strange bathrooms, especially at school, while others mimic their mother's pattern of infrequent urination and defecation (Bauer et al). Excessive neatness or a fetish for cleanliness is sometimes noted as well.

Infrequent voiding or voiding only enough to relieve the pressure of a very full bladder leads to overflow or stress incontinence, which is due to a chronically distended bladder.

Recurrent urinary infection is a frequent sequela; sometimes it is the first manifestation of the abnormal voiding pattern. Eradication of the infection may be difficult despite continuous antibiotics. Constipation and soiling with small volumes of fecal material commonly accompany this syndrome; gross perineal contamination may be another source of the recurrent infection.

Frequently the abnormal micturition pattern is detected at the time of voiding cystourethrography. A large capacity smooth-walled bladder without reflux that may or may not empty will be noted (Fig. 12–14A). Even if the child voids before any instrumentation, a significant volume of residual urine will be noted. The upper urinary tract, however, usually retains its normal appearance.

Urodynamic studies demonstrate a large-capacity hypotonic bladder with normal, ineffective (unsustained), or absent detrusor contractions (Fig. 12–14B). Straining to empty is often reported. The electromyographic activity of the external urethral sphincter is normal in configuration, as is the response of sacral reflexes to filling and emptying of the bladder. Thus, no evidence for a lower motor neuron lesion exists. The urinary flow rate may be intermittent with a normal peak flow achieved during each spurt of urine (Fig. 12–14C). Unless strongly encouraged, the child will not completely empty his or her bladder during voiding. This urodynamic picture is consistent with partial or complete myogenic failure of the bladder from chronic distention.

Treatment is based primarily on changing the child's voiding habits. A schedule of frequent and double voiding is instituted along with bethanechol chloride. If the detrusor fails to recover and the volume of residual urine remains elevated, intermittent catheterization is necessary to empty the bladder until the muscle regains its ability to empty.

PSYCHOLOGIC NONNEUROPATHIC BLADDER (NONNEUROPATHIC VOIDING DYSSYNERGIA)

There is a syndrome of voiding dysfunction that mimics a form of neurogenic bladder dysfunction but is probably an acquired disease. It was reported first in 1969 (Dorfman et al) and has been elaborated upon by Hinman and others (Johnston and Farkas; Williams et al; Allen; Allen and Bright). The syndrome has been labeled the subclinical neurogenic bladder (Dorfman et al), the occult neuropathic bladder (Martin et al; Mix; Williams et al), and the nonneurogenic neurogenic bladder (Allen), because many observers believe it represents a true but isolated neurologic abnormality involving the bladder (Johnston and Farkas; Mix). Hinman, Allen, and Bauer et al believe that this is an acquired functional disorder in which there is incoordination between the detrusor and external urethral sphincter during a bladder contraction; it therefore might best be called nonneuropathic voiding dyssynergia. Electromyographic studies of the external urethral sphincter reveal normal-appearing motor unit action potentials (Bauer et al), confirming the theory that this is an acquired disease and is not due to an anatomic defect. It has been postulated that this represents a persistence of the transitional phase in the development of micturitional control by which the child learns to prevent voiding by contracting the external urethral sphincter (Allen and Bright).

The disease usually consists of both urinary and bowel dysfunction (Table 12–8). It is characterized by infrequent voiding, urgency, urge and stress incontinence, and/or unprovoked wetting. The child may have been dry for several months or years but now has urinary accidents both during the day and at night. Urinary infection is not uncommon. The child may complain that he or she has to strain to void and the urinary stream is weak. Often one can elicit a history of infrequent bowel movements with small volume encopresis, chronic constipation, or fecal impaction. Radiographic studies of the urinary tract often reveal significant structural abnormalities (hydronephrosis) as a result of chronic retention of urine (Fig. 12–15A). Hydroureteronephrosis with or without pyelonephritic scarring occurs in about two thirds of such children (Bauer et al). Fifty per cent have severe vesicoureteral reflux (Grade III/V or greater). Almost every affected child has a grossly trabeculated bladder of large capacity with a large volume of post-void residual urine (Fig. 12–15B). Voiding films reveal a persistently narrow external sphincter area (Fig. 12–15C) in almost half the children, but the urinary flow rate is generally inadequate to evaluate the caliber of the external

Table 12-8. The Psychologic Nonneuropathic Bladder

Clinical
Wetting
  Usually day and night
Bowel dysfunction
  Encopresis
  Constipation
  Fecal impaction
Urinary infection
Social history
  Dominant parents
  Divorce
  Alcoholism
Previous surgery
  Ureteral reimplantations
  Bladder neck plasties
  Diversion

Radiologic
Hydronephrosis, with or without pyelonephritis
Reflux: III/V in degree
Large-capacity, trabeculated bladder
Large residual
Posterior urethra sometimes dilated with narrowing at external sphincter
Heavily loaded colon

Urodynamic
Elevated detrusor and voiding pressures
Ineffective detrusor contractions
High resting sphincter EMG
Unsustained sphincter relaxation during voiding
Large residual

Treatment—Individualized
Bladder retraining
  Double voiding
  Intermittent catheterization
  Biofeedback
Drugs
  Bethanechol
  Phenoxybenzamine
  Diazepam
Psychotherapy

sphincter region accurately. Finally, the scout film for the excretory urogram often shows a colon full of stool.

When one delves into the social history of these children, a recurring pattern of familial interrelationships emerges. Most parents are domineering, exacting, and intolerant of weakness or failure. Divorce or alcoholism is frequently found. One or both parents may seem intolerant of the child's wetting. After careful questioning one can usually elicit a history of punishment, both mental and physical, inflicted on the child for the inconti-

nence. The child often becomes depressed or withdrawn in fear of wetting. These children try to hold back urination and/or defecation by keeping the sphincter muscles tight. Urination is reduced to once or twice a day and defecation to every several days or once a week. The retention of urine leads to urgency and urge, stress, or overflow incontinence, or even sudden wetting when the external urethral sphincter relaxes. A similar pathophysiology accounts for the chronic constipation and fecal incontinence. In the process of learning to prevent evacuation of waste products the child develops a habitually contracted and nonrelaxed external urethral sphincter and pelvic floor musculature. This, then, becomes the usual state at the time of presentation.

Urodynamic findings reveal a bladder of large capacity with increased filling pressure, uninhibited contractions, and an ineffective detrusor contraction during voiding (Fig. 12-16A). Often a Valsalva maneuver accompanies attempts at micturition. The bethanechol supersensitivity test may be positive (increased resting pressure after administration), and it was this response that once led to the belief that these children had true neurogenic bladder dysfunction (Williams et al). Electromyographic monitoring of the external urethral sphincter reveals a normal pattern and configuration of the motor unit action potentials. There is a normal response to reflex stimulation without any evidence of denervation (Bauer et al). Although these findings tend to exclude a lower motor neuron lesion, they may also be interpreted to represent upper motor neuron dysfunction. The firing rate of the external urethral sphincter may be greater than normal at rest and during filling of the bladder. Sphincter pressure may increase with each uninhibited contraction. During attempts at voluntary voiding the external urethral sphincter may not relax but in fact may actually contract (Fig. 12-16A). The failure of effective detrusor contractility with or without complete relaxation of the sphincter is the end result of the obstruction created by the incoordination between the detrusor and the external urethral sphincter during voiding (dyssynergia). A low intermittent flow rate (Fig. 12-16B) and a significant volume of residual urine are produced.

Before this syndrome was recognized and the etiology elucidated, many children underwent multiple operations to correct reflux and

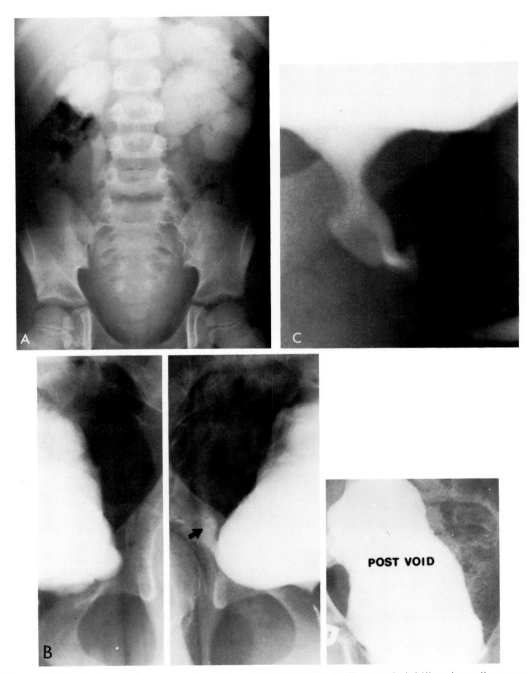

Figure 12-15. *A,* Excretory urogram in a 14-year-old boy with daytime and nighttime incontinence and encopresis. Note the large bladder. *B,* His voiding cystogram revealed trabeculation, mild right vesicoureteral reflux (*arrow*), and a large post-void residual urine volume. *C,* A film during voiding demonstrates intermittent relaxation of the external urethral sphincter area.

improve emptying of the bladder. Initially surgery may have been successful, but often the same radiologic findings reappeared. Some children were then subjected to urinary diversion.

Today, treatment is directed not only to improving the child's ability to empty his or her bladder but also to alleviating the psychosocial pressures that may have contributed to this dysfunctional voiding state (Table 12-8). A frequent voiding schedule, and even double voiding, is instituted initially. Bethanechol chloride, phenoxybenzamine, and diazepam may be prescribed to improve bladder contractility, lower bladder neck resistance, and lower external urethral sphincter resistance, respectively. Biofeedback techniques involving the external urethral sphincter may be employed to teach the child how to relax his or her external urethral sphincter and reduce the outflow obstruction caused by dyssynergia.

Psychotherapy can play a major role in the rehabilitative process. All punishments are stopped. The child is not belittled or made to feel that he or she has done something wrong when wet. Rather, the child is encouraged or rewarded when there is a satisfactory period of frequent voiding and continence. Despite these measures, some children will not overcome their symptoms or their inability to empty the bladder. Intermittent catheterization is then advocated for selected children who fail to respond to the above protocol, or as an initial form of therapy in those who have significant upper urinary tract dilatation

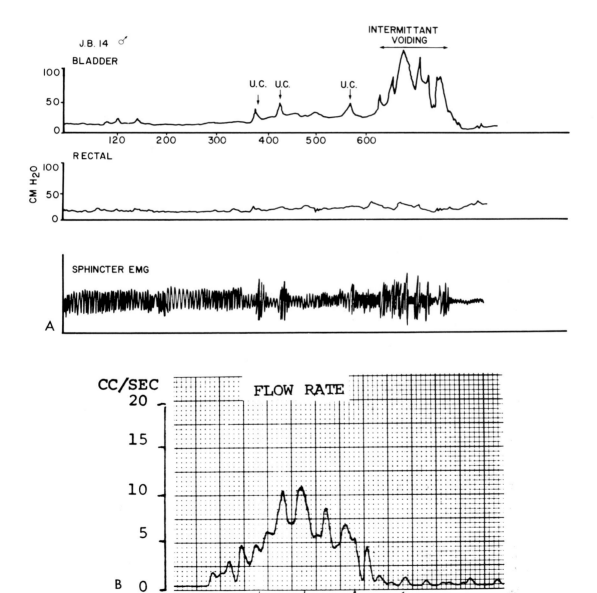

Figure 12–16. *A,* Uninhibited detrusor contractions and increases in external urethral sphincter EMG activity are noted as the bladder is filled. During voluntary voiding very high bladder pressures (above 100 cm H$_2$O) are generated owing to increased activity and then intermittent relaxation of the external sphincter. *B,* The patient's urinary flow rate reflects the voiding pattern seen on urodynamic evaluation.

requiring immediate decompression (Snyder et al). Once started, the child can undergo psychotherapy and retraining procedures with the expectation that in time the intermittent catheterization program may not be needed.

BIBLIOGRAPHY

PHYSIOLOGY OF MICTURITION

Allen TD, Bright TC: Urodynamic patterns in children with dysfunction voiding problems. J Urol 119:247, 1978.

Barrington FJF: The nervous mechanism of micturition. QJ Exp Physiol 8:33, 1914.

Bellman N: Encopresis. Acta Paediatr Scand (Suppl) 170:1, 1966.

Bors E, Comarr AE: Neurological Urology. Baltimore, University Park Press, 1971.

Bradley WE, Timm GW, Scott FB: Innervation of the detrusor muscle and urethra. Urol Clin North Am 1:3, 1974.

De Groat WC: Nervous control of the urinary bladder in the cat. Brain Res 87:201, 1975.

De Groat WC, Saum WR: Adrenergic inhibition in mammalian parasympathetic ganglia. Nature 231:188, 1971.

De Groat WC, Theobold RJ: Reflex activation of sympathetic pathways to vesical smooth muscle and parasympathetic ganglia by electrical stimulation of vesical afferents. J Physiol (Lond) 259:223, 1976.

Donker PJ, Droes JTPM, Van Ulden, BM: Anatomy of the musculature and innervation of the bladder and the urethra. *In* Scientific Foundations of Urology. Vol 2. Edited by DI Williams, GD Chisholm. Chicago, Year Book Medical Publishers, 1976, pp 32–39.

Edvardsen P: Nervous control of the urinary bladder in cats: I. The collecting phase. Acta Physiol Scand 72:157, 1968a.

Edvardsen P: Nervous control of the urinary bladder in cats: II. The expulsion phase. Acta Physiol Scand 72:172, 1968b.

El-Badawi A, Schenk EA: A new theory of the innervation of bladder musculature: I. Morphology of the intrinsic vesical innervation apparatus. J Urol 99:585, 1968.

El-Badawi A, Schenk EA: A new theory of the innervation of bladder musculature: II. The innervation apparatus of the ureterovesical junction. J Urol 105:368, 1971.

El-Badawi A, Schenk EA: A new theory of the innervation of bladder musculature: III. Innervation of the vesicourethral junction and external urethral sphincter. J Urol 111:613, 1974.

Gyermek L: Cholinergic stimulation and blockade of the urinary bladder. Am J Physiol 201:325, 1961.

Hutch JA: A new theory of the anatomy of the internal urinary sphincter and the physiology of micturition: IV. The urinary sphincter mechanism. J Urol 97:705, 1967.

Hutch JA, Rambo OA Jr: A new theory of the anatomy of the internal urinary sphincter and the physiology of micturition: III. Anatomy of the urethra. J Urol 97:696, 1967.

Khanna OP: Disorders of micturition: neuropharmaco-

logic basis and results of drug therapy. Urology 8:316, 1976.

Koelle GB: Neurohumeral transmission and the anatomic nervous system. *In* The Pharmacological Basis of Therapeutics. Fifth ed. Edited by LS Goodman, A Gilman. New York, Macmillan, 1975, pp 404–444.

Kuru M: Nervous control of micturition. Physiol Rev 45:425, 1965.

MacKeith R, Meadow SR, Turner RK: How children become dry. *In* Bladder Control and Enuresis. Edited by I Kolvin, RC MacKeith, SR Meadow. Philadelphia, JB Lippincott Co., 1973, p 3.

McNeal JE: The prostate and prostatic urethra: a morphologic synthesis. J Urol 107:1008, 1972.

Muellner SR: Development of urinary control in children. JAMA 172:1256, 1960.

Nathan PW: The central nervous system connections of the bladder. *In* Scientific Foundations of Urology. Vol 2. Edited by DI Williams, GD Chisholm. Chicago, Year Book Medical Publishers, 1976, pp 51–58.

Nyberg-Hansen R: Innervation and nervous control of the urinary bladder. Acta Neurol Scand (Suppl 20) 42:7, 1966.

Raezer DM, Wein AJ, Jacobowitz D, et al: Autonomic innervation of canine urinary bladder: cholinergic and adrenergic contributions and interaction of sympathetic and parasympathetic systems in bladder function. Urology 2:211, 1973.

Ruch TC: The urinary bladder: physiology and biophysics. *In* Physiology and Biophysics. Vol 2. Circulation, Respiration and Fluid Balance. Edited by TC Ruch, HD Patton. Philadelphia, WB Saunders Co., 1974, pp 525–546.

Tanagho EA, Smith DR: The anatomy and function of the bladder neck. Brit J Urol 38:54, 1966.

Tanagho EA, Smith DR: Mechanism of urinary continence: I. Embryologic, anatomic, and pathologic considerations. J Urol 100:640, 1968.

Tang PC: Levels of brain stem and diencephalon controlling micturition reflex. J Neurophysiol 18:583, 1955.

Woodburne RT: Anatomy of the bladder and bladder outlet. J Urol 100:474, 1968.

Yeates WK: Bladder function in normal micturition. *In* Bladder Control and Enuresis. Edited by I Kolvin, RC MacKeith, SR Meadow. Philadelphia, JB Lippincott Co., 1973a, p 28.

Yeates WK: Bladder function: increased frequency and nocturnal incontinence. *In* Bladder Control and Enuresis. Edited by I Kolvin, RC MacKeith, SR Meadow. Philadelphia, JB Lippincott Co., 1973b, p 151.

Yeates WK: Neurophysiology of the bladder. Paraplegia, 12:73, 1974.

URODYNAMIC ASSESSMENT

Abrams PH: Perfusion urethral profilometry. Urol Clin North Am 6:103, 1979.

Bates CP, Whiteside CG, Turner-Warwick RT: Synchronous cine/pressure/flow/cystourethrography with special reference to stress and urge incontinence. Brit J Urol 42:714, 1970.

Bauer SB: Pediatric neuro-urology. *In* Clinical Neurourology. Edited by RJ Krane, MB Siroky. Boston, Little, Brown & Co., 1979, p 275.

Bauer SB: Urodynamics in children: indications and methods. *In* Controversies in Neuro-urology. Edited by DM Barrett, AJ Wein. New York, Churchill-Livingston, 1983, pp 193–202.

Blaivas JG: A critical appraisal of specific diagnostic techniques. *In* Clinical Neuro-urology. Edited by RJ Krane, MB Siroky. Boston, Little, Brown & Co., 1979, p 69.

Blaivas JG, Labib KB, Bauer SB, et al: A new approach to electromyography of the external urethral sphincter. J Urol 117:773, 1977a.

Blaivas JG, Labib KB, Bauer SB, et al: Changing concepts in the urodynamic evaluation of children. J Urol 117:777, 1977b.

Bradley WE, Timm GW, Rockswold GL, et al: Detrusion and urethral electromyography. J Urol 114:891, 1974a.

Bradley WE, Timm GW, Scott FB: Sphincter electromyography. Urol Clin North Am 1:69, 1974b.

Diokno AC, Koff SA, Bender LF: Periurethral striated muscle activity in neurogenic bladder dysfunction. J Urol 112:743, 1974.

Evans, AT, Felker JR, Shank RA, et al: Pitfalls of urodynamics. J Urol 122:220, 1979.

Gierup J, Ericsson NO: Micturition studies in infants and children: intravesical pressure, urinary flow and urethral resistance in boys with intravesical obstruction. Scand J Urol Nephrol 4:217, 1970.

Gierup J, Ericsson NO, Okmian L: Micturition studies in infants and children. Scand J Urol Nephrol 3:1, 1969.

Gleason DM, Bottacini MR, Reilly, RJ: Comparison of cystometrograms and urethral profiles with gas and water media. Urology 9:155, 1977.

Gleason DM, Reilly RJ, Bottacini MR, et al: The urethral continence zone and its relation to stress incontinence. J Urol 112:81, 1974.

Maizels M, Firlit CF: Pediatric urodynamics: clinical comparison of surface vs. needle pelvic floor/external sphincter electromyography. J Urol 122:518, 1979.

Mandell J, Bauer SB, Hallett M, et al: Occult spinal dysraphism: a rare but detectable cause of voiding dysfunction. Urol Clin North Am 7:349, 1980.

Mayo ME: Detrusor hyperreflexia: the effect of posture and pelvic floor activity. J Urol 119:635, 1978.

Merrill T, Bradley WE, Markland C: Air cystometry II. A clinical evaluation of normal adults. J Urol 108:85, 1972.

Meunier MP, Mollard P: Urethral pressure profiles in children. A comparison between perfusion catheters and microtransducers, and a study of the usefulness of urethral pressure profile measurements in children. J Urol 120:207, 1978.

Scott FB, Quesada EM, Cardus D: Studies on the dynamics of micturition. J Urol 92:455, 1964.

Tanagho EA: Membrane and microtransducer catheters: their effectiveness for profilometry of the lower urinary tract. Urol Clin North Am 6:110, 1979.

Turner-Warwick RT: Some clinical aspects of detrusor dysfunction. J Urol 113:539, 1975.

Yalla SB, Rossier AB, Fam B: Vesicourethral pressure recordings in the assessment of neurogenic bladder functions in spinal cord injury patients. Urol Int 32:161, 1977.

Yalla SB, Rossier AB, Fam B, et al: Dual pressure transducer catheter for evaluating vesicourethral function. Urology 8:160, 1976.

MYELOMENINGOCELE

Bauer SB, Colodny AH, Hallett M, et al: Urinary undiversion in myelodyplasia: criteria for selection and predictive value of urodynamic testing. J Urol 124:89, 1980.

Bauer SB, Colodny AH, Retik AB: The management of vesicoureteral reflux in children with myelodysplasia. J Urol 128:102, 1982.

Bauer SB, Hallett M, Khoshbin S, et al: The predictive value of urodynamic evaluation in the newborn with myelodysplasia. JAMA, in press.

Bauer SB, Labib KB, Dieppa RA, et al: Urodynamic evaluation of boy with myelodysplasia and incontinence. Urology 10:354,1977.

Ericsson NO, Hellstrom B, Negardh A, et al: Micturition urethrocystography in children with myelomeningocele. Acta Radiol Diag 11:321, 1971.

Fry IK, McKinna JA, Simon G, et al: Some observations on the lower urinary tract in infants with spina bifida cystica. Proc Roy Soc Med 59:420, 1966.

Hobbins JC, Venus I, Tortora M, et al: Stage II ultrasound examination for the diagnosis of fetal abnormalities with an elevated amniotic fluid alpha-fetoprotein concentration. Am J Obstet Gynecol 142:1026, 1982.

Jeffs RD, Jonas P, Schillinger JF: Surgical correction of vesicoureteral reflux in children with neurogenic bladder. J Urol 115:449, 1976.

Kass EJ, Koff SA, Diokno AC: Fate of vesicourethral reflux in children with neuropathic bladders managed by intermittent catheterization. J Urol 125:63, 1981.

McGuire EJ, Woodside JR, Borden TA, et al: The prognostic value of urodynamic testing in myelodysplastic patients. J Urol 126:205, 1981.

Perlmutter AD: Experiences with urinary undiversion in children with neurogenic bladder. J Urol 123:402, 1980.

Raezer DM, Benson GS, Wein AJ, et al: The functional approach to the management of the pediatric neuropathic bladder: a clinical study. J Urol 117:649, 1977.

Shapiro SR, Lebowitz RL, Colodny AH: Fate of 90 children with ileal conduit urinary diversion, a decade later: analysis of complications, pyelography, renal function and bacteriology. J Urol 114:289, 1975.

Stark G: The pathophysiology of the bladder in myelomeningocele and its correlation with the neurologic picture. Dev Med Child Neurol (Suppl) 16:76, 1968.

Stein SC, Feldman JG, Friedlander M, et al: Is myelomeningocele a disappearing disease? Pediatrics 69:511, 1982.

Van Gool JD, Kuijten RH, Donckerwolcke RA, et al: Detrusor-sphincter dyssynergia in children with myelomeningocele: a prospective study. Z Kinderchir 37:148, 1982.

Woodside JR, McGuire EJ: Technique for detection of detrusor hypertonia in the presence of urethral sphincteric incompetence. J Urol 127:740, 1982.

SACRAL AGENESIS

Braren V, Jones W: Sacral agenesis: diagnosis, treatment and follow-up of urological complications. J Urol 121:543, 1979.

Guzman L, Bauer SB, Hallett M, et al: The evaluation and management of children with sacral agenesis. Urology 23:506, 1983.

Koff SA, DeRidder PA: Patterns of neurogenic bladder dysfunction in sacral agenesis. J Urol 118:87, 1977.

Passarge E, Lenz K: Syndrome of caudal regression in infants of diabetic mothers: observation of further cases. Pediatrics 37:672, 1966.

Thompson IM, Kirk RM, Dale M: Sacral agenesis. Pediatrics 54:236, 1974.

White RI, Klauber GT: Sacral agenesis: analysis of twenty-two cases. Urology 8:521, 1976.

OCCULT DYSRAPHISM

Anderson FM: Occult spinal dysraphism: a series of 73 cases. Pediatrics 55:826, 1975.

Dubrowitz V, Lorber J, Zachary RB: Lipoma of the cauda equina. Arch Dis Childh 40:207, 1965.

James CCM, Lassman LP: Spinal dysraphism: spina bifida occulta. New York, Appleton-Century-Crofts, 1972.

Mandell J, Bauer SB, Hallett M, et al: Occult spinal dysraphism: a rare but detectable cause of voiding dysfunction. Urol Clin North Am 7:349, 1980.

CEREBRAL PALSY

Khoshbin S, Bauer SB, Hallett M: Lower urinary tract function in children with cerebral palsy. In press.

DETRUSOR HYPERREFLEXIA

Bauer SB, Retik AB, Colodny AH, et al: The unstable bladder of childhood. Urol Clin North Am 7:321, 1980.

Firlit CF, Smey P, King LR: Micturition: urodynamic flow studies in children. J Urol, 119:250, 1978.

Kass EJ, Diokno AC, Montealegre A: Enuresis: principles of management and results of treatment. J Urol, 121:794, 1979.

MacKeith RC, Meadow SR, Turner RK: How children become dry. In Bladder Control and Enuresis. Edited by I Kolvin, RC MacKeith, SR Meadow. Philadelphia, JB Lippincott Co., 1973, p 3.

Muellner SR: Development of urinary control in children. JAMA 172:1256, 1960.

Torrens MJ, Collins CD: The urodynamic assessment of adult enuresis. Brit J Urol 47:433, 1975.

Yeates WK: Bladder function in normal micturition. In Bladder Control and Enuresis. Edited by I Kolvin, RC MacKeith, SR Meadow. Philadelphia, JB Lippincott Co., 1973, p 28.

THE INFREQUENT VOIDER

Bauer SB, Retik AB, Colodny AH, et al: The unstable bladder of childhood. Urol Clin North Am 7:321, 1980.

DeLuca FG, Swenson O, Fisher JH, et al: The dysfunctional "lazy" bladder syndrome in children. Arch Dis Childh 37:117, 1962.

PSYCHOLOGIC NONNEUROPATHIC BLADDER

Allen TD: The non-neurogenic neurogenic bladder. J Urol 117:232, 1977.

Allen TD, Bright TC: Urodynamic patterns in children with dysfunctional voiding problems. J Urol 119:247, 1978.

Bauer SB, Retik AB, Colodny AH, et al: The unstable bladder of childhood. Urol Clin North Am 7:321, 1980.

Dorfman LE, Bailey J, Smith JP: Subclinical neurogenic bladder in children. J Urol 101:48, 1969.

Hinman F: Urinary tract damage in children who wet. Pediatrics 54:142, 1974.

Johnston JH, Farkas A: Congenital neuropathic bladder, practicalities and possibilities of conservative management. Urology 5:719, 1975.

Martin DC, Datta NS, Schweitz B: The occult neurological bladder. J Urol 105:733, 1971.

Mix LW: Occult neuropathic bladder. Urology 10:1, 1977.

Snyder HM, Caldamone AA, Wein AJ, et al: The Hinman syndrome — alternatives for treatment. Presented at the Annual Meeting of the American Urological Association, Kansas City, May 16, 1982.

Williams DI, Hirst G, Doyle D: The occult neuropathic bladder. J Pediatr Surg 9:35, 1975.

13

ENURESIS

Alan D. Perlmutter

Bedwetting remains one of society's unsolved problems. Despite a voluminous literature, the causes are not clearly understood and treatment remains controversial. The writings of antiquity testify that children of our ancestors also suffered from enuresis. Enuresis is not limited to Western civilization; it has been observed in all cultures, including various African tribes and Navajo Indians (Glicklich; Louw). The variety of treatments reported through the ages to the present emphasizes the persistent enigma of this disorder and dissatisfaction with any single mode of therapy.

Bedwetting has many ramifications. When parents of enuretics are frustrated, familial relations can become strained and the child, too, may become disturbed and anxious. Enuresis can also vex the physician who must see and treat children with this common childhood complaint. The physician who feels uneasy and uncertain may reject the problem by passing it off lightly, or, conversely, he may relieve his insecurity by engaging in a rash of unnecessary studies. This review will summarize pertinent observations on the subject and will present to the practicing urologist or pediatrician a perspective that should allow for a systematic and secure approach to the problem of enuresis.

DEFINITION

Enuresis is the inappropriate or involuntary voiding of urine at an age by which control should be present; for nocturnal enuresis, this is defined as night wetting occurring beyond the age of 4 years. While the prevalence of enuresis varies somewhat among populations and according to the different authors' criteria—some including children with rare or occasional wetting—nocturnal enuresis is generally regarded as being present in 15 to 20 per cent of 5-year-old children. Bedwetting resolves with increasing age, at a fairly steady rate; between 14 and 16 per cent of the pool of enuretics stop wetting each year (Forsythe and Redmond, 1974). By the age of 10 years, the percentage falls to approximately 5 per cent and by 15 years to 1 per cent (Klackenberg; Hallgren, 1956; Oppel et al; Meadow, 1970; Bellman). While the prevalence in adults is not precisely known, it is estimated to be 1 to 2 per cent; 2 per cent of U.S. military recruits in World War II were rejected for bedwetting (Oppel et al; Thorne).

The majority of enuretics have always wet and are described as "primary enuretics." About one fourth to one third of all enuretics have had a dry period for at least several months or longer after achieving control, before starting to wet, and these children are characterized as "onset" or "secondary" enuretics (Hallgren, 1957).

About 85 per cent of enuretics wet only at night, with the remainder wetting both day and night, or days only (Hallgren, 1957). Between 10 and 25 per cent of enuretics also suffer from encopresis. While enuresis is slightly more common in males, in a ratio of three to two, encopresis is markedly more so, in a ratio of three to one. Unlike enuresis, encopresis is more commonly a daytime event (Hallgren, 1957; Bellman; Katz) and is more typically associated with overt psychological disturbances.

ETIOLOGY

Many theories of enuresis have been championed. Probably no single explanation will suffice for all cases, for enuresis is a symptom and not a disease. Also, the various etiologic factors are not necessarily mutually exclusive and in some cases have a complex interdependence. The proposed etiologies of enuresis will be discussed after a review of the acquisition of normal bladder function and control in the growing child (McGraw; Muellner; MacKeith et al; Duche; Yeates; Schmitt).

The development of normal urinary control involves a complex relationship between physiologic events dependent on maturation and behavioral influences. A useful way to understand the likelihood of normal control by a given age is to study group statistics regarding the acquisition of day and night control with increasing age. This approach however, does not distinguish environmental, social, cultural, and other behavioral influences from maturational events. The rate of maturation per se is not uniform and is influenced by a number of variables, including genetic factors.

While the details of central nervous system maturation required for the acquisition of normal bladder control are not fully understood, a useful hypothesis for viewing the steps in progressive development of cerebral functions influencing bladder function has been advanced (MacKeith et al; Yeates). From birth to about 6 months of age, voiding is frequent and uninhibited; bladder filling results in immediate voiding and complete emptying. The coordinate nature of this unconscious act suggests hypothalamic regulation. For the next 6 months, voiding tends to be less frequent, with evidence of some central nervous inhibition of the detrusor reflex, which becomes less sensitive. Sometime between 1 and 2 years of age, conscious sensation of bladder fullness appears and voiding occurs progressively less often. This awareness precedes the ability to postpone voiding any appreciable length of time. From the age of 3½ years or older, normal filling sensation is present, with both unconscious and voluntary inhibition of the desire to void. Urinary frequency is normal and the child can voluntarily initiate voiding even when the bladder is not filled. The typical sequence of acquiring bowel and bladder control in most children is as follows: (1) bowel control asleep, (2) bowel control awake, (3) bladder control awake, (4) bladder control asleep. This sequence is fairly consistent in most children; the final step— control of the bladder while asleep—follows after a variable period of time (Stein and Susser).

The behavioral aspects of bladder function include social, environmental, family, learning, and other influences that affect the timing of attainment of urinary control after the necessary maturation is present. It is further hypothesized that training and learning are important in the acquisition of normal daytime control, but that nighttime control tends to emerge spontaneously. It is felt that the emergence of bladder control, especially nighttime, cannot be accelerated but can be retarded by negative behavioral influences.

Maturational Lag and Abnormal Bladder Physiology

The most popular, although not universally accepted, hypothesis proposed for primary enuresis is delayed development of normal inhibitory control, also described as "maturational lag," consistent with delayed functional maturation of the central nervous system (Kales and Kales; Bakwin, 1961). A small bladder capacity (Muellner; Hallman; Vulliamy; Starfield, 1967; Esperanca and Gerrard, 1969a), as noted in a majority of primary enuretics, favors this explanation; this is functional and not structural, as the anatomic bladder capacity tends to be quite average when measured with the child under anesthesia (Troup and Hodgson). Bedwetting children often have diurnal frequency and urgency, with at least one fifth of those with nocturnal enuresis only and one third of day and night enuretics manifesting these symptoms (Hallgren, 1956). Other support for the concept of maturational lag comes from observations of a more generalized although not pathologic immaturity among many younger enuretics, with a tendency toward passivity, late walking, and other minor indirect evidences of developmental delay (Oppel et al; Hallgren, 1957). One recent study, however, did not demonstrate a measurable lag in neurodevelopmental maturity for enuretic boys as compared with other boys, unless encopresis also was present (Mikkelsen et al).

The cystometrogram in up to 85 per cent of bedwetting children shows persistence of an infantile pattern (detrusor instability), with a hypertonic curve, uninhibited contractions, and a small capacity (Hagglund; Linderholm; Pompeius; Johnstone; Giles et al; Mahony et al). Similarly, sleep cystometrography often shows differences between enuretics and controls (Broughton and Gastaut; Gastaut and Broughton; Spring; Kajtor et al). About one half of a group of enuretics will have an elevated intravesical pressure and spikelike detrusor contractions during filling, as is seen in the infantile bladder, whereas in nonenuretics the filling phase is relatively isotonic with a paucity of contractions, which are low pressure. Detrusor contractions that appear during sleep might subside or might cause an individual to awaken to void, either of which might normally occur, or else might, as in some enuretics, increase in magnitude with the involuntary escape of urine (Spring). These studies of bladder function suggest that subclinical bladder dysfunction ("unstable bladder") may play a role in many enuretics, whether from immaturity of the nervous system or on a neurophysiologic basis.

A neurophysiologic basis for bladder dysfunction in some bedwetters is supported by a number of observations. A urodynamic study of 50 persistent primary enuretics from 6 to 49 years of age reported that 36 of 37 nocturnal enuretics with daytime frequency, urgency, and often urge incontinence had uninhibited detrusor behavior, in contrast to those with nocturnal enuresis only, who had normal cystometry in 11 of 13 cases (Whiteside and Arnold). In addition, there are numerous reports detailing abnormal urodynamic findings in children with severe day wetting, the majority of whom also have bedwetting as well (Firlit et al; Allen and Bright; Bauer et al; Noe, 1980); in extreme cases, secondary urinary tract damage can occur (Hinman and Baumann; Hinman; Allen; Johnston et al).

More evidence for altered physiology comes from studies of adults with persistent enuresis, most of whom have urodynamic evidence of bladder dysfunction. Daytime problems are more common in adults; the majority of enuretic adults also have daytime dysfunction including urge incontinence, in contrast to approximately 15 per cent of enuretic children who also have daytime wetting. The abnormal urodynamic patterns have been found in a high percentage of both adults with nocturnal enuresis only and those with diurnal symptoms (Torrens and Collins; Hindmarsh and Byrne).

Maturation of the central nervous system in children who stop bedwetting would account for a commonly observed sequence of progressive resolution of diurnal symptoms, followed by improvement in and then cessation of bedwetting. Other neurophysiologic explanations postulated for refractory enuresis are based on investigative findings. Some defect in the sensation of bladder filling, such as a defect in the sensory receptors mediating trigonal stretch or tension, would result in persistence of inadequate or delayed recognition

of bladder filling. Cortical or subcortical dysfunction manifested by an abnormal sleep pattern could result in inadequate arousal or failure of subconscious inhibition. Uninhibited sphincter relaxation would cause involuntary leakage (Torrens and Collins; Hindmarsh).

An uncommon form of wetting, "giggle incontinence" has no apparent relationship to bedwetting. Giggle incontinence is sudden uncontrollable voiding induced by laughter, and appears distinct from stress incontinence. Tetanic bladder contraction during the event has been documented by cystometrogram. Giggle incontinence has been associated with epilepsy but can be an isolated form of recurring detrusor instability provoked centrally by uninhibited laughter, probably mediated through the hypothalamus (Cooper; Glahn; Rogers et al).

Factors in Negative Reinforcement

A transient episode of stress at a critical period of development is also postulated as the cause of enuresis (Apley and MacKeith; MacKeith). This thesis can readily explain onset enuresis; if the concept of maturational delay is incorrect, stress factors might be causal for primary enuresis as well (MacKeith). From the second to fourth year of life, and especially during the third year, there is apparently both a sensitive and a vulnerable period for the emergence of nocturnal bladder control. At that time, acute or chronic anxiety-provoking episodes can interfere with the development or emergence of normal inhibitory behavioral controls for which the neuromuscular mechanisms may already be present. In favor of such a thesis is the observation that as many as 98.5 per cent of children reared in a low-anxiety environment, with positive support and reinforcement, have achieved nocturnal bladder control by the age of 5 years (Brazelton). Conversely, the prevalence of enuresis is greater among the lower social classes, in broken homes, and after traumatic separation of child from mother (Hallgren, 1957; Stein and Susser; McKendry et al, 1968).

Genetic Factors

Genetic factors have also been implicated in enuresis (Hallgren, 1957; Frary; Bakwin, 1971). While enuresis is equally frequent in monozygotic and dizygotic twins, monozygotic twins are concordant for enuresis about twice as often as dizygotic twins, suggesting a genetic basis for the abnormality. An increased frequency of enuresis in families of bedwetters also supports a genetic factor for enuresis. Family surveys tend to be underreported, and the true familial incidence is undoubtedly even higher than that recorded. In one survey, when both parents were enuretic, 77 per cent of the children were enuretic; with one parent enuretic, 44 per cent of the children were enuretic; when neither parent was enuretic, only 15 per cent of the children were enuretic (Bakwin, 1973).

Sleep Disorders

Enuresis has also been classified as a disorder of arousal, and there is evidence from sleep research to implicate a sleep disturbance as a factor in some bedwetters (Kales and Kales; Broughton; Lowy; Anders and Weinstein; Anders et al). Sleepwalking, childhood night terrors, adult nightmares, and in some cases bedwetting, all appear to be episodic sleep disturbances, with similar disturbances of the arousal mechanism (Lowy).

Sleep is not a uniformly tranquil state but consists of cycles of varying depths, essentially an alternation of an "aroused" and an "inhibited" state. These two categories of sleep are described as rapid eye movement (REM) and nonrapid eye movement (NREM) sleep, the latter being further divided into four stages of depth. The number of sleep cycles nightly varies between four and six. In children over 2 years of age and throughout adulthood, REM sleep occupies 20 to 25 per cent of total sleep time. Children have longer periods of deep (stages 3 and 4) sleep, which progressively decrease with aging.

REM sleep is the phase of most recalled dreaming, and during REM sleep increased autonomic activity is present. In nonenuretics, any bladder contractions that might occur with a full viscus will appear only at this time, and can result in normal awakening to void (Broughton). NREM sleep is deeper sleep; autonomic activity is basal, and dreaming probably does not occur, although there is some mental activity in NREM stages 1 and 2 (Anders and Weinstein). In enuretics, any uninhibited spikelike detrusor contractions appear during the NREM phase (Gastaut and Broughton).

Bedwetting in the young child is usually

related temporally to the first sleep cycle. Early sleep studies also suggested that the "enuretic episode" generally starts in stage 4 NREM nondreaming sleep. As the sleep cycle shifts toward stage 2 or 1, voiding occurs (Broughton and Gastaut; Gastaut and Broughton). Dreams of wetting do not occur at this time, but if the subjects stay wet and are awakened during a subsequent REM period, they may describe a "wet" dream (Hallgren, 1956). In other words, dreams of wetting do not relate directly to the event but to wetness perceived subsequently. More recent sleep studies, however, have not substantiated that most enuretic events in primary enuresis are limited to NREM stages 3 and 4, but rather are related to the time of night (Kales et al; Mikkelsen et al).

For years, a role for "deep sleep" as a factor in enuresis has been claimed, but the data have been equivocal (Hallgren, 1957; McKendry et al, 1968; Braithwaite; Graham; Boyd). While reports of deep sleep being more common in enuretics are challenged on the basis of subjective bias from the increased efforts to awaken enuretics made by their parents (Graham), others present data supporting an increased difficulty in awakening enuretics. If there is a difference, the belief that it is more difficult to awaken some enuretics might be related to an exaggeration of the confusional state that can accompany any forced awakening.

Normal children who are awakened during NREM stage 4 sleep and then directed to walk and to void will be confused and will have amnesia for the episode when later normally awake. The intensity of this confusional state, which has been described as "sleep-drunkenness," seems to be greater in patients with sleep disorders (Lowy). This state, which can be stimulated in normal subjects, appears to be a necessary condition for the occurrence of a sleep disorder; arousal from slow wave sleep, with a resultant confusional or dissociative sleep state, may allow enuresis to occur. The triggering mechanism of the enuresis may be related to the higher intravesical pressures and the increased intensity and frequency of the primary detrusor contractions during NREM sleep that are observed in some enuretics (Spring; Broughton).

A group of older boys has been identified with enuresis occurring during REM sleep as an arousal event (Ritvo et al). Characteristically, these boys have significant neurotic symptoms, and Ritvo et al contrast this small group with the more typical nonarousal enuretic who has minimal evidence of maladjustment or neurotic symptomatology. They further postulate that, while psychogenic factors may not have been causative of the enuresis in arousal enuretics, these factors could be important in perpetuating it when neurotic constellations become associated with the enuretic event.

Studies of EEG's in enuretics have also shown an increased incidence of cerebral dysrhythmias (Campbell and Young; Fermaglich); in one group, 15 of 39 patients had abnormal tracings, with 13 of these showing paroxysmal spike and slow wave abnormalities (Fermaglich). These EEG abnormalities described with enuresis have been attributed to delayed functional maturation of portions of the nervous system (Kajtor et al; Edvardsen). This conclusion would correlate with the other indications previously described of a generalized maturational lag.

Psychologic Factors

Psychopathology is relatively infrequent among primary enuretics, and there is no convincing evidence that the majority of primary enuretics suffer from underlying psychoneurosis (Werry). In one study, enuretics seen in a clinical setting who were matched against nonclinical controls were noted to have a slightly higher incidence of psychologic disturbances, but when the clinical enuretics were matched to nonenuretic clinical controls both groups had a similar incidence (Hallgren, 1957). This suggests merely that patients with psychologic problems, whether enuretic or not, are more apt to seek medical help. Enuretic children do tend to be insecure and anxious (Oppel et al; Hallgren, 1957; McKendry et al, 1968), and they may display more conduct problems and immature behavior than their nonenuretic peers (Couchells et al). In some social settings a constellation of neurotic responses involving the patient and family may occur and even contribute to the persistence of the enuretic problem, but these severe responses are uncommon. Of course, primary psychopathology is seen in children who are not enuretic, and psychopathology and enuresis can coexist separately (Werry); in other situations enuresis and encopresis are among specific behavioral responses of some emotionally disturbed children (Bellman; Katz).

While some psychoanalysts have considered enuresis to be a dream substitute (Pierce), and others have regarded it as a sexual equivalent (Glicklich), there is no good evidence for either of these hypotheses. Preadolescent enuretic children were noted to masturbate no less often than nonenuretics (Hallgren, 1957), and psychological testing, including Rorschach analysis, of adolescent enuretics failed to indicate any evidence that these young people were defending against psychosexual conflicts any differently from controls (DeLuca, 1968a, 1968b).

Except for cases of obvious psychopathology, the results of psychotherapy for enuresis are not impressive (Werry and Cohrssen; Fraser) and prolonged individual treatment is required. Cures of enuresis by any of a variety of nonpsychiatric modalities do not result in symptom substitution (Werry and Cohrssen; Young and Morgan, 1973), and a long-term follow-up of young adults treated as children by medication 10 years earlier revealed no significant psychiatric disturbances (Bindelglas and Dee). These data are additional evidence that enuresis is generally a monosymptomatic disorder, and not primarily psychopathologic.

Organic Factors

Allergy was first reported as causing enuresis in 1931, but this first report of four cases was anecdotal (Bray). Other scattered reports through the years have suffered from a lack of data, as multiple therapy had been employed for the enuresis (Breneman). More recently, however, cases have been described of food allergy contributing to a reduced bladder capacity and increased vesical irritability (Esperanca and Gerrard, 1969b; Zaleski et al). In these children, dramatic improvement was obtained by elimination of the offending foods. Others, however, have not been able to demonstrate a relationship between allergy and enuresis. Serum IgE levels, which are elevated in allergic disease, were not elevated in 34 enuretic children aged 5 years or older (Kaplan). The prevalence of persistent enuresis in a group of children with respiratory allergies was similar to that of a control group without allergies (Siegel et al).

Girls with enuresis have an increased prevalence of bacteriuria. In one survey of 9411 first through third grade children, the prevalence of significant bacteriuria in the girls was 2.2 per cent overall; it was 5.6 per cent in girls who were bedwetters and 1.5 per cent in those who were not. Persistent or recurrent bacteriuria was also more common in the group of bedwetters, 65 per cent versus 21 per cent. That urinary infection can promote enuresis is well known; bacteriuria too may do so—this same study reported a 45 per cent prevalence of bedwetting in bacteriuric girls as contrasted with 17 per cent in nonbacteriuric girls (Dodge et al). In another study of 89 girls with recurrent urinary infections, 56 were enuretic when first seen. Sixteen of these 56 became dry when their infection was cured, suggesting that in this small group the enuresis was a response to the infection. However, in the other 40 the enuresis persisted after successful treatment of infection, and the bladder capacities of these girls measured during remission were considerably smaller than for the nonenuretic girls, observations consistent with underlying primary enuresis (Jones et al). These observations support the thesis that some enuretic girls may be more vulnerable to urinary infections. The reason for this is not known, although it might be related to bladder instability with abnormally elevated intravesical pressures (Lapides and Diokno). However, a past history of urinary infections does not necessarily predispose to night or day wetting; in a small series with this history, the prevalence of day or night wetting was no different from that in a control group of children (Siegel et al).

The incidence of organic urinary lesions in children with nocturnal enuresis only is as low as 1 per cent (Forsythe and Redmond, 1974). In one study of boys undergoing pressure flow voiding studies for a variety of conditions, the enuretic group had tracings no different from those of normal controls (Gierup and Ericksson). In a series of 135 enuretic children 5 years and older, 61 of whom were felt to have some outflow lesion, many of these either were minor in nature or would now be classified as variants of normal (Fisher and Forsythe; Scott). In a uroradiographic evaluation of 138 enuretic children, only 21 had a significant anatomic abnormality; all of these were in children with infection or a history of infection, or with obstructive signs or symptoms (Redman and Siebert). Another study of 115 primary enuretics concluded that children with nocturnal enuresis alone required no evaluation and that excretory urography, urodynamic studies, and endoscopy could be reserved for those with concomitant urinary infection (Kass et al).

Even among adolescent enuretics, there is a relative dearth of significant pathology. In one series of 27 adolescent enuretics, 20 of whom were evaluated urologically, half were considered to have minimal urethral or meatal "strictures," but none had severe urinary malformations (Murphy and Chapman). The authors concluded that, while these minimal lesions might possibly have contributed to the enuresis, they were not the sole cause of the enuresis. In this series of adolescent enuretics there was also no evidence for a subtle neurologic factor, excluding those few with obvious defects (Murphy et al).

Response to treatment of minor abnormalities such as meatal stenosis has been generally disappointing (Campbell and Young; Fermaglich); in one series of boys with meatal stenosis, only one of eight was dry following meatotomy (Kunin et al). The consensus among most authors is that organic urinary tract lesions rarely underlie nocturnal enuresis and that with organic lesions, other symptoms or signs are usually present in addition to the enuresis.

EVALUATION

In view of the unlikely presence of pathology in children with bedwetting, a urologic evaluation is usually unnecessary. Therefore, careful screening is essential to select those few requiring further study. Of course, urologic study should always be done when indicated, with the realization that instrumentation is unpleasant and, unless carefully explained and gently done, can be interpreted by children as punitive. Some "cures" of enuresis following urologic manipulation are temporary and may be a response to the procedure itself.

A careful history will define the pattern of enuresis. Daytime frequency despite a good stream, a family history of enuresis, and slightly delayed developmental milestones, for example, would all be suggestive of primary enuresis. The family and social history should be directed to defining intrafamilial relationships and identifying familial and sociologic problems.

Physical examination should include observation of the urinary stream, abdominal and genital examination, and evaluation for neurologic integrity. The latter can be simply done by inspecting the spinal area for dysraphism, checking peripheral reflexes, evaluating perineal sensation, and performing a careful rectal examination to evaluate anal sphincter tone and bulbocavernosus reflex response. Bimanual rectoabdominal palpation rules out significant residual urine; in the young child, only a small volume of residual urine escapes detection by this technique.

On laboratory evaluation, the urinalysis should include determination of urinary osmolality or specific gravity. An osmolality over 900 mOsm/kg or a specific gravity over 1.024 rules out significant renal disease causing obligatory polyuria. If a random urine sample has lower than the above values, then a concentrated early morning specimen should be tested. A negative urine culture excludes undetected bacteriuria. When the above evaluations are favorable in otherwise healthy children, these are "reassuring negatives," and a program of therapy can be started without additional study.

Patients with a history or findings of urinary tract infection, with a palpable urinary residual or a poor stream, or with a daytime disturbance of micturition such as dribbling and severe incontinence are candidates for further evaluation. However, children with nocturnal enuresis who have minor daytime frequency with an urgency pattern of dribbling or wetting but who have a good urinary stream or who are "supervoiders" do not require urologic study.

When urinary tract infection is detected with long-standing enuresis, wetting may not improve following evaluation and treatment of the urinary tract infection and any associated defects. In such cases, the enuresis may be primary, in contrast to the acute enuresis and urge incontinence associated with symptomatic urinary infection, which should resolve promptly after treatment. Children who also have daytime symptoms from an uninhibited bladder have a propensity to urinary infection, and here too, daytime wetting will persist despite treatment of urinary infection unless specific therapy is also directed to the bladder dysfunction.

In brief, assuming a characteristic history of nocturnal enuresis alone and a normal office examination, there is no current indication for further urologic investigation. Uroradiographic study can be reserved for those children who have had urinary infection or symptoms and signs of obstruction, with the addition of urodynamic study for those with severe daytime symptoms of bladder instability.

TREATMENT

No single therapeutic plan has been ideal, and the physician who treats enuretic children should be familiar with a variety of approaches.

A private interview with the enuretic child is often helpful. This allows the child to ventilate his or her feelings, misconceptions, and anxieties. Often this will reveal unsuspected ambivalence or strained interpersonal relationships between the patient and parents or siblings. The support of the physician is a strong part of encouraging the patient's self-confidence and an understanding that he or she is not abnormal or exceptional (Meadow, 1973). Relief of anxiety secondary to stress, by altering undesirable sociologic or environmental factors whenever possible, may improve the frequency and severity of enuresis even if a cure is not accomplished (Werry).

Lifting up the child at night, as is so frequently attempted, does not seem to cure enuresis and may even delay its disappearance (Starfield, 1972), although this may have the practical advantage of keeping the bed dry at times. However, dryness is unpredictable because there is no consistent timing between the arousal attempt and the enuretic episode, and so no conditioning occurs. The effort and discipline of this exercise may at times stimulate latent or overt hostility in the parents and anger or anxiety in the child. Diapering encourages regressive behavior; some children who have been placed for convenience in diapers at night will be dry as soon as they are placed in ordinary bed clothing.

A number of specific therapeutic programs have been utilized, including psychotherapy, hypnotherapy, diet therapy, motivational counseling, bladder training, pharmacologic therapy, and conditioning therapy; the last four programs have had the most success.

Psychotherapy

Psychotherapy has had its proponents, especially among those physicians psychoanalytically inclined. However, large scale psychotherapeutic programs are expensive and impractical for the vast numbers of enuretic children. Furthermore, since most enuresis, as previously noted in the section on Etiology, is not a manifestation of underlying psychopathology, prolonged psychoanalysis is generally an inefficient and unnecessary approach (Fraser). Therefore, psychotherapy should be limited to children with obvious psychopathology.

Hypnotherapy

While hypnotherapy has not achieved great popularity, it was remarkably effective in a group of patients with onset enuresis (Collison). In this series, those who responded all had specific precipitating stresses or a high level of family tension at the onset of the enuresis. In another group of 40 children treated by self-hypnosis, half of whom had primary enuresis, 31 were cured of bedwetting and 6 others wet less; 28 of the 31 ceased wetting in the first month of treatment (Olness). Hypnosis and self-hypnosis appear to be therapies deserving of a wider trial.

Diet Therapy

In individual instances, dramatic remissions have followed elimination of certain foods, such as dairy products, chocolate, pop and cola, egg, citrus fruits and juices, and Kool-Aid (Esperanca and Gerrard, 1969b). These items can be omitted serially from the diet to see whether and at what point enuresis will cease and a functionally reduced bladder capacity will increase. Using responders as their own controls, the evidence for a causal relationship has been convincing. However, this program appears to be effective for only a small minority of enuretics, and success has not been demonstrated by treatment of other allergies or by other investigators.

Motivational Counseling

Motivational counseling is simply an approach that encourages the child to take responsibility for the symptoms and to be actively involved in the treatment program (Schmitt) and implies a continuing relationship between a concerned and supportive physician and the child. One form of this counseling has been described as responsibility-reinforcement; this program is a combination of several approaches (Marshall et al). It offers emotional support to the patient and encourages development of a positive relationship between parents and child. The re-

sponsibility part of the technique is based on "reality therapy" as the child is encouraged to assume responsibility for his or her own learning. The positive reinforcement part, also referred to as "response shaping," is based on behavior modification therapy.

The techniques involved in responsibility-reinforcement include a progress record kept by the patient and rewards, such as a star on the calendar for a dry night. A dialogue with the physician takes place over several interviews and is part of the stepwise reinforcement. The patient is encouraged to look for feelings and factors that may influence the wetting from day to day. "Sensation awareness" is another responsibility the child assumes — an improved recognition of bladder sensation and filling. The authors of this approach emphasize that behavioral modification by response shaping requires stepwise changes toward the ultimate objective, with rewards for every level of improvement.

The cure rate from motivational therapy generally is not known but is estimated to be no better than 25 per cent (Schmitt). About 80 per cent of the patients in the responsibility-reinforcement series had a marked improvement in nocturnal enuresis — defined as a greater than 80 per cent reduction in enuresis during a 1-month period. Improvement took longer to effect than in patients treated by conditioning or by medication programs, but the relapse rate was lower — about 5 per cent (Marshall et al). Of course, the principles and techniques of motivational counseling can be incorporated into other routines of therapy, including conditioning and drug treatment.

Bladder Retention Training

The finding of a reduced functional bladder capacity in many primary enuretics leads to the obvious assumption that improvement in bladder capacity will eliminate the enuresis. While there is not an absolute bladder capacity below which enuresis will occur or above which enuresis will disappear, cessation of enuresis, whether after diet or drug therapy, bladder training, or conditioning, is associated with an increased bladder capacity and decreased diurnal frequency (Esperanca and Gerrard, 1969b; Starfield and Mellits; Starfield, 1972).

The technique of bladder retention training includes a daily log of voided volumes, forcing fluids, stream interruption, and conscious attempts to extend the times between voiding.

To establish a goal for improving the voided volumes, the appropriate bladder capacity in a child may be estimated by this formula: the bladder capacity in ounces equals the age in years plus two (Berger et al; Koff). Although many parents out of desperation limit fluids, statistical studies have not shown this to be effective, and this restriction may promote hostility between parent and child. One investigation divided enuretics into three groups (Hagglund). Twelve were fluid restricted and wakened at night; none were cured of enuresis and there was a 9 per cent mean decrease in bladder capacity in this group. Of 16 patients having supportive psychologic management only, none were cured though 7 were improved and there was a 10 per cent mean increase in bladder capacity in this group. In contrast, of 18 patients receiving forced fluids during the day without any other supportive management, 6 children were cured at 3 to 8 months follow-up, and 7 more were improved, and there was a 20 per cent mean increase in bladder capacity in this group; cystometrograms in these showed decreased vesical irritability and disappearance of involuntary contractions. Although it is difficult to convince parents that an increased fluid intake can be therapeutic, overtraining by fluid stress may help to improve the bladder capacity and, ultimately, the urinary control more rapidly. Since many enuretics have subclinical or clinical evidence of bladder instability, and since this is a demanding program, it is not surprising that the cure rate of bladder retention training is only 35 per cent (Starfield and Mellits).

Drug Therapy

Through the years, a variety of pharmacologic agents have been utilized in an attempt to eliminate enuresis. Despite the evidence that many enuretics have an uninhibited detrusor with a decreased functional bladder capacity, use of primary anticholinergic drugs such as the belladonna alkaloids or propantheline at bedtime has been equivocal and disappointing (Johnstone; Fraser; Young and Morgan, 1973; Blackwell and Currah), although some successes are described (Williams et al). Anticholinergic agents are sometimes effective for the daytime components of frequency and urge incontinence. One report does claim a distinction between primary enuresis and the enuresis associated with an uninhibited neurogenic bladder, the latter being controlled with propantheline (Diokno et al). Ephedrine, despite its mildly inhibiting effects on detrusor contractility and its alpha adrenergic stimulation of the vesical outlet, does not have a statistically demonstrable usefulness in enuresis, although individual successes are seen (Meadow, 1973). The possibility of a placebo effect for any drug having limited results must always be considered.

In 1960, the first report of a beneficial effect of imipramine (Tofranil) on enuresis appeared from a series without controlled data (MacLean). Since that time, however, numerous controlled series have been published, most of which confirm a statistically favorable effect on nocturnal enuresis (Kunin et al; Blackwell and Currah; Poussaint and Ditman; Dinello and Champelli; Kardash et al; Miller et al; Shaffer et al; Harrison and Albino; Martin, 1971). When imipramine is effective, a measurable increase in functional bladder capacity also occurs (Hagglund and Parkkulainen; Esperanca and Gerrard, 1969b).

Other tricyclic antidepressants also have a statistically favorable effect on enuresis of approximately the same magnitude as imipramine, noted in controlled studies as compared with placebo (Poussaint et al; Milner and Hills). These drugs are desipramine (Pertofrane), amitriptyline (Elavil), and nortriptyline (Aventyl), each having similar side effects and toxicity (Liederman et al). Occasional successes with one of these agents after failure with another may justify trials with different drugs in this group.

Although the degree of success from therapy with imipramine varies among the series depending upon the composition and age range of the patient populations, the methods of drug administration, and whether or not noncompliant patients are included, enuresis totally stops during therapy in up to 40 per cent of patients, with another 10 to 20 per cent "much improved." The relapse rate is high, however, with less than one third of patients being "cured" long term, once therapy is stopped. Because imipramine also can influence enuresis in the presence of organic disease (Epstein and DeQuevedo; Cole and Fried), this medication should not be started until at least an office assessment, as described in the previous section, has been completed and the patient has been found to be free of a lower urinary tract disorder.

Although the diverse pharmacologic effects of imipramine have been extensively investigated, the mechanism of action of imipramine and other tricyclic antidepressants in enuresis is unknown (Stephenson). The optimal dose of imipramine for enuresis has been calculated to be between 0.9 and 1.5 mg/kg/day (Maxwell and Seldrup). This is approximately equivalent to 25 mg for 5- to 8-year-old children and 50 to 75 mg for older children. However, the effectiveness of action of imipramine or desipramine correlates with the steady-state plasma concentration, which is the most accurate measure of appropriate dosage, but nonresponders do occur despite increasing plasma levels (Jorgensen et al; Rapoport et al). In one study, recommended doses of up to 1.5 mg/kg/day achieved therapeutic levels in only 30 per cent of children, and it was estimated that a threefold to fivefold increase in dosage would be required to achieve effective levels in all children; general use of such doses (5 mg/kg/day) would result in nearly toxic doses in some of them (Jorgensen et al). Overall, increasing dosage above recommended levels does not give a statistically significant increase in benefit but does increase side effects (The Medical Letter).

The time of administration may also alter effectiveness. Late afternoon administration seems best for children who wet before 1:00 a.m., and administration in the early evening for those who wet after 1:00 a.m., but the time seems important only when using smaller doses of the drug (Alderton).

After initiation of therapy with imipramine, a trial period of 10 to 14 days should be used before evaluating the response and making any adjustments in dosage or timing of administration. Required duration of therapy is uncertain and arbitrary and may last many months. Trial cessation therapy at 3-month intervals is recommended (Rapoport et al). Abrupt cessation of high-dose imipramine treatment as prescribed for psychopathologic conditions (5 mg/kg/day) can cause rebound symptoms of nausea, vomiting, headache, lethargy, and irritability (Petti and Law) but these are unlikely to occur with the lesser dosages used for enuresis. When relapse follows weaning, a repeat course or courses of therapy may be used. Drug dependency or long-term negative psychiatric effects after this treatment have not been observed (Bindelglas and Dee).

Side effects, although uncommon, include dry mouth, nervousness, insomnia, mild gastrointestinal disturbances, and adverse personality changes (Kardash et al; Shaffer et al;

Alderton). In children, tricyclic drugs induce a rise in diastolic blood pressure and plasma norepinephrine (Lake et al). Long-term usage results in initial weight loss followed by a decreased rate of weight gain, but no apparent effect on growth in height (Quinn and Rapoport). Overdoses can cause direct myocardial effects, such as arrhythmias and conduction blocks, with corresponding ECG changes (Fouron and Chicoine), and hypotension (Koehl and Wenzel). At therapeutic doses, however, there is no significant change in ECG (Martin, 1973). Severe symptoms from overdose can occur at 10 mg/kg and occur inevitably at 20 mg/kg, and potentially fatal toxicity occurs at 40 mg/kg (Mofenson et al). Physostigmine therapy is an effective measure for treating life-threatening manifestations of overdosage (Greene and Cromie).

Because of the hazards of overdose, the tricyclic antidepressants should always be dispensed in safety containers, and the parents must be warned of the hazards of this group of drugs. Many childhood deaths and drug poisonings have resulted from ingestion by younger siblings (Penny; Parkin and Fraser; Goel and Shanks); even some enuretics under treatment, frustrated by a poor response, have taken overdoses with severe side effects or death (Herson et al).

In brief, imipramine and other tricyclic antidepressants have been the most used adjunctive therapy for nocturnal enuresis. The response can be dramatic, but a significant failure rate, a high relapse rate, the need for prolonged therapy to maintain observed improvement, and the potential for serious side effects indicate that this family of drugs is not a panacea.

An unrelated drug, diazepam (Valium), which markedly suppresses stage 4 sleep and is helpful for other sleep disorders, apparently is not statistically useful for enuresis (Glick et al), although individual successes are encountered.

Other more recently tested medications may be useful in some wetters. Oxybutynin, an antispasmodic agent which reduces or abolishes uninhibited bladder contractions, may be beneficial in some children whose bedwetting is unresponsive to imipramine (Thompson and Lauvetz; Buttarazzi).

A very different approach to bedwetting is to alter renal function in order to provide a period of oliguria during sleep. In one report, eight adolescent bedwetters were given a diuretic in the late afternoon to provide a slight dehydration at night; seven became dry within 9 months (Scott and Morrison). Desmopressin, an analogue of vasopressin, also results in a significant reduction in the incidence of bedwetting (Birkásová et al; Aladjem et al).

Conditioning Therapy

The use of a signal alarm system triggered by the enuretic event was first described in 1938 as having dramatic success (Mowrer and Mowrer). Since then, many reports have followed, mostly in the British and Australian literature (Young and Morgan, 1973; Lovibond; McKendry et al, 1964; Young; Forsythe and Redmond, 1970; Dische; Turner). The voiding episode electrolytically triggers a buzzer intended to awaken the child, who then switches off the alarm and completes urinating in the toilet. The alarm evokes the two responses of awakening and of micturitional reflex inhibition; ultimately conditioning occurs with awakening before voiding (Young and Morgan, 1973). The results of conditioning with an alarm system appear to be considerably better than those of imipramine therapy, the average figure being somewhere around 70 per cent with relapse rates averaging about 30 per cent. Re-treatment can be given for relapse.

Although the buzzer system seems to cure almost twice as many bedwetters as the drug program, the alarm and pad system is cumbersome and requires more explanation and supervision (Forsythe and Redmond, 1970). Patient drop-out or noncompliance can be significant, from 10 to 30 per cent. Motivation is very important for success. A mean period of 16 to 17 weeks is required for the appearance of dryness (Young and Morgan, 1973; Forsythe and Redmond, 1970). When enuresis occurs during sleep, arousal by an alarm system can result in the previously described confusional state. Anxiety and fear may result until the child adjusts to the experience. It is therefore recommended that the parent stay with or near the child for the first few nights for reassurance and to help the child adjust to the use of the equipment (Dische). Some children fail to perceive the alarm and will sleep through it; this is a major cause of dropping out of the program. Increasing the intensity of the auditory stimulus is helpful and increases the success rate of this program (Finley and Wansley; Morgan).

More than simple conditioning appears to be involved; some authors classify this program as one of behavioral modification (Doleys) and note that it includes a learning component. A form of overlearning by a program of forcing fluids may temporarily increase wetting, but decreases the rate of relapse (Young and Morgan 1972, 1973; Brooksbank). Intermittent rather than continuous use of the alarm also reduces the relapse rate (Finley et al 1977; Morgan 1978), as does active and interested involvement of the physician (Close).

There is no evidence that successful use of a signal alarm for conditioning will result in the appearance of other neurotic symptoms. As a matter of fact, after cure a notable absence of substitute symptoms and a general attitudinal improvement plus increased confidence serves to emphasize the monosymptomatic nature of most enuresis (Young and Morgan, 1973; Nurnberger and Hingtgen).

Signal alarm systems are available at nominal cost through standard retail outlets in the United States and Canada. Adequately fresh batteries (Young and Morgan, 1973), a pad with recessed wires (Coote) that will minimize the likelihood of electrolysis and corrosion, and the use of no pajamas or thin cotton or nylon pajamas so that wetting through will occur rapidly, minimizing delay in triggering the alarm, are all measures to assure the most rapid conditioning response without complications (Dische).

Occasional complications occur from use of the buzzer and pad, such as "buzzer ulcers" of the skin (Borrie and Fenton; Greaves; Neal and Coote). Weakened batteries that cannot trigger the relay system allow a continuing low-voltage direct current to be applied to the moist skin, with electrolysis and eventual cell damage.

Modifications of the alarm system are available. One consists of a sensing electrode applied close to the urinary meatus for rapid detection, and skin electrodes applied to the lower abdominal region (not directly on the genitalia) to provide gentle shocking (Crosby; McKendry et al, 1972). Two other commercial devices are small, battery powered, transistorized units that avoid the complications of the pad. One has two sensors that clip to the undergarment and an alarm that fastens to the wrist. The sensor for the other fastens to a cotton pocket sewn to the undergarment; the alarm fastens to the lapel. Because both these sensing devices remain close to the source of wetting, the alarm always will be triggered rapidly, regardless of the patient's position.

In brief, the alarm system has statistically inherent advantages over the other forms of therapy, but does have certain inconveniences that make it more cumbersome to use. The explanation for its success in this group of children with a functionally immature nervous system is not clear, but it does not appear to be an avoidance reaction. It may relate to an enhanced perception of the afferent portion of the reflex arc with a resulting improvement in perception of detrusor activity.

DISCUSSION AND CONCLUSIONS

Most nocturnal enuresis is a monosymptomatic disorder of multifactorial cause. Most children with primary nocturnal enuresis seem to have a functional immaturity of the nervous system and evidence of compensated bladder instability. The enuretic disorder can become manifest following a traumatic event, usually at a critical stage of development, or can be enhanced by chronic sociologic or emotional stresses. Emotional symptoms in most bedwetters appear to be mild; no serious behavioral problems are seen in the majority. Minor changes in behavior sometimes observed usually can be adequately explained by the stresses of the disorder. Aside from a sleep disorder, which fundamentally may be due to a developmental lag, organic factors in enuresis are uncommon and may be categorized as extraurinary, such as allergy and psychopathology, or urinary, such as urinary tract infection, obstructive uropathy, and bladder instability.

Using carefully considered criteria, urologic evaluation can be selective and need not be applied to every enuretic child. Simple screening tests can distinguish most primary enuretics.

Of the multiple therapeutic modalities described, four programs are applicable for most primary enuresis: motivational counseling, bladder retention training, drug therapy, and conditioning by a signal alarm system. Most physicians will find the last two approaches most practical. Although it is simplest to start with drug treatment, its inherent dangers indicate caution with this approach. This should be supplemented with at least some of the techniques described for motivational counseling, and also with bladder retention training when there is evidence of a functionally small bladder.

The signal alarm devices are safest, with a high success rate, but require a cooperative, motivated child and an involved family and physician for best results. A combination of alarm plus imipramine has proved to be effective in a few children who do not awaken with the buzzer or who awaken frightened and confused (Gillison). Hypnosis is helpful for selected enuretic children. The occasional allergic enuretic may respond to diet elimination therapy.

Treatment of enuresis requires perception and understanding, empathy and support. A well phrased and succinct quotation from the literature (Werry) well summarizes the issue:

Since, in most cases, enuresis will prove to be unaccompanied by either demonstrable pathology or psychopathology and will be highly resistant to treatment, this represents an exercise of the highest order in the practice of good medicine. Physicians should be secure enough to be able to tolerate both etiologic ignorance and therapeutic impotence without falling into the trap of overinvestigation, overtreatment, aggression toward parents, postures of extreme somaticism or extreme psychologism or the prescription of highly impossible, impractical therapeutic regimes which because of inevitable parental omission, relieve (the physician) of further responsibility for the care of the case.

BIBLIOGRAPHY

Aladjem M, Wohl R, Boichis H, et al: Desmopressin in nocturnal enuresis. Arch Dis Child 57:137, 1982.

Alderton HR: Imipramine in childhood enuresis: further studies on the relationship of time of administration to effect. Can Med Assoc J 102:1179, 1970.

Allen TD: The non-neurogenic neurogenic bladder. J Urol 116:638, 1977.

Allen TD, Bright TC III: Urodynamic patterns in children with dysfunctional voiding problems. J Urol 119:247, 1978.

Anders TF, Carskadon MA, Dement, WC: Sleep and sleepiness in children and adolescents. Pediatr Clin North Am 27:29, 1980.

Anders TF, Weinstein P: Sleep and its disorders in infants and children: a review. Pediatrics 50:312, 1972.

Apley J, MacKeith R: The Child and His Symptoms. Second ed. Philadelphia, FA Davis Co., 1968.

Bakwin H: Enuresis in children. J Pediatr 58:806, 1961.

Bakwin H.: Enuresis in twins. Am J Dis Child 121:222, 1971.

Bakwin H: The genetics of enuresis. In Bladder Control and Enuresis. Edited by I Kolvin, RC MacKeith, SR Meadow. London, W Heinemann Medical Books Ltd., 1973, pp 73–77.

Bauer SB, Retik AB, Colodny AH, et al: The unstable bladder in childhood. Urol Clin North Am 7:321, 1980.

Bellman M: Studies on encopresis. Acta Paediatr Scand (Suppl) 170:1, 1966.

Berger RM, Maizels M, Moran GC, et al: Bladder capacity (ounces) equals age (years) plus 2 predicts normal bladder capacity aids in diagnosis of abnormal voiding patterns. J Urol 129:327, 1983.

Bindelglas PM, Dee G: Enuresis treatment with imipramine hydrochloride: a 10-year follow-up study. Am J Psychiatry 135:12, 1978.

Birkásová M, Birkás O, Flynn MJ, et al: Desmopressin in the management of nocturnal enuresis in children: a double blind study. Pediatrics 62:970, 1978.

Blackwell B, Currah J: The psychopharmacology of nocturnal enuresis. In Bladder Control and Enuresis. Edited by I Kolvin, RC MacKeith, SR Meadow. London, W Heinemann Medical Books Ltd., 1973, pp 231–257.

Borrie P, Fenton JCB: Buzzer ulcers. Br Med J 2:151, 1966.

Boyd MM: The depth of sleep in enuretic school children and in non-enuretic controls. J Psychosom Res 4:274, 1960.

Braithwaite JV: Causes of enuresis (letter). Br Med J 2:248, 1969.

Bray GW: Enuresis of allergic origin. Arch Dis Child 6:251, 1931.

Brazelton TB: A child-oriented approach to toilet training. Pediatrics 29:121, 1962.

Breneman JC: Nocturnal enuresis, a treatment regimen for general use. Ann Allergy 23:185, 1965.

Brooksbank DJ: The conditioning treatment of bed-wetting in secondary school aged children. J Adolesc 2:239, 1979.

Broughton RJ: Sleep disorders: disorders of arousal? Science 159:1070, 1968.

Broughton RJ, Gastaut H: Further polygraphic sleep studies of enuresis nocturna (intra-vesical pressure). Electroenceph Clin Neurophysiol 16:626, 1964.

Buttarazzi PJ: Oxybutynin chloride (Ditropan) in enuresis. J Urol 118:46, 1977.

Campbell EW Jr, Young JD Jr: Enuresis and its relationship to electroencephalographic disturbances. J Urol 96:947, 1966.

Close GC: Nocturnal enuresis and the buzzer alarm: role of the general practitioner. Br Med J 281(6238):483, 1980.

Cole AT, Fried FA: Favorable experiences with imipramine in the treatment of neurogenic bladder. J Urol 107:44, 1972.

Collison DR: Hypnotherapy in the management of nocturnal enuresis. Med J Aust 1:52, 1970.

Cooper C.: Giggle micturition. In Bladder Control and Enuresis. Edited by I Kolvin, RC MacKeith, SR Meadow. London, W Heinemann Medical Books Ltd., 1973, pp 61–65.

Coote MA: Apparatus for conditioning treatment of enuresis. Behav Res Ther 2:233, 1965.

Couchells SM, Johnson SB, Carter R, et al: Behavioral and environmental characteristics of treated and untreated enuretic children and matched controls. J Pediatr 99:812, 1981.

Crosby ND: Essential enuresis: successful treatment based on physiological concepts. Med J Aust 2:533, 1950.

DeLuca JN: A Rorschach study of adolescent enuretics. J Clin Psychol 24:231, 1968a.

DeLuca JN: Psychosexual conflict in adolescent enuretics. J Psychol 68:145, 1968b.

Dinello FA, Champelli J: The use of imipramine in the treatment of enuresis. A review of the literature. Can Psychiatr Assoc J 13:237, 1968.

Diokno AC, Hyndman DW, Hardy DA, et al: Comparison of action of imipramine (Tofranil) and propantheline (Probanthine) on detrusor contraction. J Urol 107:42, 1972.

Dische S: Management of enuresis. Br Med J 2:33, 1971.

Dodge WF, West EF, Bridgforth EB, et al: Nocturnal enuresis in 6- to 10-year-old children. Correlation with bacteriuria, proteinuria and dysuria. Am J Dis Child 120:32, 1970.

Doleys DM: Behavioral treatments for nocturnal enuresis in children: a review of the recent literature. Psychol Bull 84:30, 1977.

Duche DJ: Patterns of micturition in infancy. An introduction to the study of enuresis. In Bladder Control and Enuresis. Edited by I Kolvin, RC MacKeith, SR Meadow. London, W Heinemann Medical Books Ltd., 1973, pp 23–27.

Edvardsen P.: Neurophysiological aspects of enuresis. Acta Neurol Scand 48:222, 1972.

Epstein SJ, DeQuevedo A: The control of enuresis with imipramine in the presence of organic bladder disease. Am J Psychiatry 120:908, 1964.

Esperanca M, Gerrard JW: Nocturnal enuresis: studies in bladder function in normal children and enuretics. Can Med Assoc J 101:324, 1969a.

Esperanca M, Gerrard JW: Nocturnal enuresis: comparison of the effect of imipramine and dietary restriction on bladder capacity. Can Med Assoc J 101:721, 1969b.

Fermaglich JL: Electroencephalographic study of enuretics. Am J Dis Child 118:473, 1969.

Finley WW, Wansley RA: Auditory intensity as a variable in the conditioning treatment of enuresis nocturna. Behav Res Ther 15:181, 1977.

Finley WW, Wansley RA, Blenkarn MM: Conditioning treatment of enuresis using a 70% intermittent reinforcement schedule. Behav Res Ther 15:419, 1977.

Firlit CF, Smey P, King LR: Micturition urodynamic flow studies in children. J Urol 119:250, 1978.

Fisher OD, Forsythe WI: Micturating cystourethrography in the investigation of enuresis. Arch Dis Child 29:460, 1954.

Forsythe WI, Redmond A: Enuresis and the electric alarm: study of 200 cases. Br Med J 1:211, 1970.

Forsythe WI, Redmond A: Enuresis and spontaneous cure rate: study of 1129 enuretics. Arch Dis Child 49:259, 1974.

Fouron J, Chicoine R: ECG changes in fatal imipramine (Tofranil) intoxication. Pediatrics 48:777, 1971.

Frary LG: Enuresis: a genetic study. Am J Dis Child 49:557, 1935.

Fraser MS: Nocturnal enuresis. Practitioner 208:203, 1972.

Gastaut H, Broughton R: A clinical and polygraphic study of episodic phenomena during sleep. In Recent Advances in Biological Psychiatry. Edited by J. Wortis. New York, Plenum, 1965, pp 197–221.

Gierup J, Ericsson NO: Micturition studies in infants and children. Scand J Urol Nephrol 5:1, 1971.

Giles GR, Light K, Van Blerk PJP: Cystometrogram studies in enuretic children. S Afr J Surg 16:33, 1978.

Gillison TH: Enuresis again (letter). Br Med J 2:363, 1973.

Glahn BE: Giggle incontinence (enuresis risoria). A study and an aetiological hypothesis. Br J Urol 51:363, 1979.

Glick BS, Schulman D, Turecki, S: Diazepam (Valium) treatment in childhood sleep disorders. A preliminary investigation. Dis Nerv Syst 32:565, 1971.

Glicklich LB: An historical account of enuresis. Pediatrics 8:859, 1951.

Goel KM, Shanks RA: amitriptylene and imipramine poisoning in children. Br Med J 1:261, 1974.

Graham P: Depth of sleep and enuresis: a critical review. In Bladder Control and Enuresis. Edited by I Kolvin, RC MacKeith, SR Meadow. London, W Heinemann Medical Books Ltd., 1973, pp 78–83.

Greaves MW: Hazards of enuresis alarms (letter). Arch Dis Child 44:285, 1969.

Greene AS, Cromie WJ: Treatment of imipramine overdose in children. Urology 18:314, 1981.

Hagglund TB: Enuretic children treated with fluid restriction or forced drinking: a clinical and cystometric study. Ann Paediat Fenn 11:84, 1965.

Hagglund TB, Parkkulainen KV: Enuretic children treated with imipramine (Tofranil): a cystometric study. Ann Paediat Fenn 11:53, 1965.

Hallgren, B.: Enuresis. I. A study with reference to the morbidity risk and symptomatology. Acta Psychiatr Neurol Scand 31:379, 1956.

Hallgren B: Enuresis. A clinical and genetic study. Acta Psychiatr Neurol Scand 32(Suppl):114, 1957.

Hallman N: On the ability of enuretic children to hold urine. Acta Paediatr 39:87, 1950.

Harrison JS, Albino VJ: An investigation into the effects of imipramine hydrochloride on the incidence of enuresis in institutionalized children. S Afr Med J 44:253, 1970.

Herson VC, Schmitt BD, Rumack BH: Magical thinking and imipramine poisoning in two school-aged children. JAMA 241:1926, 1979.

Hindmarsh JR: Assessment of the relationship between sensation and volume, tension and compliance during the filling phase in adult enuretics. Prog Clin Biol Res 78:77, 1981.

Hindmarsh JR, Byrne PO: Adult enuresis—a symptomatic and urodynamic assessment. Br J Urol 52:88, 1980.

Hinman F: Urinary tract damage in children who wet. Pediatrics 54:142, 1974.

Hinman F, Baumann FW: Vesical and ureteral damage from voiding dysfunction in boys without neurologic or obstructive disease. J Urol 109:727, 1973.

Johnston JH, Koff SA, Glassberg KI: The pseudo-obstructed bladder in enuretic children. Br J Urol 50:505, 1978.

Johnstone JMS: Cystometry and evaluation of anticholinergic drugs in enuretic children. J Pediatr Surg 7:18, 1972.

Jones B, Gerrard JW, Shokeir MK, et al: Recurrent urinary infections in girls: relation to enuresis. Can Med Assoc J 106:127, 1972.

Jorgensen OS, Lober M, Christiansen J, et al: Plasma concentration and clinical effect in imipramine treatment of childhood enuresis. Clin Pharmacokinet 5:386, 1980.

Kajtor F, Ovary I, Zsadanyi O: Nocturnal enuresis: electroencephalographic and cystometric examinations. Acta Med Acad Sci Hung 23:153, 1967.

Kales A, Kales JD: Sleep disorders. Recent findings in the diagnosis and treatment of disturbed sleep. N Engl J Med 290:487, 1974.

Kales A, Kales JD, Jacobson A, et al: Effects of imipramine on enuretic frequency and sleep stages. Pediatrics 60:431, 1977.

Kaplan G: Allergic origin of enuresis seen possible, but unlikely. Pediatr News 7:12, 1972.

Kardash S, Hillman ES, Werry J: Efficacy of imipramine in childhood enuresis: a double blind study with placebo. Can Med Assoc J 99:263, 1968.

Kass EJ, Diokno AC, Montealegre A: Enuresis: principles of management and result of treatment. J Urol 121:794, 1979.

Katz J: Enuresis and encopresis. Med J Aust 1:127, 1972.

Klackenberg G: Primary enuresis: when is a child dry at night? Acta Paediatr 44:513, 1955.

Koehl GW, Wenzel JE: Severe postural hypotension due to imipramine therapy. Pediatrics 47:132, 1971.

Koff SA: Estimating bladder capacity in children. Urology 21:248, 1983.

Kunin SA, Limbert DJ, Platzker ACG, et al: The efficacy of imipramine in the management of enuresis. J Urol 104:612, 1970.

Lake CR, Mikkelsen EJ, Rapoport JL, et al: Effect of imipramine on norepinephrine and blood pressure in enuretic boys. Clin Pharmacol Ther 26:647, 1979.

Lapides J, Diokno AC: Persistence of the infant bladder as a cause for urinary infection in girls. J Urol 103:243, 1970.

Liederman PC, Wasserman DH, Liederman VR: Desipramine in the treatment of enuresis. J Urol 101:314, 1969.

Linderholm BE: The cystometric findings in enuresis. J Urol 96:718, 1966.

Louw JX: Nocturnal enuresis in the Bantu. S Afr Med J 42:559, 1968.

Lovibond SH: The mechanism of conditioning treatment of enuresis. Behav Res Ther 1:17, 1963.

Lowy FH: Recent sleep and dream research: clinical implications. Can Med Assoc J 102:1069, 1970.

MacKeith RC: Is maturation delay a frequent factor in the origins of primary nocturnal enuresis? Dev Med Child Neurol 14:217, 1972.

MacKeith RC, Meadow SR, Turner RK: How children become dry. In Bladder Control and Enuresis. Edited by I Kolvin, RC MacKeith, SR Meadow. London, W Heinemann Medical Books Ltd., 1973, pp 3–21.

MacLean REG: Imipramine hydrochloride (Tofranil) and enuresis. Amer J Psychiatry 117:551, 1960.

Mahoney DT, Laferte RO, Blais DJ: Studies of enuresis. IX. Evidence of a mild form of compensated detrusor hyperreflexia in enuretic children. J Urol 126:520, 1981.

Marshall S, Marshall HH, Lyon RP: Enuresis: an analysis of various therapeutic approaches. Pediatrics 52:813, 1973.

Martin GI: Imipramine pamoate in the treatment of childhood enuresis. A double-blind study. Am J Dis Child 122:42, 1971.

Martin GI: ECG monitoring of enuretic children given imipramine (letter). JAMA 224:902, 1973.

Maxwell C, Seldrup J: Imipramine in the treatment of childhood enuresis. Practitioner 207:809, 1971.

McGraw MB: Neural maturation as exemplified in achievement of bladder control. J Pediatr 16:580, 1940.

McKendry JBJ, Stewart DA, Jeffs RD, et al: Enuresis treated by an improved waking apparatus. Can Med Assoc J 106:27, 1972.

McKendry JBJ, Williams HA, Broughton, C: Enuresis—a study of untreated patients. Appl Ther 10:815, 1968.

McKendry JBJ, Williams HA, Matheson D: Enuresis: a three year study of the value of a waking apparatus. Can Med Assoc J 90:513, 1964.

Meadow RC: Childhood enuresis. Br Med J 4:787, 1970.

Meadow RC: Practical aspects of the management of nocturnal enuresis. In Bladder Control and Enuresis. Edited by I Kolvin, RC MacKeith, SR Meadow. London, W Heinemann Medical Books Ltd., 1973, pp 181–194.

The Medical Letter: Imipramine for Enuresis. Med Lett 16:22, 1974.

Mikkelsen EJ, Rapoport JL: Enuresis: psychopathology, sleep stage and drug response. Urol Clin North Am 7:361, 1980.

Mikkelsen EJ, Rapoport JL, Nee L, et al: Childhood enuresis. I. Sleep patterns and psychopathology. Arch Gen Psychiatry 37:1139, 1980.

Miller PR, Champelli JW, Dinello FA: Imipramine in the treatment of enuretic schoolchildren. Am J Dis Child 115:17, 1968.

Milner G, Hills NF: A double-blind assessment of antidepressants in the treatment of 212 enuretic patients. Med J Aust 1:943, 1968.

Mofenson HD, Greensher J, Horowitz R: Imipramine treatment of enuresis. Am J Dis Child 123:181, 1972.

Morgan RTT: Relapse and therapeutic response in the conditioning treatment of enuresis: a review of recent findings on the intermittent reinforcement, overlearning and stimulus intensity. Behav Res Ther 16:273, 1978.

Mowrer OH, Mowrer WM: Enuresis—a method for its study and treatment. Am J Orthopsychiatry 8:436, 1938.

Muellner SR: Development of urinary control in children: some aspects of the cause and treatment of primary enuresis. JAMA 172:1256, 1960.

Murphy S, Chapman W: Adolescent enuresis: a urologic study. Pediatrics 45:426, 1970.

Murphy S, Nickols J, Hammar S: Neurological evaluation of adolescent enuretics. Pediatrics 45:269, 1970.

Neal BW, Coote MA: Hazards of enuresis alarms. Arch Dis Child 44:651, 1969.

Noe, NH: Voiding dysfunction in the child with problem "wetting." Dev Behav Pediatr 1:29, 1980.

Nurnberger JI, Hingtgen JN: Is symptom substitution an important issue in behavior therapy? Biol Psychiatry 7:221, 1973.

Olness K: The use of self-hypnosis in the treatment of childhood nocturnal enuresis. Clin Pediatr 14:273, 1975.

Oppel WC, Harper PA, Rider RW: The age of attaining bladder control. Pediatrics 42:614, 1968.

Parkin JM, Fraser MS: Poisoning as a complication of enuresis. Dev Med Child Neurol 14:727, 1972.

Penny R: Imipramine hydrochloride poisoning in childhood. Am J Dis Child 116:181, 1968.

Petti TA, Law W III: Abrupt cessation of high-dose imipramine treatment in children. JAMA 246:768, 1981.

Pierce CM: Dream studies in enuresis research. Can Psychiatr Assoc J 8:415, 1963.

Pompeius R: Cystometry in pediatric enuresis. Scand J Urol Nephrol 5:222, 1971.

Poussaint AF, Ditman KS: A controlled study of imipramine (Tofranil) in the treatment of childhood enuresis. J Pediatr 67:283, 1965.

Poussaint AF, Ditman KS, Greenfield R: Amitriptyline in childhood enuresis. Clin Pharmacol Ther 7:21, 1966.

Quinn PO, Rapoport JL: One-year follow-up of hyperactive boys treated with imipramine or methylphenidate. Am J Psychiatry 132:241, 1975.

Rapoport JL, Mikkelsen EJ, Zavadil A, et al: Childhood enuresis. II. Psychopathology, tricyclic concentration in plasma, and enuretic effect. Arch Gen Psychiatry 37:1146, 1980.

Redman JF, Seibert JJ: The uroradiographic evaluation of the enuretic child. J Urol 122:799, 1979.

Ritvo ER, Ornitz EM, Gottlieb F, et al: Arousal and non-arousal enuretic events. Am J Psychiatry 126:115, 1969.

Rogers MP, Gittes RF, Dawson DM, et al: Giggle incontinence. JAMA 247:1446, 1982.

Schmitt BD: Nocturnal enuresis: an update on treatment. Pediatr Clin North Am 29:21, 1982.

Scott JES: A surgeon's view of enuresis. In Bladder Control and Enuresis. I. Kolvin, RC MacKeith, SR Meadow. London, W Heinemann Medical Books Ltd., 1973, pp 104–106.

Scott R, Morrison LM: Diuretic treatment of enuresis. J R Coll Surg Edinb 25:470, 1980.

Shaffer D, Costello AJ, Hill ID: Control of enuresis with imipramine. Arch Dis Child 43:665, 1968.

Siegel S, Rawitt L, Sokoloff B, et al: Relationship of allergy, enuresis and urinary infection in children 4 to 7 years of age. Pediatrics 57:526, 1976.

Spring WB: Sleep cystometrography: a preliminary study of bladder function during sleep. Can Med Assoc J 93:353, 1965.

Starfield B: Functional bladder capacity in enuretic and non-enuretic children. J Pediatr 5:777, 1967.

Starfield B: Enuresis: its pathogenesis and management. Clin Pediatr 6:343, 1972.

Starfield B, Mellits ED: Increase in functional bladder capacity and improvements in enuresis. J Pediatr 72:483, 1968.

Stein Z, Susser M: Social factors in the development of sphincter control. Dev Med Child Neurol 9:692, 1967.

Stephenson JD: Physiological and pharmacological basis for the chemotherapy of enuresis. Psychol Med 9:249, 1979.

Thompson IM, Lauvetz R: Oxybutynin in bladder spasm, neurogenic bladder and enuresis. Urology 8:452, 1976.

Thorne F: The incidence of nocturnal enuresis after age five. Am J Psychiatry 100:686, 1944.

Torrens MJ, Collins CD: The urodynamic assessment of adult enuresis. Br J Urol 47:433, 1975.

Troup CW, Hodgson NB: Nocturnal functional bladder capacity in enuretic children. J Urol 129:132, 1971.

Turner RK: Conditioning treatment of nocturnal enuresis: present status. In Bladder Control and Enuresis. Edited by I Kolvin, RC MacKeith, SR Meadow. London, W Heinemann Medical Books Ltd., 1973, pp 195–210.

Vulliamy D: The day and night output of urine in enuresis. Arch Dis Child 31:439, 1956.

Werry JS: Enuresis—a psychosomatic entity? Can Med Assoc J 97:319, 1967.

Werry JS: Cohrssen J: Enuresis—an etiologic and therapeutic study. J Pediatr 67:423, 1965.

Whiteside CG, Arnold EP: Persistent primary enuresis: urodynamic assessment. Br Med J 1:364, 1975.

Williams H, Jeffs R, McKendry JBJ, et al: A study of enuresis using propantheline bromide. Can Med Assoc J 82:1312, 1960.

Yeates WK: Bladder function in normal micturition. In Bladder Control and Enuresis. Edited by I Kolvin, RC MacKeith, SR Meadow. London, W Heinemann Medical Books Ltd., 1973, pp 28–36.

Young GC: The problem of enuresis. Br J Hosp Med 2:628, 1969.

Young GC, Morgan RTT: Overlearning in the conditioning treatment of enuresis. Behav Res Ther 10:147, 1972.

Young GC, Morgan RTT: Conditioning technics and enuresis. Med J Austr 2:329, 1973.

Zaleski A, Shokeir MK, Gerrard JW: Enuresis: familial incidence and relationship to allergic disorders. Can Med Assoc J 106:30, 1972.

Surgical Treatment of Urinary Incontinence

STEPHEN A. KRAMER

MECHANISMS OF URINARY CONTROL

Anatomy and Physiology of Voiding

Urinary incontinence in children results from a variety of anatomic or functional abnormalities. Methods of presentation range from simple diurnal or nocturnal enuresis to total and continuous urinary leakage. A review of the anatomy and physiology of voiding is essential before urologic investigation is undertaken on which treatment decisions are to be based (Jensen; Ganong).

Although the mechanisms of urinary control are complex, recent advances in experi-

mental and clinical research have provided us with an improved understanding of the physiology of urine storage and bladder emptying. Urinary continence and normal micturition require an integration of the autonomic, somatic spinal, and supraspinal centers (Mahony et al, 1977). Parasympathetic fibers to the bladder arise from roots of S2 through S4 and course to the bladder through the pelvic nerve, where they synapse with the postganglionic fibers in the detrusor muscle (Fig. 14–1). Sympathetic innervation to the bladder arises in the thoracolumbar cord, T11 through L2. These fibers synapse in the inferior mesenteric ganglion and provide innervation to the bladder through the hypogastric

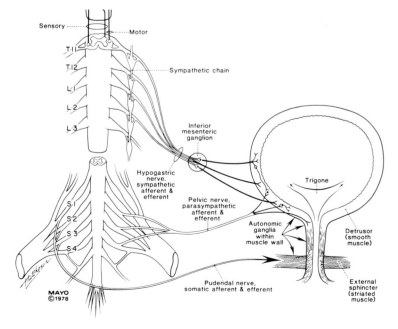

Figure 14–1. Neuroanatomy of the bladder and urethra. (From Barrett DM: Urodynamics of the lower urinary tract. *In* Transurethral Surgery. Edited by LF Greene, JW Segura. Philadelphia, WB Saunders Co., 1979, pp 353–370.)

nerve plexus (El-Badawi and Schenk, 1968, 1971).

Receptor site mapping has demonstrated that the detrusor and proximal portions of the urethra are dually innervated by the parasympathetic and sympathetic divisions of the autonomic nervous system (Benson et al, 1979). Parasympathetic receptor sites are located throughout the detrusor and proximal portions of the urethra but are most abundant in the bladder body (Taira; Raezer et al, 1973; Wein and Raezer). Stimulation of these receptors produces a detrusor contraction, which causes an increase in intravesical pressure and is the primary force for bladder emptying.

Sympathetic receptor sites are found in the bladder body, bladder neck, and proximal urethral smooth muscle (Bradley et al, 1974). Alpha adrenergic receptors from the sympathetic division of the autonomic nervous system predominate in the bladder and smooth muscle of the proximal urethra. Stimulation of these receptors results in contraction of the smooth muscle of the bladder neck and inhibits bladder emptying. Conversely, inhibition of these alpha adrenergic receptors reduces resistance at the bladder neck and proximal urethra and facilitates bladder emptying (Tulloch; Benson et al, 1976a, 1976b; Sundin et al; Tanagho, 1982). Beta adrenergic receptors are most abundant in the bladder body. Stimulation of these receptors causes relaxation of the detrusor smooth muscle and facilitates storage of urine. Inhibition of beta adrenergic receptors promotes detrusor contraction and enhances bladder emptying (Benson et al, 1976b; Tanagho, 1982).

The striated muscles of the external urinary sphincter receive somatic innervation through the pudendal nerve, arising from the sacral cord S2 through S4 (Fig. 14–1). Stimulation of this sphincter provides voluntary resistance to urine outflow, which augments bladder storage. Inhibition of striated muscular activity at the level of this sphincter reduces outflow resistance and facilitates bladder emptying (Bradley et al, 1974; Khanna; Wein and Raezer).

Maturation of Nervous System and Bladder

All children normally pass through several recognized steps as they develop urinary continence. Interestingly, in a study of 315 children who ranged in age from 1 to 7 years, Klackenberg did not find any correlation between parental "training efforts" and the development of urinary control. For about the first 6 months of life, the detrusor muscle contracts spontaneously as a result of stretch reflexes from bladder distention. In this stage of voiding, "detrusor micturition," the infant voids automatically and cannot initiate or inhibit the urinary stream voluntarily.

Between 1 and 2 years of age, the child begins to sense a full bladder and the recognition that micturition is imminent. During this interval, the child gradually acquires diurnal control. By 2 years of age, the child becomes further aware of a full bladder and begins to "hold" his urine for brief periods of time. At age 2, most children still cannot initiate voiding at will, nor can they void with less than a full bladder.

By 3 years of age diurnal control becomes well established, and by 4½ years of age the majority of children have nocturnal control as well. In Blomfield and Douglas's series, 88 per cent of children had acquired complete urinary control by 4½ years of age. There is approximately a twofold increase in bladder capacity between 2 and 4½ years of age. This enlargement in bladder size correlates extremely well with the development of urinary control (Fig. 14–2).

Mature bladder function can be represented as a cycle of filling, desire to void, postponement, initiation of sphincter relaxation and bladder contraction, and maintenance of sphincter relaxation and bladder contraction until the bladder is empty (Fig. 14–3) (Yeates). Urinary continence and normal storage of urine during bladder filling require (1) accommodation of an increase in volume of urine at a low intravesical pressure, (2) a closed bladder outlet, and (3) absence of detrusor instability — that is, absence of uninhibited bladder contractions. Intravesical pressure increases only slightly during the filling phase. The bladder outlet provides resistance to urine loss by virtue of the anatomic arrangement of the detrusor smooth muscle, the inherent tonicity of the circular smooth muscle at the bladder neck, the elastic tissue of the proximal urethra, and a sufficient length of posterior urethra within the intraabdominal position (Bradley et al, 1974; Bissada and Finkbeiner). When intravesical pressure increases as a result of standing or exertion, urethral resistance must increase to prevent loss of urine. This is accomplished through a neurally mediated reflex from the

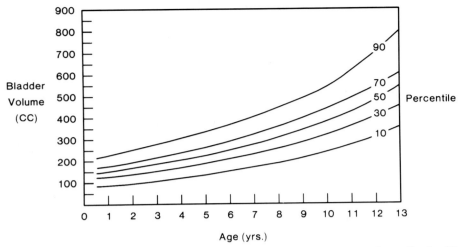

Figure 14–2. Bladder capacity in 814 children having cystoscopy under general anesthesia. (Courtesy of R. W. Geist.)

pudendal nerve to the striated muscles of the pelvic floor that causes the urethra to elongate and narrow while the vesical neck shifts anteriorly.

The desire to void is initiated by bladder distention and further accentuated by bladder contractions. Complete bladder emptying requires contraction of the detrusor body in response to activation of the parasympathetic motor fibers to the bladder. This results in an increase in intravesical pressure and sequential dilatation of the bladder neck and relaxation of the striated muscle of the external sphincter to allow a diminished pressure gradient to occur (Bradley et al, 1975; Barrett). Decreased outlet resistance at the time of detrusor contraction results from funneling of

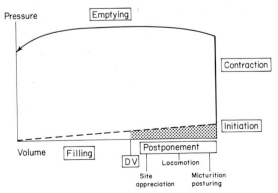

Figure 14–3. Micturition cycle. DV, desire to void. (Redrawn from Yeates WK: Disorders of bladder function. Ann R Coll Surg Engl *50*:335, 1972.)

the vesical neck and shortening of the posterior urethra.

CLASSIFICATION OF INCONTINENCE

A variety of adjectives have been used to describe urinary incontinence in children; these include urgency, stress, psychogenic, neuropathic, giggle, and paradoxic, among others. These terms are purely descriptive of the patient's symptoms and do not indicate a cause for the loss of urine. The functional classification of urinary incontinence described by Wein et al allows a logical approach on which treatment options and decisions can be based. The pathophysiology of failure of urinary storage involves increased bladder contractility or decreased outlet resistance, or both. Failure to empty the bladder occurs as a result of decreased contractility or increased outlet resistance, or both (Table 14–1).

Failure of Urinary Storage

INCREASED BLADDER CONTRACTILITY. Hyperactivity of the bladder during the filling and storage phase of micturition can be expressed as *detrusor hyperreflexia*. Detrusor hyperreflexia may occur as a result of *hypertonicity, neuropathic dysfunction, increased outflow resistance, infectious* or *inflammatory* processes in the bladder itself, or *idiopathic* causes (Table 14–1). "Hypertonicity" reflects an increase in intravesical pressure with bladder filling (poor compliance) (Raezer

Table 14–1. Classification of Urinary Incontinence

A. Failure of adequate urinary storage
   1. Increased bladder contractility (hyperreflexia)
     a. Hypertonicity
     b. Neuropathic dysfunction
       (1) Congenital—meningocele, meningomyelocele, spina bifida, sacral agenesis, spinal dysraphism, sacral teratoma
       (2) Acquired—traumatic paraplegia, transverse myelitis, osteomyelitis of the vertebral bodies, iatrogenic from excision of tumor or during surgery for imperforate anus
     c. Increased outflow resistance
       (1) Anatomic—meatal stenosis, anterior urethral diverticulum, urethral stricture, anterior or posterior urethral valves, urethral polyp, urethral calculus, vesical neck contracture, foreign body, tumor, abscess, ureterocele, labial atresia, hematocolpos, hydrocolpos, retrovesical cysts
       (2) Functional—detrusor sphincter dyssynergia, internal sphincter dyssynergia
     d. Infectious or inflammatory—acute cystitis, cystitis cystica
     e. Idiopathic
   2. Decreased outlet resistance
     a. Congenital—stress
     b. Acquired—trauma to urethra or pelvic musculature, iatrogenic from transurethral resection of vesical neck or of posterior urethral valves, Y-V plasty of vesical neck, internal urethrotomy
B. Failure of bladder emptying
   1. Decreased bladder contractility
     a. Neuropathic dysfunction
       (1) Congenital—meningocele, meningomyelocele, spina bifida, sacral agenesis, spinal dysraphism, sacral teratoma
       (2) Acquired—traumatic paraplegia, transverse myelitis, osteomyelitis of the vertebral bodies, iatrogenic from excision of tumor or during surgery for imperforate anus
   2. Increased outlet resistance
     a. Anatomic—meatal stenosis, anterior urethral diverticulum, urethral stricture, anterior or posterior urethral valves, urethral polyp, urethral calculus, vesical neck contracture, foreign body, tumor, abscess, ureterocele, labial atresia, hematocolpos, hydrocolpos, retrovesical cysts
     b. Functional—detrusor sphincter dyssynergia, internal sphincter dyssynergia
C. Congenital anatomic defects—urethral duplication, accessory urethra, absent urethra, epispadias, exstrophy, ectopic ureter
D. Psychogenic incontinence
E. Enuresis

et al, 1977). This term does not imply uninhibited bladder contractions. Hypertonic bladders are often fibrotic and of small capacity and usually are refractory to pharmacologic management. Urinary incontinence in patients with hypertonic bladders may require bladder augmentation to effect urinary control.

Vesical *neuropathic dysfunction* may be congenital or acquired (Table 14–1). Increased bladder contractility or detrusor hyperreflexia may result from destruction or bypassing of a central nervous system pathway, which is normally inhibitory to micturition. Children with "pediatric uninhibited bladders" from either maturational delays or true neurogenic disease present with urinary urgency, daytime wetting, intermittent lower abdominal pain, nocturnal enuresis, and squatting maneuvers.

In young girls with poorly developed or impaired central control centers, increased bladder contractility and urinary incontinence may be associated with *giggling* (Glahn; Rogers et al). Laughter initiates involuntary micturition that cannot be stopped, even after cessation of the laughter. Incontinence may either be partial or result in complete micturition. Giggle incontinence is distinct from stress incontinence induced by laughter. Voiding is essentially normal, and nocturnal incontinence is not present. No therapy is indicated for this group of children, and complete continence is usually achieved with further detrusor development.

Increased outflow resistance may result in increased bladder contractility and failure of urinary storage (Andersen; Hebjørn et al; Wein). The degree of incontinence is dependent upon the severity of the outlet obstruction. In the early stages of anatomic obstructive uropathy, bladder irritability is manifested by urinary urgency, frequency, and nocturnal wetting. As the obstructive process becomes more severe, detrusor decompensation occurs and is accompanied by incomplete bladder emptying, increased residual urine, and overflow incontinence.

Bladder outflow obstruction may also be secondary to functional causes such as detrusor sphincter dyssynergia and internal sphincter dyssynergia. Both of these entities are often responsible for failure of bladder emptying; however, they may also be associated with failure of adequate urinary storage. Detrusor sphincter dyssynergia results from neurologic damage that causes lack of coordination between the autonomic and somatic nervous systems, resulting in external sphincter stimulation at the time of detrusor contraction (Yalla et al). Children with this disorder void intermittently, with urinary dribbling, daytime incontinence, lower abdominal pain, and, often, squatting maneuvers. Detrusor sphincter dyssynergia may be associated with increased residual urine and may contribute to vesicoureteral reflux. Severe inappropriate pelvic floor hyperactivity may also be associated with encopresis. Recent data have shown that this symptom complex may occur in the absence of neurologic disease (Wein and Barrett). The inability to relax the sphincter during voiding may be related to unconscious inhibition of the central nervous system or straining to void.

Internal (bladder neck) sphincter dyssynergia implies a lack of coordination between the bladder neck and the detrusor muscle and is manifested by prolonged hesitancy, decreased sensation to void, weak and poor velocity of stream, urinary frequency, daytime incontinence, and frequent urinary tract infections. Lower abdominal pain or squatting postures usually do not occur in this group of patients. *Infectious* or *inflammatory* changes in the bladder may also be responsible for increased bladder contractility. Acute bacterial cystitis or cystitis cystica may produce inflammatory changes in the bladder mucosa and cause detrusor irritability, urgency, dysuria, frequency, and suprapubic pain.

The *idiopathic* form of detrusor hyperreflexia occurs in otherwise healthy children and can be particularly distressing (Turner-Warwick). Complete neurologic evaluation in this group of patients is usually negative. This entity may represent a maturational lag of delayed development of normal inhibitory control mechanisms.

DECREASED OUTLET RESISTANCE. Damage to the innervation of the smooth muscle of the bladder neck and proximal urethra or to the striated muscle of the voluntary external sphincter can be either congenital or acquired. Urinary stress incontinence is the classic example of sphincteric dysfunction and occurs when an increase in abdominal pressure causes intravesical pressure to exceed urethral resistance. Congenital childhood urinary stress incontinence is an unusual but well-documented entity that may occur in young girls. These children usually improve as they approach puberty; however, a few patients require surgery to provide support for the bladder neck and urethra.

Failure of Bladder Emptying

DECREASED BLADDER CONTRACTILITY. Inability to empty the bladder because of decreased intravesical pressure occurs as a result of *neuropathic dysfunction* of the lower motor neurons (Table 14–1). Large-capacity, hypotonic, or areflexic bladders are often associated with increased residual urine, with or without urinary tract infection. Children with this disorder are unable to establish sufficient intravesical pressure to overcome urethral resistance and experience continuous dribbling of urine because of overflow incontinence.

INCREASED OUTLET RESISTANCE. Failure to empty the bladder may be due to increased outlet resistance from either anatomic or functional causes, as previously discussed.

Congenital Anatomic Incontinence

Total urinary incontinence in children may result from congenital anomalies related to anatomic defects of the bladder or urinary sphincters (Table 14–1). These entities include urethral duplication, accessory urethra, absent urethra, epispadias, exstrophy, and ectopic ureter and are discussed elsewhere in this text.

Psychogenic Incontinence

Childhood emotional problems may be responsible for urinary incontinence. The onset of urinary leakage in a previously continent child, especially associated with a disturbing event in the child's life, is suggestive of psychogenic incontinence. Voiding patterns vary, but the child usually experiences daytime frequency and urgency unaccompanied by nocturnal enuresis. Encopresis may accompany enuresis in a psychologically disturbed child.

Enuresis

Enuresis may be diurnal or nocturnal, or both. A detailed discussion of the incidence, causes, symptoms, and treatment of this problem is provided in Chapter 13.

PATIENT EVALUATION

A thorough and detailed preoperative evaluation, including history, physical examination, renal function studies, radiographic evaluation, cystoscopy when indicated, and urodynamic investigation, is essential in determining the cause of urinary leakage. Urodynamic evaluation is discussed fully in Chapter 12 and will not be detailed here.

History

The importance of an accurate and detailed history in the child with urinary incontinence cannot be overemphasized. Incontinence varies in the amount (total, partial, or dribble) and in the pattern of urinary loss (continuous, intermittent, nocturnal, or diurnal). The character of the voided stream, such as dribbling or straining, particularly in boys, may aid in the presumptive diagnosis of bladder outlet obstruction, for example, posterior urethral valves. Urinary incontinence, from whatever cause, may be either congenital or acquired. It is important to establish at the onset whether the child has ever had urinary control. The sudden onset of urinary incontinence in a previously toilet-trained child may indicate neuropathic dysfunction, bladder outlet obstruction from either anatomic or functional causes, or incontinence due to psychogenic factors. Symptoms of urinary frequency, urgency, dysuria, fever, and chills are indicative of an associated urinary tract infection. It is important to obtain a family history, since siblings or other family members may have similar genitourinary anomalies.

Physical Examination

A thorough physical examination, including a pertinent neurologic workup, is mandatory. Abdominal sinus tracts may indicate underlying fistulas or a patent urachus. Examination of the abdomen may reveal a distended bladder consistent with chronic urinary retention. Abdominal asymmetry or associated masses may represent underlying benign or malignant neoplasms. Palpation of

the flanks will rule out nephromegaly. Transillumination of a flank mass is helpful in distinguishing cystic from solid lesions.

The back should be examined for the presence of lipomatosis, hairy patches, spinal defects, and coccygeal sinuses. The sacrum and coccyx should be palpated carefully to rule out underlying sacral abnormalities. Rectal examination is necessary to provide assessment of anal sphincter tone and to rule out pelvic mass lesions. Examination of the external genitalia is critical to the diagnosis of a variety of congenital anomalies, including epispadias, absent urethra, urethral duplication, labial adhesions, urogenital sinus abnormalities, or fistulous tracts. If possible, the child's urinary stream should be observed for both quality and character. The examiner should attempt to localize abnormal urinary leakage from extraurethral sites such as the vagina, vestibule, rectum, and perineum. Routine neurologic examination includes testing of deep tendon reflexes, perineal sensation, evaluation of anal sphincter tone, and testing for the bulbocavernous reflex. Abnormal neurologic findings indicate the need for pediatric neurologic consultation.

Renal Function Studies

Appropriate laboratory studies permit an accurate evaluation of renal function and may reveal occult renal disease. A properly collected sample for urinalysis and culture should be obtained from all children undergoing investigation for urinary incontinence. Gross or microscopic hematuria or a well-documented urinary tract infection should prompt further investigation, which should include excretory urography and voiding cystourethrography. Sterile pyuria should provide a search for acid-fast bacilli and parasitic infections. Proteinuria or glycosuria may indicate underlying systemic diseases. Determination of serum electrolytes, including blood urea nitrogen and serum creatinine, is indicated in children in whom there is radiographic evidence of renal damage. Creatinine clearance from a properly collected sample will provide an accurate index of the rate of glomerular filtration and may be indicated in selected cases.

Radiographic Evaluation

An excretory urogram and voiding cystourethrogram may be indicated in incontinent children with sterile pyuria, urinary tract infection, or gross or microscopic hematuria and in patients with abnormal physical findings suggestive of underlying congenital anomalies or neurologic disease. The scout film provides evidence of soft-tissue masses, urinary calculi, and displacement of bowel. Furthermore, the plain film of the kidney, ureter, and bladder should be scrutinized for evidence of vertebral or sacral anomalies and to rule out a widened symphysis. The presence of stool throughout the colon may be consistent with underlying neuropathic disease of bowel and bladder.

Voiding cystourethrography under fluoroscopy is obtained before excretory urography to detect any vesicoureteral reflux, bladder diverticula, trabeculation, bladder distortion from either intrinsic or extrinsic masses, and urethral pathology. The postvoiding film is important in confirming the presence of incomplete bladder emptying and in detecting any occult bladder diverticula.

Excretory urography evaluates comparative renal function and size, and it allows the diagnosis of hydronephrosis, duplication anomalies, and nonfunctional renal segments. In selected patients, radioisotopic renograms and renal scans with or without furosemide permit an accurate assessment of renal function and obstructive uropathy.

Cystourethroscopy

Technical improvements in pediatric panendoscopes allow thorough cystoscopic examination in both female and male neonates. Before the cystoscope is inserted, the urethra should be calibrated carefully with bougies to detect any anterior urethral valves or strictures. Urethroscopic examination with a 0° lens permits accurate detection of abnormalities of the anterior and posterior urethra. The bladder neck should be studied with a 0° lens while the cystoscope is being withdrawn to determine whether the vesical outlet closes appropriately. This maneuver is particularly useful in the child with epispadias, to assess the need for vesical neck reconstruction. The bladder should be examined for cystitis cystica, trabeculation, diverticula, calculi, foreign bodies, and ectopic ureteral orifices. Measurement of bladder capacity should be accomplished at the time of cytoscopy, for a decreased bladder size may contribute to incomplete urinary control.

Bimanual examination with the patient under anesthesia will indicate the presence or absence of pelvic masses. Careful study of the perineum and vestibule is important in localizing the site of abnormal urinary leakage from ectopic ureteral orifices. The administration of intravenous indigo carmine may prove extremely useful in this aspect of the examination by allowing clear delineation of the site of abnormal urinary leakage.

SURGICAL TREATMENT

Treatment options available for the child with urinary incontinence include observation, bladder training techniques, pharmacologic manipulation of the detrusor-sphincter muscles, intermittent self-catheterization, surgical reconstruction, and urinary diversion. The primary goals of surgical reconstruction in children with urinary incontinence who are deemed appropriate candidates for operative repair include (1) complete urinary control without the need for external appliances, (2) preservation and function of upper tract anatomy, (3) absence of urinary infection, (4) adequate bladder storage, (5) adequate bladder emptying at low intravesical pressures, and (6) social acceptability. The reconstructive techniques applicable to childhood urinary incontinence are listed in Table 14–2.

Techniques of Facilitating Urine Storage

DECREASE BLADDER CONTRACTILITY. Both *subarachnoid block* and bilateral anterior or posterior *sacral rhizotomy* have been used to convert hyperreflexic, hypertonic bladders into areflexic bladders, which can then be managed with intermittent self-catheterization (Wein et al). Permanent selective subarachnoid block to the sacral arcs involves instillation of a hyperbaric solution of glycerol and phenol or alcohol into the subarachnoid space. This procedure is not as selective as sacral root block and may result in impotence, perianal anesthesia, or paraparesis.

Stimulation and blockade of the individual sacral roots with the use of cystometric and sphincterometric control, before sacral rhizotomy, appear to enhance the clinical response and minimize side effects. Bilateral rhizotomy may result in loss of erectile function and temporary impairment of bowel function (Misak et al). Recently, selective sacral nerve section was used to increase bladder capacity by abolishing only the motor supply responsi-

Table 14-2. Surgery for Urinary Incontinence

A. Techniques to facilitate urine storage
  1. Surgery to decrease bladder contractility
    a. Interruption of innervation
      (1) Subarachnoid block
      (2) Sacral rhizotomy
  2. Surgery to augment bladder capacity
    a. Ileocystoplasty
    b. Ileocecocystoplasty
    c. Colocystoplasty
    d. Arap procedure
  3. Surgery to increase outlet resistance
    a. At level of bladder neck
      (1) Muscle flaps
      (2) Fascial slings
      (3) Bladder flaps
      (4) Suprapubic vesicourethral suspension
      (5) Transvaginal urethral plication
      (6) Vesical neck reconstruction
      (7) Implantation of genitourinary sphincters
    b. At level of distal mechanism
      (1) Electrical stimulation of external sphincter
      (2) Urethral compression
      (3) Periurethral Teflon injection
      (4) Implantation of genitourinary sphincters
B. Techniques to improve bladder emptying
  1. Surgery to increase bladder contractility
    a. Electrical stimulation
      (1) Directly to bladder
      (2) To nerve root or spinal cord
  2. Surgery to decrease outlet resistance
    a. At level of bladder neck
      (1) Transurethral resection
      (2) Y-V plasty
    b. At level of distal mechanism
      (1) Internal urethrotomy
      (2) External sphincterotomy
      (3) Pudendal nerve interruption
C. Urinary diversion

ble for uninhibited contractions, thus leaving sphincteric and sexual function intact (Torrens and Griffith).

AUGMENT BLADDER CAPACITY. In selected patients with small bladders, the techniques of ileocystoplasty, ileocecocystoplasty, and colocystoplasty provide attractive alternatives to urinary diversion. Arap et al have reported encouraging results with their modification of colocystoplasty to increase bladder capacity in patients with epispadias and exstrophy. These techniques are described elsewhere in this text.

INCREASE OUTLET RESISTANCE. Surgical mechanisms to increase outlet resistance at the level of the bladder neck include muscle flaps, fascial slings, bladder flaps, suprapubic vesicourethral suspension, transvaginal urethral plication, vesical neck reconstruction, and implantation of genitourinary sphincters. Surgical mechanisms to increase outlet resistance at the level of the distal mechanism in-

clude electrical stimulation of the external sphincter, urethral compression, periurethral Teflon injection, and implantation of genitourinary sphincters.

Muscle Flaps and Fascial Slings. Muscle flaps (for example, levator ani, perineal, gracilis, and pyramidalis) and fascial slings have each been utilized in efforts to provide voluntary urinary control. In 1932, Millin employed a split musculofascial strip of pyramidalis which encircled the urethra (Kaufman, 1978). Aldridge, in 1942, used fascial strips of external oblique aponeurosis passed through the rectus to encircle the urethra. The external anal sphincter has been used as a sling to provide compression and angulation of the bulbous urethra (Vergés-Flaqué; Mathisen). Most of these procedures do not allow physiologic micturition and are of little value in the treatment of childhood urinary incontinence.

Gierup and Hakelius recently reported transplantation of free autogenous muscle grafts for children with urinary incontinence. These authors achieved successful results in 10 of 16 children (63 per cent) with incontinence secondary to epispadias, exstrophy, or posterior urethral valves. The procedure involves denervation of a skeletal muscle, usually one of the short extensors of the foot, for 2 to 3 weeks. The muscle is then transplanted to the posterior urethra in close contact with normally innervated muscles, which act as reinnervation sources. The initial results with this technique are encouraging, and we eagerly await the long-term follow-up in this group of patients.

Bladder Flaps. In 1949, Barnes and Wilson described the construction of a new female urethra by means of a bladder flap. More recently, the use of bladder musculature for urethral sphincter reconstruction has been popularized by Tanagho et al, Flocks and Boldus, and Michalowski and Modelski. Detrusor loop flaps incorporate the arching fibers of the detrusor into a tubed muscular flap, which is anastomosed to the distal urethra.

The Tanagho procedure utilizes a tubularized flap made from anterior bladder wall (Tanagho et al). This concept was based on Tanagho's previous work, which demonstrated that primary sphincteric function was dependent upon the circularly oriented smooth muscle fibers surrounding the bladder neck and proximal urethra. Tanagho postulated that a flap that incorporated these circular muscle fibers of the bladder neck

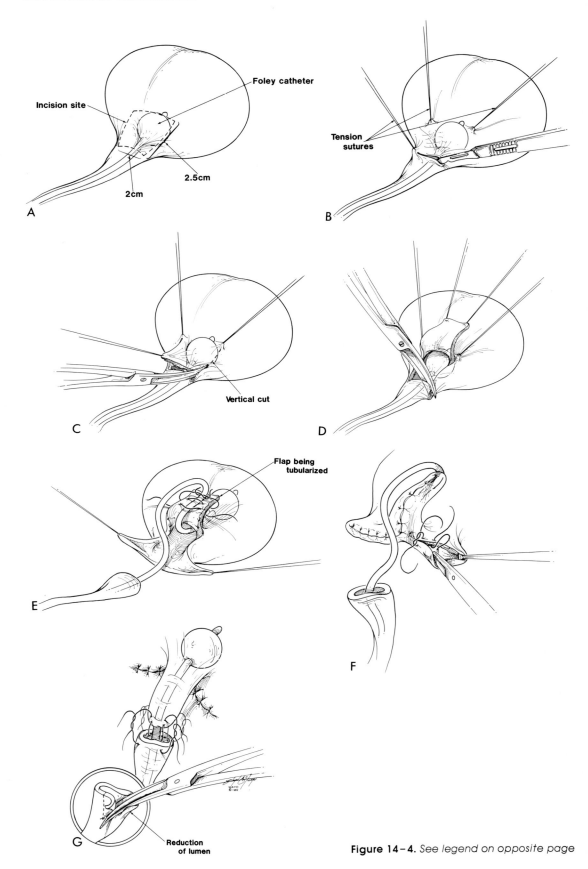

Figure 14–4. *See legend on opposite page*

would create a sphincteric mechanism in the exact anatomic location of the normal sphincteric segment. This technique was described originally for incontinence following radical prostatectomy; however, it has since been utilized for various forms of childhood congenital incontinence with an overall success rate of approximately 70 per cent (Tanagho, 1981).

The patient is placed in the supine position on the operating table, and the pelvis is extended by placing rolled towels under the sacrum. The bladder is catheterized and partially filled with sterile saline. A transverse incision is made two fingerbreadths above the pubic symphysis, and the vesical neck and anterior bladder wall are exposed by means of careful blunt and sharp dissection. In boys, the puboprostatic ligaments are transected, and the lateral aspect of the prostatovesical junction is exposed. A flap measuring 2 cm across at the vesical outlet, 2.5 cm in length, and 2.5 cm at its base is then delineated by four fixation sutures (Fig. 14–4A). It is important that the flap be measured out with the bladder only partially filled. A full-thickness transverse incision is made at the vesicourethral junction just below and beyond the stay sutures (Fig. 14–4B). Two parallel incisions are made along the bladder wall and complete formation of the flap (Fig. 14–4C). The remaining posterior attachments of the bladder and urethra are carefully transected at the vesical neck (Fig. 14–4D). In boys, the incision should be continued as deep as Denonvilliers' fascia or until the seminal vesicles and the ampulla of the vas deferens are exposed. The anterior bladder flap is then tubularized around a number 10 or 12 Foley catheter with the use of interrupted sutures of 4-0 chromic catgut (Fig. 14–4E). After closure of the tube, the apex of the trigone is approximated to the base of the tube by means of mattress sutures placed in the midline posteriorly. The bladder is closed transversely with two layers of interrupted absorbable sutures (Fig. 14–4F). The end of the tube is reanastomosed to the severed proximal urethra with interrupted 3-0

chromic catgut (Fig. 14–4G). Occasionally, excision of an anterior wedge of prostatic tissue may be necessary to reduce urethral size and thereby effect a narrowed and more satisfactory anastomosis (Fig. 14–4G). A suprapubic vesicourethral suspension (Marshall-Marchetti-Krantz) adds further support to the newly constructed vesicourethral junction. A Malecot catheter is brought through the dome of the bladder; the cystostomy tube and urethral catheter are left indwelling for 3 to 4 weeks to ensure adequate healing. The urethral catheter is removed first, and postvoiding residual urine is measured before removal of the suprapubic tube.

Suprapubic Vesicourethral Suspension. In female patients with urinary stress incontinence, the Pereyra-Stamey endoscopically controlled suspension of the bladder neck (Pereyra; Stamey) and the Marshall-Marchetti-Krantz procedures have consistently produced excellent results. The success and complication rates of these operations have been quite comparable (Stamey et al; Marshall). The Marshall-Marchetti-Krantz operation is based on the premise that elevation and fixation of the vesical neck are major factors in the maintenance of urinary control. Preoperative patient selection includes a Marshall test to confirm urinary stress incontinence. This maneuver consists of filling the bladder and demonstrating that urine is lost when abdominal pressure increases in either the supine or the erect position. The floor of the bladder is then elevated by placing ring forceps into the vagina or by placing a finger just anterior to the cervix to cause elevation and fixation of the vesical neck and urethra (Fig. 14–5A). It is important not to compress the bladder neck itself. The test is considered favorable if elevation and fixation of the vesical neck provide good urinary control with coughing and straining. Some patients have combined stress urinary incontinence and detrusor hyperreflexia. In these selected cases, preoperative urodynamic evaluation is extremely useful in identifying those patients with unstable blad-

Figure 14–4. *A,* Tanagho procedure. Flap measuring 2 cm across at vesical outlet, 2.5 cm in length and 2.5 cm at its base, is outlined. *B,* Fixation sutures delineate bladder flap. Full-thickness transverse incision is made at vesicourethral junction. *C,* Two parallel incisions are made along bladder wall which complete formation of flap. *D,* Posterior attachments of bladder and urethra are carefully transected at vesical neck. *E,* Anterior bladder flap is tubularized around Foley catheter. *F,* Tube has been formed and bladder is closed transversely. *G,* Distal end of the tube is reanastomosed to the severed proximal urethra. Excision of anterior wedge of prostate allows reduction of urethral size.

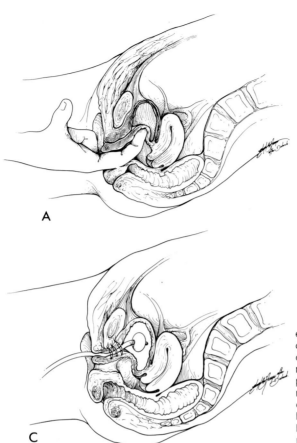

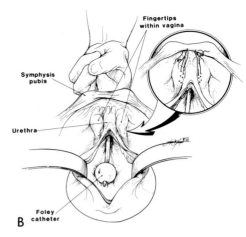

Figure 14–5. *A*, Marshall test. Floor of bladder is elevated by placing a finger just anterior to cervix and causing elevation and fixation of vesical neck and urethra. *B* In *inset*, sutures are placed approximately 1 cm from either side of the urethra into the perivaginal fascia on either side of the vesical neck. Upward displacement of the vagina by the assistant's fingers avoids tension until all sutures have been tied securely. *C*, After sutures have been tied, bladder and urethra are elevated anteriorly and superiorly.

ders who may not be candidates for surgical intervention.

The operation consists of simple elevation and immobilization of the vesical neck and urethra by suturing them to the pubis and rectus muscles. The patient is placed on the operating table in the Trendelenburg position. The bladder is catheterized and filled with sterile saline, and the Foley catheter is clamped. A transverse suprapubic incision is made 2 cm above the pubic symphysis, and the perivesical space is developed. With the use of a sponge forceps, the vesical neck and anterior urethra are exposed by blunt and sharp dissection of the loose areolar tissue on the anterior surface of the bladder. The urethra is dissected to a point 1 cm or less above the external urethral meatus. An assistant's fingers in the vagina help in palpating the Foley catheter and balloon, which correspond to the urethra and vesical neck, respectively.

A vertical cystotomy is optional and may afford better exposure for placement of the urethral and vesical neck sutures. Three absorbable sutures of 1-0 or 2-0 Vicryl or chro-

mic catgut are placed approximately 1 cm from either side of the urethra into the perivaginal fascia and on either side of the vesical neck, care being taken not to enter the urethral lumen or vagina (Fig. 14–5B). These sutures are then placed through the synchondrosis of the pubis. If this cartilaginous tissue is inadequate, holes may be drilled through the periosteum for fixation, or the perivaginal fascia may be elevated to Cooper's ligament as described by Burch. Upward displacement of the vagina by the assistant's fingers avoids undesirable tension until all sutures have been tied securely (Fig. 14–5B). Additional sutures may be used to approximate the bladder and rectus muscles to pull the bladder anteriorly into the space of Retzius (Fig. 14–5C). The wound is drained and closed in a layered fashion. The Foley catheter is removed on the fifth postoperative day.

This procedure is probably the best available for correction of urinary stress incontinence, particularly that due to cystourethrocele. Furthermore, suprapubic vesicourethral suspension can be combined with vesical neck reconstruction in children with exstrophy, epispadias, or absent urethra to enhance urinary continence. With proper patient selection, complete urinary control should be effected in 90 to 95 per cent of patients.

Transvaginal Urethral Plication. Trigonal tubed flaps incorporate the arcuate fibers of the trigonal loop and the deep transverse trigonal muscle to restore urinary continence. The vaginal approach to the trigonal loop by transvaginal urethral plication was originally described by Kelly in 1913. In 1969, King and Wendel proposed a modification of this technique for girls with total urinary incontinence due to a short patulous urethra and incompetency of the vesical neck, as in epispadias, hypospadias, or absent urethra. In their series, transvaginal plication successfully provided total urinary competence or objective improvement in more than 50 per cent of patients.

The patient is placed in the lithotomy position with the head of the operating table lowered slightly. In prepubertal girls, a small vagina may necessitate a mediolateral episiotomy to afford adequate exposure. A sponge is placed on the posterior vaginal wall, and a weighted posterior retractor is inserted. Cys-

tourethroscopy is performed with a 0° lens for adequate visualization of the vesical neck. An incompetent bladder neck fails to close and remains patulous on withdrawal of the urethroscope (Fig. 14–6A).

A Foley catheter is inserted and pulled down until the balloon is against the bladder neck. A midline incision is made through the anterior vaginal wall from 1 cm proximal to the urethral meatus to 3 to 4 cm cephalad to the vesical neck. The vaginal edges are grasped with Allis forceps, and the anterior vaginal wall is separated from the bladder base and the urethra. This maneuver allows visualization of the bladder neck and easy palpation of the Foley balloon. The vesical neck is then plicated with mattress sutures placed approximately 0.5 cm apart (Fig. 14–6B). A second layer of sutures is placed over the first row to relieve tension on the sutures at the vesical neck. This layer generally extends over the urethra and bladder base.

The catheter is withdrawn and the bladder is re-examined cystoscopically (Fig. 14–6C). The bladder neck will be narrowed and somewhat elevated, taking on the appearance of an iris diaphragm. Additional layers of plicating sutures may be necessary to narrow the vesi-

Figure 14–6. *A,* Kelly technique of transvaginal plication. Incompetent bladder neck fails to close and remains patulous on withdrawal of urethroscope. *B,* Vesical neck is plicated with mattress sutures placed approximately 0.5 cm apart. *C,* Cystoscopic examination of vesical neck after transvaginal plication demonstrates bladder neck to be narrowed and somewhat elevated, taking on the appearance of iris diaphragm. *D,* Additional layers of plicating sutures produce narrowing of vesical neck. (Redrawn from King LR, Wendel RM: A new application for transvaginal plication in the treatment of girls with total urinary incontinence due to epispadias or hypospadias. J Urol *102:* 778–782, 1969. © 1969, The Williams & Wilkins Company, Baltimore).

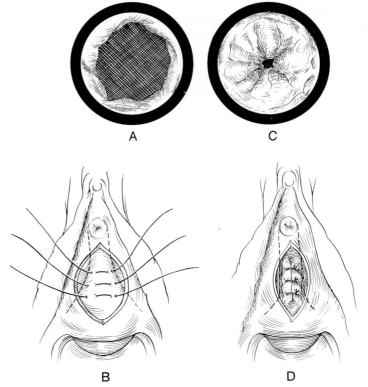

A   C

B   D

cal neck to a normal configuration (Fig. 14–6D). It is important to remove any sutures that have penetrated the bladder mucosa. When the bladder neck is competent, a Foley catheter is reinserted and the vagina is closed with running absorbable sutures. The vagina is packed with iodoform gauze, which is left in place for 2 days. The catheter is removed in 5 to 7 days.

In children in whom plication fails to establish good urinary control, tubularization of the anterior or posterior bladder wall or placement of prosthetic devices can be readily accomplished. Transvaginal plication does not violate the suprapubic tissue planes, and thus the results of subsequent surgery do not appear adversely affected.

Vesical Neck Reconstruction. In 1907, Young described the basic operative technique for reconstruction of the vesical neck for treatment of urinary incontinence. Dees introduced the modification of bilateral triangular reduction of the vesical neck and prostate in the male and the vesical neck and urethra in the female. Thompson described an operation to narrow and elongate the prostatic urethra. Leadbetter further modified the Young-Dees operation by demonstrating that proximal reimplantation of the ureters would allow more generous resection and reconstruction in the trigonal region and thereby enhance surgical success.

Initial surgical intervention should be deferred until the child is at least 3 years of age. This delay makes surgical repair technically easier and affords a greater chance of achieving a satisfactory result. Furthermore, deferring surgery until age 3 allows children to accept instruction in toilet training, which is essential to attaining a satisfactory repair. A well-developed bladder with good capacity and musculature appears to be a prerequisite for satisfactory continence after vesical neck reconstruction (Kramer and Kelalis, 1982a). In selected patients with small bladder capacities, the techniques of augmentation cystoplasty may be combined with vesical neck reconstruction to enhance the postoperative results further.

Young-Dees Procedure. The patient is placed in the supine position with the head of the operating table lowered slightly. A Pfannenstiel incision affords ready access to the perivesical space. The vesical neck and urethra are mobilized anteriorly and laterally. It is important not to mobilize the posterior aspect of the bladder base and urethra, in order to preserve the neurovascular supply to this area. The bladder is opened in the midline and the incision is extended distally into the urethra, almost to the triangular ligament. Parallel incisions are made 8 mm apart through each side of the floor of the posterior urethra. The new vesical outlet will lie midway between the verumontanum and interureteric ridge in the male and as close to the interureteric ridge as possible in the female. A triangular segment of bladder wall and trigone is excised from each side of the urethra and vesical neck. The bladder wall on each side of the central strip of mucous membrane is denuded of its mucosa (Fig. 14–7A). The urethra is constructed in two layers over a 10 or 12 F Silastic tube, which may serve as either a draining stent or a splint (Fig. 14–7B).

In boys undergoing vesical neck reconstruction, the prostatic urethra affords additional substance for closure and can further increase bladder outlet resistance. A wedge is taken from the anterior surface of the prostate; as much glandular tissue is preserved as possible (Fig. 14–7C). The neourethra is tubularized over a 10 or 12 F Silastic tube as described above.

Leadbetter Modification. The perivesical space is developed and the bladder is opened vertically as described above. Proximal reimplantation of the ureters allows more extensive tubularization of the trigone in reconstructing the bladder neck. Ureteroneocystostomy can be performed by a variety of techniques, but it usually requires combined transvesical and extravesical dissection. After ureteral reimplantation, incisions are started on the proximal urethra and extended longitudinally and posteriorly through the base of the bladder (Fig. 14–8A). Bilateral triangular flaps are made on each side of the urethra and bladder wall (Fig. 14–8B). The newly formed posterior strip of bladder should be approximately 4 to 5 cm in length and 1.5 to 2 cm in width. The mucosa on either side of the bladder wall is excised except for a central strip of mucous membrane. The neourethra is reconstructed in three layers over a 10 or 12 F Silastic tube (Fig. 14–8C). The mucosa is closed with interrupted absorbable sutures of chromic catgut or Vicryl, and the musculature is closed in an overlapping fashion.

The triangular flaps, or "dog ears," that remain after tubularization of the neourethra should be preserved to ensure adequate bladder capacity (Fig. 14–8D). The bladder is closed in two layers with interrupted absorb-

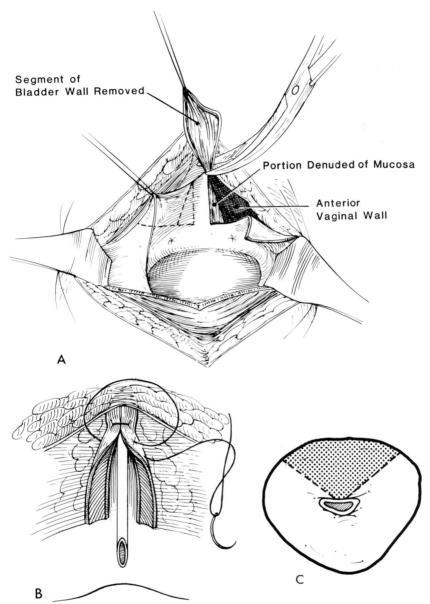

Segment of
Bladder Wall Removed

Portion Denuded of Mucosa

Anterior
Vaginal Wall

A

B

C

Figure 14-7. Young-Dees Technique. *A*, Triangular segment of bladder wall and trigone is excised from each side of the urethra and vesical neck. The bladder wall on each side of the central strip of mucous membrane is denuded of its mucosa. *B*, The urethra is constructed in two layers over a 10 or 12 French Silastic tube. *C*, Cross section of prostate shows preservation of most of lateral prostatic lobes by oblique incisions.

able sutures and a suprapubic cystostomy is brought out through the bladder dome (Fig. 14–8*E*). The urethral stent is removed in 10 to 14 days, at which time the suprapubic tube is clamped for a voiding trial. In children with urinary retention or elevated residual urines, cystostomy drainage may be maintained temporarily or the patient may be started on intermittent self-catheterization.

Postoperative Course. Complete urinary continence after vesical neck reconstruction has been established in approximately 60 to 70 per cent of males and 80 per cent of females (Kramer and Kelalis, 1982b). Urinary control may be delayed for several months postoperatively. Interestingly, urinary retention in the immediate postoperative period has often been associated with improved con-

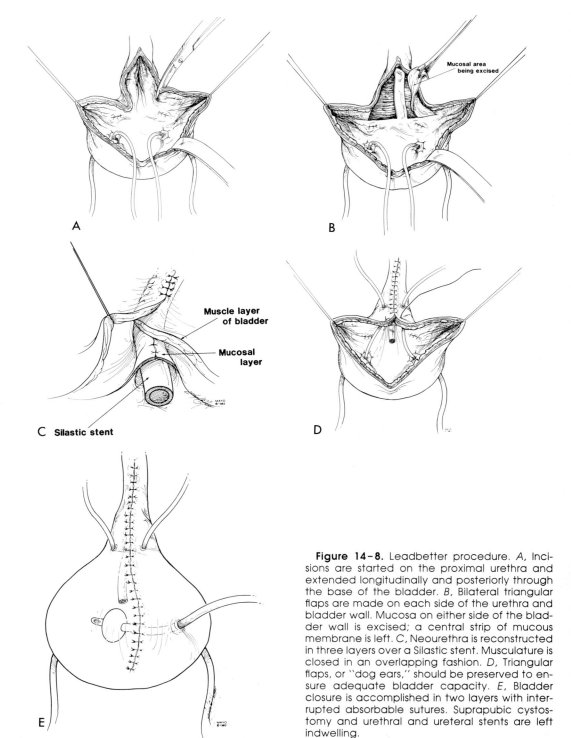

Figure 14–8. Leadbetter procedure. *A,* Incisions are started on the proximal urethra and extended longitudinally and posteriorly through the base of the bladder. *B,* Bilateral triangular flaps are made on each side of the urethra and bladder wall. Mucosa on either side of the bladder wall is excised; a central strip of mucous membrane is left. *C,* Neourethra is reconstructed in three layers over a Silastic stent. Musculature is closed in an overlapping fashion. *D,* Triangular flaps, or "dog ears," should be preserved to ensure adequate bladder capacity. *E,* Bladder closure is accomplished in two layers with interrupted absorbable sutures. Suprapubic cystostomy and urethral and ureteral stents are left indwelling.

tinence subsequent to resolution of the retention (Kramer and Kelalis, 1982a). Improved control in this group of patients appears to be related to an increased bladder capacity and enhanced detrusor function. A few patients may require intermittent self-catheterization temporarily until detrusor function develops. In males in whom continence is improved but is not complete, prostatic maturation at puberty will add additional outlet resistance and may result in complete urinary control in a significant number of children.

Electrical Stimulation of External Sphincter. Electrical stimulation of the striated muscles of the pelvic floor has been used as a method of increasing resistance at the distal mechanism (Caldwell et al, Hopkinson and Lightwood; Edwards and Malvern; Merrill et al; Wheatley et al). Successful results have been reported in children with congenital anomalies of the bladder neck (for example, epispadias) and in patients with iatrogenic incontinence due to transurethral resection of the bladder neck. Unfortunately, problems with wound infection or apparatus failure have been troublesome. Furthermore, it is difficult to achieve optimal positioning of the electrodes, and thus selective sphincter stimulation is often not achieved. These devices may have some value in providing short-term urinary continence; however, it is unlikely that this procedure will replace conventional forms of reconstructive therapy.

Urethral Compression. In 1961, Berry introduced the use of a plastic prosthesis inserted into the perineum to effect continence by pressure on the proximal bulbous urethra. A variety of procedures that provide urethral compression have been described subsequently.

In 1970, Kaufman described a technique in which the ischiocavernosus muscles were detached and crossed to provide urethral compression. This procedure was modified (Kaufman II) by bringing the crura together in the midline and inserting a propylene mesh beneath them (Kaufman, 1972). In 1973, Kaufman developed a silicone gel prosthesis, which is affixed to the crura of the corpora cavernosa. The advantage of this prosthesis is that its size, shape, and consistency can be altered by postoperative percutaneous injections. Although Kaufman and others have reported successful results in 60 to 80 per cent of adults, these procedures provide only passive resistance to the flow of urine and thus do

not act as true urinary sphincters. Furthermore, infections and urethral erosions are not infrequent. There appears to be limited indication for these devices in the treatment of childhood urinary incontinence.

Periurethral Injection of Teflon. In 1964, Politano applied a technique to increase resistance to the outflow of urine by injection of a Teflon paste into the periurethral tissues (Lim et al; Politano, 1978, 1982; Politano et al). Teflon adds bulk to the tissues and stimulates an ingrowth of fibroblasts among the small Teflon particles. In Europe, this technique has recently been applied for the correction of vesicoureteral reflux (Matouschek).

Females are placed in the lithotomy position, and cystourethroscopy is performed. A 17-gauge 4-inch needle is attached to a Lewy syringe, which is inserted at the urethral meatus and advanced periurethrally. Approximately 12 to 15 ml of the Teflon paste is injected at 1 o'clock, 4 o'clock, 7 o'clock, and 11 o'clock positions around the bladder neck and along the total length of the urethra. Injection is performed with a finger in the vagina to ensure that there is no intravaginal leakage of Teflon. The urethra is then reinspected with a panendoscope to verify that the needle has not perforated the bladder or urethra.

In males, preliminary panendoscopy is similarly performed. A 17-gauge needle with attached tubing is inserted through a modified Storz or Wolf panendoscope. The needle is inserted into the urethral mucosa just proximal to the external sphincter. Twelve to 15 ml of Teflon paste is injected circumferentially around the external sphincter. The exact sites of injection can be monitored through the panendoscope, and the blebs produced by the polytef are clearly visualized. Patients are given broad-spectrum antibiotics for approximately 1 week postoperatively. Indwelling catheters have not been used routinely; however, intermittent catheterization may be necessary in selected patients who are unable to void postoperatively.

Periurethral Teflon injections have been applied to both male and female children with urinary incontinence, including patients with epispadias, neuropathic bladder, ectopic ureter, and patulous urethra. Complications have been minimal, and good to excellent results have been obtained in approximately 80 per cent of cases. It is noteworthy, however, that approximately two thirds of patients will require a second injection of Teflon 6 months after the initial procedure to achieve complete urinary control. It appears advisable to wait 4 to 6 months before repeating injections because some patients will acquire continence during this interval. The use of polytef paste does not appear to exclude subsequent open surgical procedures such as vesical neck reconstruction or placement of a genitourinary sphincter.

Although the urologic use of Teflon paste has been widespread, recent data from animal experiments demonstrated migration of small Teflon particles beyond the injection site. Malizia et al showed that periurethral injections of Teflon paste were associated with distant migration of Teflon particles to pelvic lymph nodes, lungs, kidneys, and brains of laboratory animals. These injections have also been noted to cause foreign body granuloma reactions in host animals. Histologic analysis in short-term animal experiments (10 to 70 days) revealed particle migration to the pelvic lymph nodes in six of seven animals and to the lungs in four of seven animals. In long-term animal experiments ($10\frac{1}{2}$ months), particles were found in pelvic nodes, lungs, and brains in seven of seven animals; in the kidneys in four of seven; and in the spleens in two of seven. The migrating particles ranged in size from 4 to 80 μm. Particle diameter in currently marketed polytef paste ranges from 4 to 100 μm. These findings raise concern about the use of Teflon paste in children and young adults until more information is gained about migration and the long-term tissue reaction to this material. At the date of this writing, the Food and Drug Administration had not approved Teflon paste for urologic use.

Techniques to Improve Bladder Emptying

INCREASE BLADDER CONTRACTILITY. In patients with hypotonic, areflexic bladders as a result of decreased contractility, *electrical stimulation* directly to the bladder itself (Bradley et al, 1963; Boyce et al; Hald et al) or via direct stimulation to the spinal cord (Grimes et al, 1973, 1975) has been attempted. Unfortunately, the increase in intravesical pressure is not coordinated with bladder neck opening or relaxation of the pelvic floor, and thus concomitant measures to decrease resistance at the bladder neck or distal mechanism levels may also be required. The

application of these techniques has been met with little enthusiasm and only partial success, and they are rarely indicated for childhood urinary incontinence.

DECREASE OUTLET RESISTANCE. Historically, *transurethral resection of the vesical neck* was performed in children with presumed "vesical neck contracture." The rarity of this entity has now been well established. A diagnosis of congenital vesical neck contracture must be supported by accurate urodynamic evaluation. There must be anatomic or functional obstruction at the level of the bladder neck and proximal urethra that prevents bladder emptying even with sustained detrusor contraction. In children with bladder hypotonicity as a result of neuropathic vesical dysfunction, transurethral resection of the vesical neck has been performed in an attempt to improve bladder emptying. It would appear that most of these children can be managed with nonoperative therapy, such as intermittent self-catheterization and pharmacologic manipulation; this would eliminate the risk of iatrogenic total urinary incontinence from inappropriate surgical intervention. This procedure may have a limited indication in boys with acquired vesical neck contracture due to traumatic or iatrogenic causes. Transurethral resection of the vesical neck should not be performed in females, because of the increased risk of total urinary incontinence postoperatively.

There are limited indications for *Y-V plasty* in children; this procedure has often resulted in total urinary incontinence. In selected patients, Y-V plasty of the bladder neck has been used to convert a hypotonic, poorly emptying bladder into one with essentially no outlet resistance. An artificial genitourinary sphincter may then be placed to achieve urinary continence and control of micturition, as described in the other article in this chapter.

Patients with congenital or acquired urethral strictures may acquire increased residual urine and overflow incontinence. In these patients, direct-vision *internal urethrotomy* has proved extremely useful. In selected patients with prune-belly syndrome, transurethral incision of the external sphincter has been used successfully to lower urethral resistance and decrease residual urine (Snyder et al). In patients with detrusor sphincter dyssynergia and increased residual urine, *external sphincterotomy* has improved bladder emptying in approximately 70 to 90 per cent of cases (Koontz et al; Schellhammer et al). This is most often seen in children with traumatic injury to the suprasacral spinal cord or injury from neurologic disease such as multiple sclerosis. Recent data indicate that a single deep incision through the skeletal muscle at the 12 o'clock position minimizes both postoperative hemorrhage and impotence and is sufficient to decrease outflow resistance. The incision is performed with either a Collin knife or the resectoscope loop.

Relief of functional obstruction at the level of the striated external sphincter can also be achieved by *pudendal neurectomy* (Stark; Mulholland et al). Lidocaine (Xylocaine), 1 per cent, is injected into the area of the pudendal nerve medial to the ischial tuberosity. Objective methods of assessing the effectiveness of the pudendal block include (1) urethral pressure profilometry before and after injection of the pudendal nerve and (2) studying the voiding pattern under fluoroscopy before and after the injection (Raz et al). A reduction in external sphincter pressure associated with a concomitant rise in urinary flow would indicate that permanent pudendal block should decrease outflow resistance and thereby improve bladder emptying. Permanent pudendal block may be accomplished with phenol or alcohol or by pudendal neurectomy. Unilateral pudendal nerve interruption is recommended over bilateral pudendal neurectomy, since the latter procedure may be associated with impotence and fecal incontinence (Engel and Schirmer). The advent of effective transurethral external sphincterotomy has essentially eliminated the use of pudendal neurectomy.

Urinary Diversion

In selected patients, urinary diversion may be the only surgical option available. These techniques are thoroughly reviewed in Chapter 17.

BIBLIOGRAPHY

Aldridge AH: Transplantation of fascia for relief of urinary stress incontinence. Am J Obstet Gynecol 44:398, 1942.

Andersen JT: Detrusor hyperreflexia in benign infravesical obstruction: a cystometric study. J Urol 115:532, 1976.

Arap S, Martins Giron A, Menezes de Góes G: Initial results of the complete reconstruction of bladder exstrophy. Urol Clin North Am 7:477, 1980.

Barnes RW, Wilson WM: Reconstruction of the urethra with a tube from bladder flap. Urol Cutan Rev 53:604, 1949.

Barrett DM: Pharmacologic management of lower urinary tract emptying failure. *In* Pharmacology of the Urinary Tract and the Male Reproductive System. Edited by AE Finkbeiner, GL Barbour, NK Bissada. New York, Appleton-Century-Crofts, 1982, pp. 217–235.

Benson GS, Jacobowitz D, Raezer DM, et al: Adrenergic innervation and stimulation of canine urethra. Urology 7:337, 1976a.

Benson GS, McConnell JA, Wood JG: Adrenergic innervation of the human bladder body. J Urol 122:189, 1979.

Benson GS, Wein AJ, Raezer DM, et al: Adrenergic and cholinergic stimulation and blockade of the human bladder base. J Urol 116:174, 1976b.

Berry JL: A new procedure for correction of urinary incontinence: preliminary report. J Urol 85:771, 1961.

Bissada NK, Finkbeiner AE: Neuropharmacology of the lower urinary tract. *In* Pharmacology of the Urinary Tract and the Male Reproductive System. Edited by AE Finkbeiner, GL Barbour, NK Bissada. New York, Appleton-Century-Crofts, 1982, pp 199–216.

Blomfield JM, Douglas JWB: Bedwetting: prevalence among children aged 4–7 years. Lancet 1:850, 1956.

Boyce WH, Lathem JE, Hunt LD: Research related to the development of an artificial electrical stimulator for the paralyzed human bladder: a review. J Urol 91:41, 1964.

Bradley WE, Chou SN, French LA: Further experience with the radio transmitter receiver unit for the neurogenic bladder. J Neurosurg 20:953, 1963.

Bradley WE, Timm GW, Scott FB: Innervation of the detrusor muscle and urethra. Urol Clin North Am 1:3, 1974.

Bradley WE, Timm GW, Scott FB: Cystometry. II. Central nervous system organization of detrusor reflex. Urology 5:578, 1975.

Burch JC: Urethrovaginal fixation to Cooper's ligament for correction of stress incontinence, cystocele, and prolapse. Am J Obstet Gynecol 81:281, 1961.

Caldwell KPS, Flack FC, Broad AF: Urinary incontinence following spinal injury treated by electronic implant. Lancet 1:846, 1965.

Dees JE: Congenital epispadias with incontinence. J Urol 62:513, 1949.

Edwards L, Malvern J: Electronic control of incontinence: a critical review of the present situation. Br J Urol 44:467, 1972.

Elbadawi A, Schenk EA: A new theory of the innervation of bladder musculature. Part 1. Morphology of the intrinsic vesical innervation apparatus. J Urol 99:585, 1968.

Elbadawi A, Schenk EA: A new theory of the innervation of bladder musculature. Part 2. The innervation apparatus of the ureterovesical junction. J Urol 105:368, 1971.

Engel RME, Schirmer HKA: Pudendal neurectomy in neurogenic bladder. J Urol 112:57, 1974.

Flocks RH, Boldus R: The surgical treatment and prevention of urinary incontinence associated with disturbance of the internal urethral sphincteric mechanism. J Urol 109:279, 1973.

Ganong WF: Review of Medical Physiology. Eighth ed. Los Altos, Cal., Lange Medical Publications, 1977, pp 32–37.

Gierup HJW, Hakelius L: Further experience of free muscle transplantation in children with urinary incontinence. Br J Urol 55:211, 1983.

Glahn BE: Giggle incontinence (enuresis risoria): a study and an aetiological hypothesis. Br J Urol 51:363, 1979.

Grimes JH, Nashold BS, Anderson EE: Clinical application of electronic bladder stimulation in paraplegics. J Urol 113:338, 1975.

Grimes JH, Nashold BS, Currie DP: Chronic electrical stimulation of the paraplegic bladder. J Urol 109:242, 1973.

Hald T, Meier W, Khalili A, et al: Clinical experience with a radio-linked bladder stimulator. J Urol 97:73, 1967.

Hebjørn S, Andersen JT, Walter S, et al: Detrusor hyperreflexia: a survey on its etiology and treatment. Scand J Urol Nephrol 10:103, 1976.

Hopkinson BR, Lightwood R: Electrical treatment of incontinence. Br J Surg 54:802, 1967.

Jensen D: The Principles of Physiology. New York, Appleton-Century-Crofts, 1976, pp 113–155.

Kaufman JJ: A new operation for male incontinence. Surg Gynecol Obstet 131:295, 1970.

Kaufman JJ: Surgical treatment of post-prostatectomy incontinence: use of the penile crura to compress the bulbous urethra. J Urol 107:293, 1972.

Kaufman JJ: Urethral compression operations for the treatment of post-prostatectomy incontinence. J Urol 110:93, 1973.

Kaufman JJ: History of surgical correction of male urinary incontinence. Urol Clin North Am 5:265, 1978.

Kelly HA: Incontinence of urine in women. Urol Cutan Rev 17:291, 1913.

Khanna OP: Disorders of micturition: neuropharmacologic basis and results of drug therapy. Urology 8:316, 1976.

King LR, Wendel RM: A new application for transvaginal plication in the treatment of girls with total urinary incontinence due to epispadias or hypospadias. J Urol 102:778, 1969.

Klackenberg G: Primary enuresis: when is a child dry at night? Acta Paediatr Scand 44:513, 1955.

Koontz WW Jr, Smith MJV, Currie RJ: External sphincterotomy in boys with meningomyelocele. J Urol 108:649, 1972.

Kramer SA, Kelalis PP: Assessment of urinary continence in epispadias: review of 94 patients. J Urol 128:290, 1982a.

Kramer SA, Kelalis PP: Surgical correction of female epispadias. Eur Urol 8:321, 1982b.

Leadbetter GW Jr: Surgical correction of total urinary incontinence. J Urol 91:261, 1964.

Lim KB, Ball AJ, Feneley RCL: Periurethral Teflon injection: a simple treatment for urinary incontinence. Br J Urol 55:208, 1983.

Mahony DT, Laferte RO, Blais DJ: Integral storage and voiding reflexes: neurophysiologic concept of continence and micturition. Urology 9:95, 1977.

Malizia AA Jr, Reiman HM, Myers RP, et al: Polytef (Teflon) injected periurethrally: migration and granulomatous reaction. JAMA, in press.

Marshall VF: Suprapubic vesicourethral suspension for stress incontinence (Marshall-Marchetti-Krantz). In Campbell's Urology. Vol 3. Fourth ed. Edited by JH Harrison, RF Gittes, AD Perlmutter, et al. Philadelphia, WB Saunders Co., 1979, pp 2294–2298.

Marshall VF, Marchetti AA, Krantz KE: The correction of stress incontinence by simple vesicourethral suspension. Surg Gynecol Obstet 88:509, 1949.

Mathisen W: A new operation for urinary incontinence. Surg Gynecol Obstet 130:606, 1970.

Matouschek E: Die Behandlung des vesikorenalen Refluxes durch transurethrale Einspritzung von Teflonpaste. Urologe [Ausg A] 20:263, 1981.

Merrill DC, Conway C, DeWolf W: Urinary incontinence: treatment with electrical stimulation of the pelvic floor. Urology 5:67, 1975.

Michalowski E, Modelski W.: The replacement of the urethral musculature by detrusor flap: contribution to the operative treatment of incontinence. J Urol 107:791, 1972.

Misak SJ, Bunts RC, Ulmer JL, et al: Nerve interruption procedures in the urologic management of paraplegic patients. J Urol 88:392, 1962.

Mulholland SG, Yalla SV, Raezer DM, et al: Primary external urethral sphincter hyperkinesia in a boy. Urology 4:577, 1974.

Pereyra AJ: A simplified surgical procedure for the correction of stress incontinence in women. West J Surg Obstet Gynecol 67:223, 1959.

Politano VA: Periurethral Teflon injection for urinary incontinence. Urol Clin North Am 5:415, 1978.

Politano VA: Periurethral polytetrafluoroethylene injection for urinary incontinence. J Urol 127:439, 1982.

Politano VA, Small MP, Harper JM, et al: Periurethral Teflon injection for urinary incontinence. J Urol 111:180, 1974.

Raezer DM, Benson GS, Wein AJ, et al: The functional approach to the management of the pediatric neuropathic bladder: a clinical study. J Urol 117:649, 1977.

Raezer DM, Wein AJ, Jacobowitz D, et al: Autonomic innervation of canine urinary bladder: cholinergic and adrenergic contributions and interaction of sympathetic and parasympathetic nervous systems in bladder function. Urology 2:211, 1973.

Raz S, Magora F, Caine M: The evaluation of pudendal nerve block by measurements of urethral pressure. Surg Gynecol Obstet 133:453, 1971.

Rogers MP, Gittes RF, Dawson DM, et al: Giggle incontinence. JAMA 247:1446, 1982.

Schellhammer PF, Hackler RH, Bunts RC: External sphincterotomy: an evaluation of 150 patients with neurogenic bladder. J Urol 110:199, 1973.

Snyder HM, Harris NW, Whitfield HN, et al: Urodynamics in the prune belly syndrome. Br J Urol 48:663, 1976.

Stamey TA: Endoscopic suspension of the vesical neck for urinary incontinence. Surg Gynecol Obstet 136:547, 1973.

Stamey TA, Schaeffer AJ, Condy M: Clinical and roentgenographic evaluation of endoscopic suspension of the vesical neck for urinary incontinence. Surg Gynecol Obstet 140:355, 1975.

Stark G: Pudendal neurectomy in management of neurogenic bladder in myelomeningocele. Arch Dis Child 44:698, 1969.

Sundin T, Dahlström A, Norlén L, et al: The sympathetic innervation and adrenoreceptor function of the human lower urinary tract in the normal state and after parasympathetic denervation. Invest Urol 14:322, 1977.

Taira N: The autonomic pharmacology of the bladder. Annu Rev Pharmacol 12:197, 1972.

Tanagho EA: Bladder neck reconstruction for total urinary incontinence: 10 years of experience. J Urol 125:321, 1981.

Tanagho EA: Anatomy and physiology of the lower urinary tract. In Pharmacology of the Urinary Tract and the Male Reproductive System. Edited by AE Finkbeiner, GL Barbour, NK Bissada. New York, Appleton-Century-Crofts, 1982, pp 175–197.

Tanagho EA, Smith DR, Meyers FH, et al: Mechanisms of urinary continence. II. Technique for surgical correction of incontinence. J Urol 101:305, 1969.

Thompson IM: Incontinence following prostatectomy. J Urol 86:130, 1961.

Torrens MJ, Griffith HB: The control of the uninhibited bladder by selective sacral neurectomy. Br J Urol 46:639, 1974.

Tulloch AGS: Sympathetic activity of internal urethral sphincter: in empty and partially filled bladder. Urology 5:353, 1975.

Turner-Warwick R: Observations on the function and dysfunction of the sphincter and detrusor mechanisms. Urol Clin North Am 6:13, 1979.

Vergés-Flaqué A: Flaqué-Lowsley operation for urinary incontinence: preliminary report. J Urol 65:427, 1951.

Wein A, Barrett DM: Etiologic possibilities for increased pelvic floor electromyography activity during cystometry. J Urol 127:949, 1982.

Wein AJ: Pharmacologic management of lower urinary tract storage failure. In Pharmacology of the Urinary Tract and the Male Reproductive System. Edited by AE Finkbeiner, GL Barbour, NK Bissada. New York, Appleton-Century-Crofts, 1982, pp 237–272.

Wein AJ, Raezer DM: Physiology of micturition. In Clinical Neuro-Urology. Edited by RJ Krane, MB Siroky. Boston, Little, Brown, 1979, pp 1–33.

Wein AJ, Raezer DM, Benson GS: Management of neurogenic bladder dysfunction in the adult. Urology 8:432, 1976.

Wheatley JK, Woodard JR, Parrott TS: Electronic bladder stimulation in the management of children with myelomeningocele. J Urol 127:283, 1982.

Yalla SV, Blunt KJ, Fam BA, et al: Detrusor–urethral sphincter dyssynergia. J Urol 118:1026, 1977.

Yeates WK: Disorders of bladder function. Ann R Coll Surg Engl 50:335, 1972.

Young HH: Suture of the urethral and vesical sphincters for the cure of incontinence of urine, with a report of a case. Trans South Surg Gynecol Assoc 20:210, 1907.

Artificial Urinary Sphincter in Children

DAVID M. BARRETT AND WILLIAM L. FURLOW

Although many incontinent children have improved urinary control through the use of clean intermittent catheterization, bladder training techniques, and pharmacologic manipulation of the detrusor and sphincter muscles, there remains a group of children with persistent, significant urinary incontinence. Conventional surgical techniques may help many of these children; however, others should be considered for some type of proximal urinary diversion. The social pressures of wetness, especially for the child entering school, can be devastating. Eventually, significant alterations in social behavior render the patient irreparably scarred psychologically. This reality, along with the need to avoid urinary diversion, has given impetus for the use of a totally implantable artificial urinary sphincter (Barrett and Furlow, 1982).

Not until the introduction of the AS 721 artificial sphincter by Scott et al in 1973, which allowed for the placement of an inflatable cuff around the bladder neck, was there an implantable sphincter that could be used in both male and female children. During the last 10 years, various design changes in the sphincter mechanism have evolved. However, the basic concept of an inflatable cuff used to create circumferential compression at the bladder neck has persisted (Artificial Urinary Sphincter Investigational Study Group; Furlow, 1980).

MECHANICAL DESIGN

The currently used device is the AS 791/792 artificial urinary sphincter (Fig. 14–9).* This ingenious design concept, made of a silicone elastomer and stainless steel, employs an elastic balloon reservoir that regulates the fluid pressure within the system. The pressure within the system is established by the manufacturer so that a constant pressure is produced when a given volume of fluid is

---

* American Medical Systems, 11001 Bren Road, Minnetonka, MN 55343.

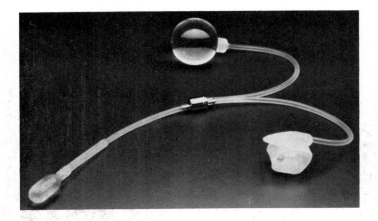

Figure 14–9. AS 792 artificial urinary sphincter with inflatable snap-on cuff, pressure balloon reservoir, deflate pump, and stainless steel control assembly.

inserted (Fig. 14–10). The amount of pressure in the system is of critical concern, as theoretically enough pressure must be transferred from the inflatable cuff to the bladder neck to produce continence, but not so much pressure that the underlying tissue develops ischemic necrosis and cuff erosion ensues. This particular point has been the nemesis of most sphincter design concepts. However, the AS 791/792 mechanism appears to have established the optimal balance of pressures, with available balloon pressures ranging between 41 to 50 cm and 81 to 90 cm of water.

The inflatable cuff can be snapped on, which has obviated the need for cumbersome sutures. The outer backing allows for inward expansion only and, thus, much more uniform transfer of pressures to the area of the bladder neck. The single deflate pump has a

volume of approximately 1 ml and is used to propel fluid out of the cuff into the pressure balloon reservoir when the patient desires to void. This fluid transfer is directed and regulated by a control assembly of stainless steel to which all sphincter components are attached (Fig. 14–11). When the pump is compressed, fluid passes from the cuff into the pressure balloon reservoir through a series of unidirectional check valves. The intrinsic pressure within the balloon automatically directs the fluid back into the cuff. However, the rate of cuff filling is regulated by a flow resistor between the balloon and the cuff (Fig. 14–12). The time required for cuff repressurization is 2 to 5 minutes, depending on cuff size.

There are numerous advantages and one distinct disadvantage with the AS 791/792 design. Its advantages include (1) constant,

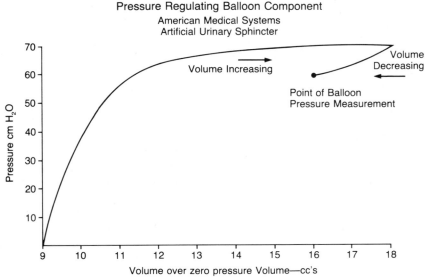

Figure 14–10. Pressure-volume curve for 60 to 70 cm H$_2$O.

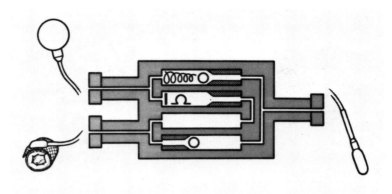

Figure 14–11. AS 791/792 control assembly design, which directs fluid through the system and provides for delayed refilling of the cuff.

predetermined pressure within the system, (2) simple one-pump operation, (3) dip-coated construction to prevent leaks, (4) a "snap-on" cuff, (5) a control assembly with only three tubing connections, and (6) multiple cuff sizes and balloon pressures from which to select. The main disadvantage is the constant pressure within the system and on the bladder neck or urethra immediately after implantation, with no built-in mechanism for deactivation.

PATIENT SELECTION

All children selected for implantation of an artificial sphincter should first be treated with the more conservative methods of managing incontinence. Selected surgical procedures also may be attempted, with care taken to select the patient who has a reasonable opportunity to become dry by that surgery. For example, children with neurologic defects in-

volving the detrusor and bladder neck are unlikely to have an optimal result from a tubularization procedure. Conversely, a patient with exstrophy or epispadias may benefit from a Young-Dees-Leadbetter procedure and thus become dry by virtue of normal tissue. After all measures have been tried, including conventional reasonable surgical procedures, the child may be considered for an artificial sphincter in lieu of a proximal urinary diversion.

Criteria have been established to ensure optimal success and little risk to the upper urinary tract (Table 14–3). Patient and parent motivation is the initial factor that must be assessed. An overwhelming desire to be dry must be expressed by the child, with full acceptance of the mechanical nature of the sphincter mechanism. Both child and parent must be willing to accept the potential for mechanical failure and be fully aware that additional surgery may be necessary to make repairs. The child should be at least 5 or 6

Figure 14–12. Diagrams showing deflation (cuff open on left) and deflation (cuff closed on right).

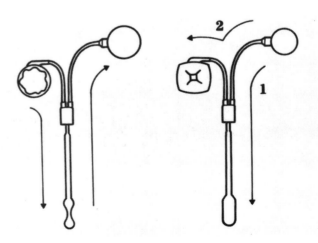

Table 14-3. Criteria for Patient Selection for Pediatric Artificial Sphincter

Motivated, cooperative patient, at least 5 years of age

Sphincteric incontinence

Minimal residual urine by voiding or capability for intermittent self-catheterization

Absence of, or pharmacologically manageable, detrusor hyperreflexia

Absence of significant vesicoureteral reflux

Technical feasibility

Sterile urine

years of age, not only because of anatomic considerations but also because younger children rarely are sufficiently responsible to carry out regular sphincter operation.

A neurourologic evaluation is undertaken, including excretory urography, voiding cystourethrography, endoscopy, and urodynamic study. All tests are designed to define adequately the type of incontinence and the status of the upper urinary tract. Ultimately, some children will be deemed unsuitable for implantation of the artificial sphincter and others will need to undergo surgical procedures that will make them more suitable candidates. For instance, significant vesicoureteral reflux (grades II to V) should be corrected before implantation. Similarly, the management of bladder neck or urethral strictures, urolithiasis, undescended testis, and hernias should be undertaken.

It is also tempting to try to convert patients who have excessive residual volumes to more ideal candidates by rendering them totally incontinent surgically. In general, this option is not recommended, and instead nothing should be done that would make the child clinically worse in the event the artificial sphincter failed, thus leaving no alternative other than urinary diversion. Children with multiple previous bladder neck operations may not be candidates, as it is technically difficult to dissect through scar tissue between the bladder neck and the rectum or vagina.

TECHNICAL CONSIDERATIONS

The numerical designations AS 791 and AS 792 refer mainly to the location of the inflatable cuff. AS 792 is used in bladder neck cuff placement, and the AS 791 is placed around the male bulbous urethra (Scott).

In all prepubertal males and all females, the inflatable cuff is implanted around the bladder neck (AS 792). The urethra of the prepubertal male may be easier to dissect than the bladder neck. However, the small diameter of the urethra makes it unsuitable for cuff placement. The urethra of the male child is also extremely thin and is relatively poorly vascularized, making failure due to cuff erosion or stricture formation more likely. Placement of the bladder neck cuff has the advantage of creating continence resistance in its normal location, where there is abundant tissue under the cuff, making injury less likely if catheterization or instrumentation becomes necessary.

Of concern also is the sexual function of the patient, and ejaculation is probably not impaired with the cuff at the bladder neck.

Great care is taken to prevent infection. Antibiotics, usually cephalosporins, are administered preoperatively and are designed to provide prophylaxis against infection of the wound and around the prosthesis. Children with urinary bacilluria have antibiotics administered commensurate with sensitivity studies well in advance of the date of implantation. At surgery, a liberal 10-minute iodophor preparation is used, which includes the perineum and external genitalia. The vagina is also prepared so that the surgeon may introduce the examining hand or instruments to facilitate pelvic dissection. Unnecessary traffic in the operating theater is discouraged, and all operating room personnel wear hats or hoods designed to cover exposed hair.

The child is placed on the operating table in the supine position with the legs slightly apart. Draping is done so that easy intraoperative access may be gained to the urethral area without contamination. A rectal tube is inserted and draped out of the operative area. Any anterior abdominal incision designed to provide easy access to the retropubic space may be used, but there is no need to open the peritoneal cavity. With blunt instruments, the plane of cleavage between the lateral aspect of the bladder neck and the underlying rectum or vagina is defined. The endopelvic fascia need not be opened. However, this dissection should begin distal to the trigone area (Fig. 14-13).

In patients who have had previous retropubic, vaginal, or bladder neck trauma or surgery, such dissection may be difficult, if not impossible. Urethral catheters, rectal tubes, and vaginal packs will make the identification of tissue planes much easier, but it may be necessary to open the bladder to define the plane of dissection more adequately.

After dissection of the bladder neck, a cuff

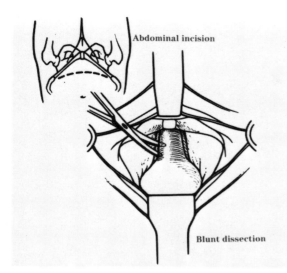

Figure 14–13. Diagram showing abdominal incision (*inset*) and blunt dissection for preparation of artificial urinary sphincter procedure.

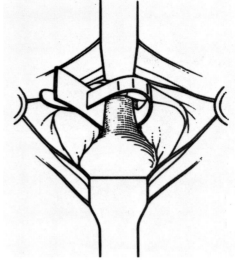

Figure 14–14. Diagram showing measurement of bladder neck.

sizer is used to measure the outer circumference (Fig. 14–14). The appropriate length of inflatable cuff is passed around the bladder neck and is snapped in place (Fig. 14–15). The deflate pump is placed in a subcutaneous tunnel created by a blunt instrument, such as

a Hegar dilator, down into the scrotum or labia majora.

The selection of pressure for the balloon reservoir is of concern because excessive pressure may lead to cuff erosion and inadequate pressure allows for persistent incontinence.

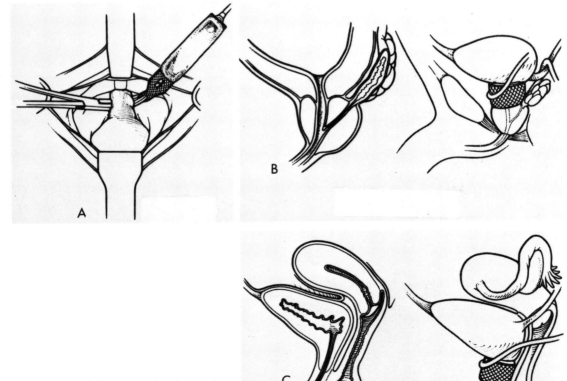

Figure 14–15. Diagrams showing positioning cuff (*A*) and sagittal view of cuff site (*B* and *C*).

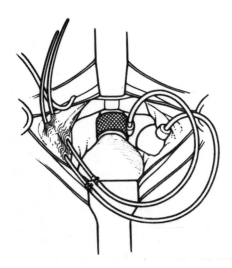

Figure 14–16. Diagram showing positioning of balloon and routing of component tubing.

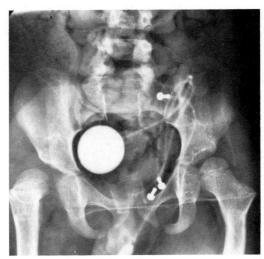

Figure 14–17. AS 792 urinary sphincter with primary deactivation in a 7-year-old boy with sphincteric incontinence as a result of meningomyelocele. Note that all components have been implanted, with the exception of the control assembly, and the tubings are occluded with stainless steel plugs.

Unfortunately, assessments of intraoperative urethral pressure or bladder neck pressure have not been helpful in this selection. Experience has shown that balloon pressures between 60 and 80 cm of water are best, and most frequently balloon pressures between 60 and 70 cm of water have been used (Scott et al, 1981). The balloon is placed in the prevesical space, and its tubing, along with the cuff tubing, is brought through the rectus muscle and fascia on the same side as the pump (Fig. 14–16).

The inherent design of this sphincter mechanism provides for constant pressure under the cuff after activation. The pressure applied to freshly operated bladder neck tissue may potentiate the risk of cuff erosion due to pressure necrosis. This is especially true of bladder necks that have previously been operated on or of bladder necks that have been injured or opened at the time of dissection. Thus, initial deactivation is recommended (Barrett and Furlow, 1981; Furlow, 1981). Deactivation is accomplished by filling all of the sphincter components with the recommended volume of contrast medium (11.7 per cent Cysto-Conray II), except the cuff, which is not inflated. Instead of insertion of the control assembly, each tube is occluded with a stainless steel plug (Fig. 14–17). The ends of the tubes are placed in the deep subcutaneous tissue, and the incision is closed (Fig. 14–18). After a healing period of 8 to 12 weeks, during which time revascularization under and around the cuff occurs, the patient returns and secondary

activation is done. The corner of the incision is opened and, using the electrocautery with the "cut" mode, each tube can be dissected free without injury. With the appropriate fluid volume in the balloon (16 to 18 ml), the cuff is pressurized and the control assembly is inserted (Fig. 14–19). An added benefit of the delayed activation concept is the lack of tenderness around the pump, which allows the child to begin deflating the cuff immediately without discomfort.

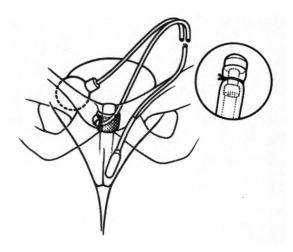

Figure 14–18. Diagram showing implanted device (primary deactivation).

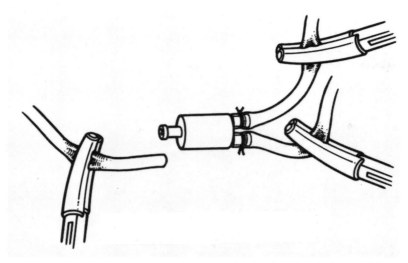

Figure 14–19. Diagram showing the connecting of the control assembly.

At activation, urethral pressure profiles may be used to confirm cuff function. However, the magnitude of urethral closing pressure has not generally been useful in predicting continence. Roentgenograms are taken on the operating table to substantiate device function during inflation and deflation (Fig. 14–20).

POSTOPERATIVE CARE

At the completion of the primary deactivation procedure, a small, closed system drain may be placed in the retropubic space. Not all patients require drainage, but in those whose bladder has been opened, drainage is recommended. The antibiotic prophylaxis is continued for 4 days and then is replaced with suppressive urinary tract medication for an additional 2 weeks.

The child and parents are advised to apply gentle, downward traction to the deflate pump three or four times daily during the next 2 weeks. This ensures a dependent location for the pump in the scrotum or labia. Hospitalization is usually 6 to 8 days for the initial implantation and 2 to 3 days for activation.

Because the patient's incontinence persists until secondary activation is done, external

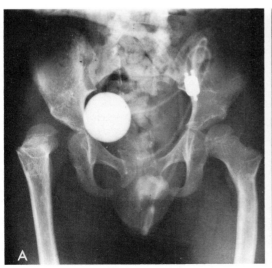
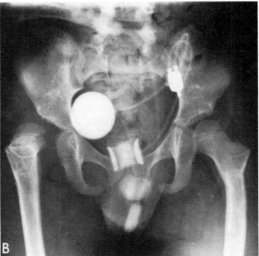

Figure 14–20. AS 792 urinary sphincter activation. *A*, Cuff deflated. *B*, Cuff inflated.

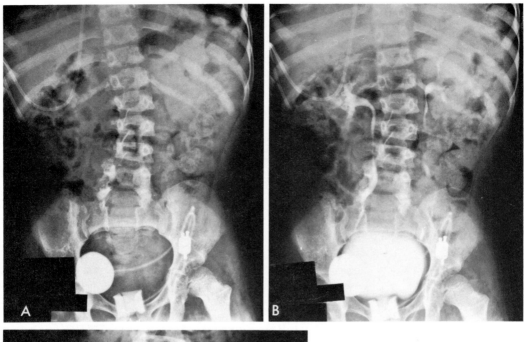

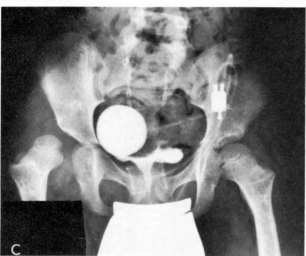

Figure 14–21. *A,* Kidney-ureter-bladder study showing activated AS 792 urinary sphincter. *B,* Excretory urogram showing location of AS 792 sphincter and confirming the status of the kidneys, ureters, and bladder. *C,* Excretory cystogram after voiding film, confirming minimal residual urine volume.

catheters or pads are advised, but permanent internal catheters should be avoided. If the child uses intermittent catheterization, this may be continued as before surgery.

When the child returns for secondary activation, a roentgenogram of the lower abdomen is taken to identify the location of the sphincter component. Sterile urine and antibiotic prophylaxis are required as before. A small Foley catheter is used after secondary activation and is removed when the child has recovered from general anesthesia. Pump deflation is undertaken initially every 3 hours, even with the catheter in place. After catheter removal, attempted voiding or intermit-

tent catheterization should continue every 3 hours, until the process of voiding becomes a reality to the patient. In children who are unable to empty completely and who require intermittent self-catheterization, the pump is compressed just before the catheter is inserted. Dryness will be complete in most patients. However, if the intravesical volume is excessive, overflow leaking may occur, thus signaling the need for intermittent catheterization. Excretory urography is recommended to be done approximately 3 months after activation. This time interval allows for evaluation of the upper tracts and confirms complete bladder emptying (Fig. 14–21).

COMPLICATIONS

There are three main possibilities for post-operative complications: infection, cuff erosion, and mechanical malfunction.

Infection of the sphincter components or wound has not been a major problem in more than 40 cases, with only one child developing a localized *Staphylococcus epidermidis* abscess around the deflate pump. The abscess was drained, and a new pump was inserted in the opposite hemiscrotum. Most infections, including infections related to all types of genitourinary prostheses, have involved *S. epidermidis* organisms. Although the prophylactic regimen is a broad-spectrum one, extreme care should be exercised in skin preparation and operating room sterility. If infection develops, the principles of incision and drainage are recommended. The sphincter may be salvaged if small, closed system drains are inserted into the infected area and are irrigated with antibiotic solutions during the healing period.

Throughout the evolution of the artificial urinary sphincter, the main cause for total failure has been erosion of the inflatable cuff into the lumen of the bladder neck or urethra (Bruskewitz et al). Such erosion becomes clinically evident if fever, lower abdominal pain, or unexplained incontinence develops. The diagnosis is established by retrograde urethrocystography and endoscopic inspection of the bladder neck. Unfortunately, the treatment for cuff erosion is removal of the cuff, intubation of the urethra and bladder neck with a silicone catheter, and retropubic drainage.

The main cause for erosion is ischemic necrosis from excessive pressure on the tissue under the cuff. Technical changes designed to eliminate erosion have been the use of delayed activation and lower pressures within the balloon reservoir.

Mechanical problems consist of leaks, tubing kinks, and dysfunction of the control assembly. Because of the simple design and dip-coated construction, these malfunctions have been very infrequent, with a reliability rate of 95 per cent during a 36-month period (Barrett and Furlow, 1983). Incontinence and failure of the pump to reinflate are clinical signs of potential mechanical problems. Confirmation is established by taking roentgenograms during inflation and deflation. Absence of the contrast medium within the device suggests the presence of a leak, while failure of the cuff to inflate or deflate implies the presence of a kink or control assembly problems.

Repair of a mechanical problem requires general anesthesia, antibiotic prophylaxis, and sterile urine. The incision is opened over the control assembly, and each component is tested for leaks or kinks and appropriately replaced. Dissection of the sphincter components is facilitated by using the electrocautery cutting instrument, as the silicone tubing will be preserved. In the event that a cuff leak is identified, a new cuff should be placed in the same sheath formed by the old. Whether or not to reactivate the sphincter mechanism at that time depends on the difficulty of dissection and the quality of tissue under the cuff.

FUTURE CONSIDERATIONS

We are encouraged by the short-term clinical results and the mechanical reliability of the AS 791/792 urinary sphincter. There remain several questions that will be answered only with the passage of time:

1. What effect will patient growth have on the sphincter, and will changes be required to compensate for an increase in body size?
2. Will the upper urinary tracts change?
3. Will sexual function be altered?
4. What degree of long-term mechanical reliability can be expected?
5. Can changes and repairs be made without complication?

As the reliability of the sphincter becomes established, there may be other applications for the device. Theoretically, nonrefluxing conduits could be attached to the urethra and the sphincter cuff placed around the distal end of the conduit, thus providing the patient with a continent bladder substitute. The sphincter cuff could be placed around the bladder neck at the time of an anti-incontinence tubularization procedure, with the cuff being available if the tubularization failed to produce continence. Another alternative would be the use of the sphincter mechanism with bladders made of synthetic materials.

The main deficiency with the earlier sphincter designs using the pressure balloon reservoir concept was the inability to deactivate and activate cuff pressurization without surgery. The new AS 800 sphincter incorporates the inflate-deflate pump and the control assembly into a single housing (Fig. 14–22). A small button on the side of the pump-control

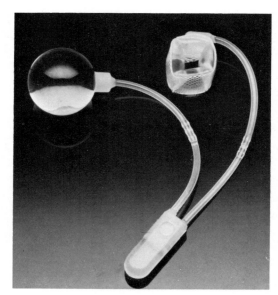

Figure 14–22. AS 800 urinary sphincter design, which provides an "on" and "off" button built into the control assembly mechanism located in the pump.

assembly allows for manual activation and deactivation of the device. We have now begun using this device exclusively and maintain the cuff in an unpressurized configuration for 6 to 8 weeks after implantation.

The versatility introduced by the AS 800 sphincter allows for (1) unhurried intermittent catheterization, (2) deactivation at night or during periods when incontinence is likely to be a problem, and (3) deactivation indefinitely if urinary tract status is in doubt or infection is suspected.

BIBLIOGRAPHY

Artificial Urinary Sphincter Investigational Study Group. Minneapolis, American Medical Systems, 1980.

Barrett DM, Furlow W: Implantation of a new semi-automatic artificial genitourinary sphincter: experience with patients utilizing a new concept of primary and secondary activation. Prog Clin Biol Res 78:375, 1981.

Barrett DM, Furlow WL: The management of severe urinary incontinence in patients with myelodysplasia by implantation of the AS 791/792 urinary sphincter device. J Urol 128:484, 1982.

Barrett DM, Furlow WL: Radical prostatectomy incontinence and the AS 791 artificial urinary sphincter. J Urol 129:528, 1983.

Bruskewitz R, Raz S, Smith RB, et al: AMS 742 sphincter: UCLA experience. J Urol 124:812, 1980.

Furlow WL: Artificial sphincter. *In* Surgery of Female Incontinence. Edited by SL Stanton, EA Tanagho. New York, Springer-Verlag, 1980, pp 119–134.

Furlow WL: Implantation of a new semiautomatic artificial genitourinary sphincter: experience with primary activation and deactivation in 47 patients. J Urol 126:741, 1981.

Scott FB: The artificial sphincter in the management of incontinence in the male. Urol Clin North Am 5:375, 1978.

Scott FB, Bradley WE, Timm GW: Treatment of urinary incontinence by implantable prosthetic sphincter. Urology 1:252, 1973.

Scott FB, Light JK, Fishman I, et al: Implantation of an artificial sphincter for urinary incontinence. Contemp Surg 18:11, 1981.

15

VESICOURETERAL REFLUX

Natural History, Classification, and Reflux Nephropathy

SELWYN B. LEVITT AND ROBERT A. WEISS

Vesicoureteral reflux (VUR) is the regurgitation of bladder urine into the upper urinary tract. This review focuses upon the diagnosis, etiology, and pathogenesis of VUR, emphasizing recent observations on the mechanisms whereby VUR results in renal damage. In addition, the controversy of operative intervention versus antibiotic prophylaxis will be presented.

HISTORICAL REVIEW

The subject of VUR continues to occasion intense interest. More than 1500 publications related to this subject appeared in the medical literature during a single decade studied by Ehrlich (1982a). Leonardo Da Vinci described abnormal urinary tract anatomy possibly in association with VUR (Lines). Semblinow, in 1883, first demonstrated reflux experimentally. He injected a colored solution under moderate pressure into the bladder of anesthetized rabbits and followed its course up the ureter. Pozzi, in 1893, observed reflux for the first time in man when he noted urine flow from the cut end of the distal ureter following nephrectomy. However, in experiments with human cadavers in 1898, Young was unable to make urine flow backward from the bladder into the ureter. Sporadic experimental and clinical reports on VUR subsequently appeared in the literature, but Hutch's pioneering studies on the pathophysiology of reflux in paraplegics and its deleterious effect on the kidney ushered in the modern era of interest

in reflux. This work occasioned more widespread use of the voiding cystourethrogram (VCU) in the evaluation of patients with unexplained hydronephrosis and of those with a proclivity to recurrent urinary tract infection (UTI).

Reflux is virtually always present in the rat and might be considered a normal phenomenon. Reflux is often encountered in rabbits and dogs (Winter). When absent, it can be produced by incising the trigone (Tanagho et al), crushing a part of the bladder and introducing bacteria causing chronic cystitis (Schoenberg et al, 1964), or by interfering with the innervation of the trigone as is seen following lumbar sympathectomy (Tanagho et al). Resection of the roof of the submucosal tunnel also will result consistently in reflux. When VUR is produced surgically, its presence or absence is influenced by posture (Winter) and anesthesia (Friedland). The adage that "reflux, if present, may be demonstrated only intermittently" is probably even more true in animals than in humans (Winter).

Jeffs and Allen, as well as Kaveggia et al, induced acute pyelonephritis by the introduction of bacteria via a nephrostomy tube and were able to produce VUR without direct manipulation of the ureterovesical junction. These investigators suggested that reflux could be caused by pyelonephritis and bacteriuria in the absence of disease of the bladder or urethra. Boyarski's demonstration of the toxic effect of bacteriuria on the ureter, which interferes with normal peristalsis, may explain this effect, since normal peristalsis is known to be one of the defense mechanisms that protects against reflux into the renal pelvis.

In the past three decades, the frequency of reflux in children with UTI has become apparent. At first, reflux was thought to be secondary to bladder pathology. Relative narrowing at the bladder neck in relation to the proximal urethra as seen on voiding films, overinterpretation of residual urine seen on postvoiding films, and the frequently observed fine bladder trabeculation seen cystoscopically in children with UTI and reflux were interpreted as indicative of obstruction at the bladder neck. This formulation occasioned widespread use of bladder neck Y-V plasty for the treatment of reflux during the 1950's and early 1960's. A decade passed before this notion was dispelled and the current view of reflux as a primary and congenital abnormality of the ureterovesical junction in most affected children was established.

EPIDEMIOLOGY

The prevalence of VUR in the noninfected general population is not well established because, for obvious reasons, few studies have been done in healthy children. In a compilation of 535 VCUs performed in apparently normal neonates, infants, and children, only 7 instances of reflux were noted (Ransley). Three of these were from children with abnormalities outside of the genitourinary tract, and one other was from a child suspected of having obstruction of the bladder neck. These data suggest that the prevalence of VUR in healthy children is less than 1 per cent. When UTI has been the indication for investigation of the urinary tract, VUR has been discovered in 29 to 50 per cent of children (Walker et al, 1977; Williams, 1974; Shopfner, Smellie and Normand, 1966; Kunin; Savage et al, 1969; Wein and Schoenberg). In children with UTI, the prevalence of VUR is inversely proportional to age (Smellie et al, 1975; Smellie; Baker et al). Infants are more commonly found to have VUR in association with UTI. With growth, the submucosal ureter elongates, and the ratio between the length of the submucosal tunnel and the diameter of the ureter increases (King et al; Stephens and Lenaghan), making the disturbance of the valve mechanism less likely.

There is a high prevalence of VUR in the siblings of children with VUR. In a review by Jerkins and Noe, 104 siblings of 78 patients with VUR were screened cystographically without anesthesia. Thirty-four (33 per cent) were found to have VUR. Seventy-three per cent (25 of 34) of this group had no history of UTI, nor any abnormal voiding symptoms. VUR was more likely to be detected in siblings of those patients with urologic evidence of renal damage, regardless of patient gender. The prevalence of both reflux and renal scarring is estimated to be at least ten times higher in siblings of school-age children with known VUR than in an unselected age-matched population (Lancet Editorial, 1978). The pattern of genetic transmission is undetermined. Most investigators favor a polygenic or multifactorial mode of inheritance (Lancet Editorial, 1982). However, an autosomal dominant or sex-linked pattern is suggested in some families (Lewy and Belman). The genetic predisposition of numerous congenital and acquired disorders has recently been shown to be closely linked to cell surface markers. These histocompatibility antigens (HLA) are present on the sixth chromosome at the A & B (or BW) locus and can be identified and typed by serologic testing of peripheral blood lymphocytes.

A review of 88 families at Christ Church Hospital in New Zealand revealed an increased frequency of HLA A9 and B12 in patients with end-stage renal disease (ESRD) due to VUR-associated renal scarring (Bailey RR, personal communication, 1982). In addition, Torres et al have found HLA B8 and BW15 more frequently in such patients. Also of interest from a genetic standpoint is the observation that VUR is perhaps one tenth as prevalent in a black population of girls with UTI as compared with a similar white population (Askari and Belman).

DIAGNOSIS

The diagnosis of VUR is most accurately established by performance of the VCU with radiocontrast material and fluoroscopy. The methodology employed varies, and this may account for the differences that are reported in the rate of prevalence. A comprehensive review of confounding variables in the performance of the VCU has been offered by Friedland, who suggests that instillation of contrast material at room temperature rather than body temperature is irritating to the trigone and may produce reflux. Concentrations of contrast material greater than 15 per cent (McAlister et al) and large urethral catheters have been shown to irritate the trigone in experiments in rats. Friedland postulates that trigonal irritation due to these factors may result in transient VUR in humans.

The level of intravesical pressure is also an important consideration. Mild degrees of reflux may be evident only at higher intravesical pressures, as occurs with detrusor contraction. More severe reflux is usually detected during both bladder filling and voiding. Although there is universal agreement that contrast should be introduced by gravity flow rather than with a syringe (McAlister et al), the optimal hydrostatic pressure is still debated. Most radiologists favor a pressure of no more than 100 cm (controlled by the height of the infusion bottle above the bladder).

Reflux occurring only during voiding generally is less severe than that seen during both bladder filling and voiding, and is termed high-pressure reflux. However, since all children who are awake during voiding cystourethrography are anxious, bladder pressure may be artificially elevated by straining to resist bladder filling (King). In addition, voiding against a closed bladder neck, especially when a Foley catheter is used, may contribute to this phenomenon (King). Conway et al have observed reflux during bladder filling three times more frequently than during voiding in the course of performing radionuclide cystography (see below). The interpretation of reflux during filling as being "low pressure," thereby implying a more severe grade, must be critically questioned (King).

Another often uncontrolled variable in VCU is the rate of urine flow. A high rate is associated with an increase in the frequency and magnitude of ureteral peristalsis (Briggs et al), which prevents VUR. Conversely, low rates of flow, consequent to either dehydration or poor renal function, may increase the possibility of detecting VUR.

Sedation and general anesthesia influence the prevalence of reflux by their effect on urinary flow. Anesthesia results in a reduction in glomerular filtration rate and consequently in urinary flow rate (Mazze et al). Infants and children undergoing general anesthesia may be dehydrated, also causing a reduction in urine flow. Conversely, the diagnosis of VUR in an unanesthetized child who is tense and

may be unable to void may be missed, since in a proportion of cases VUR can be demonstrated only during voiding (Poznanski and Poznanski; Colodny AH, personal communication, 1979). Timmons et al found that in 23 of 67 refluxing ureters, reflux was detected only when the patient was awake, whereas in 5, reflux was detected only when the patient was anesthetized. The remaining ureters refluxed under both conditions, but in 20 the grade of VUR was more severe under anesthesia. In a similar study, Lyon (1977) observed VUR in the awake state only in 30 per cent of children with reflux. Another 30 per cent demonstrated VUR solely when anesthetized. Woodard and Filardi confirmed Lyon's observations. Reflux in either the awake or the anesthetized state only was observed in a similar proportion of children with VUR.

The dynamic voiding study in the awake child delineates the bladder neck and urethral anatomy more accurately and allows for a better estimation of true bladder size. Therefore, a VCU performed in the awake state is recommended as the preferred study when VUR is suspected and the lower urinary tract is being evaluated for the first time. The expression cystogram performed with the patient under anesthesia should be reserved for special circumstances, such as the extremely anxious child. An isotope study (see below) may be more helpful when reflux is suspected but not demonstrated on the usual x-ray cystogram.

The timing of the VCU in relationship to the presence of UTI must also be taken into consideration, since edema at the ureterovesical junction may result in transient VUR. There is also evidence that intravesical pressure is elevated during acute UTI (Van Gool and Tanagho). This pressure may be transmitted to the upper tracts when VUR is present. Therefore, a bacteriuria-free interval of at least 2 and preferably 4 weeks is recommended before the VCU is performed.

Isotope cystography is an attractive alternative to the conventional cystogram with radiopaque contrast material (Conway et al; Weiss and Conway). A dose of 0.5 millicurie of technetium-99m pertechnetate, instilled into the bladder in saline, provides a gonadal radiation dose of only 4 to 5 millirads, which is significantly less than the exposure with conventional VCU with fluoroscopy (Blaufox et al). In addition to minimizing the risk from radiation, the technique allows for prolonged

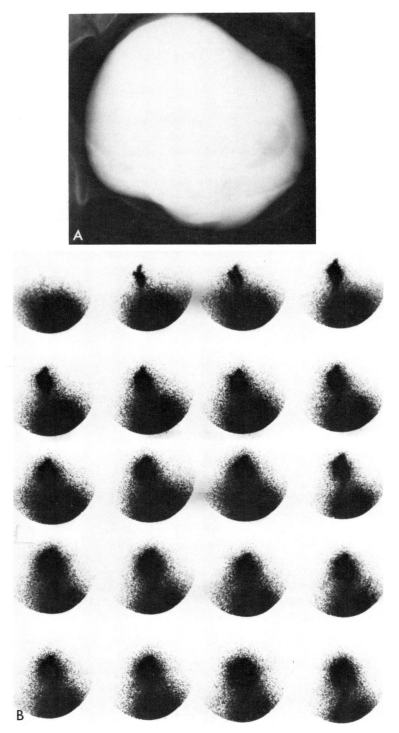

Figure 15–1. 15-year-old girl with recurrent clinical left pyelonephritis with three Hypaque cystograms showing no reflux. (*A*) Representative film of filling phase of Hypaque cystogram. Patient unable to void during study. (*B*) Isotope cystogram performed 1 hour later shows obvious left reflux during filling, already evident by the second frame. (Courtesy of Dr. Stanley J. Kogan.)

observation under the gamma camera, thereby enhancing the sensitivity of the test by providing all of the advantages of the delayed cystogram (Stewart). Intermittent reflux or suspected reflux that cannot be demonstrated by conventional cystography may be detected using this technique (Fig. 15–1). The radionuclide cystogram is especially useful for follow-up patients with known reflux (Nasrallah et al) and for confirming the absence of reflux after surgical correction.

Another radionuclide technique involves the use of technetium-99m diethylenetriaminepentaacetic acid injected intravenously (Pollet et al). This radiopharmaceutical agent is cleared by glomerular filtration and most of the radionuclide is in the bladder within 20 minutes. The child may then be scanned for VUR, thereby avoiding bladder catheterization. When compared with conventional voiding cystourethrography, this method appears to have all the advantages of the radionuclide VCU and, in addition, obviates the need for bladder catheterization. However, Kass et al observed a 50 per cent false negative rate using indirect radionuclide cystograms in children when compared with direct radionuclide cystography. This method is particularly unreliable with milder grades of reflux. Moreover, the method is dependent upon patient cooperation, and the children must have bladder control. Finally, estimates of gonadal radiation exposure were calculated to be higher with indirect radioisotope cystography than with the direct radioisotope cystogram. Radiation exposure increases further when a prolonged period is required to induce voiding.

Ultrasonography has been proposed for the detection of VUR. The diameter of the pelvi-calyceal system can be measured accurately by this technique and would be expected to increase during moderately severe VUR. Tremewan et al reported detection of reflux in three patients with severe VUR. Pfister et al instilled a carbonated solution into the bladder and was able to detect CO_2 bubbles in the upper urinary tract by sonography. With further advances in ultrasonography, this method may prove to be ideal as a screening technique in selected high-risk infants for detection of VUR before renal damage occurs. Although the absence of ionizing radiation is attractive, ultrasound for detection of VUR at present must be considered a research tool.

GRADING OF VUR

There is a strong inverse correlation between the severity of VUR at the time of initial diagnosis and the likelihood of spontaneous resolution. Several grading schemes have been proposed, based upon the severity of reflux as seen on the contrast VCU (Rolleston et al, 1970; Dwoskin and Perlmutter; Heikel and Parkkulainen). Some authors emphasize ureteral caliber as well as pelvicalyceal dilatation (Howerton and Lich; Bridge and Roe; Edelbrook and Mickelson), while others grade VUR according to bladder pressure (i.e., filling versus voiding) (Lattimer et al; Melick et al; Smellie et al, 1975). Duckett and Bellinger, in a recent literature review, described no less than nine grading schemes. The five most commonly used systems are compared in Table 15–1.

Recently, an international grading system

Table 15–1. Classification of Severity of Vesicoureteral Reflux

Rolleston et al	Smellie	Dwoskin & Perlmutter	Heikel & Parkkulainen	Hodson
Mild	I	I	I	I
Moderate (no dilation)	II voiding only III filling and voiding	IIa	II	II III
Severe				
Some dilation	IV	IIb	III	IV
Moderate dilation	IV	III	IV	IV
Gross dilation	IV	IV	V	IV

From Duckett JW, Bellinger MF: A plea for standardized grading of vesicoureteral reflux. Eur Urol 8:74, 1982. By permission of S Karger AG, Basel.

has been proposed (see Fig. 7–45) that aims at providing a standard classification for more objective comparison of therapeutic modalities. This system can best be communicated by describing the degree of reflux present in comparison with the maximum to avoid confusion, e.g., II/V or IV/V, as cardiologists symbolize heart murmurs.

ETIOLOGY AND PATHOGENESIS OF PRIMARY VUR

The anatomic features that characterize the normal valve mechanism of the ureterovesical junction include an oblique entry of the ureter into the bladder (Harrison; Winter), an adequate length of the intramural ureter, especially of its submucosal segment (Johnston, 1962; King, et al), and support of the detrusor muscle (King) (Fig. 15–2). With bladder filling, the ureteral lumen is flattened between the bladder mucosa and the detrusor muscle, thereby creating a flap valve mechanism that prevents VUR. The ratio of the submucosal tunnel length to the ureteral diameter is the main factor that determines the effectiveness of this mechanism (Stephens and Lenaghan). The length of the intravesical ureter (intramural plus submucosal segments) has been estimated to average 1.3 cm in adults and 0.5 cm in neonates (Hutch, 1961).

The "valve" is mainly passive (Young and Wesson; Tanagho et al, 1965), although there is an active component that includes the ureterotrigonal longitudinal muscles, which, during a detrusor contraction, closes the ureteral meatus and submucosal tunnel (Winter; Stephens and Lenaghan). Active ureteral peristalsis, as is noted during diuresis, also acts to prevent reflux (Fairley; Ekman et al).

Primary VUR is regarded as a congenital condition resulting mainly from a deficiency of the longitudinal muscle of the submucosal ureter. The severity of this disturbance can be assessed cystoscopically from the degree of lateral displacement of the ureteral orifice (Fig. 15–3) as well as from its shape (Fig. 15–4), the degree of patulousness, and the length of the submucosal tunnel.

Lyon et al (1969) meticulously assessed the configuration of the ureteral orifice in infants and children. They found only a 4 per cent prevalence of VUR in patients with a normal configuration, 28 per cent in those with a stadium orifice, 83 per cent in those with a horseshoe shape, and 100 per cent when the orifice was golf-hole in appearance. Stephens has described an additional orifice configuration that he termed the "lateral pillar defect." It falls between a horseshoe and golf-hole type of orifice (Fig. 15–4). Heale et al, in an independent survey of ureteric orifice position and configuration, confirmed Lyon's ob-

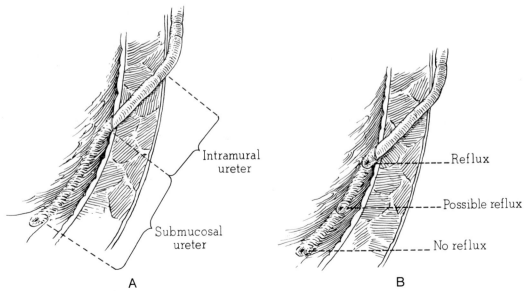

A   B

Figure 15–2. *A,* Normal ureterovesical junction. Demonstration of length of intravesical submucosal ureteral segment. *B,* Refluxing ureterovesical junction. Same anatomic features as nonrefluxing orifice, except for inadequate length of intravesical submucosal ureter, are shown. Some orifices reflux intermittently with borderline submucosal tunnels. (From Glenn J (editor): Urologic Surgery. Second ed. New York, Harper & Row, 1975.)

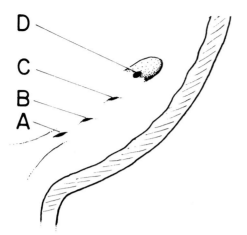

Figure 15–3. Diagram showing four different orifice positions. *A*, Normal position. *B*, Moderately lateral. *C*, Very lateral. *D*, Orifice at the mouth of a diverticulum. (From Glassberg KI: Vesicoureteral reflux. In Practice of Surgery. Urology. Edited by HS Goldsmith, New York, Harper & Row, 1982.)

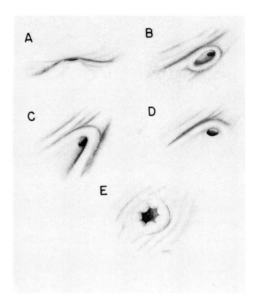

Figure 15–4. Orifice morphology. *A*, Normal cone or volcanic orifice. *B*, Stadium orifice. *C*, Horseshoe orifice. *D*, Lateral pillar defect orifice. *E*, Golf-hole orifice. (From Glassberg KI: Vesicoureteral reflux. In Practice of Surgery. Urology. Edited by HS Goldsmith. New York, Harper & Row, 1982.)

servations. The higher prevalence and grade of VUR, as well as renal scarring, were seen with the more laterally placed and abnormally shaped orifices.

The degree of bladder filling must also be taken into account in describing the cystoscopic shape of the orifice and its position. Progressive bladder filling displaces the orifice laterally and changes its appearance toward a more abnormal type.

King has emphasized submucosal tunnel length as an important prognostic measurement for predicting the likelihood of spontaneous resolution of VUR. The length of the submucosal tunnel can best be measured with a graduated ureteral catheter (Fig. 15–5). An

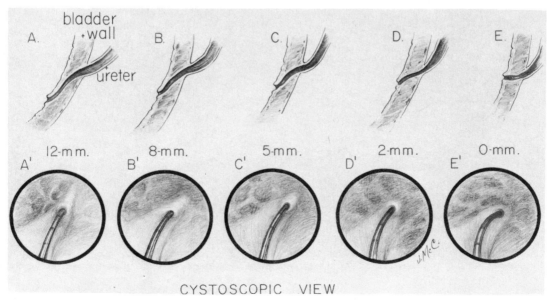

CYSTOSCOPIC VIEW

Figure 15–5. The cystoscopic appearance of the ureterovesical junction. A ureteral catheter is used to estimate the length of the submucosal tunnel. The ureter is drawn as normal in diameter to emphasize the appearance of the flap elevated by the catheter.

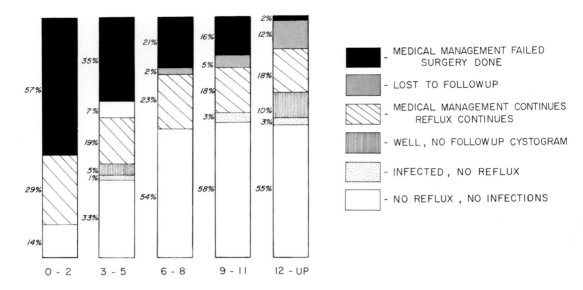

LENGTH OF INTRAMURAL URETER IN MILLIMETERS

Figure 15–6. This graph depicts the relationship between the estimated length of the intravesical ureter at the time of diagnosis and the outcome of a trial of nonoperative management in 247 refluxing units in which the tunnel length was estimated in patients followed 4 to 10 years. There is a nearly linear relationship between original tunnel length and eventual cessation of reflux, indicating the importance of this parameter.

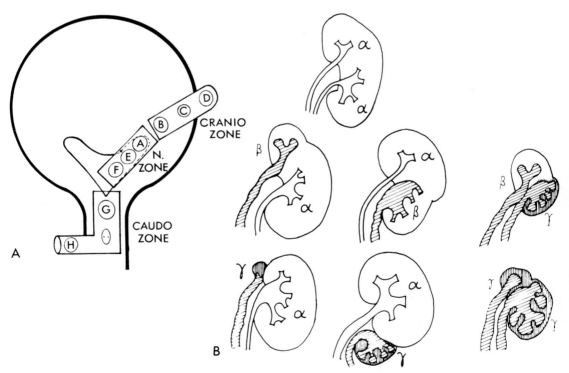

Figure 15–7. A, Possible sites of ureteral orifices. In dissection of stillborn material, orifices on the trigone in the normal position A or in the E and F positions are associated with normal (alpha) kidneys. Refluxing orifices in the B, C, or D positions are associated with hypoplastic (beta) or dysplastic (gamma) kidneys shown in B. The more lateral the orifice, the worse the renal segment, as development in utero is apparently impaired if the ureteral bud arises from an abnormal position.

B, The renal segment in duplicated systems. A shaded ureter indicates reflux. (From Mackie GG, Awang H, Stephens FD: The ureteric orifice: the embryologic key to radiologic status of the ureter. J Pediatr Surg 10:473, 1975.)

almost linear relationship between tunnel length at time of diagnosis and likelihood of eventual cessation of reflux was noted in this study, indicating the importance of this factor (Fig. 15–6).

Abnormal location and configuration of the ureteral orifice may also be associated with developmental renal anomalies. Mackie and Stephens have proposed the "ureteral bud theory" to explain this observation. Autopsy studies were done on 36 neonates and 7 children up to age 6 with duplex collecting systems. Renal morphology, based upon a quantitative scale of hypoplasia (decreased number of glomeruli) and dysplasia (abnormal metanephric differentiation), was correlated with the position of the ureteric orifice. The more severe degrees of displacement of the orifice correlated well with high scores on the hypoplasia/dysplasia scale (Fig. 15–7). Stephens postulated that when the ureteral bud does not arise from the appropriate segment of the wolffian duct, the ureteral orifice will be located in an abnormally lateral position on the bladder base. The eventual point of contact of the bud with the nephrogenic cord will be similarly ectopic and closer to the tail of the cord, which has less nephrogenic mesenchyme and more stromagenic tissue, making it less likely to differentiate normally. Anomalies of renal differentiation may explain the poorly functioning kidney with diffuse parenchymal thinning that is seen in infants with severe VUR but no evidence of UTI.

More recent work by Sommer and Stephens examined the role of position of the orifice associated with dysplasia and renal scarring in children with VUR compared with that in children with partial ureteral obstruction without reflux. Both groups were considered to have comparable degrees of caliectasis. Histologic examination of those with partial ureteric obstruction revealed obstructive atrophy but not dysplasia. Only those refluxing renal units with ureteral ectopia and caliectasis contained dysplastic elements. The authors contended that these findings support the concept of renal parenchymal maldevelopment occurring pari passu with VUR rather than secondary to the hydrodynamic effects of VUR.

Opponents of the "ureteral bud" theory have not found a high prevalence of dysplasia in refluxing scarred kidneys drained by single collecting systems. Ambrose et al, using the Bernstein criteria of renal dysplasia, were able to find only a 3 per cent prevalence of dysplasia in 61 patients with reflux and renal atrophy when the 4 cases of obstructive uropathy in their series were excluded. Duckett (1981) observed in an editorial comment that there were more examples that failed to fit the theory than those that confirmed the hypothesis. The Stephens' hypothesis, therefore, seems most plausible when applied to duplex systems and those with the most severe degrees of reflux. Further studies, with exact anatomic definitions, are needed to document the role of dysplasia in the atrophic kidney associated with reflux.

INFECTION AND THE URETEROVESICAL JUNCTION

Transient reflux may occur in a marginally competent ureterovesical orifice secondary to bladder inflammation. Bacterial and viral cystitis, as well as an indwelling catheter, can produce edema of the trigone, rendering the flap valve mechanism temporarily ineffective. This is particularly true in neonates and infants, in whom the ratio of submucosal tunnel length to the ureteral diameter is low. However, this type of reflux generally will resolve spontaneously with treatment of the infection and disappearance of the inflammatory changes at the ureterovesical junction. Most authors, therefore, advocate delaying the VCU for at least 2 to 4 weeks after the urine has been sterilized, as discussed earlier in this chapter.

Whether VUR itself predisposes children to UTI remains debatable. Conventional theory holds that refluxed urine returns to the bladder after voiding, contributing to urinary stasis and acting as a fertile incubation medium for urinary pathogens in susceptible children. In support of the role of VUR predisposing to UTI, Govan and Palmer have shown that children with reflux develop UTI at an earlier age than their anatomically normal counterparts. Following successful antireflux surgery, 70 to 80 per cent of children are cured of their propensity to develop UTI (Willscher et al, 1976a and b). Conversely, most children with recurrent UTI do not have reflux.

DETRUSOR DYSFUNCTION

VUR secondary to severe obstruction of the bladder outlet, such as with posterior urethral valves, is a well-known entity (Williams, 1974; Johnston, 1979). Dysfunctional voiding is also an important secondary cause of VUR. Hinman and Baumann first called attention to this problem in 1973. Both Allen and Koff et al observed VUR in approximately 50 per cent of children undergoing urodynamic evaluation for an abnormal voiding pattern. In many of these children, VUR was initially thought to be the predominant problem, but reimplantation surgery proved unsuccessful. Five of Allen's patients had a previously normal VCU, suggesting that VUR due to dysfunctional voiding can be an acquired phenomenon.

Dysfunctional voiding secondary to detrusor-sphincter dyssynergia and uninhibited detrusor contractions may result in high intravesical pressure, thereby predisposing to VUR (Kondo et al). Van Gool has demonstrated that UTI alone can produce high intravesical pressure secondary to inflammation by similar mechanisms. Appropriate diagnosis and treatment of dysfunctional voiding is an integral part of the management of VUR in such children. Surgical correction of reflux should not be attempted until the detrusor dysfunction is properly controlled. Postoperative management may include drug therapy for the unstable bladder.

ASSOCIATION OF VUR AND RENAL SCARRING

Clinical Studies

The impact of VUR on the prognosis for children with urinary tract infection is considered to be deleterious. In 1960, Hodson and Edwards first demonstrated the association of VUR with renal scarring. The renal damage associated with VUR takes three forms on urography: (1) focal pyelonephritic scarring where the contracted parenchyma is associated with calyceal clubbing, (2) generalized calyceal dilatation and parenchymal atrophy, and (3) renal growth failure, associated with either focal scarring or generalized atrophy. Reflux nephropathy has been suggested as a preferable term for the scarred kidney associated with VUR, where hypertension, proteinuria, and reduced renal function in any combination, may also be present.

Radiologic evidence of scarring is almost always accompanied by VUR; conversely, between 30 and 60 per cent of children with VUR have renal scarring (Smellie et al, 1975). The higher figure is derived from data originating in surgical clinics (Williams and Eckstein), and the lower from medical clinics (Smellie and Normand, 1968).

It has been suggested that sterile VUR alone may be sufficient to cause renal scarring (Rolleston et al, 1975). Nevertheless, the appearance of fresh scars or the extension of established scars, in the absence of obstruction or a neuropathic bladder, has been documented satisfactorily only in children with urinary infection. Smellie et al (1979) reported no new scars in 150 normal or scarred kidneys in children with uncomplicated primary VUR in whom continuous low-dose chemoprophylaxis was successful in maintaining a sterile urine. Only 2 developed new scarring on continuous low-dose chemoprophylaxis over a 7- to 15-year follow-up period. Both of these cases were associated with breakthrough infection, and in both there was a moderate to severe degree of VUR.

Lenaghan and Stephens used intermittent short courses of antibacterial drugs for the treatment of recurrent infections in 120 children with VUR. In 76 kidneys that were initially normal, scarring developed in 16 (21 per cent). Of 44 kidneys with established scars, 29 developed additional scarring (66 per cent). All patients with new or progressive scarring had intercurrent infections. In an addendum to this report, Stephens suggested that continuous prophylaxis would have prevented these changes.

Filly et al observed 2 new scars in 16 initially normal kidneys with VUR while the children were on "intermittent" therapy. However, scars developed in 2 of 15 (13 per cent) initially normal kidneys in which VUR was not demonstrated. Cystoscopic examination of these latter children demonstrated widely separated and poorly muscularized ureteral orifices, suggesting that reflux may have been present at some time in the past. Fifteen of 24 (62 per cent) initially scarred kidneys showed progression of scarring.

A history of bacteriuria often can be elicited in children with VUR and renal scarring. The higher the grade of reflux, the more likely is the occurrence of new or progressive scarring associated with urinary tract infection (Rolleston et al, 1970). The typical radiographic appearance of renal scarring requires a period of at least 8 months to develop (Hodson). It is difficult to determine whether scars in fact progress or simply become more obvious as the surrounding healthy renal parenchyma grows.

When present, scarring is usually seen at the time of the initial excretory urogram in the child with VUR and UTI. Some investigators claim that scars rarely, if ever, occur de novo in normal kidneys beyond infancy and that, when present, they do not progress even when both reflux and infection coexist (Blank).

It should be noted that the clinical studies cited included all degrees of VUR. In addition, assessment of the severity and progression of renal scarring was often ill-defined. These factors make comparison between studies difficult.

Experimental Studies

Most of the recent experimental work regarding the pathogenesis of renal scarring has centered on the concept of intrarenal reflux (IRR). This is defined as the extension of refluxed urine into the collecting tubules of the nephrons and provides a readily apparent mechanism by which urinary microorganisms may gain access to the renal parenchyma and produce renal scarring.

Roberts et al produced IRR in primates with a bacterial inoculum in order to define the precise mechanism of tubular damage secondary to bacterial infection. Phagocytosis of bacteria by invading neutrophils produces superoxide, an enzyme toxic to renal tubular cells. Administration of superoxide dismutase, an antagonist of superoxide, was successful in preventing tubular cell damage histologically but did not interfere with phagocytosis of bacteria. Thus, Roberts' work suggests that the inflammatory response itself, while eliminating invading bacteria by neutrophil phagocytosis, may produce irreversible damage to renal tissue.

Besides inflammation of the parenchyma due to bacterial infection, other mechanisms have been proposed to explain the pathogenesis of scar formation. Cotran and colleagues have investigated the role of Tamm-Horsfall protein (THP). This mucoprotein is produced in high concentration by the tubular epithelial cells of the loop of Henle and distal nephron and is a primary constituent of renal tubular casts. Immunofluorescence techniques have demonstrated extratubular THP in the interstitium of kidneys with IRR. Extratubular THP, therefore, may serve as a marker of urinary extravasation. Such deposits of THP are associated with inflammatory infiltrates as well as fibrosis. Further investigations regarding the role of THP and extratubular urinary extravasation are necessary before this phenomenon can be given a role in the genesis of pyelonephritic scarring.

Other studies (Ransley and Risdon, 1978; Tamminen and Kaprio) indicate that the areas of renal parenchyma susceptible to IRR and subsequent scarring are drained by flat or concave papillae, which occur predominantly in the polar regions of the kidney (Fig. 15-8). The pig possesses renal papillary morphology similar to that in the human. Thus, this animal model is ideal to elucidate the mechanism of IRR and renal scarring.

Hodson et al, also using the pig model, demonstrated that focal scarring can be produced by sterile IRR, but only in the presence of a sustained increase in intravesical pressure. Additional experimental work by Ransley and Risdon (1978) has attempted to address the issue of whether or not sterile reflux can produce renal damage. Using three strains of pigs and sophisticated urodynamic monitoring, they found that parenchymal scarring occurred only when there was sufficient bladder outlet obstruction (due to a ring applied surgically to the urethra) to result in bladder decompensation. They concluded that during the relatively brief interval (days) of high intravesical pressure without bladder decompensation no lesions were produced, but that once bladder decompensation supervened, lesions of coarse scarring were noted. Thus, if

Figure 15-8. Papillary factors in intrarenal reflux: *A,* Convex papilla (nonrefluxing papilla)—crescentic or slitlike openings of collecting ducts opening obliquely onto the papilla; *B,* concave or flat papilla (refluxing papilla)—round collecting ducts opening at right angles onto flat papilla. (From Ransley PG, Risdon RA: Reflux and renal scarring. Br J Radiol Suppl *14,* 1978.)

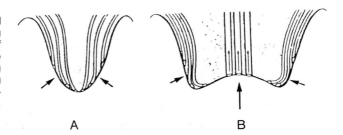

A   B

the results of such studies in pigs can be extrapolated to humans, it would seem unlikely that sterile VUR results in renal damage in the absence of severe obstruction.

More recent studies in the pig suggest that *in the presence of infected urine,* IRR results in the development of scarring in less than 4 weeks. However, antimicrobial treatment, introduced after 1 week of urinary tract infection, significantly reduces the extent of scar formation (Ransley and Risdon, 1981).

Clinical Importance of IRR

In the clinical context, IRR has been defined radiologically as the appearance of contrast material in the renal parenchyma during voiding cystourethrography (Fig. 15–9). However, visualization of IRR may be difficult when the upper tracts are dilated and filled with nonopacified urine, which dilutes the contrast.

The radiologic detection of IRR almost certainly underestimates its true prevalence. IRR has been observed in 5 to 15 per cent of neonates and infants with VUR (Rolleston et al, 1974; Rose et al). Rolleston et al studied VCUs of several hundred children with VUR. IRR was detected only in children under the age of 5 years, and it was seen only with moderate to severe degrees of VUR. In addi-

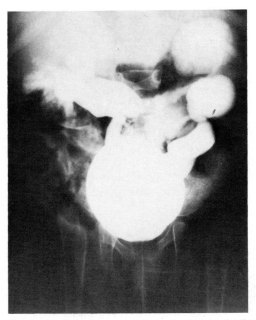

Figure 15–9. Hypaque cystogram demonstrating gross bilateral intrarenal reflux in an infant with grade V VUR, international classification.

tion, there was a significant correlation between the presence of IRR and the subsequent development of renal scarring in the affected area.

The more frequent detection of IRR in neonates and infants with VUR can be explained by the relatively large size of the collecting ducts, allowing better visualization of contrast in the renal parenchyma (Tamminen and Kaprio). In older children in whom scarring has already occurred, parenchymal fibrosis may prevent IRR into affected segments.

Studies of papillary morphology in human kidneys indicate that at least two thirds possess papillae of the type that allow IRR (Ransley and Risdon, 1978; Tamminen and Kaprio). Controversy exists concerning the clinical significance of IRR in the production of renal scars. Since most VCUs are performed with UTI as the indication, data concerning the occurrence of VUR and IRR in children with sterile urine are unavailable.

Ransley and Risdon have attempted to reconcile the clinical, radiologic, and pathologic features of IRR-related renal scarring. In the majority of infants and children with VUR and renal scarring, the scarring is already present on the initial urogram (Rolleston et al, 1974). The hypothesis that this is the result of an episode of previous pyelonephritis has been called the "big bang" theory (Williams, 1977). Ransley and Risdon suggest that the initial UTI in the infant with VUR and nonconical papillae results in pyelonephritic scarring, which occurs most frequently at one or both poles. Since all susceptible segments of the kidney are affected simultaneously, sequential scar formation is unusual. However, on occasion, marginally refluxing papillae may be transformed to the refluxing variety, rendering them susceptible to IRR and to subsequent scarring with recurrent infections. This sequence of events would account for the diffusely contrasted kidney sometimes seen on urography.

Despite the very impressive evidence that the combination of moderate to severe VUR, IRR, and bacteriuria results in pyelonephritic scarring, 30 to 40 per cent of patients investigated for renal insufficiency and found to have the radiographic features of reflux nephropathy (RN) have no definite history of UTI (Bakshandah et al). Family surveys of index patients with VUR regularly report individuals with advanced RN and no urinary tract symptomatology or history of UTI. In addition, RN is often detected during the course of diagnostic evaluation for hypertension or proteinuria in the older child. The explanation for this would appear to rest on the fact that UTI in infants and children may be underdiagnosed. Transient febrile illnesses with nonspecific symptomatology are generally not considered indications for urine culture in the usual pediatric practice. The Ransley-Risdon "big bang" theory of acute, severe, but unrecognized pyelonephritis in infancy may account for those individuals with RN who have no documented history of UTI.

Bailey has proposed a number of possible pathogenetic mechanisms other than infection to account for this observation. Young infants with severe VUR presumably have had reflux in utero, and, therefore, the generalized parenchymal scarring present at the time of their presentation with UTI may be secondary to hydrodynamic factors. Alternatively, Stephens' ureteral bud theory of renal parenchymal malformation (dysplasia) associated with severe (grade V) VUR could account for the generalized rather than focal nature of the renal damage seen in some young infants, without the need to invoke bacteriuria and IRR.

Nevertheless, the development of new renal scars in the clinical setting has been clearly documented only in the presence of UTI (Edwards et al). Experimental and clinical evidence suggests that in the vast majority of instances the combination of VUR, IRR, and UTI is necessary for the production of renal scarring.

VUR AND RENAL GROWTH

VUR, with or without associated infection, may interfere with the normal growth of the kidney. Sequential measurements of renal length alone on the excretory urogram have been used to assess renal growth. The length of normal kidneys has been shown to be affected by numerous factors (Hernandez et al). When the renal parenchyma is undergoing scar formation, total renal mass is reduced. This may not be reflected accurately by simple measurement of renal length. Hypertrophy of the intervening normal renal parenchyma and the predominantly polar distribution of renal scars make interpretation of renal size using renal length alone inaccurate and unreliable. Most studies of renal growth in kidneys with VUR suffer from this methodologic deficiency (Redman et al).

Claësson et al (1981b) have critically addressed the issue of renal parenchymal thickness. They have devised a nomogram to compare observed and expected renal mass derived from linear measurements on the urogram. The distance in millimeters from the upper surface of the first to the lower edge of the third lumbar vertebra is used to correct for body size. Total bipolar length, the distance from the upper pole calyx to the upper renal margin, and the distance from lower pole calyx to the lower renal margin are measured in addition to mid-zone thickness. The nomogram allows one to determine whether or not a particular kidney or segment of kidney has appropriate mass for somatic size (Fig. 15–10).

Further work by Claësson's group has produced the technique of computerized planimetry to measure total renal parenchymal area in units of square centimeters. A standard urogram of high quality is submitted to a computerized method of tracing the renal parenchymal outline as well as that of the calyceal system. Thus, not only is there anatomic detail, but areas of compensatory hypertrophy are visualized and sequential measurements can be compared.

Radionuclide renal scans have added another facet to the study of renal anatomy and function in the patient with VUR. Individual renal function can be calculated from the uptake of iodine-131 Hippuran (effective renal plasma flow) or technetium-99m diethylenetriaminepentaacetic acid (glomerular filtration rate).

2,3 Dimercaptosuccinic acid (DMSA), a recently available cortical imaging agent, provides good anatomic detail when compared with the two aforementioned agents and can reveal small areas of diminished renal function not detected by conventional urography. This sensitive method for the determination of renal damage may prove especially beneficial in the longitudinal evaluation of children with reflux. In addition, DMSA uptake can be used to calculate unilateral renal function. However, each isotope method has problems with interpretation and limits with respect to accuracy and reproducibility. At present, no ideal technique for measurement of renal mass is available.

Given the shortcomings of bipolar renal length measurements, Lyon (1973) and Redman et al observed a subnormal rate of renal growth in the presence of VUR without documented urinary infection. Kelalis, on the other

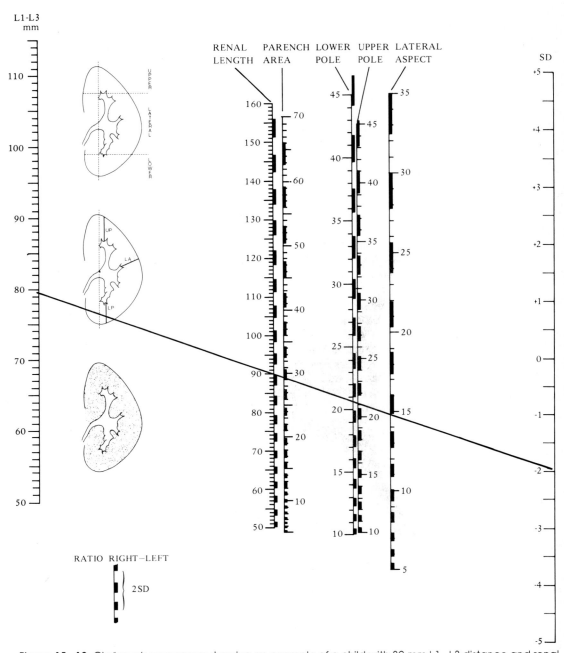

Figure 15–10. Claësson's nomogram showing an example of a child with 80 mm L1–L3 distance and renal length of 90 mm. A straight line between these two points falls within two standard deviations (SD) of normal on the far right column. A similar linear relationship allows comparison of lower pole, upper pole, and lateral parenchymal thickness to expected norms using the appropriate ordinates. Parenchymal area is measured separately by planimetry and can also be related to norms using the same methodology. One SD is denoted by one filled segment plus one unfilled segment. Normal values lie within two SD. (From Claësson I, Jacobsson B, Olsson T, et al: Assessment of renal parenchymal thickness in normal children. Acta Radiol Diagn 22:305, 1981.)

Table 15-2. Renal Growth in 111 Kidneys with Vesicoureteral Reflux Related to Recurrence of Infection during 791 Kidney-Years of Observation

Renal Growth	Infection	No Infection	Total
Normal	20	80	100
Slow	10	1	11

$x^2 = 25.3$, df = 1, p 0.001.

From Smellie JM, Edwards D, Normand ICS, et al: Effect of VUR on renal growth in children with UTI. Arch Dis Child 56:593, 1981.

hand, reported resumption of renal growth in kidneys with VUR after infection had been eliminated.

Longitudinal measurements of bipolar renal length were used by Smellie et al (1981) to monitor the effects of VUR on the kidney in a series of 76 children with persistent VUR of varying grades. Renal growth was impaired (bipolar length less than half of the increment expected for the child's linear growth) in only 5 of 93 kidneys drained by undilated ureters. Of the 18 kidneys drained by a dilated ureter, 6 had growth impairment; 5, however, were already scarred at the time of presentation. The sixth developed de novo renal scarring. All patients had episodes of documented UTI. The overall relationship between the grade of VUR, the presence of UTI, and the rate of renal growth can be seen in Tables 15-2 and 15-3. The extent of damage on the refluxing side, the presence of a normal or abnormal contralateral kidney, infection of the urinary tract, and the grade of VUR all may influence growth of the affected kidney. Although pat-

Table 15-3. Renal Growth in 111 Kidneys with Vesicoureteral Reflux, Related to Grade of Reflux on First Diagnosis

| Renal Growth | Vesicoureteral Reflux | | Total |
	Grades 1-3	Grade 4	
Accelerated or normal	88	12*	100
Slow	5	6†	11

$x^2 = 13.20$, df = 1, p 0.001.

* Three kidneys were scarred.

† Five kidneys were scarred; all six were exposed to infection.

From Smellie JM, Edwards D, Normand ICS, et al: Effect of VUR on renal growth in children with UTI. Arch Dis Child 56:593, 1981.

terns of renal growth differ from case to case over a period of time, with prolonged follow-up through puberty there may be no ultimate difference in rates of renal growth whether VUR is treated medically or surgically (Claësson et al, 1981a).

The effect of antireflux surgery on renal growth has been examined by several investigators. McRae et al reported accelerated growth after successful surgery. Babcock et al, considering the effects of unilateral VUR, observed neither radiographic improvement nor a change in the ratio of the size of the refluxing kidney to the normal contralateral organ after elimination of VUR. On the other hand, Willscher et al (1976b) demonstrated normal rates of growth in unscarred kidneys with severe VUR. However, these kidneys showed accelerated growth after surgical elimination of VUR. When renal scarring was present, this accelerated pattern of growth following surgery was seen only when scarring was bilateral. Murnaghan observed significant focal nodular parenchymal hypertrophy in two postpubertal patients following successful antireflux surgery.

In addition, somatic growth of prepubertal children with VUR has been observed to accelerate after successful surgical correction (Merrell and Mowad). However, physical growth alone, particularly during puberty, may account for the increased renal growth rate (Claësson et al, 1981b) that has been observed by some investigators.

VUR AND RENAL FUNCTION

The morphologic appearance of kidneys drained by ureters with moderate to severe reflux is often one of reduced size and one or more areas of contracted parenchyma. The function of such kidneys has been examined by Aperia et al, utilizing the technique of external ureteral compression to collect urine from each kidney separately. Above the age of 6, those refluxing renal units with dilated ureters demonstrated a significant decline in glomerular filtration rate (GFR). In cases of unilateral reflux with a dilated ureter, when the GFR of the damaged kidney was below 25 ml/min/1.73 m², there was a supranormal GFR in the contralateral normal kidney.

Claësson et al have confirmed these observations in children with unilateral renal scarring and reflux, using computerized renal planimetry to estimate unilateral GFR. In fol-low-up studies for periods of up to 15 years, compensatory hypertrophy was usually quite efficient and overall GFR was normal by ado-lescence.

The concept of renal functional damage associated with VUR usually refers to GRF. However, the pathologic lesion is one of a chronic tubulo-interstitial nephritis, in which glomerular scarring may be a relatively late finding. Aperia has examined unilateral tubu-lar function by comparing glucose reabsorp-tion and sodium excretion in kidneys dam-aged by reflux with that in the normal contralateral organ. While glucose reabsorp-tion was appropriate in both kidneys, dam-aged kidneys had higher salt excretion. Walker et al (1983) have examined maximal concentrating capacity (a tubular function) in reflux patients with and without renal scar-ring. During a mean follow-up interval of 3.5 years, they found that renal growth was better in patients without a concentrating defect than in those with a concentrating defect. They speculate that the presence of a concen-trating defect may represent either a physio-logic disturbance or a pathologic lesion, with adverse implications for renal growth.

HYPERTENSION

Hypertension, occasionally of such magni-tude as to be classified malignant, is a well-known long-term complication encountered in children and young adults with VUR and coarse renal scarring. An analysis of 100 children with severe hypertension (diastolic BP > 100 mm Hg) revealed 14 children with RN, all of whom presented between the ages of 6 and 15 years (Gill et al). Pyelonephritic scarring was second in frequency only to chronic glomerulonephritis as the etiology of hypertension in this age group. Holland has reviewed 177 cases of hypertension with scarred, atrophic kidneys under various diag-nostic terms in 16 series (Table 15–4). She suggests that all of these terms, in fact, refer to the same pathologic entity.

Smellie's long-term follow-up study of a large population of children with VUR showed progression of renal damage in those patients who developed hypertension. The prevalence of hypertension in patients with renal scarring associated with VUR is un-known, but it is a significant feature of those developing end-stage renal failure. In Smel-lie's series, hypertension was detected in 20 per cent of children with established scars. Six of the 17 hypertensive children had malig-nant hypertension, and 8 had some degree of renal insufficiency. However, more than half had normal or near normal renal function, indicating that the appearance of hyperten-sion in these patients is not necessarily related to the development of renal failure, but rather to the associated vascular lesions (Kincaid-Smith). In favor of such a mechanism is the finding of high plasma renin activity in two girls with hypertension and reflux nephropa-thy in whom serum creatinine levels were 0.6 and 1.2 mg/dl (Siegler).

Savage et al (1978) studied 100 normoten-sive children with reflux nephropathy and found 8 with raised renin plasma levels. A longitudinal study is in progress to determine whether these hyperreninemic patients are at greater risk of developing hypertension. After 5 years of follow-up, 2 of these 8 children have developed hypertension (Dillon, MJ,

Table 15–4. Hypertension Associated with Reflux and Renal Scarring

Diagnosis	No. Cases	F:M Ratio	Prior Hx UTI %	Prevalence VUR No. with VUR/No. VCUs done	
Chronic pyelonephritis	99	4:1	66	36/43	(84%)
Segmental hypoplasia	49	5:1	8	9/21	(43%)
Primary interstitial nephritis	15	4:1	—	10/11	(91%)
Reflux nephropathy	8	8:0	75	8/8	(100%)
Ask-Upmark kidney	6	6:0	50	2/2	(100%)

From Holland N: Reflux nephropathy and hypertension. *In* Reflux Nephropathy. Edited by J Hodson, P Kincaid-Smith. © 1979, Masson Publishing USA, Inc., New York.

personal communication, 1982). From the same center, an additional 51 patients with hypertension and coarse renal scarring were examined. Almost all of these had evidence of VUR; 36 had elevated plasma renin activity.

Smellie has suggested that hypertension associated with VUR and renal scarring is an age-related phenomenon with increasing risk above age 15. Thus, the long-term outcome of patients with renal scarring needs to be determined. Wallace et al reported hypertension in 18.5 per cent of children with bilateral renal scars more than 10 years following surgery for VUR. Hypertension was observed in 11.3 per cent of cases with unilateral renal scarring. Stecker et al reported hypertension in 3 of 70 children 1 to 19 years after ureteral reimplantation and stated that elimination of reflux does not protect against the development of hypertension. Stickler et al found no improvement in hypertension in two patients following antireflux surgery. On the other hand, two of eight patients in a series by Hicks et al had elevated blood pressures that returned to normal or became easily controllable following successful ureteral reimplantation as the only surgical procedure.

In addition to pharmacologic antihypertensive therapy, unilateral nephrectomy has been advocated for relief of hypertension associated with VUR when the affected kidney has very poor function. Dillon performed 46 renal vein renin (RVR) studies in 44 hypertensive patients with renal scarring. Ten patients with unilateral scars underwent nephrectomy, with RVR ratio of >1.5 in nine. Eight were cured of their hypertension and two were improved.

Six patients with asymmetric bilateral involvement, with RVR ratios of >1.5, underwent surgery. Five had unilateral nephrectomy and one had unilateral nephrectomy and contralateral partial nephrectomy. Three were cured of their hypertension and three were improved. Of special interest is the observation that approximately half of these 44 patients required *segmental* RVR studies in order to determine the source of their hypertension.

A prospective trial at Christ Church Hospital in New Zealand is attempting to examine the role of nephrectomy in hypertensive patients with severe unilateral renal damage (GFR < 10 ml/min in the affected kidney) (Table 15–5). These patients are being randomly allocated to either nephrectomy or

Table 15–5. Role of Nephrectomy in Treatment or Prevention of Hypertension with Severe Unilateral Reflux Nephropathy

		No. Hypertensive at Follow-Up (At Least 2 Years)
Hypertensive Patients		
Drug therapy	5	5
Nephrectomy	6	3
Normotensive Patients		
Observation	8	2
Nephrectomy	6	1

From Bailey RR: Reflux nephropathy and hypertension. *In* Reflux Nephropathy. Edited by J Hodson, P Kincaid-Smith. © 1979, Masson Publishing USA, Inc., New York.

drug therapy. In addition, because of the known long-term risk of hypertension with reflux nephropathy, normotensive patients with unilateral disease are also being randomly allocated to either nephrectomy or observation in an effort to determine whether surgery can successfully forestall or prevent the development of hypertension. Nephrectomy in patients already hypertensive was curative in only 50 per cent. Only one of six patients in the normotensive group developed hypertension after nephrectomy. Whether prophylactic nephrectomy in normotensive patients will significantly reduce the incidence of later hypertension cannot be determined at this time, since the follow-up is too brief and the number of patients in each group is small (Bailey, 1979a; Bailey, RR, personal communication, 1983).

MEDICAL VERSUS SURGICAL MANAGEMENT OF VUR

The ultimate therapeutic goal of therapy for VUR, whether medical or surgical, aims at protecting the kidney from scarring and allowing the fulfillment of renal growth potential. The latter may be defined as the achievement of maximal GFR and concentrating capacity, as well as the prevention of hypertension associated with such renal damage. In addition, UTI and its symptoms must be prevented.

Medical Management

The case for medical management of VUR is based upon the observations that there is a natural tendency for VUR to improve or cease with time (Edwards et al) and that antibiotic chemoprophylaxis of UTI will protect the kidney from damage due to infection. Such an approach assumes that sterile reflux is not harmful. As discussed previously, this assumption is currently undergoing intense investigation in animal models as well as in prospective, randomized clinical trials (International Reflux Study Committee).

Smellie and Normand (1979) have followed 75 children up to 15 years and have observed disappearance of VUR in 80 per cent of kidneys with undilated ureters on cystogram (grades I and II, international classification), but in only 41 per cent of kidneys with ureteral dilatation (grades III, IV, and V, international classification). Thus, dilatation of the ureter at initial presentation with VUR appeared to be an important factor affecting the outcome. Configuration of the ureteral orifice and length of the submucosal tunnel are also thought by many investigators to be important factors in determining whether or not spontaneous resolution of reflux will occur. In a surveillance study of children with VUR followed 4 to 10 years, King noted no cases of spontaneous cure of reflux when the orifice was golf-hole in shape and there was no vestige of an intravesical ureter.

It has been suggested that spontaneous resolution of VUR is most likely to occur within the first months or years following diagnosis (Scott). However, it now appears that the rate at which VUR disappears remains constant throughout childhood, being 20 to 30 per cent for each 2-year period (Normand and Smellie). Reflux was as likely to disappear in children who had recurrent urinary infections as in those who had no further infection. Puberty was not associated with an increased rate of spontaneous cessation of VUR (Edwards et al).

Even VUR associated with paraureteric diverticula has been observed to undergo spontaneous resolution. Colodny observed eight children, all with grade III/V or IV/V international classification VUR and paraureteric diverticula of up to 2 cm in diameter. All had cessation of VUR without surgery, and in seven of eight the diverticula also disappeared. However, when the ureter actually enters the diverticulum, VUR cannot be expected to resolve spontaneously (Fig. 15–11).

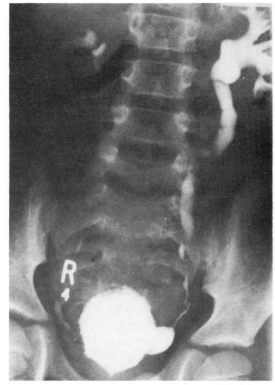

Figure 15–11. Refluxing ureter with sizable diverticulum. If the ureter enters the diverticulum, reflux cannot stop with growth, and surgical correction is required.

Reflux into the lower-pole moiety of a completely duplicated collecting system may also resolve with medical management. As with primary VUR, one may advocate an individualized approach in duplicated systems based upon grading of reflux and the cystoscopic findings. However, Kaplan et al observed spontaneous resolution of reflux in only 5 of 23 such ureters (22 per cent) followed nonoperatively over a 13-year observation period.

The basis of medical management consists of continuous low-dose chemoprophylaxis administered until the disappearance of VUR is documented. There should be no interruption of this prophylaxis, such as to obtain a urine culture. Chemoprophylactic agents should meet the following criteria: achievement of high urinary concentrations, activity against a broad spectrum of urinary pathogens, nondisturbance of periurethral and bowel bacterial flora, minimal side effects, convenience of administration, and low cost. Equally important is strict compliance with the regimen and careful follow-up with periodic urine cultures, which may be performed at home with dip slides. Nonpharmacologic management, such as frequent voiding (some suggest double voiding) and avoidance of constipation, is also recommended. In addition, infants and toddlers should be allowed to develop normal bladder maturation without overemphasis on early toilet training.

In summary, the observation that mild to moderate grades of VUR tend to undergo spontaneous resolution during childhood justifies a trial of medical management in many patients (Fig. 15–12). A careful explanation of

the goal of medical management to well-motivated parents is a prerequisite for initiating such a treatment plan (Table 15–6).

Surgical Management

Ureteral reimplantation surgery is a highly successful procedure, with elimination of VUR in more than 95 per cent of operated cases (Lyon, 1977). It should be noted that these statistics all apply to reports in which lesser grades of reflux predominate. Those

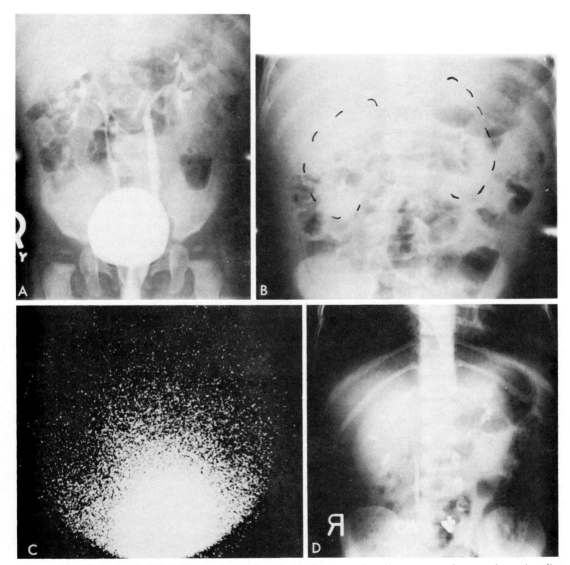

Figure 15–12. *A*, Grade III/IV VUR in a 2-month-old girl, discovered on Hypaque cystogram 6 weeks after resolution of acute UTI. *B*, Excretory urogram performed at the time, while technically suboptimal, showed no obvious scars or apparent pelvicalyceal abnormalities. *C*, Following 4 years of medical management with continuous low-dose antibiotic chemoprophylaxis and interval urine cultures, reflux has resolved. *D*, Follow-up excretory urogram demonstrates no scarring and normal renal growth. Renal function remains normal.

Table 15-6. Suggested Guide for Surveillance Studies in Medical Management of Vesicoureteral Reflux

---

Urine Culture—monthly for first 3 months after UTI, then once every 3 months.

Cystogram—isotope cystogram at 1 to 2 year intervals.

*Excretory Urogram—limited study (2 to 3 films) at 1 to 2 year intervals to monitor renal growth and scars.

Renal Function Tests
  BUN and serum creatinine—yearly, especially if VUR bilateral.
  GFR—can be estimated (Schwartz and Haycock) by the formula

$$\frac{\text{height in cm} \times 0.55}{\text{serum creatinine}} = \text{GFR in ml/min/1.73 m}^2$$

  Maximum urinary osmolality—yearly.

Height, Weight and Blood Pressure—yearly.

Cystoscopy—rarely necessary in patients with grades I/V or II/V VUR unless other abnormalities are noted on the VCU or if a history of significant voiding disturbance is obtained (see below). However, cystoscopy with ureteral tunnel calibration is very helpful in patients with grades III/V and IV/V reflux. The finding of a golf-hole orifice with short or absent submucosal tunnel is rarely associated with spontaneous resolution of reflux. Grade V/V reflux is generally considered to be best treated by reimplantation surgery and the cystoscopy is done at the time of operation to complete the evaluation.

Urodynamic Evaluation—indicated if there is a history of voiding dysfunction. Appropriate therapy for dysfunctional voiding symptoms is an essential adjunct to the successful management of reflux in children. This is true for the medically treated group as well as for those who require surgical correction. In fact, premature surgical correction of VUR without appropriate therapy of associated voiding dysfunction can result in disastrous sequelae (Hinman and Baumann; Allen).

---

* Ultrasound, DMSA, or glucoheptinate scans can be substituted for the excretory urogram.

---

who tend to operate on grades IV and V alone do *not* have 95 per cent success. The best results are obtained by surgeons with pediatric urologic experience. A rigidly standardized operative technique need not be used; the surgical procedure should be tailored to the needs of the individual patient (Randel). Surgical complications include postoperative VUR for a period of time on the unoperated side, which usually disappears within the first year after surgery (Willscher et al, 1976a and b; Scott). Ureteral obstruction requiring reoperation occurs in 1.2 to 4 per cent of cases (Willscher et al, 1976a and b; Scott; Randel); most obstructions are temporary and do not require reoperation. Widespread use of the cross-trigonal reimplant, employing the old bladder hiatus, has virtually eliminated this complication (Ehrlich, 1982b).

VUR and Compromised Renal Function

The role of antireflux surgery in patients with advanced reflux nephropathy and compromised renal function remains controversial. Torres et al (1980b) reported continued renal deterioration in 11 patients with bilateral VUR and renal scarring. Mean serum creatinine values were greater than 2.75 mg/dl, and progression to renal failure occurred despite successful surgical correction of VUR. In children with bilateral severe VUR, Berger et al suggested that proteinuria and a creatinine clearance of less than 25 ml/min/m² portend progressive renal insufficiency, regardless of therapy.

Salvatierra, however, continues to recommend surgical correction of bilateral VUR even in older children and adolescents with reflux nephropathy and compromised renal function. This recommendation seems at variance with his published report in 1973 of patients with serum creatinine values varying between 1.7 and 4.2 mg/dl who, despite successful antireflux surgery, progressed inexorably to end-stage renal failure (ESRF). However, this retrospective analysis, as he points out, reflects only those patients who progressed to ESRF. It does not follow that all patients in similar circumstances who undergo successful antireflux surgery derive no benefits from reflux correction. Indeed, successful surgical correction of VUR does seem to retard the rate of progression toward ESRF in some patients (Salvatierra, O, Jr, personal communication, 1982). In children with glomerular filtration rates of 25 ml/min/1.73 m² or greater, this may be important for maximizing somatic growth potential. Murnaghan's report of significant compensatory hypertrophy following surgical correction of reflux in two patients with severe reflux nephropathy lends added support to the concept that VUR correction may be beneficial in some patients. Reflux correction may also prevent the accelerated deterioration that sometimes occurs in patients with reflux nephropathy following an episode of acute pyelonephritis. This residual renal function allows for a more liberal fluid intake concurrent with maintenance dialysis either before transplant or following a failed transplant. Anemia in patients on dialysis is also less severe in patients who retain their native kidneys, and blood transfusions are less frequently required. No increased morbidity or increased proclivity to urinary tract infections has been reported in transplant patients with ESRF secondary to reflux nephropathy where reflux has been corrected and the native kidneys have been left in situ. In contrast, VUR with secondary urinary tract infection in an immunosuppressed patient represents a significant threat. Moreover, reflux correction obviates the need for bilateral nephroureterectomies in preparation for renal transplantation when ESRF ensues. Transabdominal bilateral nephroureterectomy, if complicated by small bowel obstruction in the dialysis patient or immunosuppressed patient, is a difficult management problem associated with significant risk and morbidity.

In summary, bilateral ureteral reimplantation for moderate to gross VUR even in the presence of renal impairment (not ESRF) when done by an experienced urologic surgeon is a simpler and safer procedure than bilateral nephroureterectomy. It obviates the need for nephroureterectomies in most potential transplant recipients and may retard the progression toward ESRF in some patients.

VUR AND PREGNANCY

Surgical correction of VUR is generally recommended when reflux persists beyond puberty. The rationale for this recommendation is to protect the sexually active woman from pregnancy-related pyelonephritic episodes, possible premature delivery, and increased perinatal loss.

Hutch (1961) demonstrated VUR during pregnancy in 5 of 12 woman in whom gestation was complicated by pyelonephritis. He also showed a disproportionately high incidence of pyelonephritis during pregnancy among 23 women known to have recurrent bacteriuria and a radiologic diagnosis of chronic pyelonephritis with VUR.

Heidrick et al performed 200 cystograms in the last trimester of pregnancy, in an unselected population; 7 studies revealed VUR (3.5 per cent). An additional 121 women underwent cystography within 30 hours of delivery; 2 of these showed VUR (1.6 per cent). Three of these 9 women with VUR had developed pyelonephritis earlier in their pregnancy, compared with only 4.8 per cent in those without reflux. The prevalence of reflux in these studies was unaffected by the presence of asymptomatic bacteriuria.

Williams et al evaluated 100 women with asymptomatic coliform bacteriuria during pregnancy (Table 15–7). All were treated with an acute course of antibiotic therapy. They were studied radiographically 4 to 6 months post partum. Cystography demonstrated VUR in 21, and coliform bacteriuria at the time of the study was found in 13 of these (62 per cent) as compared with only 16 per cent of the women without VUR. Ten of the 21 patients (48 per cent) with VUR had renal scarring, compared with 9 per cent of the nonrefluxing group. Two thirds of those with VUR, compared with one fourth of those without VUR, required two or more courses of

Table 15–7. Postpartum Evaluation of 100 Women with Asymptomatic Bacteriuria during Pregnancy

	Reflux		No Reflux	
	n = 21		n = 79	
Bacteriuria post-delivery	13/21	(62%)	13/79	(16%)
Renal scarring	10/21	(48%)	7/79	(9%)
Bacteriuria cleared with one course of antibiotics	7/21	(33%)	61/79	(77%)
Bacteriuria required two or more courses of antibiotics	14/21	(67%)	18/79	(23%)

From Williams GL, Davies DKL, Evans KT, et al: Vesicoureteral reflux in patients with bacteriuria in pregnancy. Lancet 2:1202, 1968.

antibiotics to clear their bacteriuria. These data suggest that bacteriuria in pregnant women with VUR is more difficult to eradicate than bacteriuria during pregnancy without VUR. Moreover, bacteriuria during pregnancy appears to identify a population of women with a high prevalence of VUR and previous renal scarring.

The prevalence of asymptomatic bacteriuria during pregnancy is generally quoted as 4 to 6 per cent. Although there is controversy concerning the prevalence of VUR in bacteriuric pregnant women, the finding of bacteriuria, especially when it persists, suggests VUR.

Pyelonephritis, which is observed in only 1 to 2 per cent of all pregnancies, occurs in 30 per cent of pregnant women with asymptomatic bacteriuria (Whalley and Cunningham). Previous predictions of a high incidence of prematurity as a result of asymptomatic bacteriuria were not substantiated in subsequent studies (Cunningham et al). Mattingly and Borkowf reported only one case of prematurity among 23 pregnant women with untreated asymptomatic bacteriuria. In addition, they noted no prematurity in their nine patients with VUR, three of whom had acute pyelonephritis early in their pregnancy.

In summary, a careful analysis of the sparse available literature suggests that women with VUR and bacteriuria may be more susceptible to acute pyelonephritis during pregnancy. Bacteriuria, when it occurs in pregnant women with VUR, may be more difficult to eradicate with a single course of antibiotics and tends to persist more frequently post partum. Although there is a suspicion that VUR during pregnancy does predispose to bacteriuria, the lack of a longitudinal study from a population of women with known VUR prior to pregnancy does not permit a definitive statement concerning this issue. Since we cannot predict which women will develop bacteriuria during pregnancy, most authors continue to recommend surgical correction of VUR when it persists beyond puberty.

PROBLEM OF CHOOSING CORRECT MANAGEMENT IN CHILDREN WITH VUR

More than 20 years after Hodson and Edwards' observation of the association between VUR and renal scarring, many questions remain unanswered. Can VUR alone, or infection alone, precipitate progressive renal damage? Are both necessary for its occurrence?

It has become apparent that most cases of VUR not accompanied by ureteral dilatation will disappear with time. If continuous antibacterial therapy is administered, most children with VUR can be maintained in an uninfected state, which will result in limited, if any, parenchymal scarring or progression of already established scars.

Those with higher grades of VUR, however, in whom ureteral and pelvicalyceal dilatation is present (grades IV and V in the international classification) must be considered separately. Scars are commonly present on the initial urogram; spontaneous resolution of the VUR is less likely in this group. Medical management may be chosen for these children provided that their urine can be maintained sterile. This requires compliance on the part of both parents and child, serial urine cultures, and careful observation with radiographic re-evaluation at regular intervals. Progression of scars, or the development of new scars, even in these patients, has been documented only following pyelonephritic episodes. Thus, the prevention of such insults is the aim of both medical and surgical treatment.

Surgery offers immediate correction of the abnormality and greatly reduces the risk of pyelonephritis. At present, neither mode of treatment offers a clear advantage in terms of prevention of hypertension or with respect to renal growth. Whatever form of treatment is used, long-term observation is essential in order to identify potential sources of morbidity (such as new pyelonephritic episodes when VUR persists), the development of hypertension, and the rare instance of late obstruction after surgery. Detection of the latter complication, more than 5 years after apparently successful ureteral reimplantation, was heralded by recurrent UTI in the two cases reported by Weiss et al.

The only absolute indications for surgical correction of reflux would appear to be: (1) pyelonephritic episodes despite antibiotic chemoprophylaxis, (2) noncompliance with the regimen of medical management, (3) a refluxing ureter that opens into a bladder diverticulum, and (4) ureteral obstruction in association with reflux. In addition, the cystoscopic observation of a golf-hole orifice with no submucosal tunnel virtually guarantees that spontaneous resolution of VUR will not occur.

CLINICAL TRIALS OF MEDICAL VERSUS SURGICAL MANAGEMENT OF VUR

It is clear that a great deal remains unknown about the natural history of VUR, and that only randomized prospective trials of medical versus surgical management can determine which therapy is preferable. Moreover, the issue of sterile reflux and its potential deleterious effect on the kidney can be examined only in such a context.

In the only published prospective randomized trial (Scott and Stansfeld) comparing the results of early surgical correction of VUR with prophylactic antibiotic therapy, renal growth in children in whom the reflux was surgically cured exceeded that observed in those children in whom the reflux was still present. Unfortunately, the population sampled was small and the follow-up short. In view of the accelerated renal growth rate observed during puberty in medically treated patients with VUR, this difference may not be significant in the long term (Claësson et al, 1981a).

Recently, the Birmingham Reflux Study Group published their observations on 96 children (135 refluxing renal units) who were randomly allocated to either surgery or antibiotic prophylaxis. Two groups of patients were included in the trial according to the severity of reflux and the presence or absence of renal scarring on the urogram. If, on the VCU, the contrast material reached the renal pelvis but did not distend the calyces, this was considered grade II VUR. Among this group, only those with renal scarring were randomized. A second group comprised those in whom the VCU demonstrated distention of the calyceal system. This was considered grade III VUR, and all patients in this group were randomized, whether or not renal scarring was present on the urogram. Renal growth was analyzed by comparing renal length with L1 to L3 intervertebral distance. The preliminary results (2 year follow-up) indicate that there was no significant difference between the two treatment groups with respect to renal growth, the development of new scars, or progression of pre-existing scars.

In 1980, an international prospective randomized clinical trial was initiated among a group of major teaching hospitals in the United States and Europe. Because children with moderate to severe VUR present the most difficult management problem, it was this group that were selected for study. All patients with primary grade IV (international classification) VUR are accepted into the trial, as well as patients with grade III VUR beyond infancy in the European branch. The American collaborative group will study only grade IV VUR. The specific aims of the study are to compare the effects of successful antireflux surgery performed at the time of diagnosis, with effective continuous low-dose antibiotic prophylaxis. This therapeutic trial is designed to test (1) whether sterile, high-grade VUR is harmful in itself, and (2) whether a difference exists between early successful surgery and effective medical management in preventing the possibly deleterious effect of VUR on the renal growth rate, the development of new scars, and the progression of established scars. In addition, this study will establish the incidence of recurrent urinary tract infection and hypertension in surgically versus medically treated patients.

The prospective approach, the random allocation of patients to the surgical or medical management groups, the precise definitions used to select patients, the standardization of diagnostic, therapeutic, and follow-up procedures, and the advance identification of reliable and recognizable end points should permit an accurate comparison between these two therapeutic approaches. Preliminary results may be available by the middle of this decade.

Acknowledgments

We would like to acknowledge the editorial assistance of Dr. Chester M. Edelmann, Jr., and the secretarial help of Mrs. Gloria Muscarella.

REFERENCES

Allen TD: Vesicoureteral reflux as a manifestation of dysfunctional voiding. In Reflux Nephropathy. Edited by J Hodson, P Kincaid-Smith. New York, Masson Publishing USA, 1979, pp 171–180.

Ambrose SS, Parrott TS, Woodard JR, et al: Observations on the small kidney associated with vesicoureteral reflux. J Urol 123:349, 1980.

Aperia A, Broberger O, Ericsson NO, et al: Effect of

vesicoureteral reflux on renal function in children with recurrent urinary tract infections. Kidney Int 9:418, 1976.

Arant BS Jr, Sotelo-Avila C, Bernstein J: Segmental "hypoplasia" of the kidney (Ask-Upmark). J Pediatr 95:931, 1979.

Askari A, Belman AB: Vesicoureteral reflux in black girls. J Urol 127:747, 1982.

Ask-Upmark E: Über juvenile maligne Nephrosklerose und ihr Verhältnis zu Störungen in der Nierenentwicklung. Acta Pathol Microbiol Scand 6:383, 1929.

Babcock JR, Keats GK, King LR: Renal changes after an uncomplicated antireflux operation. J. Urol 115:720, 1976.

Bailey RR: Reflux nephropathy and hypertension. In Reflux Nephropathy. Edited by J Hodson, P Kincaid-Smith. New York, Masson Publishing USA, 1979a, pp 263–267.

Bailey RR: Sterile reflux: is it harmless? In Reflux Nephropathy. Edited by J Hodson, P Kincaid-Smith. New York, Masson Publishing USA, 1979b, pp 334–339.

Baker R, Maxted W, Maylath J, et al: Relation of age, sex and infection to reflux: data indicating high spontaneous cure rate in pediatric patients. J Urol 95:27, 1966.

Bakshandah K, Lynne C, Carrion H: Vesicoureteral reflux and end-stage renal disease. J Urol 116:557, 1976.

Berger RE, Ansell JS, Shurtleff DB, et al: Vesicoureteral reflux in children with uremia. JAMA 246:56, 1981.

Birmingham Reflux Study Group: Prospective trial of operative vs. non-operative treatment of severe vesicoureteral reflux: two years observation in children. Brit Med J 287:171, 1983.

Blank E: Caliectasis and renal scars in children. J Urol 110:255, 1973.

Blaufox MD, Gruskin A, Sandler P, et al: Radionuclide scintigraphy for detection of vesicoureteral reflux in children. J Pediatr 79:239, 1971.

Boyarski S, Labay P: Ureteral Dynamics. Baltimore, Williams & Wilkins, 1972, p 354.

Bridge RAC, Roe CW: Grading of vesicoureteral reflux. J Urol 101:821, 1969.

Briggs EM, Constantine CE, Govan DE: Dynamics of the upper urinary tract: IV. The relationship of urine flow rate and rate of ureteral peristalsis. Invest Urol 10:56, 1972.

Claësson I, Jacobsson B, Jodal U, et al: Compensatory kidney growth in children with UTI and unilateral renal scarring: an epidemiologic study. Kidney Int 20:759, 1981a.

Claësson I, Jacobsson B, Olsson T, et al: Assessment of renal parenchymal thickness in normal children. Acta Radiol Diagnosis 22:305, 1981b.

Conway JJ, King LR, Belman AB, et al: Detection of vesicoureteral reflux with radionuclide cystography. A comparison study with roentgenographic cystography. Am J Roentgenol Radium Ther Nucl Med 115:720, 1972.

Cotran RS, Pennington JE: Urinary tract infection, pyelonephritis, and nephropathy. In The Kidney. Vol. II. Second ed. Edited by BM Brenner, RC Rector Jr. Philadelphia, WB Saunders Co., 1981, pp 1571–1632.

Cunningham FG, Morris GB, Mickal A: Acute pyelonephritis of pregnancy: a clinical review. Obstet Gynecol 42:112, 1973.

De Vargas A, Evans K, Ransley P, et al. A family study of vesicoureteric reflux. J Med Genet 15:85, 1978.

Duckett JW: Editorial comment. J Urol 125:71, 1981.

Duckett JW, Bellinger MF: A plea for standardized grading of vesicoureteral reflux. Eur Urol 8:74, 1982.

Dwoskin JY: Sibling uropathology. J Urol 115:725, 1976.

Dwoskin JY, Perlmutter AD: Vesicoureteral reflux in children: a computerized review. J Urol 109:888, 1973.

Edelbrook HH, Mickelson JC: Selection of children for vesicoureteroplasty. J Urol 104:342, 1970.

Editorial: Screening for reflux. Lancet 2:23, 1978.

Edwards D, Normand ICS, Prescod N, et al: Disappearance of reflux during long-term prophylaxis of urinary tract infection in children. Br Med J 2:285, 1977.

Ehrlich RM: Soc Pediatr Urol Newsletter, December, 1982a.

Ehrlich RM: Success of the transvesical advancement technique for VUR. J Urol 128:554, 1982b.

Ekman H, Jacobsson B, Kock NG, et al: High diuresis: a factor in preventing vesicoureteral reflux. J Urol 95:511, 1966.

Fairley KF: The effects of a diuresis on vesicoureteric reflux. In Reflux Nephropathy. Edited by J Hodson, P Kincaid-Smith. New York, Masson Publishing USA, 1979, p 102.

Filly RF, Friedland GW, Govan F, et al: Development and progression of clubbing and scarring in children with recurrent urinary tract infection. Radiology 113:145, 1974.

Friedland GW: The voiding cystourethrogram: an unreliable examination. In Reflux Nephropathy. Edited by J Hodson, P Kincaid-Smith. New York, Masson Publishing USA, 1979, pp 93–99.

Gill DG, Mendes da Costa B, Cameron JS, et al: Analysis of 100 children with severe and persistent hypertension. Arch Dis Child 51:951, 1976.

Govan DE, Palmer JM: Urinary tract infection in children: the influence of successful antireflux operations in morbidity from infection. Pediatrics 44:677, 1969.

Habib R, Courtecuisse V, Ehrensperger J, et al: Hypoplasie segmentaire du rein avec hypertension arterielle chez l'enfant. Ann Pediatr (Paris) 12:262, 1965.

Harrison R: On the possibility and utility of washing out the pelvis of the kidney and the ureters through the bladder. Lancet 1:463, 1888.

Heale WF: In Reflux Nephropathy. Edited by J Hodson, P Kincaid-Smith. New York, Masson Publishing USA, 1979, p 120.

Heidrick WP, Mattingly RF, Amberg JR: Vesicoureteral reflux in pregnancy. Obstet Gynecol 29:571, 1967.

Heikel PE, Parkkulainen KV: Vesico-ureteric reflux in children: a classification and results of conservative treatment. Ann Radiol 9:37, 1966.

Hernandez RJ, Poznanski AK, Kuhns LR, et al: Factors affecting measurement of renal length. Radiology 130:653, 1979.

Hicks CC, Woodward JR, Walton KW, et al: Hypertension as complication of vesicoureteral reflux in children. Urology 7:587, 1976.

Hinman F, Baumann FW: Vesical and ureteral damage from voiding dysfunction in boys without neurologic or obstructive disease. J Urol 109:727, 1973.

Hodson CJ: The radiological contribution toward the diagnosis of chronic pyelonephritis. Radiology 88:857, 1967.

Hodson CJ, Edwards D: Chronic pyelonephritis and vesicoureteric reflux. Clin Radiol 11:219, 1960.

Hodson CJ, Maling TMJ, McManamon PH, et al: Pathogenesis of reflux nephropathy. Br J Radiol Suppl 13:1, 1975.

Holland N: Reflux nephropathy and hypertension. In Reflux Nephropathy. Edited by J Hodson, P Kincaid-Smith. New York, Masson Publishing USA, Inc, 1979, pp 257–262.

Howerton LW, Lich R Jr: The cause and correction of ureteral reflux. J Urol 89:672, 1963.

Hutch JA: Theory of maturation of the intravesical ureter. J Urol 86:534, 1961.

Hutch JA: Ureteric advancement operation: anatomy, technique and early results. J Urol 89:180, 1963.

International Reflux Study Committee: Medical versus surgical treatment of primary vesicoureteral reflux. Pediatrics 67:392, 1981.

Jeffs RD, Allen MS: Relationship between ureterovesical reflux and infection. J Urol 88:691, 1962.

Jerkins GF, Noe HN: Familial vesicoureteral reflux: a prospective study. J Urol 128:774, 1982.

Johnston JH: Vesicoureteral reflux: its anatomical mechanism, causation, effects and treatment in the child. Ann R Coll Surg Engl 30:324, 1962.

Johnston JH: Vesicoureteral reflux with urethral valves. Br J Urol 51:100, 1979.

Johnston JH, Mix LW: The Ask-Upmark kidney: a form of ascending pyelonephritis? Br J Urol 48:393, 1976.

Kaplan WE, Nasrallah P, King LR: Reflux in complete duplication in children. J Urol 120:220, 1978.

Kass J, Majd M, Belman BA: The accuracy of the indirect radionuclide cystogram in children. Presented at the Urologic Section of the American Academy of Pediatrics meeting, October 6, 1982.

Kaveggia L, King LR, Grana L, et al: Pyelonephritis: a cause of vesicoureteral reflux? J Urol 95:158, 1966.

Kelalis PP: Subject review: proper perspective on vesicoureteric reflux. Mayo Clin Proc 46:807, 1971.

Kincaid-Smith P: Glomerular and vascular lesions in chronic atrophic peylonephritis and reflux nephropathy. Adv Nephrol 5:3, 1975.

King LR: Vesicoureteral reflux: history, etiology and conservative management. In Clinical Pediatric Urology. PP Kelalis, LR King. Philadelphia, WB Saunders Co., 1976, pp 342–366.

King LR, Zami SO, Belman AB: Natural history of vesicoureteral reflux: outcome of a trial of non-operative therapy. Urol Clin North Am 1:441, 1974.

Koff SA, Lapides J, Piazza DH: The uninhibited bladder in children: a cause for urinary obstruction, infection and reflux. In Reflux Nephropathy. Edited by J Hodson, P Kincaid-Smith. New York, Masson Publishing USA, 1979, pp 161–170.

Kondo A, Kobayashi M, Otani T, et al: Children with unstable bladder: clinical and urodynamic observation. J Urol 129:88, 1983.

Kunin CM, Deutscher R, Paquin A Jr: Urinary tract infection in school children: an epidemiologic, clinical and laboratory study. Medicine 43:91, 1964.

Lattimer JK, Appearson JW, Gleason DM, et al: The pressure at which reflux occurs: an important indicator of prognosis and treatment. J Urol 89:395, 1963.

Lenaghan JD, Whitaker G, Johnson F, et al: The natural history of reflux and long-term effects of reflux on the kidney. J Urol 115:728, 1976.

Lewy PR, Belman AB: Familial occurrence of nonobstructive, noninfectious vesicoureteral reflux with renal scarring. J Pediatr 86:851, 1975.

Lines D: 15th century ureteric reflux. Lancet 2:1473, 1982.

Lyon RD: Discussion. Birth Defects 13:364, 1977.

Lyon RP: Renal arrest. J Urol 109:707, 1973.

Lyon RP, Halverstadt D, Tank ES, et al: Vesicoureteral reflux. Dial Ped Urol 1:1, 1978.

Lyon RP, Marshall S, Tanagho EA: The ureteric orifice: its configuration and competency. J Urol 102:504, 1969.

Mackie GG: Stephens FD: Duplex kidneys: a correlation of renal dysplasia with position of the ureteral orifice. J Urol 114:274, 1975.

Mattingly RF, Borkowf HI: Clinical implications of ureteral reflux in pregnancy. Clin Obstet Gynecol 21:863, 1978.

Mazze RI, Schwartz FS, Slocum HC, et al: Renal function during anesthesia and surgery. Anesthesiology 24:279, 1963.

McAlister WH, Shackelford GS, Kissane L: The histological effects of 30% Cystokon, Hypaque 25% and Renografin-30 in the bladder. Radiology 104:563, 1972.

McRae CU, Shannon FT, Utley WLF: Effect on renal growth of reimplantation of refluxing ureters. Lancet 1:1310, 1974.

Melick WF, Brodeur AE, Darellos DN: A suggested classification of ureteral reflux and suggested treatment based on cineradiographic findings and simultaneous pressure recordings by means of the strain gauge. J Urol 88:35, 1962.

Merrell RW, Mowad JJ: Increased physical growth after successful antireflux operation. J Urol 122:523, 1979.

Middleton GW, Howards SS, Gillenwater JY: Sex-linked familial reflux. J Urol 114:36, 1975.

Murnaghan GF: Urologists correspondence. March 1980.

Nasrallah PF, Conway JJ, King LR, et al: Quantitative nuclear cystogram. Urology 12:654, 1978.

Normand C, Smellie J: Vesicoureteral reflux: the case for conservative management. In Reflux Nephropathy. Edited by J Hodson, P Kincaid-Smith. New York, Masson Publishing USA, 1979, pp 281–286.

Pfister RR, Biber RJ, Rose JS, et al: Monitoring ureteral reflux with ultrasound. Presented at the Urologic Section of the 51st American Academy of Pediatrics meeting, October 6, 1982.

Pollet JE, Sharp PF, Smith RW, et al: Intravenous radionuclide cystography for the detection of vesicorenal reflux. J Urol 125:75, 1981.

Poznanski E, Poznanski AK: Psychogenic influences on voiding: observations from voiding cystourethrography. Psychosomatics 10:339, 1969.

Pozzi S: Ureteroverletzung bei Laparatomie. Zentralbl Gynäk 17:97, 1893.

Randel DR: Surgical judgement in the management of vesicoureteral reflux. J Urol 119:113, 1978.

Ransley PG: Vesicoureteral reflux: continuing surgical dilemma. Urology 12:246, 1978.

Ransley PG, Risdon RA: Reflux and renal scarring. Br J Radiol Suppl 14, 1978.

Ransley PG, Risdon RA: Reflux nephropathy: effects of antimicrobial therapy on the evolution of the early pyelonephritic scar. Kidney Int 20:733, 1981.

Redman JF, Scriber LJ, Bissad NK: Apparent failure of renal growth secondary to vesicoureteral reflux. Urology 3:704, 1974.

Roberts JA, Roth JK Jr, Domingue G, et al: Immunology of pyelonephritis in the primate model. V. Effect of superoxide dismutase. J Urol 128:1394, 1982.

Rolleston GL, Maling TMJ, Hodson CJ: Intrarenal reflux and the scarred kidney. Arch Dis Child 49:531, 1974.

Rolleston GL, Shannon FJ, Utley WLF: Relationship of infantile vesicoureteral reflux to renal damage. Br Med J 1:460, 1970.

Rolleston GL, Shannon FT, Utley WLF: Follow up of vesicoureteric reflux in the newborn. Kidney Int 8:59, 1975.

Rose JS, Glassberg KI, Waterhouse K: Intrarenal reflux and its relationship to renal scarring. J Urol 113:400, 1975.

Salvatierra O, Jr, Kountz SL, Belzer FO: Primary vesicoureteral reflux and end stage renal disease. JAMA 226:1454, 1973.

Salvatierra O, Jr, Ransley P, Dwoskin J: Reflux. Panel discussion at Society for Pediatric Urology. SB Levitt, moderator. 77th Annual Meeting of American Urologic Association, Kansas City, May, 1982.

Savage DCL, Wilson MI, Ross EM, et al: Asymptomatic bacteriuria in girl entrants to Dundee Primary School. Br Med J 3:75, 1969.

Savage JM, Shah V, Dillon MJ, et al: Renin and blood pressure in children with renal scarring and vesicoureteric reflux. Lancet 2:441, 1978.

Schoenberg HW, Beisswanger P, Howard WJ, et al: Effect of lower urinary tract infection upon ureteral function. J Urol 92:107, 1964.

Schwartz GJS, Haycock G: A simple estimate of glomerular filtration rate in children derived from body length and plasma creatinine. Pediatrics 58:249, 1976.

Scott JES: The role of surgery in the management of vesicoureteric reflux. Kidney Int 8:73, 1975.

Scott JES, Stansfeld JM: Ureteric reflux and kidney scarring in children. Arch Dis Child 43:468, 1968.

Semblinow VI: Zur Pathlogie der durch Bacterien bewinkten ambsteifenden Nephritis. 1883 Dissertation quoted by Alksne J: Folia Urol 1:338, 1907.

Shopfner CE: Vesicoureteral reflux. Radiology 95:637, 1970.

Siegler RL: Renin dependent hypertension in children with reflux nephropathy. Urology 7:474, 1976.

Smellie JM: The disappearance of reflux in children with urinary tract infection during prophylactic chemotherapy. In Proceedings of the 4th International Congress on Nephrology (Stockholm). Vol. 3. Basel, S Karger, 1969, p 357.

Smellie JM, Edwards D, Hunter N, et al: Vesicoureteric reflux and renal scarring. Kidney Int 8(Suppl 4):S65, 1975.

Smellie JM, Edwards D, Normand ICS, et al: Effect of VUR on renal growth in children with UTI. Arch Dis Child 56:593, 1981.

Smellie JM, Normand ICS: The clinical features and significance of urinary infection in childhood. Proc R Soc Lond 59:415, 1966.

Smellie JM, Normand ICS: Experience of follow-up of children with urinary tract infection. In Urinary Tract Infection. Edited by F O'Grady, W Brumditte. London, Oxford University Press, 1968, p 123.

Smellie JM, Normand ICS: Reflux nephropathy in childhood. In Reflux Nephropathy. Edited by J Hodson, P Kincaid-Smith. New York, Masson Publishing USA, 1979, pp 14–20.

Sommer JT, Stephens FD: Morphogenesis of nephropathy with partial ureteral obstruction and vesicoureteral reflux. J Urol 125:67, 1981.

Stecker JR, Read PB, Poutasse EF: Pediatric hypertension as a delayed sequela of reflux induced pyelonephritis. J Urol 118:644, 1977.

Stephens FD: Ureteric configurations and cystoscopy schema. Soc Pediatr Urol Newsletter Jan. 23, 1980, p 2.

Stephens FD, Lenaghan D: Anatomical basis and dynamics of vesicoureteral reflux. J Urol 87:669, 1962.

Stewart CM: Delayed cystograms. J Urol 70:588, 1953.

Stickler GB, Kelalis PP, Burke EC, et al: Primary interstitial nephritis with reflux—a cause of hypertension. Am J Dis Child 122:144, 1971.

Tamminen TE, Kaprio EA: The relation of the shape of renal papillae and of collecting duct openings to intrarenal reflux. Br J Urol 49:345, 1977.

Tanagho EA, Hutch JA, Meyers FH, et al: Primary vesicoureteral reflux: experimental studies of its etiology. J Urol 93:165, 1965.

Timmons JW, Watts FB, Perlmutter AD: A comparison of awake and anesthesia cystography. Birth Defects 13:364, 1977.

Torres VE, Moore SB, Kurtz SB, et al: In search of a marker for genetic susceptibility to reflux nephropathy. Clin Nephrol 14:217, 1980a.

Torres VE, Velosa JA, Jolly KE, et al: The progression of vesicoureteral nephropathy. Ann Int Med 92:776, 1980b.

Tremewan RN, Bailey RR, Little TMJ, et al: Diagnosis of gross vesico-ureteric reflux using ultrasonography. Br J Urol 48:431, 1976.

Van Gool JD: Bladder infection and pressure. In Reflux Nephropathy. Edited by J Hodson, P Kincaid-Smith. New York, Masson Publishing USA, 1979, pp 181–189.

Van Gool J, Tanagho EA: External sphincter activity and recurrent urinary tract infections in girls. Urology 10:348, 1977.

Walker DR III, Richard GA, Fennell RS, et al: Renal growth and scarring in kidneys with reflux and a concentrating defect. J Urol 129:784, 1983.

Walker RD, Duckett J, Bartone F, et al: Screening school children for urologic disease. Pediatrics 60:239, 1977.

Wallace DMA, Rothwell DL, Williams DI: The long-term follow-up of surgically treated vesicoureteric reflux. Br J Urol 50:479, 1978.

Wein HA, Schoenberg HW: A review of 402 girls with recurrent urinary tract infections. J Urol 107:329, 1972.

Weiss S, Conway JJ: The technique of direct radionuclide cystography. Appl Radiol 4:133, 1975.

Weiss RM, Schiff M Jr, Lytton B: Late obstructions after ureteroneocystostomy. J Urol 106:144, 1971.

Whalley PJ, Cunningham FG: Short-term vs. continuous antibiotic therapy for asymptomatic bacteriuria in pregnancy. Obstet Gynecol 49:292, 1977.

Williams DI: Commentary at International Pediatric Nephrology Association Meeting, Helsinki, Finland, 1977.

Williams DI: Obstructive uropathy: the urethra. In Urology in Childhood. Edited by DI Williams. Berlin, Springer-Verlag, 1974, pp 207–229.

Williams DI: The ureter, the urologist and the pediatrician. Proc R Soc Lond 63:595, 1970.

Williams DI, Eckstein HB: Surgical treatment of reflux in children. Br J Urol 37:12, 1965.

Williams GL, Davies DKL, Evans KT, et al: Vesicoureteral reflux in patients with bacteriuria in pregnancy. Lancet 2:1202, 1968.

Willscher MK, Bauer SB, Zammuto PJ, et al: Infection of the urinary tract after antireflux surgery. J Pediatr 89:743, 1976.

Willscher MK, Bauer SB, Zammuto PJ, et al: Renal growth and urinary tract infection following antireflux surgery in infants and children. J Urol 115:722, 1976.

Winter CC: Vesicoureteral Reflux and Its Treatment. New York, Appleton-Century-Crofts, Meredith Corp., 1969.

Woodard JR, Filardi G: The demonstration of vesicoureteral reflux under general anesthesia. J Urol 116:501, 1976.

Young HH, Wesson MB: The anatomy and surgery of the trigone. Arch Surg 3:1, 1921.

Surgical Correction of Vesicoureteral Reflux

PANAYOTIS P. KELALIS

There is now universal agreement about the role of surgery in the treatment of vesicoureteral reflux, at least in the majority of cases. Such surgical treatment is necessary to correct some of the deformities that cause incompetence of the ureterovesical angle, even though the degree of incompetence that justifies such treatment is still, to a small extent, a matter of debate.

It is now well established that the role that infection plays in causing incompetence of the ureterovesical junction (and thereby causing secondary reflux) has been overestimated in the past—reflux persists in most children long after infection has been eliminated. Furthermore, a natural tendency exists for vesicoureteral reflux to improve or cease with time (Aladjem et al, Edwards et al). Among children followed for 9 to 15 years, reflux disappeared in 80 per cent of those in whom ureteral dilatation was absent but in only 41 per cent of those with dilatation; the conclusion was that dilatation of the ureter is an important factor affecting the outcome of nonoperative treatment (Smellie and Normand, 1979). Thus, reflux is likely to cease when it is mild and the kidneys are unscarred, but scarring of the kidneys per se does not appear to have an adverse influence on the resolution of reflux. Accumulating clinical and experimental data suggest that, in the absence of infection or obstruction, such reflux is a benign phenomenon producing neither anatomic nor functional derangement of the kidney involved, at least for several years (King et al, 1972). Exceptions to this have rarely been recorded.

However, evidence has been presented that the water hammer effect of reflux, even in the absence of infection, may have a detrimental effect on renal function (Helin et al). Significant improvement after antireflux surgery in children with impaired renal function also was recorded (Mundy et al), but such conclusions are not generally supported by similar studies (Torres et al). Improvement in renal concentrating ability also can occur after successful antireflux surgery (Uehling and Wear).

Stickler et al described a group of children who had reflux without evidence of urinary infection and who had progressive renal deterioration. These children were said to have interstitial nephritis rather than chronic pyelonephritis. Experience with this small fraction of the large number of children with vesicoureteral reflux can hardly be extrapolated as evidence that sterile reflux has a damaging effect on the kidney, especially when the cause-and-effect relationship between the reflux and the changes in the kidney has not been conclusively demonstrated and the probability exists that other factors may be involved, including the likelihood of unrecognized urinary infection in early childhood. Nonetheless, the prevalence of hypertension in patients with renal scarring secondary to reflux is a significant feature in those in whom end-stage renal failure develops (Smellie and Normand, 1976). Of greater significance is the finding by Savage et al that, in normotensive children with reflux nephropathy, plasma renin levels are increased. A disturbing number of children with renal scars—up to one fifth of those who underwent antireflux surgery—were hypertensive 10 years later (Wallace et al). Others reported return of blood pressure to normal levels after ureteroneocystostomy, at least in some cases (Hicks et al).

According to Murnaghan (1972, 1974), any patient who reaches adulthood with persistent reflux caused by an immature or incompetent ureterovesical junction is likely to demonstrate evidence of renal damage on roentgenologic examination. This may be a somewhat exaggerated view, not necessarily confirmed by others, but even a cursory review of recent reports of reflux in adults establishes that most of these patients have renal damage demonstrable by excretory urography and that in many instances they have functional derangement as well (Estes and Brooks; Markland and Kelly; Salvatierra et al). Clearly, then, if the potential of reflux for causing renal damage is to be accurately assessed, it is in the adult that one must examine the problem. Once this is done, the conclusion is inescapable: Permanent reflux places the kidney at great risk. This leads to the question, How does one distinguish those children in whom reflux is of a temporary kind (and therefore self-terminating and not damaging to the kidney) from those who have permanent reflux? The former can be treated non-operatively. For the latter, surgical correction is justified.

The urologist can become increasingly adept at predicting the eventual outcome on the basis of cystographic and endoscopic findings, the former relating to the degree of reflux (Winberg et al) and the latter to the morphology of the ureterovesical junction (Lyon et al). In this way, one can distinguish permanent reflux from temporary reflux with reasonable accuracy. Early reports lauding the nonoperative approach — the so-called expectant treatment of reflux — have been overoptimistic, and the reported success rate for this approach appears to be decreasing as the follow-up period lengthens (Fisher and Darling; King et al, 1972).

A patient cannot be considered cured on the basis of a single negative follow-up cystourethrographic study. Reflux frequently appears on subsequent examinations, without any symptoms or urinary infection, and therefore the evanescent nature of reflux must always be taken into consideration in the planning of rational therapy. In the light of recent reports, it appears that a significant group of children with reflux will have it permanently (Blight and O'Shaughnessy; King et al, 1972). Therefore, in this group, expectant treatment is neither definitive nor advisable, because the probability of eventual damage to the kidney is high. A child who, upon careful overall evaluation, is considered unlikely to outgrow the reflux should be a candidate for early surgical correction (Kelalis, 1974).

ANATOMIC CONSIDERATIONS: URETEROVESICAL JUNCTION

Many anatomic and physiologic studies have attempted to elucidate the delicate mechanism of the ureterovesical junction by attempting to define both its structural features and its functional characteristics. The conclusions of the many observers who have studied this problem often conflict and diverge. However, there is enough uniformity of opinion — at least as to the major factors that affect the competence of the ureterovesical angle — to allow some valid conclusions (Hutch et al, 1961; Tanagho and Hutch;

Woodburne, 1964). The anatomic features that are characteristic of the normal valve mechanism of the ureterovesical junction include an oblique entry of the ureter into the bladder, an adequate length of its submucosal segment, and, especially, the ratio of the length to the diameter of the ureter (Stephens and Lenaghan).

All agree that the arrangement of muscle fibers in the intravesical ureter is solely longitudinal. These fibers continue beyond the ureteral orifice into the trigone, where they meet fibers from the opposite side. Thus, a ureterotrigonal continuity (or complex) is formed. It has been shown that this complex acts as a single functional unit; experimental interruption of the unit leads to incompetence and vesicoureteral reflux (Tanagho et al, 1965). The longitudinal fibers of the ureter are probably the most significant firm attachment of the ureter to the bladder, a point of utmost surgical significance. Other connections between the ureter and the bladder in the forms of slings or fascia have been suggested (Hutch, 1958), but their existence has been questioned by other investigators (Woodburne, 1964).

The well-established continuity between the ureter and the trigone prevents excessive mobility of the orifice by fixing it in position. The submucosal tunnel is thus enabled to persist or elongate with progressive filling of the bladder, and the valvelike action of the structure is thereby maintained or enhanced. At the beginning of micturition, further stress is put on the region of the ureterovesical junction because of contraction of the bladder detrusor and subsequent increase in intravesical pressure. This stress can at times herniate the ureteral orifice through the wall of the bladder, especially when the ureterotrigonal continuity is deficient or compromised by maldevelopment of the trigonal region and lateral placement of the ureteral orifice. Such herniation cannot occur when the ureterovesical junction is in a normal state, because the ureter is then firmly attached.

The factor most important in maintaining the one-way characteristic of the ureterovesical junction is the occlusion of the ureteral lumen as the increase in intravesical pressure presses it against the detrusor muscle. For this to occur, it is essential that the orifice be immobile (to allow persistence of the submucosal tunnel) and that detrusor support be adequate. Paraureteral diverticula amply demonstrate the dynamics of the ureterovesical angle because, as the bladder fills, they tend to enlarge and obliterate the tunnel by extravesically displacing the intramural ureter and at times the orifice.

Thus, the ureterovesical angle appears to be a simple one-way flap that functions in a passive manner. Other factors also may have a bearing on its competence. For example, the longitudinal fibers of the ureter may contract, acting as a ureteric sphincter that occludes the ureteral lumen and thus prevents retrograde flow of urine. In this regard, Tanagho et al (1969) described muscular deficiency of the wall of the intravesical ureter in patients with primary reflux; the degree of deficiency was variable and usually correlated with the degree of incompetence of the ureterovesical junction.

Increases in both the frequency and the amplitude of ureteral peristalsis as a response to an increase in intravesical pressure generate sufficient pressures to empty the distal ureter (Scott and De Luca, 1960a; 1960b) and therefore may play a part in the early stages of the development of reflux, but it is unlikely that this can prevent reflux for prolonged periods if the ureterovesical angle is deranged.

In the final analysis, there is divergence of opinion as to the functional characteristics of the ureterovesical junction, but this is of little clinical significance. All are agreed that if reflux is to be prevented, the ureter must have a firm fixation. Furthermore, the passive nature of the mechanism of the ureterovesical angle is well demonstrated by the fact that reflux cannot be produced in the postmortem specimen.

From the foregoing discussion, one can surmise that the revised ureterovesical junction should not be expected to function as precisely or adaptably as the normal structure would, but it should permit urine to drain freely from the ureter into the bladder without allowing reflux or causing hydronephrosis.

Ideally, therefore, ureteroneocystostomy should produce a straight ureteral course, a submucosal ureter within a well-developed tunnel of a length commensurate with the size of the ureter, a ureteral hiatus located in an immobile portion of the bladder base, and, most important, a good fixation of the ureter without undue tension on the anastomosis. Removing the distal end of the ureter should not be necessary as a routine measure and probably is best reserved for those cases in which there is reflux along with some func-

tional or anatomic obstruction (Weiss and Lytton).

DIAGNOSTIC EVALUATION

One should defer routine diagnostic evaluation until the child has recovered from any episode of active urinary infection, because it is possible that the reflux may be secondary to the infection. Bacteriuria in itself is not considered a contraindication to such evaluation, even though sterile urine is preferable. In addition to a careful taking of the history, physical examination, investigation of renal function, and bacteriologic studies of the urine, cystourethrography with fluoroscopy and excretory urography should be axiomatic. Cystography need not be postponed when infection fails to respond to therapy. Knowing that reflux is present may change the therapeutic approach, and a catheter is helpful for a few days if reflux is recognized and the fever does not abate.

RADIOGRAPHIC EVALUATION. Even though it is invaluable in demonstrating the state of the renal parenchyma, the excretory urogram simply shows the anatomic caliber of the collecting system. In contrast, cystourethrography displays the functional and dynamic characteristics of the urinary tract during voiding. Frequently, a minimal ureteral dilatation seen on excretory urography may convert to gross ureteral dilatation during reflux, a most important prognostic consideration regarding the outcome of antireflux surgery (Fig. 15 – 13).

If reflux is demonstrated, ureteral peristalsis should be observed under fluoroscopy. Retrograde peristalsis is normal when reflux occurs and is not a contraindication to surgery. Any evidence of delayed emptying of the ureteral contents into the bladder after voiding suggests an abnormal distal ureteral segment and concomitant ureterovesical obstruction. Weiss and Lytton observed that in approximately 10 per cent of ureters with reflux, some degree of associated ureterovesical junction obstruction was also present. In this situation, the ureter is narrowed in its most distal portion, and microscopic examination may reveal an increase of fibrous tissue with muscular disruption. The resultant rigidity of the distal segment permits reflux and also provides an element of obstruction.

Cystourethrography also may furnish evidence of infravesical obstruction in boys, al-

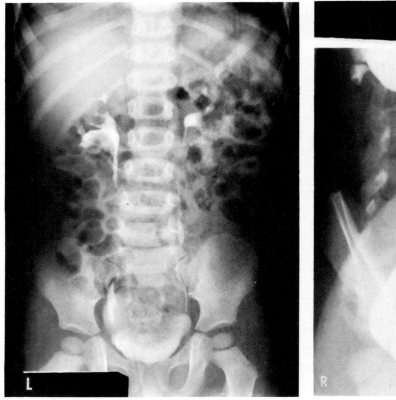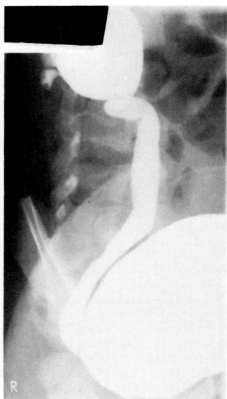

Figure 15 – 13. *Left,* Excretory urogram, showing minimal dilatation of right ureter. *Right,* Cystourethrogram showing reflux in same ureter with gross dilatation. (From Kelalis PP: Proper perspective on vesicoureteral reflux. Mayo Clinic Proc 46:807, 1971.)

though it has been disappointing in this respect when used in girls (Shopfner). No reliable correlation of bladder pressure with the appearance of reflux has been established.

CYSTOSCOPIC EVALUATION. Cystoscopy serves to exclude the presence of vesical diverticula, neuropathy, dyssynergia manifested by trabeculation, and infravesical obstruction. By this examination, measurable deficiencies of the submucosal tunnel can be noted, but this fails to take into consideration the diameter of the ureter involved (Ireland and Cass). The position and shape of the orifice also have a bearing on the competence of the ureterovesical angle.

Thus, cystourethrography can be used to establish some of the functional characteristics of the upper urinary tract and, to a lesser degree, of the bladder and urethra per se. Cystoscopy can exclude obstruction and can confirm that the neural mechanism of micturition appears intact. Primary reflux is most likely to be associated with some degree of ureterovesical angle incompetence evidenced by lateral ectopy of an abnormal ureteral ori-

fice or with measurable deficiencies of the submucosal tunnel or with both.

On the basis of these examinations, one can predict with fairly good accuracy which child is likely to have permanent reflux and is therefore unlikely to be benefited by a trial of nonoperative management.

Selection of Patients for Ureteroneocystostomy

Vesicoureteral reflux in an undilated system (grade I or II, international classification) is likely to cease, and therefore it is not a surgical problem unless, of course, the urine is chronically infected. Nonetheless, the clear understanding at all times that surgery can be elected when nonoperative treatment fails is an important aspect of such expectant treatment.

In general, factors pointing to lifelong reflux should suggest the need for early surgery. These are largely anatomic and include paraureteral diverticula large enough to displace the orifice with bladder filling and ureteral ectopia, especially when they are associated with lack of a discernible submucosal tunnel (a golf-hole orifice). Even though vesicoureteral reflux into only the lower segment of a complete duplication is not in itself an absolute indication for surgery when the anatomic derangement of the ureterovesical angle is relatively mild, early surgical intervention is often preferable. Because spontaneous resolution of reflux in a dilated system is unlikely in most cases, it can be argued that early surgery is the more "conservative" approach because it eliminates the need for continuous antibiotic treatment for many years. Reflux in a grossly dilated and tortuous system is a surgical problem, as is the identification of concomitant reflux and obstruction. Renal scarring in itself is not an indication for surgery, but the rare appearance of new renal scars or the progression of an old one suggest recurrent infection, which usually should be further prevented by antireflux surgery. Intrarenal reflux in association with urinary infection is an important indication for surgery unless the infection is readily controlled (Fig. 15-14).

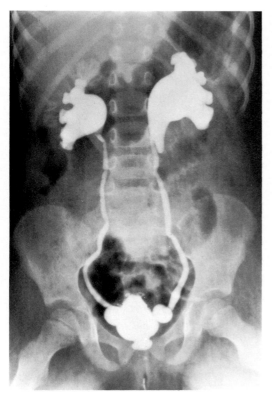

Figure 15-14. Reflux and caliceal-tubular backflow on right side.

Irrespective of the grade of reflux, repeated failure of medical treatment to control infection also points to the need for surgery.

The hazards of continuous prolonged chemotherapy coupled with constant supervision and frequent examinations and visits to the physician may produce severe psychologic problems, which should be weighed against the benefits of early surgery. Poor compliance in taking antibiotics or returning for urine examinations is a definite indication for surgery, and children in families who, because of social or geographic situations, are not likely to follow a strict medical regimen are probably often best served by early surgery. Lastly, the disappearance of reflux at puberty does not occur often enough to justify delay of surgical treatment in the hope of spontaneous cure (Edwards et al).

URETERONEOCYSTOSTOMY

General Surgical Principles

The multiplicity of antireflux procedures available and the countless variations employed by individual surgeons reflect the intense interest evoked by the problem and not the inadequacy of any one method. The various techniques employed are generally concerned with intravesical or extravesical lengthening of the intramural ureter (suprahiatal repair) or with advancing the ureteral orifice toward the vesical neck (infrahiatal repair). A combination of these maneuvers seems ideal. Some procedures are more popular than others, but all are acceptable, provided that comparable results can be achieved by the surgeons who are using them. A rigid, standardized technique should not be followed.

It is preferable that ureteroneocystostomy be done in the absence of infection and not sooner than several weeks after an acute urinary infection has been eliminated. If the procedure is done too soon after a urinary infection, edema of the mucosa adds to the difficulties of an already delicate operation.

A Pfannenstiel incision is preferable, but a midline suprapubic incision may be used, especially when extensive work on the ureters, such as straightening or caliber reduction, is contemplated.

If the bladder is opened transversely, care should be taken not to extend the incision too far laterally, lest it interfere with the creation

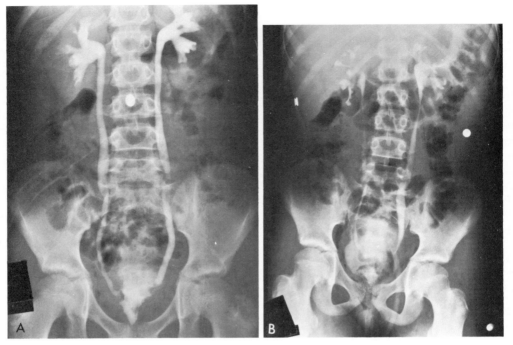

Figure 15–15. *A*, Ten-minute excretory urogram on fourth postoperative day. *B*, Same, 3 months later.

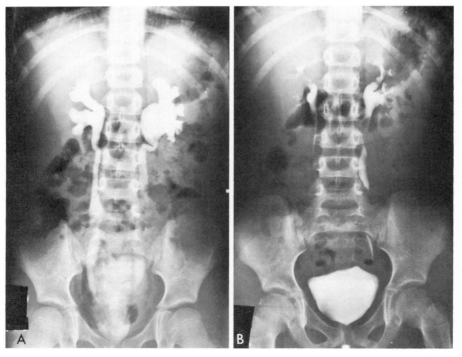

Figure 15–16. Bilateral distal ureteral advancement and tunneling. *A*, Twenty-minute excretory urogram on fifth postoperative day. Note edema of bladder wall. *B*, Same, 4 weeks later.

of the submucosal tunnels. If, rarely, preoperative evaluation suggests obstruction or dysfunction at the vesical neck, raising the possibility of its revision, the bladder incision should be in the form of a V, with the apex exactly at the vesical neck for possible revision. Careful dissection of the ureter with preservation of its adventitia is essential; it should not be handled with forceps.

Fine chromic catgut, 5-0 or possibly 6-0, should be used for the anastomosis of the ureter to the bladder. If a suprapubic catheter is used, it should be placed high in the dome of the bladder to avoid irritation of the base. Prior to its removal, the catheter can be clamped in order to test bladder function. Some surgeons prefer to use a urethral catheter only, especially in girls, in whom a large size can be inserted.

A single 10-minute excretory urogram before dismissal will assure satisfactory drainage through the reconstructed ureterovesical junction. Minimal ureterectasis is usually present. In most cases, definitive urographic and cystographic re-evaluation is deferred for several months (Figs. 15 – 15 and 15 – 16). Occasionally the postoperative study shows considerable dilatation. In such instances, urographic re-evaluation within weeks is essential to assure that regression of the hydronephrosis has occurred. Koff et al suggested the diuretic radionuclide urogram as an alternative means of assessing both early and late drainage characteristics of the ureterovesical anastomosis. If results of the initial postoperative study within the first postoperative year are satisfactory, serial urographic examinations are scheduled at 18 months, 3 years, and 5 years from the time of surgery. Renal sonography is an alternative method of follow-up in these children. If the early postoperative urogram shows no obstruction, development of obstruction in later years is unlikely. Reappearance of reflux many years after an apparently successful operation occasionally occurs; therefore, periodic cystographic examinations are necessary. A single postoperative cystographic study is inadequate evidence that the reflux has been permanently arrested. Nuclear cystographic examinations — to diminish exposure to radiation, especially if symptoms recur — are advisable.

Suppressive chemotherapy for several weeks to 3 months, until healing has been completed, is desirable.

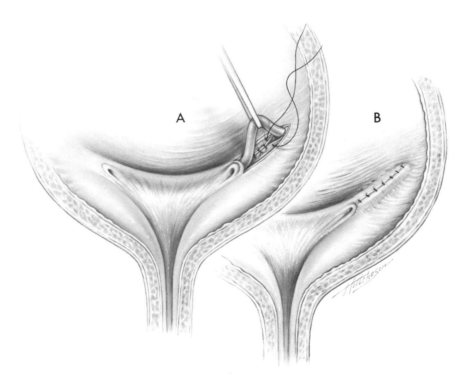

Figure 15 – 17. Hutch-1 technique of ureteroneocystostomy.

Suprahiatal Repair

Hutch-I Technique

In the transvesical approach of the Hutch-I technique, the mucosa covering the roof of the ureter is incised and then undermined on each side. The detrusor musculature alone is closed behind the ureter; next, the mucosa is closed over it (Fig. 15–17). This technique has been criticized because (1) it leaves the orifice in an abnormal lateral position, and (2) it does not strengthen the weak fixation of the ureter to the trigone. Also, it cannot possibly correct any kinks, adhesions, or redundancy. It can be applied only to the normal or slightly dilated ureter, because ureteral caliber reduction is not possible.

If rigid criteria are applied in the selection of patients, however, excellent results can be achieved (Palken). It is particularly useful in the presence of severe bladder trabeculation due to obstruction or neuropathic bladder, since trabeculation may interfere with proper tunnel creation. Because distal ureteral continuity (and blood supply) is not interrupted, it is also useful when the blood supply of the ureter has been compromised above by the performance of pyelostomy or ureterostomy.

Lich-Grégoir Technique

Revision of the ureterovesical angle also may be accomplished extravesically, without opening the bladder, by the Lich-Grégoir technique. The ureter is dissected down to the ureteral hiatus, and the vesical musculature is incised for 2 to 3 cm upward. The ureter is embedded under the mucosa, and the vesical musculature is closed behind it. The tunnel must be fashioned vertically on the posterior bladder wall, and the incision must not interfere with ureterotrigonal continuity (Marberger et al). The operation achieves the same objectives as the Hutch-I, and the final arrangement is identical (Fig. 15–18). Even though the results are variable and the reports conflicting, it is the preferred operation at several medical centers (Arap et al, 1971, 1981; Grégoir and Schulman).

Politano-Leadbetter Technique

Both one of the most widely used and one of the most successful techniques of ureteroneocystostomy is the Politano-Leadbetter technique. A circular incision around the ureteral orifice frees it from the trigone. Dissection of the intravesical ureter is carried transvesically and then brought inside the bladder via a generous new hiatus above and lateral to the original one.

A submucosal tunnel is developed from the site of the new hiatus down to the original one, and the ureteral orifice is sutured back to its previous position. Many urologists discard the ureteral orifice and terminal ureter, particularly when an obstructive component may be present. They then simply anastomose the cut end of the ureter to the mucosa of the bladder. Thus, a long intravesical ureteral segment lies submucosally and is supported by intact and unincised vesical detrusor (Fig. 15–19). This technique achieves most of the basic objectives of ureteroneocystostomy and can be applied to almost any situation requiring revision of the ureterovesical junction. It lends itself to straightening of kinks, excision of redundancy, and reduction of the caliber of the ureter.

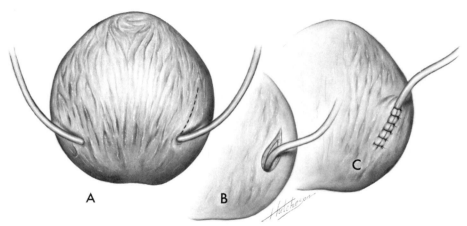

Figure 15–18. Lich-Grégoir technique of ureteroneocystostomy.

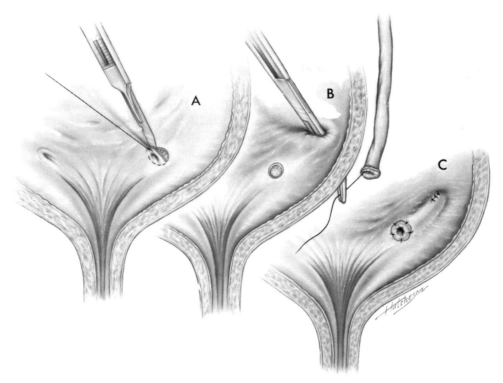

Figure 15–19. Politano-Leadbetter technique of ureteroneocystostomy.

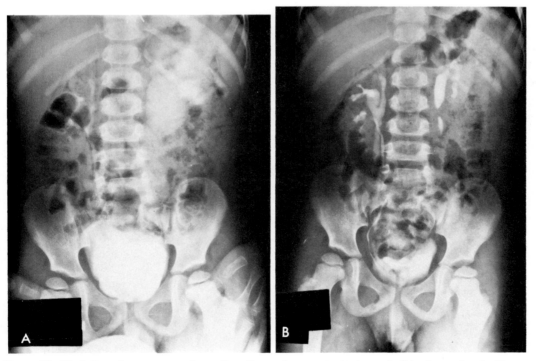

Figure 15–20. *A,* Excretory urogram 3 months after ureteroneocystostomy. Left hydronephrosis. At operation, left ureter was found to traverse lumen of sigmoid. Secondary ureteroneocystostomy. *B,* Postoperative urogram.

One hazardous aspect (and criticism) of the Politano-Leadbetter procedure is that it is done completely intravesically, and kinking of the ureter therefore can occur at the level of the new hiatus, which is developed blindly. In addition, the ureter may be inadvertently transposed through the peritoneal cavity and, at times, through bowel (Fig. 15–20), or it may be wrapped around a vessel such as the uterine artery. Many surgeons therefore prefer combining an extravesical with an intravesical approach to make certain that a straight, uninhibited course of the ureter results (Tocci et al).

The Politano-Leadbetter procedure is difficult to perform in the severely trabeculated or inflamed bladder because the mucosal flap is hard to raise under such circumstances.

Paquin Ureteroneocystostomy

The Paquin ureteroneocystostomy procedure (Fig. 15–21) combines transvesical and extravesical approaches and allows correction of any type of problem in this area, congenital or acquired. It is ideal for use when revision of the ureterovesical angle is necessary after failure of ureteroneocystostomy (Fig. 15–22).

The Paquin technique differs from the Politano-Leadbetter in that the vesical wall is split open to the chosen site of the new hiatus. The terminal ureter may be severed and left in place. A submucosal tunnel is developed from the ureter's new superior point of entry to just below and medial to the original ureteral orifice. The cut end of the ureter is everted to form a cuff or a nipple before it is sutured into place, but this is rarely practiced. A stent is advisable. Excellent results have been reported with this operation (Woodard and Keats).

We frequently use this technique in secondary procedures, so that extravesical mobilization is necessary. The ureter is often short. A vesicopsoas hitch is an important adjunct to the technique, allowing a long intravesical

Figure 15–21. Paquin procedure.

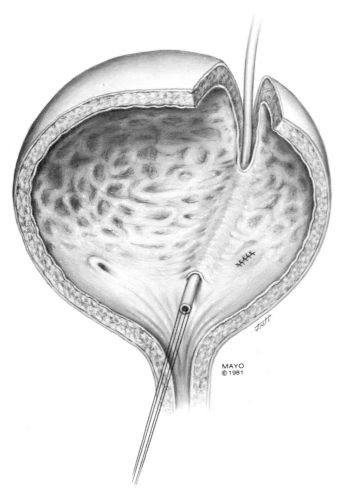

MAYO
© 1981

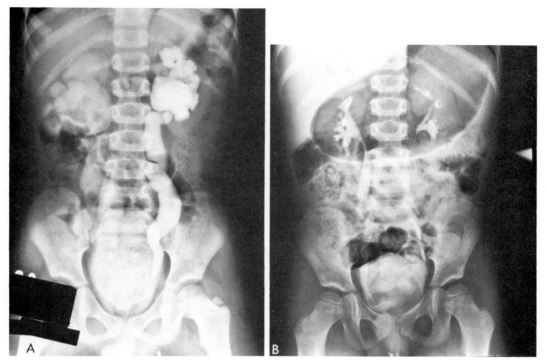

Figure 15–22. *A*, Failed bilateral ureteroneocystostomy. Bilateral distal ureteral stenosis. *B*, Excretory urogram after bilateral revision of ureterovesical junction. Paquin technique.

ureter so that reflux is avoided and holding the new ureteral hiatus at a fixed point so that both kinking and obstruction are prevented (Cukier et al, 1981). When a psoas hitch is contemplated, the bladder should be opened obliquely on its anterolateral surface. The corresponding site of the bladder is simply

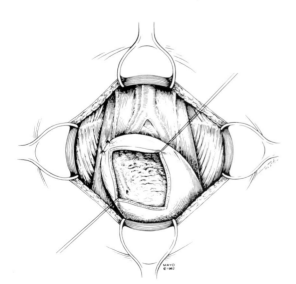

Figure 15–23. Psoas hitch.

brought up and sutured with chromic catgut to the psoas muscle lateral to the iliac vessels (Prout and Koontz) (Fig. 15–23).

Infrahiatal Repair

Glenn-Anderson Technique

The advantage of the Glenn-Anderson advancement technique is that the ureter enters the bladder via the normal hiatus, and therefore the chance of kinking or obstruction — so-called J-hooking — of the ureter because of a high ureteral hiatus is virtually eliminated. The infrahiatal principle is applicable only when the ureteral orifices are laterally placed and space exists between the original ureteral hiatus and the vesical meatus for the new intravesical ureter. It is also applicable in situations in which the ureters have been reimplanted high in the bladder wall rather than on the base.

In these procedures, submucosal ureteral length is gained by freeing the intravesical ureter and then advancing the ureteral orifice and simply fixing it closer to the vesical neck. Once the ureter is freed transvesically, a submucosal tunnel can be developed from the

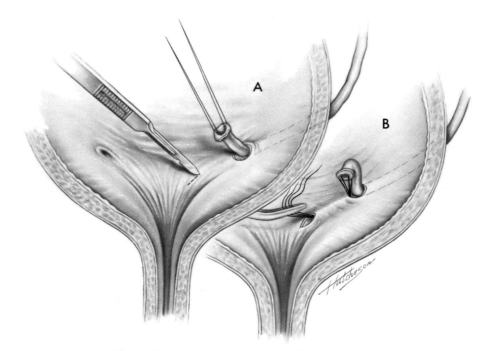

Figure 15–24. Glenn-Anderson technique of ureteroneocystostomy.

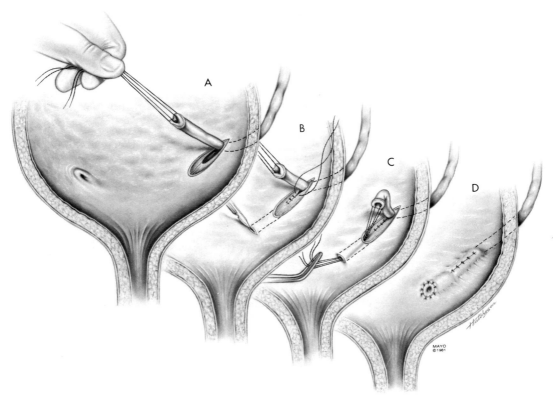

Figure 15–25. Modification of Glenn-Anderson technique.

ureteral hiatus toward the vesical neck. Creation of the tunnel distally is sometimes difficult. In some cases, it is prudent to incise the bladder mucosa in the direction of the tunnel and elevate flaps laterally by simple dissection. The ureter can then be placed on the muscular bed and the mucosa sutured over it. The ureter is sutured onto the raw trigonal muscular edge as described by Glenn and Anderson (1967) (Fig. 15–24). No attempt should be made to narrow the internal hiatus unless it has been severely traumatized or has been widened by inept dissection; doing so might produce angulation at this point. This technique is simple, can be accomplished rapidly, avoids extravesical dissection, and places the ureter in a proper physioanatomic position. The results have been highly satisfactory (Gonzales et al, 1972; Glenn and Anderson, 1977).

Figure 15–25 shows a modification of the above technique. The entrance of the ureter is moved posterolaterally, thus increasing the length of the submucosal tunnel.

Cohen Advancement Procedure

This surgical technique, most widely used in Europe, has also gained popularity elsewhere. Sufficient mobilization of the ureters is accomplished transvesically. Separate submucosal tunnels are created for each ureter across the bladder base, so that each ureter opens on the opposite side from its hiatus (Fig. 15–26). Because of this positioning, problems may arise if retrograde ureteral catheterization becomes necessary (Lamesch). This difficulty can be bypassed by Cystocath puncture of the bladder, which permits ureteral catheterization. This technique is simple, safe, and reliable for prevention of reflux (Cukier et al, 1975), and, in our experience, it is particularly applicable when reimplantation of the ureters is required after trigonal tubularization for urinary incontinence.

Combined Suprahiatal and Infrahiatal Repair

If the new ureteral hiatus is placed posterolaterally on the mobile portion of the vesical base or bladder wall during a suprahiatal repair, it may be stretched or displaced when the bladder fills. The result is intermittent, and at times permanent, ureteral obstruction —J-hooking of the ureter. Liberal mobilization of the ureter does not prevent this. Rather, the hiatus must be created posteromedially on a relatively immobile part of the

Figure 15–26. Cohen advancement procedure.

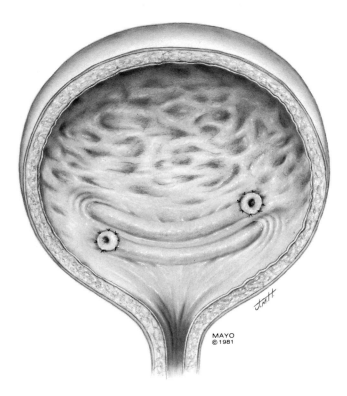

MAYO
©1981

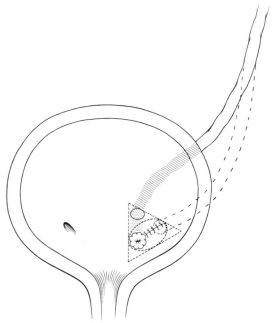

Figure 15–27. Principle of combined suprahiatal and infrahiatal repair. (From Kelalis PP: The present status of surgery for vesicoureteral reflux. Urol Clin North Am 1:457, 1974.)

bladder, and the submucosal tunnel can be lengthened by advancing the ureteral orifice. Because a tunnel in this position has good support and changes little with bladder filling, a shorter than usual length suffices (Kelalis, 1974). The length of the tunnel should bear an approximately 3 : 1 ratio to the anticipated diameter of the ureter. This principle is depicted diagrammatically in Figure 15–27.

The operation should be performed transvesically so that the nerve supply to the bladder is compromised as little as possible. When there is any doubt about the proper position of the ureter, extravesical exploration should be resorted to. From Figure 15–27 it can be clearly seen that unless the ureter is sufficiently mobilized, an acute angulation may occur in its new course into the bladder.

The ureter is catheterized, and traction sutures of two different materials (silk and catgut) are placed inferomedial and supralateral to the orifice. The purpose of the sutures is twofold: (1) by applying slight tension on them, the operator can raise the mobile ureter from the base of the bladder, and (2) they

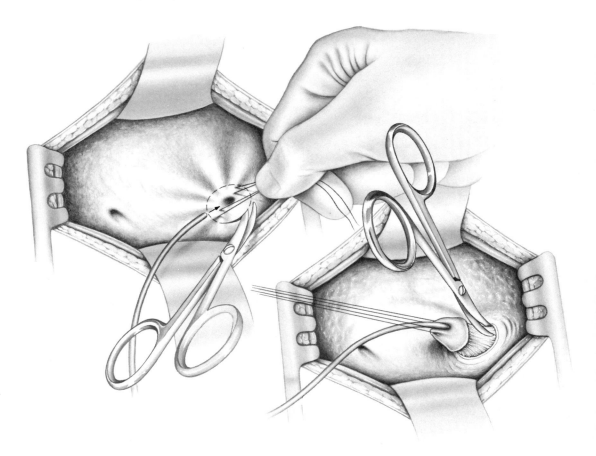

Figure 15–28. Combined suprahiatal and infrahiatal technique of ureteroneocystostomy.

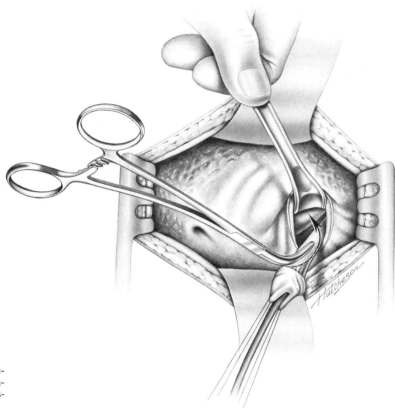

Figure 15–29. Combined suprahiatal and infrahiatal technique of ureteroneocystostomy.

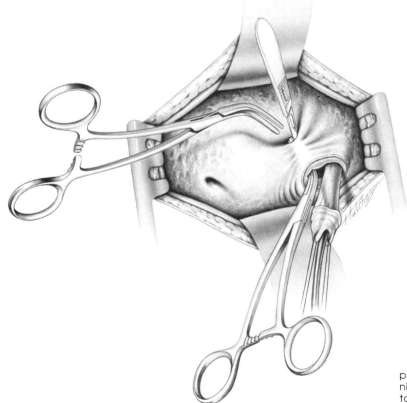

Figure 15–30. Combined suprahiatal and infrahiatal technique of ureteroneocystostomy.

help the operator to identify proper anatomic orientation of the orifice and thus avoid twisting the ureter after its transposition into the bladder.

The mucosal cuff around the orifice is outlined by a circumferential incision, and a plane of cleavage is established between the adventitia of the ureter and the fibers of the bladder (Fig. 15–28). Once this plane is identified, sufficient mobilization of the ureter is easily achieved by using both sharp and blunt dissection.

The base of the bladder is elevated with a vein retractor, and the peritoneal reflection is pushed away from the bladder base, thus ensuring that there is no obstructive element in the new course of the ureter toward its neocystostomy (Fig. 15–29). A right-angle clamp is passed from the old ureteral hiatus outside the bladder to the point where the new hiatus is to be created (Fig. 15–30). Once the tip of this clamp appears in the bladder and the new hiatus is stretched to avoid subsequent narrowing, a second clamp is attached to its tip and guided into the bladder to such a position that it can grasp the traction

sutures and pull the ureter into the bladder via the new hiatus (Fig. 15–31).

The defect of the original hiatus is firmly closed (Fig. 15–32), and a submucosal tunnel is then constructed. The ureter is brought through this tunnel to its final position, which is the most distal (or anteromedial) portion of the mucosal defect. Submucosal injection of saline facilitates the creation of the tunnel.

The ureteral catheter removed after the dissection of the ureter was completed is reinserted and advanced all the way to the kidney to exclude any obvious anatomic obstruction. (The distal end of the ureter is removed only if it has shown functional evidence of obstruction at cystourethrography, in which case it also will be stenotic and will fail to propagate peristaltic activity, or if it has been traumatized during the dissection. In such instances, it is a good policy to use an indwelling ureteral stent for 48 to 72 hours.)

The mucosal cuff of the ureter is sutured to the mucosa of the bladder (Fig. 15–33). The distal sutures should encompass muscle as well as mucosa at the bladder wall, because they serve to anchor the ureter into position

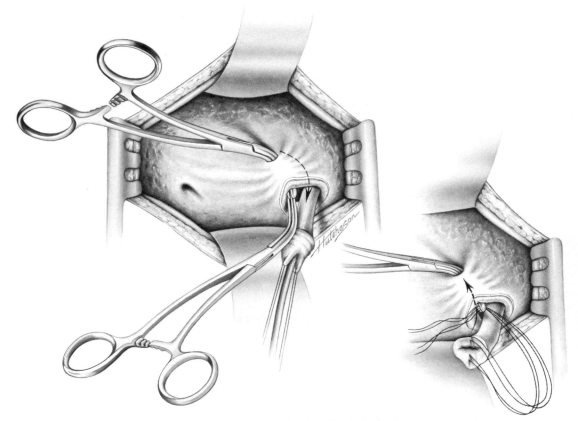

Figure 15–31. Combined suprahiatal and infrahiatal technique of ureteroneocystostomy.

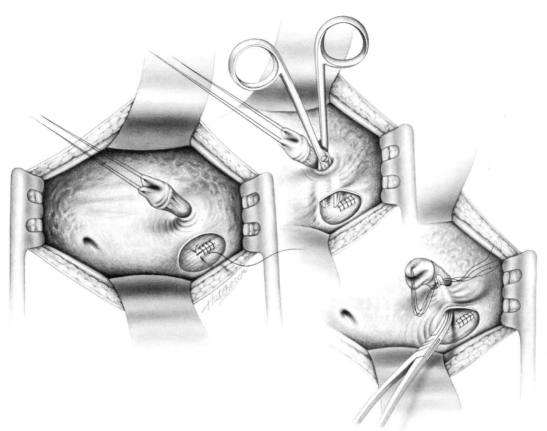

Figure 15–32. Combined suprahiatal and infrahiatal technique of ureteroneocystostomy.

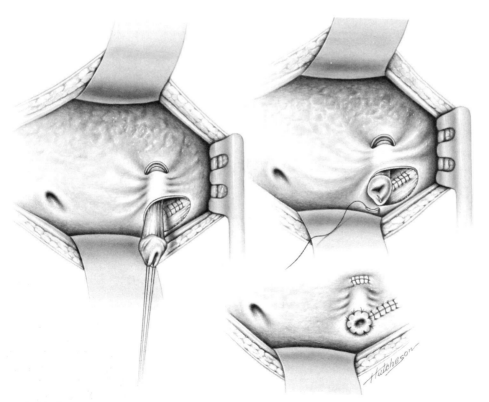

Figure 15–33. Combined suprahiatal and infrahiatal technique of ureteroneocystostomy. (From Kelalis PP: The present status of surgery for vesicoureteral reflux. Urol Clin North Am 1:457, 1974.)

and establish ureterotrigonal continuity. The mucosa at the bladder overlying the original ureteral hiatus is closed in a linear fashion, as is the proximal end of the tunnel. The length of the latter need not exceed 2 to 3 cm, provided that it has been positioned on the base of the bladder, close to the vesical neck.

After appropriate diuresis, the ureteral catheter is removed. If spurts of urine are seen issuing from the reimplanted orifice or orifices, the operation is completed by closure of the bladder.

Use of Catheters and Stents

Gonzalez et al (1978) advocated removal of the urethral catheter within 48 hours of surgery. They thought that with use of this method, bladder spasms would be diminished and patients would therefore receive less medication. Early removal of the catheter would appear to lower the incidence of nosocomial infections, and, most importantly, hospital stay is shortened considerably. So et al carried this a step further, using neither vesical catheters nor ureteral stents, but simply paravesical drainage, postoperatively. None of the postoperative complications in their study were directly attributed to the absence of catheters.

If vesical drainage is used, bladder spasms are prevented by antispasmodics and sedatives. Belladonna and opium suppositories are quite effective, as is oxybutynin chloride (Ditropan) given at regular intervals.

The use of stents in ureteroneocystostomy, as in other types of ureteral surgery, is a matter of debate. Indwelling ureteral catheters are used to avoid possible obstruction by circumventing the effect of edema at the orifice and to maintain ureteral fixation and defunctionalization temporarily. If, on completion of the corrective procedure, the ureteral orifice is seen to spurt clear urine at regular intervals, use of a stent probably is not indicated. Small stents are troublesome because the lumen may become occluded and they may then occlude the ureter, but stenting is probably advisable if the operation is performed in the presence of intractable urinary infection.

The possibility of excessive dissection of or trauma to the ureter, angulation at the ureteral hiatus, diminished ureteral peristalsis secondary to a dilated ureter, or compromised vacularity in the terminal ureter justifies the use of stents. These conditions are likely to be present during reoperation on the ureter. If in doubt, one had probably best use a stent. Silastic tubing of appropriate size and length or small feeding tubes are quite suitable. Stents seldom do harm but may lengthen the hospitalization and will not in themselves prevent subsequent complications when a suitable anatomic reconstruction cannot be achieved.

Preliminary Drainage

When there is a dilated, refluxing aperistaltic ureter with diminished renal function, azotemia, and possibly infection, it is desirable to provide temporary drainage prior to operation on the ureterovesical junction. The use of a suprapubic or urethral catheter for a few days has decided advantages. Otherwise, if drainage for a longer period is required, it is better to divert by cutaneous vesicostomy.

Preliminary drainage should be maintained as long as is necessary to obtain maximal improvement in renal function. The preliminary diversion will also reduce the caliber of the ureter and allow a technically more satisfactory procedure on the ureterovesical angle.

In some infants with severe dilatation and urinary infection, cutaneous vesicostomy for several months to years has decided advantages because it allows the child to reach a size at which surgical correction can be accomplished with a greater degree of success. It is preferable to close the vesicostomy, allow the bladder wall to return to normal, and then proceed with ureteroneocystostomy. Despite the unsatisfactory stoma, this procedure is fully acceptable in the diaper-wearing infant.

At present, the most common indication for supravesical urinary diversion is the obstructed ureteroneocystostomy with rapidly progressing hydroureteronephrosis or unremitting infection in an obstructed megaureter; in this situation, several months must elapse before the reaction subsides enough to permit reoperation. During this time, a temporary supravesical diversion preserves the function of the involved kidney. The advantages of nephrostomy in this situation are that the tube can be inserted percutaneously and can be clamped immediately after reconstruction of the ureterovesical angle, so that urine flow is reestablished promptly after the operation. In doubtful cases, ureteral flow pressure studies can be easily obtained to measure the degree

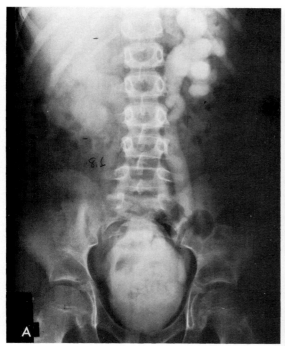

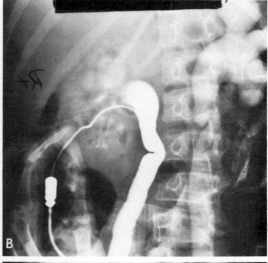

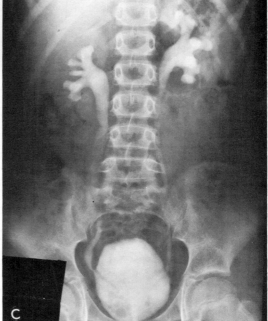

Figure 15–34. A, Bilateral ureteroneocystostomy. Distal ureteral obstruction. B, Right percutaneous nephrostomy. C, Bilateral revision of ureterovesical angles after 5 months with nephrostomy.

of obstruction (or patency) of the junction by objective means (Fig. 15–34).

Postoperative Results

Postoperative results should be judged in the context of the objectives of antireflux surgery, namely, to protect the kidney from the ravages of reflux of infected urine from the bladder and to eliminate residual urine in the upper urinary tract. The two criteria most often considered to judge whether a given procedure is satisfactory are (1) its technical success, i.e., whether reflux has been eliminated without producing hydronephrosis, and (2) its effect on the course of urinary infection (Fig. 15–35).

Surgery offers a reasonable guarantee of success in children with primary vesicoureteral reflux. Experiences in large recent series show that well over 90 per cent and even more than 95 per cent of such surgical procedures are successful technically after a single operation (Gonzales et al, 1972; Palken; Politano, 1963; Woodard and Keats). However,

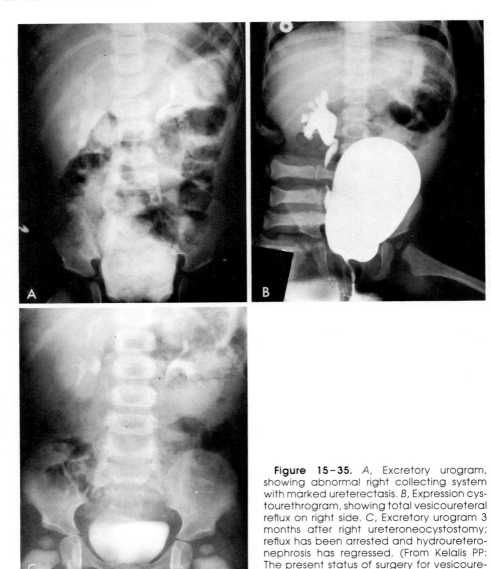

Figure 15-35. *A,* Excretory urogram, showing abnormal right collecting system with marked ureterectasis. *B,* Expression cystourethrogram, showing total vesicoureteral reflux on right side. *C,* Excretory urogram 3 months after right ureteroneocystostomy; reflux has been arrested and hydroureteronephrosis has regressed. (From Kelalis PP: The present status of surgery for vesicoureteral reflux. Urol Clin North Am 1:457, 1974.)

bacteriuria reportedly recurs postoperatively in 10 to 30 per cent of patients. This is approximately the same incidence of bacteriuria as is found in children with no reflux and in those with reflux who are being treated nonoperatively. Girls are affected almost exclusively. Such observations suggest that reflux is not the major or even a minor factor in causing recurrent bacteriuria.

The incidence of clinical pyelonephritis, however, is markedly decreased after antireflux surgery. In the series reported by Govan and Palmer, it decreased from approximately 50 per cent to less than 10 per cent. Willscher et al (1976b) reported that even though infection recurred postoperatively in 21 per cent of their patients, less than 2 per cent had clinical pyelonephritis. In these series, the incidence of postoperative infections, one third of which occurred within 6 months of surgery and while the patient was still receiving antibiotics, did not correlate with either the preoperative urographic appearance or the severity of reflux. Thus, elimination of reflux obviates antibiotic therapy in most children who would otherwise receive continuous prophylaxis, a particularly important point when reflux is associated with significant dilatation because at best the long-term chance of spontaneous resolution is small—less than 40 per cent.

Almost all reports on the surgical treatment

of reflux deal with selected series in which only those patients who have been resistant to medical treatment or have some abnormal features are chosen. In the only published prospective randomized trial between medical and surgical treatments, reported by Scott and Stansfeld (1968a), the authors found a small but significant overall advantage with surgical treatment in decreasing the number of recurrent infections and in stimulating renal growth. Unfortunately, the population sampled was small and probably selective, and the follow-up was short. Because of the accelerated renal growth observed during puberty in medically treated patients with vesicoureteral reflux, this difference may not be significant in the long term. McRae et al suggested that surgery may be more beneficial in patients with gross reflux, in that resumption of normal renal growth follows a successful operation, whereas, with lesser degrees of dilatation, surgical treatment is not likely to affect subsequent events, although the kidneys will grow normally irrespective of the presence or absence of reflux.

Babcock et al considered the effects of unilateral ureteroneocystostomy in unilateral reflux but observed neither radiographic improvement nor a change in the ratio of the size of the refluxing kidney to the normal contralateral kidney after surgery. Surgical correlation of reflux failed to prevent progression of renal scarring in the study by Filly et al (1974b). However, infants with intrarenal reflux showed no progression of renal scarring when surgically treated, whereas progression or development of scars was observed in medically treated patients (Rolleston et al, 1974). This observation is not uniformly accepted, however.

As a result of a carefully conducted retrospective study, Willscher et al (1976b) reported on the effect of antireflux surgery on renal growth. Their series included 94 children (188 kidneys) whose radiographic studies provided adequate urographic data for purposes of comparison. When unilateral reflux without pyelonephritis was present, the refluxing kidney was longer than expected after surgery. When unilateral reflux was associated with pyelonephritis, expected normal renal length was seen, with no accentuated growth. When bilateral reflux and normal kidneys were present, postoperative renal length on both sides was greater than expected. Finally, when bilateral reflux was associated with bilateral pyelonephritis, the

length of each kidney following surgery was greater than expected, as a result of accelerated growth. Therefore, all refluxing kidneys that showed no radiographic evidence of pyelonephritis demonstrated accelerated growth postoperatively. However, the growth of the pyelonephritic kidney was greater than usual postoperatively only when such changes were present bilaterally.

The same authors suggested, in view of these findings, that renal growth in the child with reflux is dependent on a physiologic balance between the two kidneys. Indeed, there is evidence to suggest the existence of a serum factor (renotropin) that could stimulate damaged refluxing units to faster than normal growth after removal of the injury stimulus (Lowenstein and Stern; Silk et al). It would appear from these data that when unilateral pyelonephritis is present, compensation for nephron loss occurs primarily in the opposite kidney.

It should be emphasized now that most studies to date, including those cited, assess renal growth by measurement of renal length alone on the excretory urogram, a determination affected by numerous factors (Hernandez et al). Total mass may be reduced by scar formation, which is not completely reflected by renal length (Fig. 15–36). Hypertrophy of normal parenchyma and the predominantly polar distribution of scars make interpetation of renal size on the basis of renal length unreliable.

Lastly, Merrell and Mowad pointed out that

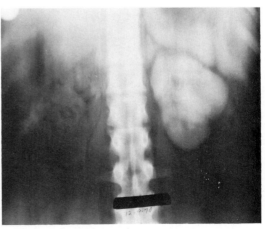

Figure 15–36. Difficulty in interpretation of renal length and growth of kidney. Asymmetrical lateral growth of kidney with reflux nephropathy.

physical growth of prepubertal children with vesicoureteral reflux is accelerated after successful antireflux surgery, a finding that may have a direct relationship to renal size.

Complications

It is clear that surgical treatment offers a good chance of eliminating reflux, but it is not entirely free of risk. In a small but significant number of patients, reflux (although sometimes of a lesser degree than preoperatively) may persist, or obstruction with hydronephrosis may ensue.

Rather surprisingly, reflux appearing on the cystogram made shortly after surgery does not always signify failure. It seems likely that those ureters that reflux postoperatively and then stop represent marginal reimplantations in which the presence of postoperative infection may play a deciding role. Once inflammation subsides, the pliability of the submucosal ureter improves, and the antireflux flap valve mechanism may then become competent, usually within the first postoperative year (Willscher et al, 1976a). However, delayed reappearance of reflux after initial successful outcome has also been observed (Amar, 1978).

Obstruction probably results from acute angulation in the supravesical segment, especially as it enters into the bladder via its newly created orifice. Such angulation is a consequence of the surgeon's failure to free the ureter from its vascular and adventitial connections sufficiently (Fig. 15–37).

Minimal degrees of obstruction may regress with time (Figs. 15–38 and 15–39). Although devascularization of the lower ureter with subsequent stricture can occur, the obstruction or angulation most often appears to be at the new entrance of the ureter into the bladder. Frequently it is intermittent, and it results from angulation of the ureter at its new entrance into the bladder—J-hooking—when the entrance is too far posterolateral. Clearly, infrahiatal repairs eliminate this difficulty, which may at times require revision of the ureterovesical junction. In such instances, a film taken with the bladder empty will show regression of hydroureteronephrosis (Figs. 15–40 to 15–42).

Rarely, obstruction first appears several years after ureteroneocystostomy. This may be the effect of growth on the ureterovesical angle, and the fact that it sometimes appears clearly stresses the need for careful follow-up of the kidneys. However, Broaddus et al, in a study of this problem, concluded that obstructions after antireflux surgery are evident early in the postoperative period and questioned the need for periodic urographic investigation for many years when obstruction is absent in the immediate postoperative period. With the present refinement in techniques, the general incidence of obstruction requiring reoperation ranges between 1.2 and 4 per cent of cases (Randel; Scott, 1977). Revision of the ureterovesical angle, possibly preceded by supravesical diversion in such cases, may be necessary. Surprisingly, the results of reoperation on the ureter are quite satisfactory, probably because of the enrichment of the ureteral blood supply secondary to obstruc-

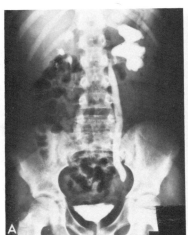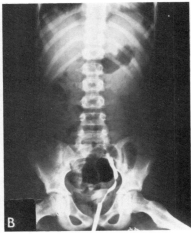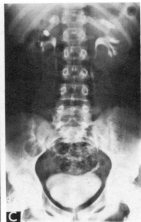

Figure 15–37. Postoperative ureteroneocystostomy. Left ureter hooks around uterine vessels. A, Preoperative excretory urogram. B, Preoperative retrograde ureterogram. C, After revision.

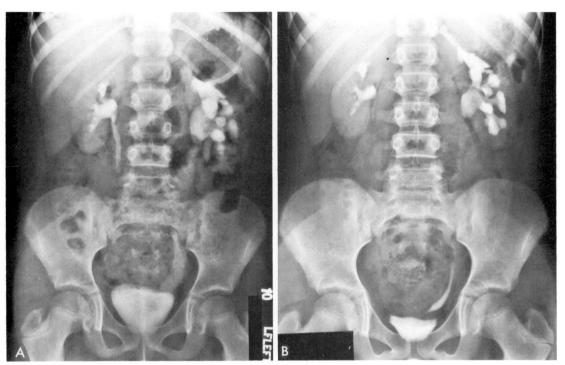

Figure 15–38. Left ureteroneocystostomy. Spontaneous improvement over a 3-year period. Regression of left ureterectasis.

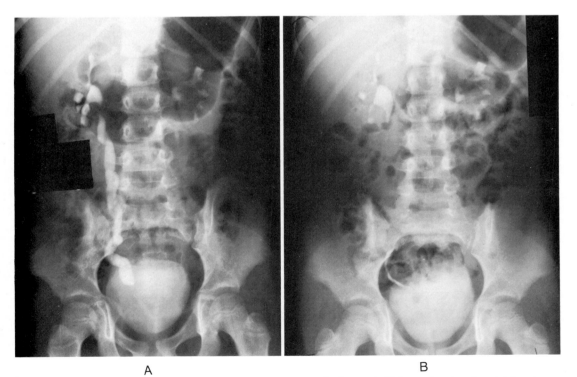

A   B

Figure 15–39. Excretory urograms after right ureteroneocystostomy. *A,* At 6 months, showing right ureterectasis. *B,* Spontaneous improvement 6 months later.

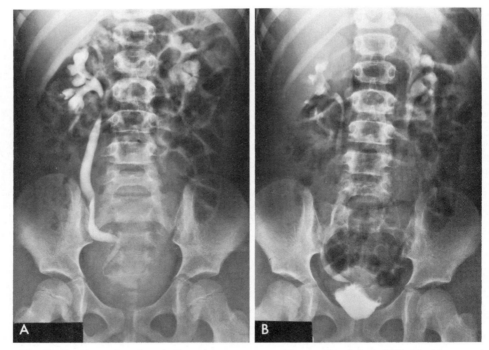

Figure 15–40. Hooking of ureter. *A,* Excretory urogram with bladder full. *B,* With bladder empty. Note regression of dilatation of ureter and straightening of its course.

tion (Hendren, 1974). A triangular flap technique is also quite satisfactory (Manley and Ferrell).

In some children, progressive ureteral dilatation takes place after antireflux surgery, but obstruction cannot be demonstrated in either a retrograde or an antegrade fashion; in these children, reflux is also absent. A possible explanation in these instances is that one is dealing with a form of ureterovesical incoor-

dination resulting in a functional type of obstruction. It is unlikely that a secondary procedure would be of benefit in these instances. When the disorder is unilateral, anastomosis of the dilated ureter to the normal ureter (transureteroureterostomy) should be regarded at least as favorably as, if not in preference to, secondary ureteroneocystostomy (Figs. 15–43 and 15–44).

Persistence of reflux in the reimplanted ure-

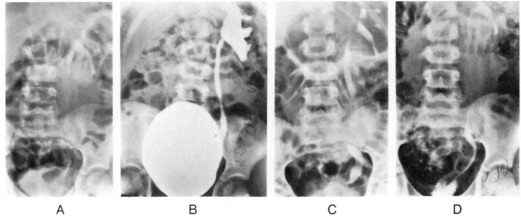

| A | B | C | D |

Figure 15–41. Intermittent ureteral obstruction after ureteroneocystostomy. *A,* Preoperative excretory urogram, showing solitary left kidney. *B,* Cystogram shows total left vesicoureteral reflux. *C,* At 3 months postoperatively, excretory urogram shows ureterectasis. *D,* During same study there is regression of ureteral dilatation with bladder empty.

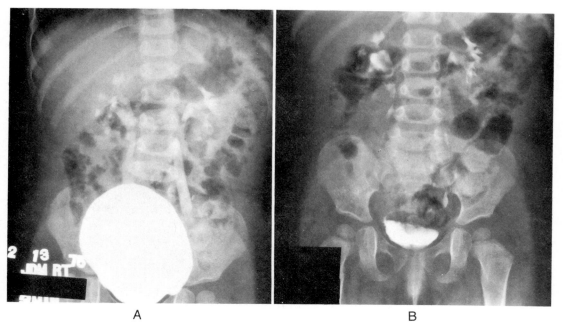

Figure 15–42. Postureteroneocystostomy excretory urograms with bladder full (*A*) and empty (*B*). Note difference in ureteral dilatation. (No reflux demonstrated.)

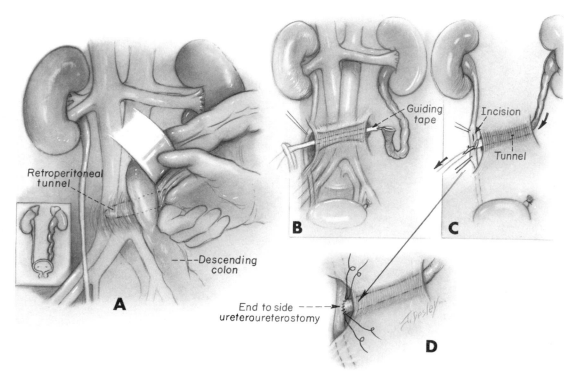

Figure 15–43. Transureteroureterostomy.

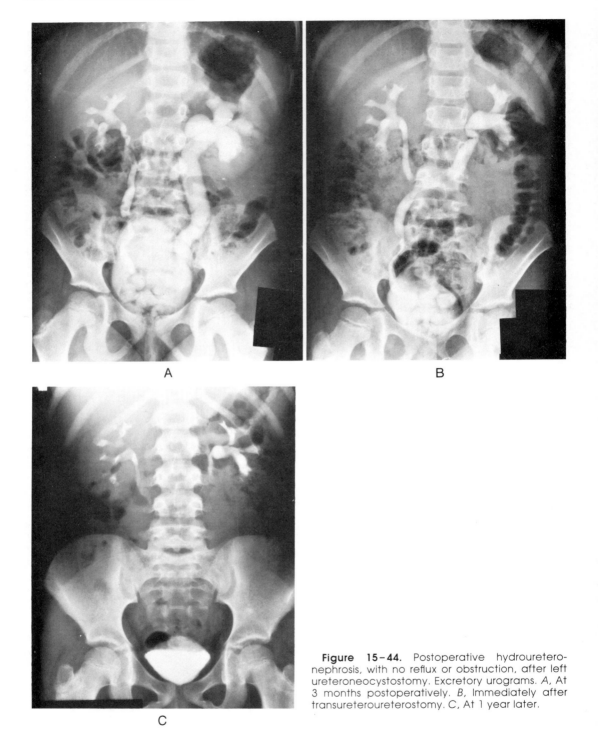

A

B

C

Figure 15–44. Postoperative hydroureteronephrosis, with no reflux or obstruction, after left ureteroneocystostomy. Excretory urograms. *A,* At 3 months postoperatively. *B,* Immediately after transureteroureterostomy. *C,* At 1 year later.

terovesical angle is perhaps slightly more common than obstruction. It is probably related to an inadequate tunnel, especially with ureteral dilatation, retraction of the implanted ureter, or reimplantation of the ureter into a bladder affected by neuropathic dysfunction.

According to Willscher et al (1976b), who observed reflux on the operated or ipsilateral side in 10 of 342 ureters (3 per cent), such reflux subsides spontaneously in the majority of cases.

When unilateral ureteroneocystostomy is

performed, contralateral reflux may appear subsequently in 15 to 20 per cent of children (Bauer et al; Parrott and Woodard; Warren et al). Elimination of the safety valve and readjustment of bladder pressure may precipitate reflux in a marginally incompetent ureterovesical junction on the contralateral side, or this may simply be the result of failure to demonstrate reflux on that side preoperatively. It is unlikely that this results from injury of the reflux prevention mechanism (ureterotrigonal continuity) of the opposite side, because it can also occur after extravesical ureteroplasty (Marberger et al). In most cases, such contralateral reflux is likely to abate spontaneously. In patients in whom reflux was shown to have taken place at some time or another before surgery in the now nonrefluxing side, bilateral reimplantation should be considered (Harty and Howerton).

Antireflux Surgery in the Neuropathic Bladder

"Occult" neuropathy of the bladder is an infrequent cause of failure of antireflux surgery. Admittedly, the detection of minor vesical dysfunction in the absence of objective neurologic findings is difficult, but the unexplained failure of such an operation should point to the need for urodynamic investigation in an effort to uncover the subtle defect. Radiographic abnormalities of bladder silhouette, increase in capacity, vesical irritability, and a thick-walled, trabeculated bladder may suggest such diagnosis (Bucy and Carlin).

Hinman and Baumann pointed out the need to recognize voiding dysfunction before embarking on surgical treatment of the reflux, since dysfunction may lead to failure. Preoperative recognition and correction of the problem by retraining or even hypnotherapy are essential.

Because the true neuropathic bladder is generally both hypertrophied and sacculated and the ureters are often thick-walled, dilated, and adherent to paraureteral tissues, reimplantation is more difficult and the results are quite variable and in general less satisfactory than is the case with surgery for primary reflux. Methods to improve bladder emptying, such as administration of phenoxybenzamine, endoscopic incision of the external sphincter or bladder outlet to lower urethral resistance, and the institution of a course of clean intermittent catheterization, may improve the success rate of antireflux surgery (Kass et al). Contralateral reflux after unilateral reimplantation in the neuropathic bladder occurs in up to 50 per cent of cases (Johnston et al). In general, techniques that require bringing the ureter through a new hiatus (suprahiatal ureteroneocystostomy) should be avoided. Advancement procedures are generally preferred. The results of such surgery vary from poor (Hirsch et al) to quite satisfactory (Johnston et al; Jeffs et al; Belloli et al). These differences in results may be attributed not only to choice of technique but also to attempts to effect better emptying of the bladder before surgery.

DUPLEX KIDNEY

More than 10 per cent of children undergoing antireflux surgery have complete or almost complete duplication of the collecting system (Devine et al). This condition requires special considerations, and several surgical procedures are available for its correction.

In rare cases, the duplicated ureters unite in the juxtavesical region; in this instance, reflux occurs by means of a common orifice but affects both components of the duplication. If operative treatment is indicated, it is preferable that the two ureters be converted into complete duplication by resecting the common stem and reimplanting both ureters as a unit through a single submucosal tunnel. Simple reimplantation without distal ureteral excision may accentuate the functional obstruction at the union of the two ureters, worsen the ureteroureteral reflux, and, possibly, lead to hydroureteronephrosis (Scott, 1963).

When complete duplication is present, reflux nearly always takes place in the lower segment orifice (see Fig. 15–47A). Several alternatives are available for correcting this problem. Removal of the involved renal segment may be the most conservative procedure when damage is severe, but total nephrectomy is almost never justified. In the management of the involved ureter, subtotal distal ureterectomy to the point where the ureter becomes intimately involved with its mate can also be accomplished via the same flank incision. Whether the ureter should be removed totally or a short stump should be left behind remains a controversial point. As a rule, troublesome infection continues only if

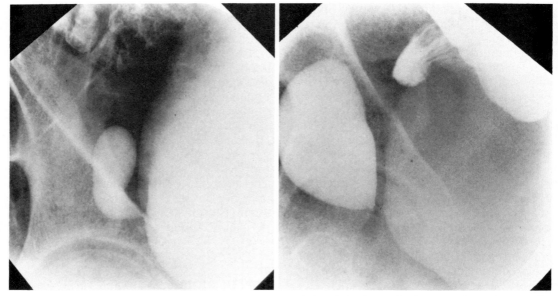

Figure 15–45. Reflux after heminephrectomy and subtotal ureterectomy. Cystograms show stump acting as vesical diverticulum with progressive distention during voiding.

the ureteral stump is left too long or drains poorly because of concomitant obstruction, becoming increasingly dilated and therefore acting as a vesical diverticulum (Fig. 15–45). In such instances, total excision through a second incision suprapubically is necessary in a small percentage of cases. To prevent complications, the ureteral stump may be left

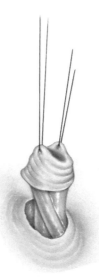

Figure 15–46. Ureteroneocystostomy in complete ureteral duplication. (From Fehrenbaker LG, Kelalis PP, Stickler GB: Vesicoureteral reflux and ureteral duplication in children. J Urol *107*:862–864, 1972. © 1972, The Williams & Wilkins Company, Baltimore.)

open with appropriate paravesical drainage for a few days or the ureter may be split open down to the bladder.

Reimplanting the ureters via a common submucosal tunnel after the two ureters have been mobilized in their common sheath generally gives satisfactory results, provided that the ureter responsible for the reflux is not greatly dilated relative to its normal ipsilateral mate (Fig. 15–46) (Fehrenbaker et al). This method effectively eliminates the reflux in the lower ureter without disturbing the function of the upper segment. Disadvantages of this procedure are that the larger ureter may obstruct the smaller one and that the procedure does not allow examination of the kidney.

In the presence of ureteral dilatation and reflux, an attractive alternative is pyeloureterostomy (Fig. 15–47C). A flank approach is necessary, so the procedure also allows examination and biopsy of the involved renal segment (Belman et al). Distal anastomosis of the two ureters has also been reported by Lytton et al, but this procedure creates the theoretical possibility of ureteroureteral reflux and resultant stasis (Fig. 15–47B). Bracci et al and Duthoy et al prefer ureteroureterostomy, citing as advantages the simple nature of the procedure and the high degree of success even in the presence of a dilated ureter. It also allows removal of the refluxing ureteral stump, and everything can be accomplished through a single incision. Thus, when there is

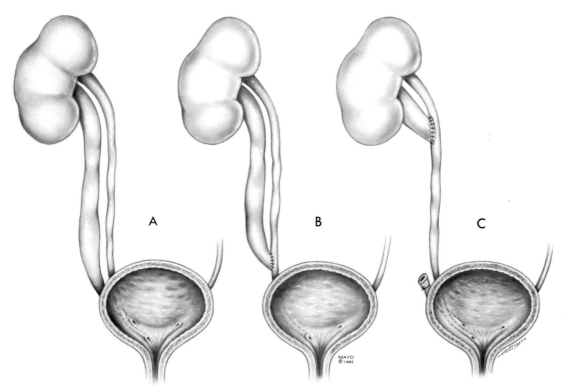

Figure 15–47. *A,* Complete duplication with reflux in lower segment. *B,* Ureteroureterostomy. *C,* Pyeloureterostomy.

ureteral dilatation, bypassing the ureterovesical junction is often preferable; pyeloureterostomy has many theoretical advantages over low ureteral anastomosis.

For a successful pyeloureterostomy or ureteroureterostomy, there must be one normally draining nonrefluxing unit in a pair of duplicated ureters. However, this anastomosis can be difficult if the caliber of the recipient ureter is small. The pelvis or upper ureter of the lower segment is anastomosed to the side of the upper ureter with fine interrupted chromic catgut, as shown in Figure 15–47C, and the anastomotic area is drained. Important surgical details should be noted. The anastomosis must be correctly angled, about 2 cm long, and placed so that the end result is similar to the naturally occurring bifid renal pelvis. This is better accomplished if the kidney is not mobilized excessively. An anterior flank incision, as described for ureteropelvic obstruction, is used.

Irrespective of the method used for correction of reflux in the duplicated system at either the bladder or renal level, the results are highly satisfactory (Barrett et al; Belman et al; Fehrenbaker et al).

SURGICAL TREATMENT OF MEGAURETER (REDUCTIVE URETEROPLASTY; URETERAL CALIBER REDUCTION-MODELAGE)

Revision of the ureterovesical junction in the refluxing or the congenital megaureter or in the grossly dilated ureter associated with urethral valves entails reduction of the ureteral caliber in addition to reimplantation. This is done to achieve an adequate length-to-width ratio in the new intravesical ureter, to relieve ureteral dilatation, to allow effective ureteral peristalsis, and to eliminate large pools of residual urine. The advantages as well as the disadvantages of this procedure are discussed in Chapter 16. It should be stressed that, although spectacular results have been achieved, great problems and disastrous consequences have also been encountered. Irrespective of the underlying pathologic condition, if the problem is bilateral with severe upper tract damage and the bladder is very abnormal, it is a very difficult procedure indeed.

Reflux in a very dilated ureter is unlikely to cease spontaneously, and it is therefore a surgical problem. Also, ureters that show both reflux and obstruction should be given the benefit of prompt surgery (Whitaker and Flower). Indications for the surgical correction of congenital megaureter or for revision of the ureterovesical junction obstruction associated with urethral valves will be described elsewhere (Chapter 16). This section deals mostly with the technique of ureteral caliber reduction, in which some points are of paramount importance.

As a rule, ureters that are more than 1 cm in diameter after transection almost certainly will require reduction in caliber, particularly if they are relatively aperistaltic (Tanagho, 1971). If the musculature of the wall of the dilated ureter produces active peristalsis capable of occluding the lumen, however, the dilatation is likely to regress after simple correction of reflux or obstruction. Therefore, in addition to the diameter of the ureter or the severity of ureteral dilatation, the ureteral musculature as it relates to peristaltic activity is an important factor. The refluxing megaureter shows gross dilatation, and it is elongated and tortuous with infrequent poor peristaltic waves even with the bladder empty.

In general, analysis of the results with respect to the underlying pathologic entity responsible for the massive ureteral dilatation indicates clearly that the cause is a crucial factor in the success or failure of surgery. A selective approach is therefore necessary. In short, the obstructive megaureter responds well to surgical reconstruction (Rabinowitz et al, 1978), whereas surgical results in the refluxing type are less satisfactory (Johnston and Farkas).

Procedures to decrease the volume of the upper urinary tract are sometimes necessary in the management of megaureter. Bischoff (1961), Johnston (1967), and Hendren (1969) all have advocated segmental management of the dilated upper urinary tract, and it would appear that the response to this approach is good.

Irrespective of the procedure used, maintaining the blood supply of the ureter is absolutely essential. It presents as a medial mesentery from the kidney to the pelvic brim but actually is a lateral blood supply in the true pelvis. In segmental ureteroplasty, reduction of the ureteral caliber should always begin with the distal third of the ureter; excessive length is discarded. This is a good anatomic principle as well as a good surgical one, because this portion of the ureter receives most of its blood supply from below and therefore

it is most likely to be rendered ischemic when disconnected from the bladder.

Technique

The ureter is freed in the same fashion as in simple ureteroneocystostomy and, after mobilization for 5 to 10 cm has been achieved transvesically, it is transposed to the paravesical space. Straightening the tortuous ureter to the extent that the blood supply will allow is advantageous. The redundant lower portion is discarded. Reduction of the caliber of the ureter not only should include the portion that will occupy the submucosal tunnel but also should extend for a few centimeters proximal to this point to the pelvic brim (Fig. 15–48A to C) (Johnston, 1967). Bischoff (1961) advocates a more extensive caliber reduction in order to bring the ureter down to normal caliber in greater length, but this is probably unnecessary. One-stage total remodeling of the dilated and tortuous ureter, when indicated, has also been accomplished with success (Hanna).

The portion of the ureter to be removed can be marked by using special clamps (Hendren, 1969) or by placing sutures to trap the ureteral catheter (usually 10 or 12 F) in the ureter that is left behind. Reduction in caliber is achieved by excising the side of the ureter farthest from its blood supply (antimesenteric) (Fig. 15–48D). The ureter that is left behind is subsequently closed with fine continuous or interrupted chromic catgut sutures (Fig. 15–48E).

Once the ureteroneocystostomy has been accomplished, any excessive length of tapered ureter is removed (Fig. 15–48 F and G), and its distal end, if so desired, is everted to create a nipple, but this is not generally necessary. The transition between the reduced ureter and the dilated ureter should be gradual, and in general the ureter should fit loosely over the catheter (Tanagho, 1971) (Fig. 15–49). Anchoring the bladder wall to the psoas muscle is an added safety feature to prevent angulation of the ureter at its entrance into the bladder. This measure is especially useful if the ureter is short and therefore under some tension (Prout and Koontz).

A second-stage procedure to reduce the caliber of the upper ureter may rarely be necessary several months later if improvement of the collecting system and the upper ureter is not apparent urographically (Johnston, 1967). Except in a small number of cases with sec-

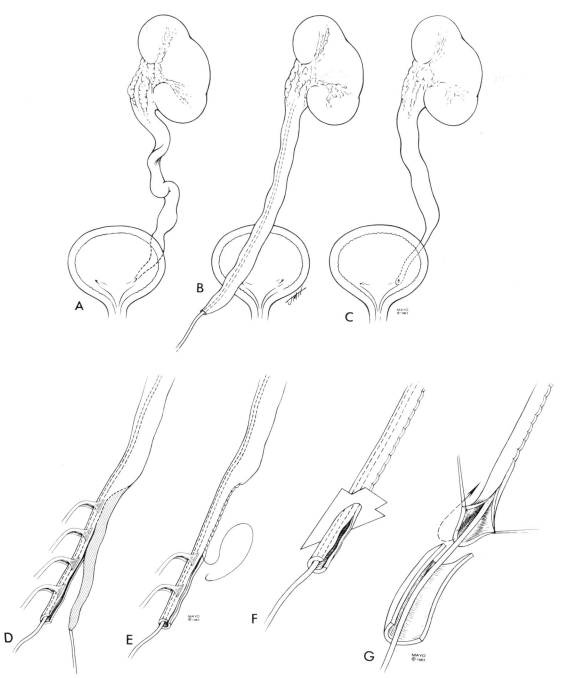

Figure 15–48. Technique of ureteral caliber reduction.

ondary ureteropelvic obstruction, however, once obstruction of the lower end is removed and the lower end is remodeled, spontaneous regression of the upper part occurs (Hendren, 1977).

In 1975, Hodgson and Thompson described an innovative technique of reductive ureteroplasty that yielded excellent results, with the distinct advantage that no instru-

ments were used on the ureter to risk damage of its wall and blood supply. After the ureter is detached from the bladder, an indwelling Silastic tube is inserted all the way to the renal pelvis; then, a running horizontal mattress suture of chromic catgut is placed on the antimesenteric border of the ureter to mold the lumen to the catheter (Fig. 15–50A). The redundant ureter is then excised, and a second

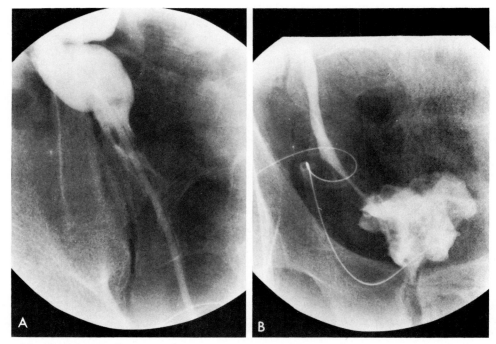

Figure 15–49. Ureteral caliber reduction. Ureterograms on 10th postoperative day before (*A*) and immediately after (*B*) removal of ureteral stent. No extravasation.

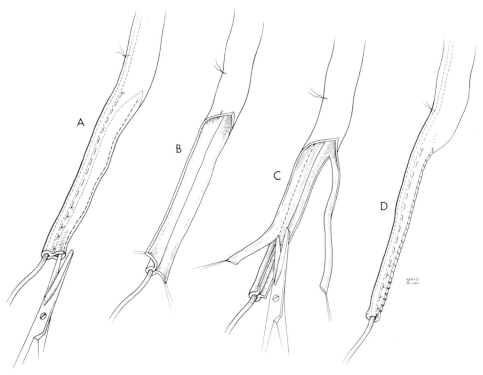

Figure 15–50. Ureteral caliber reduction.

layer of running chromic catgut suture is used for hemostasis and sealing (Fig. 15–50B to D). A ureteroneocystostomy is performed in the usual fashion. This method provides flexibility and safety in the tailoring of the ureter in that it avoids the possibility of excessive removal of its wall.

Ureteral Folding Technique

Tapering the dilated ureter without incision or excision of its wall (Figs. 15–51 and 15–52) has decided advantages, since possible interference with its blood supply is thereby avoided. First reported by Kalicinski et al and used with modification by Politano (1981) and by Starr, this technique is appealing because it accomplishes tapering without excision. A running absorbable suture is used for modeling an appropriate width of ureter. The lateral excluded (unused) lumen is folded under posteriorly with multiple interrupted sutures along the medial wall. The procedure can be performed intravesically, thus avoiding the hazards of extravesical dissection. As in other types of tailoring, the reduction of ureteral caliber should extend for a few centimeters proximal to the bladder wall.

A ureteroneocystostomy by one of the accepted techniques is next performed. The bulk of the folded ureter does not interfere with its placement in the submucosal tunnel but, should difficulty be experienced in transpos-

ing the ureter through the tunnel, the bed can be prepared by incising the mucosa and dissecting it from the muscularis. Once the ureter is placed in position, the tunnel can be formed by closing the mucosa over it. The attraction of this technique is that it obviates suture line leakage, and therefore the need for prolonged ureteral stenting is avoided. Instead, the stents are removed within 48 to 72 hours. Ureteral folding appears to have a very low incidence of complications (Ehrlich).

Evaluation of Results

Evaluating the results of ureteral caliber reduction and ureteroneocystostomy is at best difficult. The difficulty is compounded in that in some series all types of megaureter have been grouped together (Lockhart and Politano). Often the condition is referred to as decompensated ureter. Even in those series in which the various types have been distinguished or selected, the surgical treatment has not been uniform, and, in many instances, simple ureteroneocystostomy without ureteral caliber reduction was done with uniformly unsuccessful results. Furthermore, it should be stressed that the results of the operation should not be evaluated solely on the basis of urographic improvement (Figs. 15–53 and 15–54). One also should consider renal growth and function (information fre-

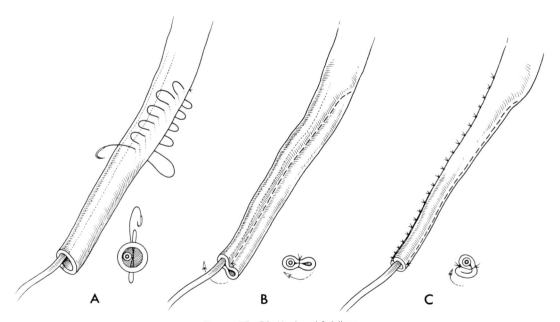

Figure 15–51. Ureteral folding.

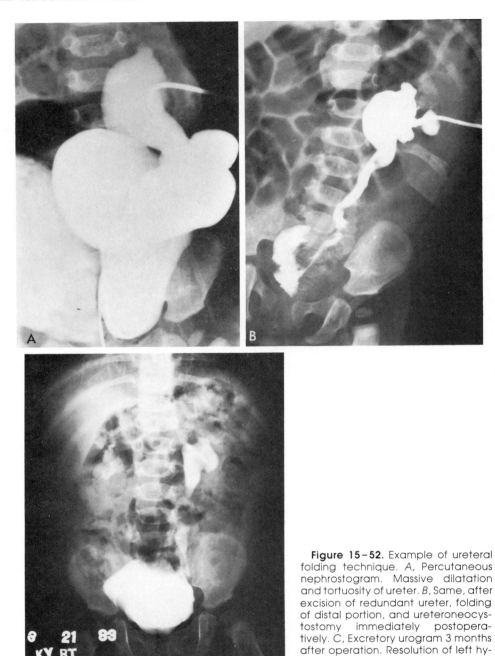

Figure 15–52. Example of ureteral folding technique. *A*, Percutaneous nephrostogram. Massive dilatation and tortuosity of ureter. *B*, Same, after excision of redundant ureter, folding of distal portion, and ureteroneocystostomy immediately postoperatively. *C*, Excretory urogram 3 months after operation. Resolution of left hydroureteronephrosis with good function.

quently lacking in most series attempting to evaluate such procedures). Long-term radiologic follow-up is essential, because definite improvement and stabilization can occur up to 2 years later (Retik et al).

Complications of this more extensive antireflux operation consist of varying degrees of persistence of obstructive dilatation or reflux. In general, the results vary from excellent to poor (Bruezierre; Derrick; Hendren, 1970; Johnston, 1967; Rabinowitz et al, 1979). The reasons for failure include ureteral fistula or stricture as a result of compromised ureteral blood supply (Hendren, 1970), persistence of reflux due to inadequate antireflux mechanism at the newly created ureterovesical junction, and absence of urographic improvement. Even though the results of such

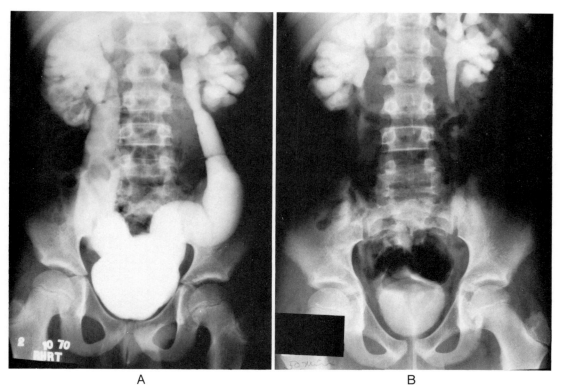

A   B

Figure 15-53. Reflux megaureter. Excretory urograms before (A) and 1 year after (B) ureteral caliber reduction.

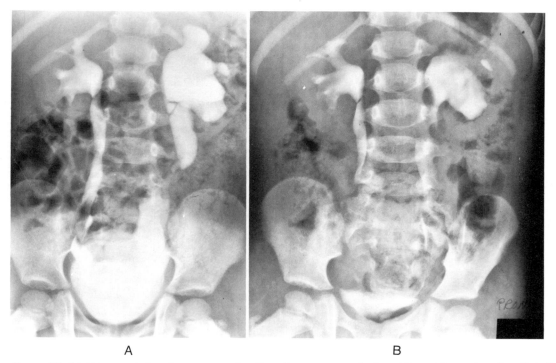

A   B

Figure 15-54. Primary obstructive megaureter. Excretory urograms before (A) and 5 months after (B) left ureteral reduction.

procedures have varied widely, technical success can be expected in at least 3 of 4 patients overall. Especially in infants, initial reconstruction with ureteral tailoring and reimplantation should be performed by experienced surgeons familiar with the entity, expert anesthesia, and supportive postoperative intensive care.

BIBLIOGRAPHY

Ahmed S: Ureteral reimplantation by the transverse advancement technique. J Urol 119:547, 1978.

Ahmed S, Smith AJ: Results of ureteral reimplantation in patients with intrarenal reflux. J Urol 120:332, 1978.

Aladjem B, Boichis H, Hertz M, et al: The conservative management of vesicoureteral reflux: a review of 21 children. Pediatrics 65:78, 1980.

Amar AD: Reflux in duplicated ureters. Br J Urol 40:385, 1968.

Amar AD: Reimplantation of completely duplicated ureters. J Urol 107:230, 1972a.

Amar AD: Vesicoureteral reflux associated with congenital bladder diverticulum in boys and young men. J Urol 107:966, 1972b.

Amar AD: Delayed recurrence of reflux after initial success of antireflux operation. J Urol 119:131, 1978.

Amar AD, Chabra K: Reflux in duplicated ureters: treatment in children. J Pediatr Surg 5:419, 1970.

Ambrose SS: Reflux pyelonephritis in adults secondary to congenital lesions of the ureteral orifice. J Urol 102:302, 1969.

Ambrose SS, Nicolson WP: Ureteral reflux in duplicated ureters. J Urol 92:439, 1964.

Ansell JS: The Bischoff submucosal ureteroplasty: a clinical evaluation. J Urol 95:768, 1966.

Arap S, Abrão G, Menezes de Góes G: Treatment and prevention of complications after extravesical antireflux technique. Eur Urol 7:263, 1981.

Arap S, Cabral AD, De Campos Freire JG, et al: The extravesical antireflux plasty: statistical analysis. Urol Int 26:241, 1971.

Babcock JR, Keats GK, Kind LR: Renal changes after an uncomplicated antireflux operation. J Urol 115:720, 1976.

Bailey RR: The relationship of vesico-ureteric reflux to urinary tract infection and chronic pyelonephritis: reflux nephropathy. Clin Nephrol 1:132, 1973.

Barrett DM, Malek RS, Kelalis PP: Problems and solutions in surgical treatment of 100 consecutive ureteral duplications in children. J Urol 114:126, 1975.

Bauer SB, Willscher MK, Zammuto PJ, et al: Long-term results of antireflux surgery in children. In Reflux Nephropathy. Edited by J Hodson, P Kincaid-Smith. New York, Masson Publishing USA Inc, 1979, pp 287–298.

Belloli GP, Musi L, Campobasso P, et al: Ureteral reimplantation in children with neurogenic bladder. J Pediatr Surg 14:119, 1979.

Belman AB, Filmer RB, King LW: Surgical management of duplication of the collecting system. J Urol 112:316, 1974.

Bernstein J: Development of abnormal renal parenchyma. Pathol Ann 3:213, 1968.

Bettex M, Kummer-Vago M, Kuffer F: Ureteroneocystostomy in refluxing ureteric duplication: indications, techniques and results. J Pediatr Surg 5:622, 1970.

Bischoff P: Megaureter. Br J Urol 29:416, 1957.

Bischoff P: Operative treatment of megaureter. J Urol 85:268, 1961.

Bischoff PF, Busch HG: Origin, clinical experiences and treatment of urinary obstructions of the lower ureter in childhood. J Urol 85:739, 1961.

Blank E: Calicectasis and renal scars in children. J Urol 110:255, 1973.

Blank E, Girdany BR: Prognosis with vesicoureteral reflux. Pediatrics 48:782, 1971.

Blight EM, O'Shaughnessy EJ: Vesicoureteral reflux in children: a prospective study. J Urol 102:44, 1969.

Bracci U, Miano L, Laurenti C: Ureteroureterostomy in complete ureteral duplication. Eur Urol 5:347, 1979.

Broaddus SB, Zickerman PM, Morrisseau PM, et al: Incidence of later ureteral obstruction after antireflux surgery in infants and children. Urology 11:139, 1978.

Bruezierre J: Les mega-ureteres primitifs chez le nourrisson. Chirurgie 100:712, 1974.

Bucy JG, Carlin R: The silent neurogenic bladder. J Urol 114:296, 1975.

Cohen SJ: Ureterozystoneostomie: Eine neue antireflux technik. Aktuel Urol 6:1, 1975.

Cukier J, Beurton D, Vacant J, et al: Correction of malformative vesicorenal reflux through the advancement of the ureteral submucosa. Acta Urol Belg 43:345, 1975.

Cukier J, Cabane H, Michel FR, et al: The psoas bladder: experience with 88 operations (author's translation). J Urol (Paris) 87:507, 1981.

Derrick FC Jr: Management of the large, tortuous, adynamic ureter with reflux. J Urol 108:153, 1972.

De Sy W, Oosterlinck W, Verbaeys A: Revaluation of the advancement operative technique for the care of vesicorenal reflux. Eur Urol 5:18, 1979.

Devine PC, Davis CS Jr, Devine CD Jr, et al: Vesicoureteral reflux in children: indications for surgical and nonsurgical treatment. Urology 3:315, 1974.

DeWeerd JH, Farsund T, Burke EC: Ureteroneocystostomy. J Urol 101:520, 1969.

Diaz-Ball FL, Fink A, Moore CA, et al: Pyeloureterostomy and ureteroureterostomy: alternative procedures to partial nephrectomy for duplication of the ureter with only one pathological segment. J Urol 102:621, 1969.

Dodson AI: Some improvements in the technique of ureterocystostomy. J Urol 55:225, 1946.

Dwoskin JY, Perlmutter AD: Vesicoureteral reflux in children: a computerized review. J Urol 109:888, 1973.

Duthoy EJ, Soucheray JA, McGroarty BJ: Ipsilateral ureteroureterostomy for vesicoureteral reflux in duplicated ureters. J Urol 118:826, 1977.

Edwards D, Normand ICS, Prescod N, et al: Disappearance of reflux during long term prophylaxis of urinary tract infection in children. Br Med J 2:285, 1977.

Ehrlich RM: Ureteral folding technique for megaureter surgery. Soc Pediatr Urol Newsletter, May 5, 1982, pp 56–57.

Estes RC, Brooks RT: Vesicoureteral reflux in adults. J Urol 103:603, 1970.

Fehrenbaker LG, Kelalis PP, Stickler GB: Vesicoureteral reflux and ureteral duplication in children. J Urol 107:862, 1972.

Filly RA, Friedland GW, Fair WR, et al: Late ureteric obstruction following ureteral reimplantation for reflux: a warning. Urology 4:540, 1974a.

Filly R, Friedland GW, Govan DE, et al: Development and progression of clubbing and scarring in children with recurrent urinary tract infections. Radiology 113:145, 1974b.

Fisher JH, Darling DB: The course of vesicoureteral reflux associated with urinary tract infection in children. J Pediatr Surg 2:221, 1967.

Glenn JF, Anderson EE: Distal tunnel ureteral reimplantation. J Urol 97:623, 1967.

Glenn JF, Anderson EE: Technical considerations in distal tunnel ureteral reimplantation. Trans Am Assoc Genitourin Surg 69:23, 1977.

Gonzales ET, Glenn JF, Anderson EE: Results of distal tunnel ureteral reimplantation. J Urol 107:572, 1972.

Gonzales ET Jr, Caffarena E, Carlton CE Jr: The advantages of short-term vesical drainage after antireflux operation. J Urol 119:817, 1978.

Govan DE, Fair WR, Friedland GW, et al: Urinary tract infection in children. II. The child with refluxing bacteriuria. West J Med (in press).

Govan DE, Palmer JM: Urinary tract infection in children: the influence of successful antireflux operations in morbidity from infection. Pediatrics 44:677, 1969.

Grégoir W, Schulman CC: Die extravesikale Antirefluxplastik (extravesical antirefluxplasty). (authors translation) Urologe A 16:124, 1977.

Grégoir W, Van Regemorter G: Le reflux vésico-urétéral congénital. Urol Int 18:122, 1964.

Gutierrez J, Chang CY, Nesbit RM: Ipsilateral ureteroureterostomy for vesicoureteral reflux in duplicated ureter. J Urol 101:36, 1969.

Halpern GN, King LR, Belman AB: Transureteroureterostomy in children. Trans Am Assoc Genitourin Surg 64:99, 1972.

Hanna MK: New surgical method for one-stage total remodeling of massively dilated and tortuous ureter: tapering in situ technique. Urology 14:453, 1979.

Harty JI, Howerton LW Jr: Bilateral or unilateral ureteroneocystostomy for unilateral reflux. Urology 18:241, 1981.

Helin I: Clinical and experimental studies on vesicoureteric reflux. Scand J Urol Nephrol (Suppl) 28:1, 1975.

Helin I, Okmian L, Olin T: Renal blood flow and function in vesico-ureteric reflux: an experimental study in the pig. Scand J Urol [Suppl] 28:71, 1975.

Hendren WH: Ureteral reimplantation in children. J Pediatr Surg 3:649, 1968.

Hendren WH: Operative repair of megaureter in children. J Urol 101:491, 1969.

Hendren WH: Functional restoration of decompensated ureters in children. Am J Surg 119:477, 1970.

Hendren WH: Reoperation for the failed ureteral reimplantation. J Urol 111:403, 1974.

Hendren WH: Technical aspects of megaureter repair. Birth Defects 13:21, 1977.

Hernandez RJ, Poznanski AK, Kuhns LR, et al: Factors affecting the measurement of renal length. Radiology 130:653, 1979.

Hicks CC, Woodard JR, Walton KN, et al: Hypertension as complication of vesicoureteral reflux in children. Urology 7:587, 1976.

Hinman F Jr, Baumann FW: Complications of vesicoureteral operations from incoordination of micturition. J Urol 116:638, 1976.

Hirsch S, Carrion H, Gordon J, et al: Ureteroneocystostomy in the treatment of reflux in neurogenic bladders. J Urol 120:552, 1978.

Hodgson NB, Thompson LW: Technique of reductive ureteroplasty in the management of megaureter. J Urol 113:118, 1975.

Hutch JA: The Ureterovesical Junction: The Theory of Extravesicalization of the Intravesical Ureter. Berkeley, University of California Press, 1958.

Hutch JA: Theory of maturation of the intravesical ureter. J Urol 86:534, 1961.

Hutch JA: Ureteric advancement operation: anatomy, technique and early results. J Urol 89:180, 1963.

Hutch JA, Amar AD: Politano-Leadbetter operation. In Vesicoureteral Reflux and Pyelonephritis. New York, Appleton-Century-Crofts, 1972a.

Hutch JA, Amar AD: Techniques of antireflux. In Vesicoureteral Reflux and Pyelonephritis. New York, Appleton-Century-Crofts, 1972b.

Hutch JA, Ayres RD, Loquvam GS: The bladder musculature with special reference to the ureterovesical junction. J Urol 85:531, 1961.

Hutch JA, Bunge RG, Flocks RH: Vesicoureteral reflux in children. J Urol 74:607, 1955.

Hutch JA, Smith DR, Osborn R: Review of a series of ureterovesicoplasties. J Urol 100:285, 1968.

International Reflux Study Committee: Medical versus surgical treatment of primary vesicoureteral reflux. Pediatrics 67:392, 1981.

Ireland GW, Cass AS: The clinical measurement of the ureteral submucosal tunnel. J Urol 107:564, 1972.

Jeffs RD, Jonas P, Schillinger JF: Surgical correction of vesicoureteral reflux in children with neurogenic bladder. J Urol 115:449, 1976.

Johnston JH: Urinary tract duplication in childhood. Arch Dis Child 36:180, 1961.

Johnston JH: Reconstructive surgery of mega-ureter in childhood. Br J Urol 39:17, 1967.

Johnston JH, Farkas A: The congenital refluxing megaureter: experiences with surgical reconstruction. Br J Urol 47:153, 1975.

Johnston JH, Shapiro SR, Thomas GG: Anti-reflux surgery in the congenital neuropathic bladder. Br J Urol 48:639, 1976.

Kalicinski H, Kansy J, Kotarbińska B, et al: Surgery of megaureters — modification of Hendren's operation. J Pediatr Surg 12:183, 1977.

Kaplan WE, Nasrallah P, King LR: Reflux in complete duplication in children. J Urol 120:220, 1978.

Kass EJ, Koff SA, Diokno AC: Fate of vesicoureteral reflux in children with neuropathic bladders managed by intermittent catheterization. J Urol 125:63, 1981.

Kelalis PP: Proper perspective on vesicoureteral reflux. Mayo Clin Proc 46:807, 1971.

Kelalis PP: The present status of surgery for vesicoureteral reflux. Urol Clin North Am 1:457, 1974.

King LR, Kazmi SO, Campbell JA, et al: The case for nonsurgical management of vesicoureteral reflux. In Current Controversies in Urologic Management. Edited by R Scott Jr, HL Gordon, CE Carlton, et al. Philadelphia, WB Saunders Co., 1972, pp 200–215.

Koff SA, Kogan B, Kass EJ et al: Early postoperative assessment of the functional patency of ureterovesical junction following ureteroneocystostomy. J Urol 125:554, 1981.

Lamesch AJ: Retrograde cathetarization of the ureter after antireflux plasty by the Cohen technique of transverse advancement. J Urol 125:73, 1981.

Lich R Jr, Howerton LW, Davis LA: Recurrent urosepsis in children. J Urol 86:554, 1961.

Lockhart JL, Politano VA: Management of massively dilated ureters in children. Urology 18:229, 1981.

Lockhart JL, Singer AM, Glenn JF: Congenital megaureter. J Urol 122:310, 1979.

Lowenstein LM, Stern A: Serum factor in renal compensatory hyperplasia. Science 142:1479, 1963.

Lyon RP, Marshall S, Tanagho EA: The ureteral orifice: its configuration and competency. J Urol 102:504, 1969.

Lyon RP, Tanagho EA: Distal urethral stenosis in little girls. J Urol 93:379, 1965.

Lytton B, Weiss RM, Berneike RR: Ipsilateral ureteroureterostomy in the management of vesicoureteral reflux in duplication of upper urinary tract. J Urol 105:507, 1971.

MacKellar A, Stephens FD: Vesical diverticula in children. Aust NZ J Surg 30:20, 1960.

Mackie GG, Awang H, Stephens FD: The ureteric orifice: the embryologic key to radiologic status of duplex kidneys. J Pediatr Surg 10:473, 1975.

Mackie GG, Stephens FD: Duplex kidneys: a correlation of renal dysplasia with position of the ureteral orifice. J Urol 114:274, 1975.

Manley CG, Ferrell JM: Management of ureteral obstruction after an antireflux operation: triangular flap ureteroplasty. J Urol 113:121, 1975.

Marberger M, Altwein JE, Straub E, et al: The Lich-Grégoir antireflux plasty: experience with 371 children. J Urol 120:216, 1978.

Markland C, Kelly WD: Experiences with the severely damaged urinary tract. J Urol 99:327, 1968.

Mathisen W: Vesicoureteral reflux and its surgical correction. Surg Gynecol Obstet 118:965, 1964.

McGovern JH, Marshall VF: Reimplantation of ureters into the bladders of children. Trans Am Assoc Genitourin Surg 59:116, 1967.

McRae CU, Shannon FT, Utley WLF: Effect on renal growth of reimplantation of refluxing ureters. Lancet 1:1310, 1974.

Merrell RW, Mowad JJ: Increased physical growth after successful antireflux operation. J Urol 122:523, 1979.

Mitchell TS: Development of surgical treatment for vesicoureteral reflux. Contemp Surg 6:53, (May), 1975.

Mundy AR, Kinder CH, Joyce MRL, et al: Improvement in renal function following ureteric reimplantation for vesicoureteral reflux. Br J Urol 53:542, 1981.

Murnaghan GF: The physiology of megaureter. Proc R Soc Med 51:776, 1958.

Murnaghan GF: Indications for surgical treatment of primary vesicoureteral reflux. Urol Digest, July 1972, 17–19.

Murnaghan GF: Indications for surgical treatment of primary vesicoureteric reflux (abstract). Br J Urol 46:113, 1974.

Murnaghan GF, et al: In Renal Infection and Renal Scarring. Edited by P Kincaid-Smith, KF Fairley. Melbourne, Australia, Mercedes Publishing Services, 1970, pp 315–325.

Nanninga J, King LR, Downing J, et al: Factors affecting the outcome of 100 ureteral reimplantations done for vesicoureteral reflux. J Urol 102:772, 1969.

Palken M: Surgical correction of vesicoureteral reflux in children: results with the use of a single standard technique. J Urol 104:765, 1970.

Paquin AJ Jr: Ureterovesical anastomosis: the description and evaluation of a technique. J Urol 82:573, 1959.

Parrott TS, Woodard JR: Reflux in opposite ureter after successful correction of unilateral vesicoureteral reflux. Urology 7:276, 1976.

Pitts WR Jr, Muecke EC: Congenital megaloureter: a review of 80 patients. J Urol 111:468, 1974.

Politano VA: One hundred reimplantations and five years. J Urol 90:696, 1963.

Politano V: Poster Session, American Urological Association, Boston, 1981.

Politano VA, Leadbetter WF: An operative technique for the correction of ureteric reflux. J Urol 79:932, 1958.

Prout GR Jr, Koontz WW Jr: Partial vesical immobilization: an important adjunct to ureteroneocystostomy. J Urol 103:147, 1970.

Rabinowitz R, Barkin M, Schillinger JF, et al: The influence of etiology on the surgical management and prognosis of the massively dilated ureter in children. J Urol 119:808, 1978.

Rabinowitz R, Barkin M, Schillinger JF, et al: Surgical treatment of the massive dilated primary megaureter in children. Br J Urol 51:19, 1979.

Randel DE: Surgical judgment in the management of vesicoureteral reflux. J Urol 19:113, 1978.

Retik AB, McEvoy JP, Bauer SB: Megaureters in children. Urology 11:231, 1978.

Reule GR, Ansell JS: Reimplantation of double ureters. J Urol 102:172, 1969.

Rolleston GL, Maling TMJ, Hodson CJ: Intrarenal reflux and the scarred kidney. Arch Dis Child 49:531, 1974.

Rolleston GL, Shannon FT, Utley WLF: Relationship of infantile vesicoureteric reflux to renal damage. Br Med J 1:460, 1970.

Salvatierra O Jr, Kountz SL, Belzer FO: Primary vesicoureteral reflux and end-stage renal disease. JAMA 226:1454, 1973.

Savage JM, Shah V, Dillon MJ, et al: Renin and blood-pressure in children with renal scarring and vesicoureteric reflux. Lancet 2:441, 1978.

Scott JE: Ureteric reflux in the duplex kidney. Acta Urol Belg 31:73, 1963.

Scott JE: Results of anti-reflux surgery. Lancet 2:68, 1969.

Scott JE: The role of surgery in the management of vesicoureteric reflux. Kidney Int [Suppl] 4:S73, 1975.

Scott JE: The management of ureteric reflux in children. Br J Urol 49:109, 1977.

Scott JE, De Luca FG: An experimental study of the lower end of the ureter and ureterovesical junction in dogs. Br J Urol 32:216, 1960a.

Scott JE, De Luca FG: Further studies on the ureterovesical junction of the dog. Br J Urol 32:320, 1960b.

Scott JE, Stansfeld JM: Treatment of vesico-ureteric reflux in children. Arch Dis Child 43:323, 1968a.

Scott JE, Stansfeld JM: Ureteric reflux and kidney scarring in children. Arch Dis Child 43:468, 1968b.

Shopfner CE: Cystourethrography: an evaluation of method. Am J Roentgenol Rad Ther Nucl Med 95:776, 1966.

Silk MR, Homsy GE, Merz T: Compensatory renal hyperplasia. J Urol 98:36, 1967.

Smellie JM, Normand ICS: Urinary tract infection with and without anatomic malformations. In Clinical Pediatric Nephrology. Edited by E Lieberman. Philadelphia, JB Lippincott Co., 1976, p 194.

Smellie JM, Normand ICS: Reflux nephropathy in childhood. In Reflux Nephropathy. Edited by J Hodson, J Kincaid-Smith. New York, Masson Publishing USA, 1979, p 14.

So EP, Brock WA, Kaplan GW: Ureteral reimplantation without catheters. J Urol 125:551, 1981.

Starr A: Ureteral plication: a new concept in ureteral tailoring for megaureter. Invest Urol 17:153, 1979.

Stephens FD: Treatment of megaureters by multiple micturition. Aust NZ J Surg 27:130, 1957.

Stephens FD: Congenital Malformations of the Rectum,

Anus and Genitourinary Tracts. Edinburgh, E & S Livingstone, 1963.

Stephens FD: Idiopathic dilatations of the urinary tract. J Urol 112:819, 1974.

Stephens FD, Lenaghan D: The anatomical basis and dynamics of vesicoureteral reflux. J Urol 87:669, 1962.

Stevens AR, Marshall VF: Reimplantation of the ureter into the bladder. Surg Gynecol Obstet 77:585, 1943.

Stickler GB, Kelalis PP, Burke EC, et al: Primary interstitial nephritis with reflux. A cause of hypertension. Am J Dis Child 122:144, 1971.

Tanagho EA: Surgical revision of the incompetent ureterovesical junction: a critical analysis of techniques and requirements. Br J Urol 42:410, 1970.

Tanagho EA: Ureteral tailoring. J Urol 106:194, 1971.

Tanagho EA, Guthrie TH, Lyon RP: The intravesical ureter in primary reflux. J Urol 101:824, 1969.

Tanagho EA, Hutch JA: Primary reflux. J Urol 93:158, 1965.

Tanagho EA, Hutch JA, Meyers FH, et al: Primary vesicoureteral reflux: experimental studies of its etiology. J Urol 93:165, 1965.

Tanagho EA, Meyers FH, Smith DR: The trigone: anatomical and physiological considerations. I. In relation to the ureterovesical junction. J Urol 100:623, 1968.

Tanagho EA, Pugh RCB: The anatomy and function of the ureterovesical junction. Br J Urol 35:151, 1963.

Tocci PE, Politano VA, Lynne CM, et al: Unusual complications of transvesical ureteral reimplantation. J Urol 115:731, 1976.

Torres VE, Velosa JA, Holley KE, et al: The progression of vesicoureteral reflux nephropathy. Ann Intern Med 92:776, 1980.

Uehling DT, Wear JB Jr: Concentrating ability after antireflux operation. J Urol 116:83, 1976.

Walker D, Richard G, Dodson D, et al: Maximum urine concentration: early means of identifying patients with reflux who may require surgery. Urology 1:343, 1973.

Wallace DMA, Rothwell DL, Williams DI: The long-term follow-up of surgically treated vesicoureteric reflux. Br J Urol 50:479, 1978.

Warren MM, Kelalis PP, Stickler GB: Unilateral ureteroneocystostomy: the fate of the contralateral ureter. J Urol 107:466, 1972.

Weiss RM, Lytton B: Vesicoureteral reflux and distal ureteral obstruction. J Urol 111:245, 1974.

Weiss RM, Schiff M Jr, Lytton B: Late obstruction after ureteroneocystostomy. J Urol 106:144, 1971.

Weiss RM, Schiff M Jr, Lytton B: Reflux and trapping. Radiology 118:129, 1976.

Wesson MB: Anatomical, embryological and physiological studies of the trigone and neck of the bladder. J Urol 4:279, 1920.

Whitaker RH, Flower CD: Ureters that show both reflux and obstruction. Br J Urol 51:471, 1979.

Williams DI, Eckstein HB: Surgical treatment of reflux in children. Br J Urol 37:13, 1965.

Williams DI, Rabinovitch HH: Cutaneous ureterostomy for the grossly dilated ureter in childhood. Br J Urol 39:696, 1967.

Williams DI, Scott J, Turner-Warwick RT: Reflux and recurrent infection. Br J Urol 33:435, 1961.

Willscher MK, Bauer SB, Zammuto PJ, et al: Infection of the urinary tract after anti-reflux surgery. J Pediatr 89:743, 1976a.

Willscher MK, Bauer SB, Zammuto PJ, et al: Renal growth and urinary infection following antireflux surgery in infants and children. J Urol 115:722, 1976b.

Winberg J, Larson H, Bergström T: Comparison of the natural history of urinary infection in children with and without vesico-ureteric reflux. In Renal Infection and Renal Scarring. Edited by P Kincaid-Smith, KF Fairley. Melbourne, Australia, Mercedes Publishing Services, 1970, pp 293–302.

Woodard JR, Keats G: Ureteral reimplantation: Paquin's procedure after 12 years. J Urol 109:891, 1973.

Woodburne RT: Anatomy of the ureterovesical junction. J Urol 92:431, 1964.

16

OBSTRUCTIVE UROPATHY

Pathophysiology and Diagnosis

Robert M. Weiss

Under normal conditions, ureteral peristaltic activity begins with the origin of electrical activity at pacemaker sites located in the proximal portion of the collecting system (Bozler; Weiss et al, 1967; Gosling and Dixon). The electrical activity is propagated distally from one muscle cell to another across areas of close cellular apposition, intermediate junctions (Notley; Libertino and Weiss). The similarity of these close cellular contacts to low resistance intercellular pathways in other smooth muscles suggests that they may play an important role in the propagation of the peristaltic wave (Barr et al). The electrical activity results in changes in the calcium concentration in the region of the contractile proteins and thereby triggers the peristaltic contraction wave that propels the urinary bolus from the kidney to the bladder. Peristaltic contraction waves occur at a frequency of 2 to 6 per minute (Edmond et al) and are propagated at a rate of 2 to 6 cm/sec (Kobayashi; Kuriyama et al). Efficient propulsion of the urinary bolus in a distal direction is dependent upon complete coaptation of the ureteral walls during the peristaltic contraction (Woodburn and Lapides). Normal resting or baseline ureteral pressure is approximately 0 to 5 cm H_2O and peristaltic contraction waves of 20 to 60 cm H_2O are superimposed on this baseline pressure (Edmond et al).

EFFECT OF OBSTRUCTION ON URETERAL FUNCTION

The effect of obstruction on ureteral function is dependent on the degree and duration of the obstruction, on the rate of urine formation, and on the presence or absence of infec-

tion. Subsequent to the onset of an obstruction, there is a backup of urine within the urinary collecting system proximal to the site of obstruction. This is associated with an increase in baseline ureteral pressure and dimensions (Rose and Gillenwater, 1973; Biancani et al, 1976) (Fig. 16–1). The dimensional changes—increase in ureteral length and diameter—are manifested clinically by ureteral dilatation and tortuosity. The increase in baseline intraluminal pressure is dependent on the continued production of urine by the kidney which cannot pass beyond the obstruction, while the increase in ureteral dimensions results from the increased ureteral intraluminal pressure and the increase in the volume of urine retained within the ureter. Associated with these initial dimensional and ureteral baseline resting pressure changes, there is a transient increase in the amplitude and frequency of the peristaltic contraction waves (Rose and Gillenwater, 1978). With time as the ureter fills with urine and baseline pressure increases, the contraction waves become smaller and are unable to coapt the walls of the dilated ureter. Urine transport at that time becomes dependent on the hydrostatic forces generated by the kidney (Rose and Gillenwater, 1973). Fluid within the wide ureter in which peristalsis is not effective tends to move in a to-and-fro manner with no systematic onward progression and without bolus formation (Whitaker, 1975). Chronic obstruction has also been shown to alter the hierarchical organization of the multiple coupled pacemakers within the renal calyces and pelvis that normally coordinate peristaltic activity. Such disruption causes discoordination of pelvic contractility with resultant incomplete emptying of the renal pelvis (Djurhuus

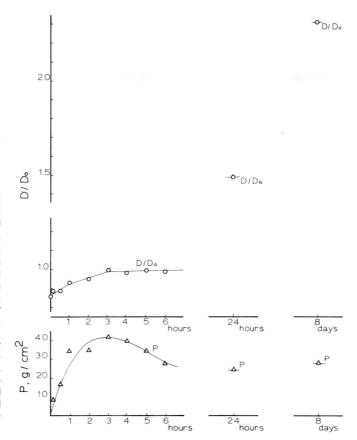

Figure 16-1. Changes in intraluminal pressure and diameter following obstruction of rabbit ureter. Time from onset of obstruction is on abscissa. Change in diameter (D/D_O) is on upper ordinate; pressure (P) is on lower ordinate. During initial 3 hours of obstruction, intraluminal pressure increases to reach maximum and is associated with an increase in dimensions. Between 3 and 6 hours after onset of obstruction, pressure declines, although deformational changes persist. After 6 hours, pressure remains essentially unchanged, although diameter continues to increase. D_O, initial diameter; D, diameter during deformation; P, intraluminal pressure. (From Biancani P, Zabinski MP, Weiss RM: Time course of ureteral changes with acute and chronic obstruction. Am J Physiol *231*:393, 1976.)

and Constantinou). Superimposed infection results in a complete absence of contractions in the obstructed ureter and causes even more severe impairment of urine transport.

A few hours following the onset of obstruction, intraluminal baseline ureteral pressure reaches a peak and then begins to decline. The dimensions that had previously increased from normal remain stable during the time in which the intraluminal pressure is decreasing. The decrease in intraluminal baseline pressure can be attributed to changes in intrarenal dynamics, such as reduction in renal blood flow (Vaughan et al, 1971), which is reflected in a decrease in glomerular filtration rate and in intratubular hydrostatic pressure (Gottschalk and Mylle). Reabsorption of urine into the venous and lymphatic systems and a decrease in wall tension also may play a role in the reduction in baseline ureteral pressure (Rose and Gillenwater, 1978). The persistence of dimensional changes despite a decrease in intraluminal pressure is dependent on the hysteretic properties of the viscoelastic ureteral structure. That is, at any given pressure, ureteral dimensions are larger during unload-

ing than at comparable pressures during loading (Biancani et al) (Fig. 16-2).

Over time, intraluminal baseline ureteral pressure decreases to a level only slightly higher than the normal baseline pressure and then remains stable. As obstruction persists, there is a gradual increase in ureteral length and diameter to considerable dimensions in the face of this relatively low constant intraluminal pressure. This phenomenon can be explained by creep of the viscoelastic ureteral structure (Fig. 16-3). A continued, albeit small, urine production is required for this increase in intraureteral volume. These changes account for the relatively low intrapelvic pressures observed in the massively dilated, chronically obstructed upper urinary tracts (Vela-Navarrete; Backlund et al; Struthers; Djurhuus and Stage) and in experimentally produced obstruction (Schweitzer; Vaughan et al, 1970; Koff and Thrall, 1981a).

One could postulate that with prolonged complete obstruction, total cessation of urine output ultimately occurs. Subsequent decrease in ureteral dimensions would depend on whether urine is reabsorbed, and on the

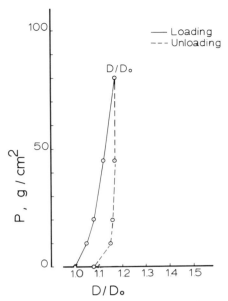

Figure 16–2. Demonstration of hysteretic properties of ureter showing that dimensional changes are dependent on intraluminal pressure and on the direction of change of that pressure. At comparable pressures, deformations are greater during ureteral emptying than during ureteral filling. Solid line shows data obtained during loading; interrupted line, data obtained during unloading. D_o, initial diameter; D, diameter during deformation; P, intraluminal pressure in g/cm². (From Biancani P, Zabinski MP, Weiss RM: Time course of ureteral changes with acute and chronic obstruction. Am J Physiol 231:393, 1976.)

mechanical properties of the ureteral wall at that time.

In order to determine the effect of obstruction on the contractile properties of the ureteral musculature, a rabbit model, in which the ureter had been totally obstructed for 2 weeks, has been extensively studied (Hausman et al; Biancani et al, 1982). Following the onset of obstruction, the ureteral muscle, at least initially, undergoes hypertrophy. After 2 weeks of obstruction, cross-sectional muscle area increases by 250 per cent, ureteral length by 24 per cent, and ureteral outer diameter by 100 per cent. In addition to undergoing muscle hypertrophy, in vitro segments from obstructed ureters develop greater contractile forces, in both longitudinal and circumferential directions, than do segments from control ureters. Since obstruction results in an increase in muscle mass, these changes in force could have resulted from either an increase in muscle mass alone or from an actual increase in contractility. Stress measurements, that is, force per unit area of muscle, provide a better

means of assessing actual changes in contractility. When analyzed in this manner, the increases in force were associated with an increase in maximum active circumferential stress but no change in maximum active longitudinal stress (Fig. 16–4). The sum of these stresses (total stress) or overall contractility thus increases following 2 weeks of obstruction. In order to account for these differences in longitudinal and circumferential stresses occurring following obstruction, rotation of muscle bundles must occur; otherwise, longitudinal and circumferential stress would increase equally. This rotation could result from the greater increase in diameter than in length following obstruction, from remodeling of the muscle fibers, or from both.

The dilated ureter following 2 weeks of obstruction thus is not mechanically decompensated, but rather undergoes changes that result in an increase in contractility. However, despite muscle hypertrophy and despite increase in contractility, it is evident in the clinical situation and from in vivo experimental studies (Rose and Gillenwater, 1973) that the obstructed ureter's ability to develop the intraluminal pressures required for urine transport decreases. The decrease in intraluminal pressure despite an increase in contractility results from the increase in ureteral diameter following obstruction and can be explained by the Laplace relationship:

$$\text{Pressure} = \text{stress} \times \frac{\text{wall thickness}}{\text{radius}}$$

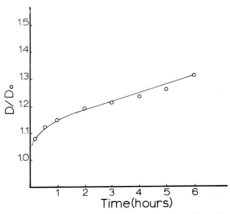

Figure 16–3. Change in diameter as a function of time after the sudden application of a pressure of 20 g/cm². Diameter increases gradually over a 6-hour period. D_o, initial diameter; D, diameter during deformation. (From Biancani P, Zabinski MP, Weiss RM: Bidimensional deformation of acutely obstructed in vitro rabbit ureter. Am J Physiol 225:671, 1973.)

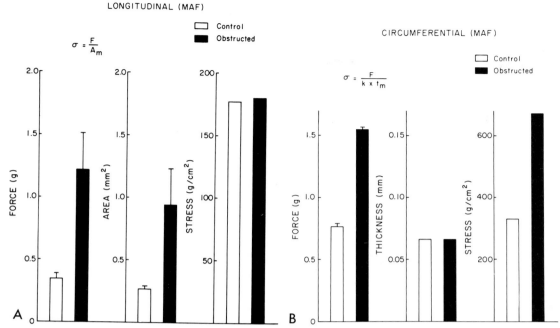

Figure 16–4. A, Longitudinal force, cross-sectional muscle area, and longitudinal stress at length of maximum active force development. B, Circumferential force, average muscle thickness, and circumferential stress at length of maximum active force development. σ, stress; F, force; A_m, cross-sectional muscle area; t_m, average thickness of muscle layer; k, a constant related to width of cut rings. (From Weiss RM, Biancani P: A rationale for ureteral tapering. Urology 20:482, 1982.)

Although stress increases following 2 weeks of obstruction, the decrease in the ratio of wall thickness to radius resulting from the marked increase in intraluminal diameter and thinning of the muscle layer results in a decrease in pressure. It must be realized that longer durations of obstruction or the presence of infection could alter these relationships (Rose et al).

Figure 16–5 is a diagrammatic attempt to elucidate the Laplace relationship as it pertains to changes observed with obstruction.

Figure 16–5. Diagrammatic representation of changes that occur with obstruction. F, force developed by each half of the ureter; W, blocks or weights representing load proportional to force; A, area over which force is distributed; P, pressure. (From Weiss RM, Biancani P: A rationale for ureteral tapering. Urology 20:482, 1982.)

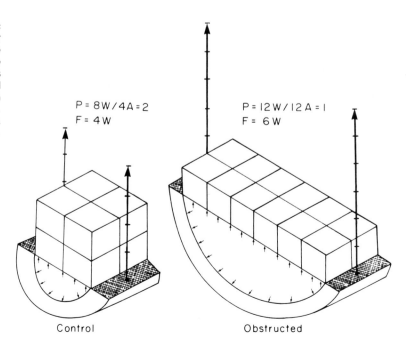

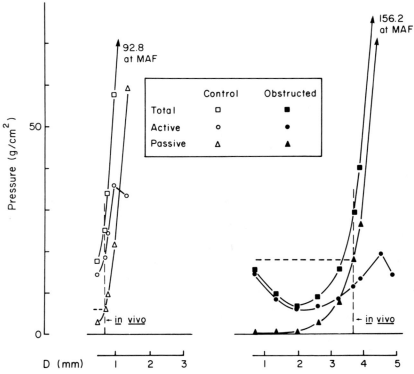

Figure 16–6. Pressure-diameter relationships of control and obstructed ureters. Calculated total, active, and passive pressures are shown as a function of calculated intraluminal diameters, D. In vivo passive pressures are indicated by horizontal dashed lines and in vivo dimensions by vertical dashed lines. (From Biancani P, Hausman M, Weiss RM: Effect of obstruction on ureteral circumferential force-length relations. Am J Physiol 243:F204, 1982.)

With obstruction, there is an increase in diameter and an increase in developed force. The increase in force is represented by an increase in the height of the arrows which equilibrate the weight of the blocks. Pressure is proportional to the height of the pile of blocks. An increase in diameter permits a wider distribution of the blocks, thus reducing the pressure. Intraluminal pressure therefore decreases in obstruction in spite of an increase in force and contractility.

Estimates of intraluminal pressures can be made from in vitro force-length contractility data (Biancani et al, 1982; Weiss and Biancani, 1982) (Fig. 16–6) and correspond to in vivo measurements (Rose and Gillenwater, 1973; Biancani et al, 1976). The obstructed ureter at in vivo dimensions has a higher resting (baseline) pressure and a lower contractile (active) pressure than control ureters. In control ureters, the total (active plus passive or resting) pressure developed at all diameters exceeds the passive pressure shown by the dotted line, and thus the generated active or contractile pressures are able to coapt the ureteral lumen

and propel the urine bolus. This information is readily apparent from direct observation.

In the obstructed ureter, however, the calculated active pressure is not synonymous with the pressure measured in a peristaltic contraction wave, but rather estimates the pressure that would develop if the whole ureter contracted simultaneously and uniformly throughout its whole length. In reality, this is not the case and only a small segment of the ureter contracts at any given time. Since at diameters less than 3.3 mm the passive pressure shown by the dotted line exceeds the total pressure, the contraction ring is incapable of contracting below this diameter and the pressure in the whole ureter remains approximately uniform and equal to the passive pressure. The principal effect of the contraction wave in the obstructed dilated ureter is to reduce slightly the ureteral volume and thereby raise slightly the overall resting pressure. Thus, although the obstructed ureter is able to develop greater circumferential contractile forces than control ureters, the expected intraluminal pressure generated by the obstructed ureter would be little different from resting pressure, and the contraction occurring during propagation of peristalsis would be incapable of coapting the ureteral lumen and propelling the urine bolus in an effective manner. This is in accord with observed changes in the clinically obstructed ureter. If, however, the urine were removed, for instance by relieving the obstruction, the ureter obstructed for 2 weeks would be able to immediately coapt and produce pressure comparable to control ureters. As shown in Figure 16–6, the total pressure in the control ureter near zero diameter is comparable to the total pressure in the obstructed ureter at a similar diameter.

Thus, 2 weeks of obstruction results in an increase in ureteral contractility but a decrease in contractile intraluminal pressures. This decrease in the ability to generate an active intraluminal pressure and the associated inability to coapt the ureter lumen impairs urine transport in the obstructed ureter.

Lastly, it should be noted that dilatation of the upper urinary tract resulting from obstruction may alter the response of the muscle to neurotransmitters and other pharmacologic agents (Kinn and Nergardh). Such changes may have some significance in the physiologic response of the upper urinary tract to obstruction.

DIAGNOSIS OF OBSTRUCTION

Dilatation of the upper urinary tract may occur secondary to obstruction or vesicoureteral reflux or may occur as a primary process without the presence of either obstruction or vesicoureteral reflux. Dilatation may persist following relief of obstruction even though urine transport is adequate. The excretory urogram can indicate whether hydroureteronephrosis exists, but it cannot be used to determine whether obstruction is present and therefore whether the function of the dilated upper urinary tract will improve following surgery. When attempting to determine the cause of dilatation in children, one must first consider whether or not vesicoureteral reflux is present. If vesicoureteral reflux is the cause of the dilatation, it can be readily determined by a voiding cystourethrogram. Occasionally, obstruction can coexist with vesicoureteral reflux and be a salient factor in the development of upper urinary tract dilatation (Weiss and

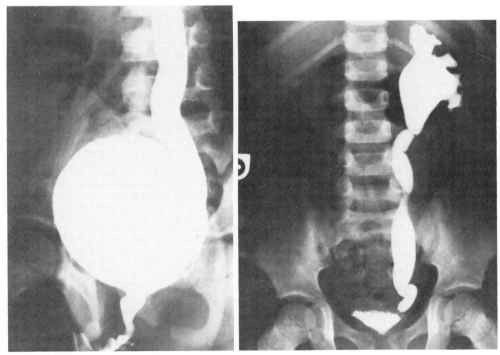

Figure 16–7. Voiding and postvoiding films from cystogram. (Adapted from Weiss RM, Lytton B: Vesicoureteral reflux and distal ureteral obstruction. J Urol *111*:245, 1974. © 1974, The Williams & Wilkins Co., Baltimore.)

Lytton; Whitaker and Flower) (Fig. 16–7). Such a process can be recognized on the postvoiding drainage film. If vesicoureteral reflux is not present, there are then two further possibilities to consider: Either there is upper urinary tract dilatation with obstruction or there is upper urinary tract dilatation without obstruction (Whitaker, 1975). Differentiating between these two entities may be difficult at times and has important clinical and therapeutic implications.

If ureteral dilatation in a nonrefluxing system extends to the level of the ureterovesical junction, it is important to determine whether abnormal bladder emptying or increased intravesical pressure is the cause of the dilatation. Under normal conditions ureteral contractile pressure exceeds intravesical pressure, resulting in passage of urine into the bladder. Since there is no evidence that the ureterovesical junction relaxes (Weiss and Biancani, 1983), it is this relationship between ureteral intraluminal pressure and intravesical pressure that determines the efficacy of urine passage across the ureterovesical junction. In the dilated, poorly contracting ureter or in the ureter during extreme flows, as observed with perfusion, it is the baseline pressure of the column of urine within the ureter that must exceed intravesical pressure for efficient transport. Intravesical pressure during storage is the most important parameter, since this is the pressure that the ureter works against over the greatest period of time. With filling of the normal bladder, the viscoelasticity of the bladder wall and sympathetic impulses inhibit the intravesical pressure rise of the tonus limb and maintain a relatively low intravesical pressure (McGuire). In some forms of neuropathic vesical dysfunction, and in some scarred bladders, the bladder is autonomous and relatively small increases in bladder volume are associated with large increases in intravesical pressure with resultant impairment of ureteral emptying and the development of ureteral dilatation (Fig. 16–8). The ureter has been shown to decompensate when intravesical pressures approach 40 cm H_2O (McGuire et al).

In addition to urodynamic testing of the lower urinary tract, an excretory urogram with an indwelling catheter within the bladder will often help to determine whether the bladder accounts for ureteral dilatation. Bladder drainage will decrease the degree of ureteral dilatation observed with the excretory urogram if the bladder is the cause of the hydroureteronephrosis. If the bladder is elim-

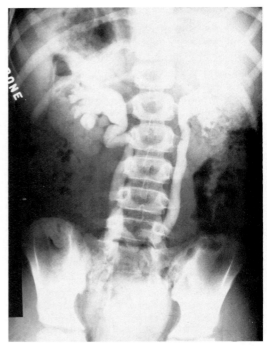

Figure 16–8. Excretory urogram in child with high pressure neurogenic bladder, showing bilateral upper urinary tract dilatation. A cystogram showed no reflux. Such bladders are often said to be "non-compliant" and may also be encountered in boys with severe obstruction from urethral valves, or after undiversion. (From Weiss RM: Clinical implications of ureteral physiology. J Urol 121:401, 1979. © 1979, The Williams & Wilkins Co., Baltimore.)

inated as a cause for dilatation, attention must be directed more proximally to differentiate obstructive from nonobstructive ureteral and renal pelvic dilatation in the nonrefluxing upper urinary tract.

Retrograde and/or antegrade pyelograms may aid in defining the site of urine holdup, but only in the most severe cases will these examinations alone determine whether obstruction exists. Retrograde and antegrade pyelography are not tests of function and do not provide the important physiologic information that will differentiate obstructive from nonobstructive dilatation. Cineradiography of the ureter also is of limited value in assessing function. Movement of fluid can be observed within the ureter, but quantitative assessment of the efficacy of urine transport to the bladder or the functional capacity of the ureteral wall cannot be obtained. Cineradiography also may aid in defining anatomic abnormalities in selected cases, but a standard excretory urogram usually will provide the same information with far less radiation exposure.

Measurements of basal or resting intraluminal pressures do not help in differentiating an obstructive from a nonobstructive dilatation. As previously noted, basal pressures are elevated significantly for only a short time following the onset of obstruction. Pressures are obviously low in the nonobstructive system, but also may be low in the presence of obstruction (Vela-Navarrete; Struthers). Baseline pressure is also influenced by the state of hydration, the degree of renal function, the severity and duration of obstruction, and the compliance of the system. The static reading of baseline ureteral or renal pelvic pressure, therefore, is not of diagnostic value. Nor are alterations in the amplitude of ureteral peristaltic pressure waves.

Evaluation

The best available methods for differentiating obstructive from nonobstructive dilatation of the ureter and renal pelvis in nonrefluxing systems depend on assessing the efficacy of urine transport. The upper urinary tract can transport a predetermined maximum amount of fluid per unit of time. When transport is inadequate, urine stagnates, and dilatation results. Dilatation is dependent on the compliance of the system and can result either from too much fluid entering the system per unit of time or too little fluid exiting the system per unit of time. The balance between input and output determines the adequacy of transport. The properly functioning upper urinary tract should transport urine over the entire range of physiologically possible flow rates without undergoing marked deformational changes or increases in intraluminal pressure of a magnitude that would be deleterious to the function of the smooth muscle of the ureter and renal pelvis or to renal function itself. With minor degrees of obstruction, urine transport may not be significantly impeded at low flow rates but may be inadequate at high flow rates with resultant development of dilatation. More marked degrees of obstruction may impede urine transport regardless of the flow rate. These relationships hold for both anatomic and functional obstructions.

Diuretic Urograms

Diureteric urograms determine whether the upper urinary tract can handle increases in flow without undergoing marked increases in dimensions. Significant dimensional changes with diuresis are indicative of the upper urinary tract's inability to transport fluid efficiently over a range of physiologic flow rates and implies that at these high flow rates, elevated intraluminal pressures are present that may adversely affect renal function and structure (Fig. 16–9). In order for such

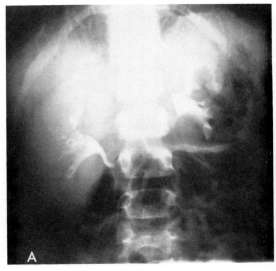
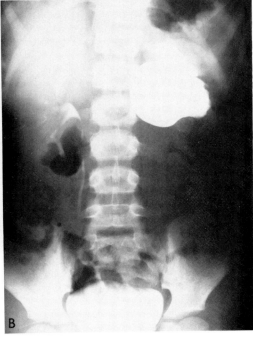

Figure 16–9. A, Excretory urogram showing essentially normal upper tracts. B, Film taken from same child immediately after massive diuresis induced by cardiac angiogram. (From Weiss RM: Clinical implications of ureteral physiology. J Urol 121:401, 1979. © 1979, The Williams & Wilkins Co., Baltimore.)

changes to be observed, renal function must be such that the kidney responds to the diuretic stimulus with a significant increase in urine output and that the system be adequately compliant. Whitfield et al (1977) quantified changes on the excretory urogram, both before and after furosemide-induced diuresis, to diagnose ureteropelvic junction obstruction. A 22 per cent increase in renal pelvic area following diuresis correlated with other objective urodynamic evidence of obstruction.

Diuretic Radionuclide Renogram

The diuretic radionuclide renogram is another modality that has been used to differentiate the obstructed from the nonobstructed dilated upper urinary tract in nonrefluxing systems (O'Reilly et al; Koff et al, 1979; Stage and Lewis). The hypothesis upon which the method is based is that the prolonged retention of isotope in the nonobstructed dilated system is due to a reservoir effect and that increased urine flow following diuretic administration should cause a prompt washout of activity from the dilated structure, whether it be renal pelvis or ureter. Conversely, in a dilated obstructed system, administration of a diuretic is unable to cause a significant washout of retained isotopic tracer. In this technique, either iodine-131 hippuran or technetium-99m diethylenetriaminepentaacetic acid is injected intravenously. A gamma scintillation camera is used for imaging, and counts per unit of area of the dilated system are accumulated on a nuclear medicine computer. Fifteen to 30 minutes after injection of the radionuclide, at a time at which there is holdup of nuclide in the dilated upper urinary tract on the renogram curve, furosemide (0.3 to 0.5 mg/kg) is injected intravenously and computer data collection is continued for an additional 15 to 20 minutes. The dosage must be standardized, as increasing amounts produce an increased diuretic effect. Similar response patterns are observed if the diuretic is given prior to administration of the radiotracer (O'Reilly et al).

Four categories of response have been described (Fig. 16–10). Response 1 or the normal pattern is characterized by a rapid uptake of radionuclide and a subsequent prompt spontaneous washout of the excreted radionuclide without the administration of furosemide. Response 2 or the obstructed pattern consists of an initial slow uptake and then gradual accumulation of the radioactive tracer in the dilated system. The curve may plateau or continue to increase progressively. Administration of a diuretic does not result in a significant washout of tracer. Response 3a is the dilated but nonobstructive pattern. The renogram curve initially following the injection of the radionuclide is similar to that observed with obstruction. There is a slow uptake and gradual accumulation of tracer in the dilated system. However, in contrast to the pattern observed with obstruction, there is a prompt effective washout of radionuclide following the administration of furosemide. Response 3b is an equivocal pattern. Initially

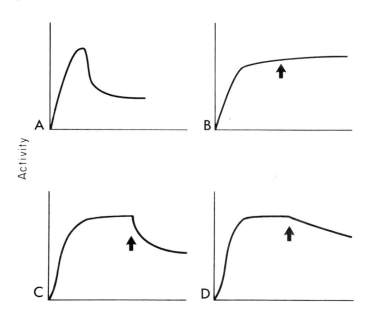

Figure 16–10. Schematic representation of response categories observed with diuretic radionuclide renograms. *A,* Response 1 or normal pattern. *B,* Response 2 or obstructed pattern. *C,* Response 3a or dilated nonobstructed pattern. *D,* Response 3b or equivocal pattern. Arrows indicate time of furosemide administration. (From Weiss RM: Clinical correlations of ureteral physiology. Am J Kid Dis 2:409, 1983. © 1983, National Kidney Foundation, Inc.)

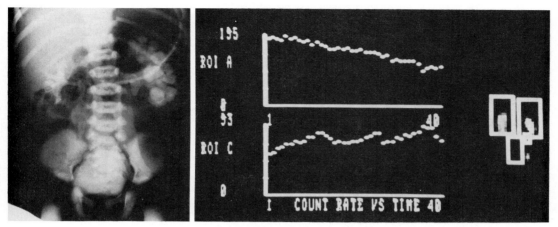

Figure 16–11. Excretory urogram of child with left ureterovesical junction obstruction. Renogram curves are shown from the time of furosemide administration. Top curve obtained with counter over left renal pelvis; bottom curve with counter over distal left ureter. Renogram was obtained with catheter in the bladder and draining.

after injection of the radionuclide, the pattern is similar to that observed with obstruction; that is, there is a slow uptake and gradual accumulation of tracer in the dilated system. Following the administration of the diuretic, there is only a minimal or moderate washout of radionuclide, rendering interpretation of the test difficult or impossible. Further quantitative studies such as a Whitaker test are required before one will be able to determine whether a given case with this pattern is obstructed or not (see Chapter 8). This pattern may be observed in unobstructed patients when renal function is very poor or the collecting system is extremely dilated.

There are several pitfalls in the use of diuretic renography. Severe renal impairment may prevent sufficient clearance of isotope to provide an accurate renogram. A flat curve could mean either that there is inadequate function to effect a diuresis or that severe obstruction exists (Koff et al, 1980). On the other hand, definite washout of tracer sometimes still can effectively rule out obstruction even if renal function is poor. It also is important when performing diuretic renography to select the area of interest in the region of the suspected obstruction (Koff et al, 1979; Thrall et al). For instance, if obstruction is in the region of the ureterovesical junction, administration of a diuretic may result in washout of tracer from the renal pelvis into the ureter. If only the renal pelvis was monitored for data analysis, an erroneous opinion that obstruction was not present might be obtained. Appropriate placement of the probe in the region of the ureterovesical junction would reveal

the failure of tracer washout and lead to the correct diagnosis of obstruction at that level (Fig. 16–11). Furthermore, when a lower ureteral obstruction is suspected or when the kidney is low-lying or in the pelvis, it is important to drain the bladder with a catheter so that tracer in the bladder does not overlap the field of interest.

To understand the clinical application for the diuretic excretory urogram and the diuretic renogram, one should consider the following possibilities. An upper urinary tract at low flows may be: (1) normal, that is, nonobstructed and nondilated; (2) nonobstructed and capacious or dilated; (3) obstructed but not stressed and thus nondilated; or (4) obstructed and dilated. If the system is nonobstructed and nondilated, then the standard excretory urogram at low flows will be, by definition, nondilated. Following diuresis, this nonobstructed upper urinary tract should be able to handle the increased flow. Thus, any increase in dimensions should be minor, producing less than a 20 per cent increase in area (Whitfield et al, 1977; Bratt et al; Nilson et al). In such a system, the renogram should show a prompt spontaneous washout of isotope even at low flows. It is unnecessary to administer a diuretic to washout counts that have already been dissipated.

If a system is nonobstructed but dilated at low flows, the excretory urogram will show a dilated system. Since the system is not obstructed, it should be able to handle higher flows; thus, induced diuresis should either wash out the contrast material and decrease the dimensions, or at least not result in a significant increase in the area of retained contrast material. The renogram in such a system should show retention of tracer in the capacious system and subsequent washout or decrease in counts following diuresis. The diuretic renogram has its greatest value in excluding obstruction in this type of system.

If a system is obstructed but nondilated at low flows, diuresis may precipitate dilatation and thus demonstrate the presence of obstruction. Such a system can handle low but not high flows. A diuretic excretory urogram would show a significant increase in the area of retained contrast material, since diuresis would precipitate dilatation. Diuretic urograms have their greatest value in such a system.

If a system is truly obstructed and dilated at low flows, then diuresis should increase the magnitude of the dilatation. Diuresis will then increase the dimensions of the collecting system on an excretory urogram if the system had not been maximally dilated prior to the administration of the diuretic. A renogram in this situation should show a slow and gradual accumulation of radioactive tracer with dilated system, and tracer washout should be inadequate following administration of a diuretic.

Deconvolution analysis is another radioisotopic technique that has been used to assess the significance of upper urinary tract dilatation (Whitfield et al, 1978). This technique allows one to differentiate isotope transport in the parenchyma from that in the renal pelvis. In the dilated nonobstructed system, parenchymal transit time remains normal although whole kidney (parenchyma plus pelvis) transit time is increased. In significantly obstructed systems, the isotope transit time in the parenchyma also is prolonged when compared with that in normal or dilated nonobstructed systems. This technique is somewhat complex and not as widely employed as the diuretic renogram.

Perfusion Studies

Perfusion studies are widely used in an attempt to differentiate dilated systems that are obstructed from those that are not obstructed, particularly when the diuretic renogram is equivocal (Whitaker, 1973, 1978; Backlund and Reuterskiold, 1969a and b; Reuterskiold, 1969, 1970). Following nephrostomy or percutaneous puncture of the dilated upper urinary tract, the system is per-

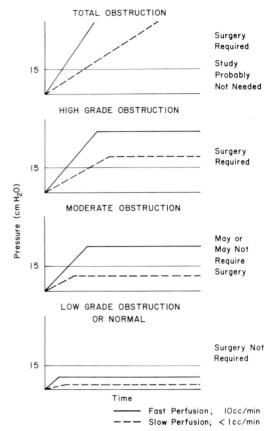

Figure 16–12. Schematic representation of data obtained with perfusion studies. Fast perfusion rate, 10 ml/min, is used in standard examinations. Slow perfusion rate, less than 1 ml/min, is more physiologic. (From Weiss RM: Clinical implications of ureteral physiology. J Urol *121*:401, 1979. © 1979, The Williams & Wilkins Co., Baltimore.)

fused at 10 ml/min and pressures are measured continuously after achievement of steady state conditions, which is assumed to occur when an equilibrium is reached between the constant flow into and out of the system. Such an equilibrium would not be reached with a total obstruction (Fig. 16–12), but perfusion studies are usually not required under such conditions. The basic premise in the perfusion studies is that if the dilated upper urinary tract can transport 10 ml/min —a fluid load greater than would ever be expected during usual physiologic states— without an inordinate increase in pressure, no physiologic obstruction is present. From a large clinical experience, Whitaker (1978) concluded that under these flow conditions a pressure less than 15 cm H_2O correlated with a nonobstructive state, whereas pressures greater than 22 cm H$_2$O invariably correlated with obstruction. With this definition, minor degrees of obstruction could be undetected. However, the presumption is that if at high flows the hydrostatic pressure in the system is not at a level that would produce renal deterioration, then lower physiologic flows surely should be well tolerated. It must be emphasized that high perfusion pressures at flows of 10 ml/min do not necessarily mean that the hydrostatic pressure within the system would be elevated at lower or more physiologic flow rates. The higher flows are used to stress the system and thus to detect the slightest propensity to obstruction. The interpretation of data obtained by perfusion studies is schematically shown in Figure 16–12.

In performing perfusion studies, strict ad-

herence to detail is imperative in order to obtain relevant information. The resistance to flow that is related to needle size and position, length and compliance of extrinsic tubing, viscosity of perfusion fluid, temperature, and flow rate must be taken into account in obtaining quantitative data (Toguri and Fournier). Care must be taken to assure that an equilibrium state has been reached prior to obtaining pressure measurements. Furthermore, the bladder needs to be continuously drained to eliminate the bladder's effect on urine transport. Fluoroscopic monitoring aids in interpretation of data (Coolsaet et al; Whitfield et al, 1976).

Perfusion studies are invasive procedures and require, in many instances, a percutaneous puncture of the upper urinary tract. The

Figure 16–13. A, Intravenous pyelogram in newborn showing nonvisualization of right kidney secondary to ureteropelvic junction obstruction and mild left ureteropelvic junction obstruction (arrow). B, Three months later, subsequent to a right nephrectomy, there is progression of the left hydronephrosis.

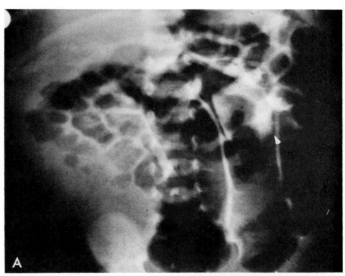
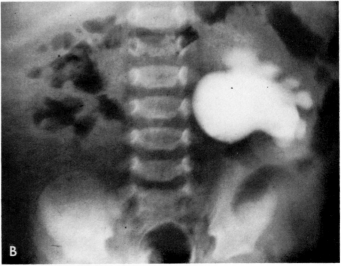

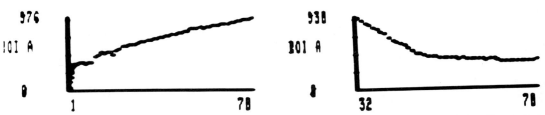

Figure 16–14. Diuretic renogram on patient demonstrated in Figure 16–13 showing nonobstructive pattern following injection of furosemide. Renogram was performed at the time at which Figure 16–13B was obtained. Tracing on left is prior to injection of furosemide, tracing on right following injection of furosemide.

examination is not indicated in instances in which the diagnosis can be made with standard radiographic or isotopic techniques or in instances in which the data obtained would not directly affect therapy. However, the study can, if performed and interpreted properly, show important and clinically relevant information in selected cases. It is helpful in determining whether the dilated system remaining after surgical repair of a long-standing obstruction is still obstructed. The potential risks of the procedure are less in those patients who have a nephrostomy or loop ureterostomy. In cases with retained stone fragments in which it is planned to irrigate with renacidin through a nephrostomy tube, the same principle can be used to determine a rapid and yet safe flow rate for renacidin infusion.

Although the perfusion study is presently the standard for distinguishing the obstructed from the nonobstructed system, the invasive nature of the procedure has led many to adopt the diuretic renogram as the initial method of determining whether a nonrefluxing dilated system is obstructed and to reserve the pressure flow study for the equivocal case in which precise knowledge is essential. The basic problem in the interpretation of data obtained with either of these methodologies is the definition of "clinically relevant obstruction," that is, just how much holdup to flow or increase in pressure is required to result in renal functional or anatomic deterioration over time taking into account the compliance of the system (Koff and Thrall, 1981b). Furthermore, false positive and false negative conclusions are possible with either of these studies. Figure 16–13 shows progressive changes with time secondary to a ureteropelvic junction obstruction, and yet the diuretic renogram (Fig. 16–14) performed at the time of the second pyelogram was normal, as was a perfusion study. This could be interpreted as a

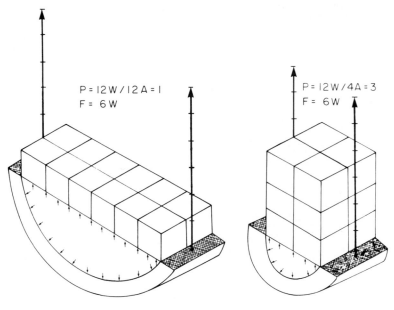

Figure 16–15. Diagrammatic representation of changes that occur with ureteral tapering. F, force developed by each half of ureter; W, blocks or weights representing load proportional to force; A, area over which force is distributed; P, pressure. (From Weiss RM, Biancani P: A rationale for ureteral tapering. Urology 20:482, 1982.)

$P = 12W/12A = 1$
$F = 6W$

$P = 12W/4A = 3$
$F = 6W$

Obstructed

Tapered

failure of the studies to detect a clinically significant obstruction or could be consistent with an intermittent obstructive process that defied detection.

Lastly, it is theoretically possible that the wide and/or weakly contracting ureter may by itself, with urine bolus flow, result in an obstructive process, even if the ureterovesical junction and lower ureter are normal (Griffiths). Such changes would not be detected by perfusion studies. Perhaps this provides an indication for ureteral tapering (Hendren), a procedure that to date has been shown to improve radiographic appearance, although the question remains as to whether it aids in preserving renal function when anatomic or functional obstruction does not exist at the ureterovesical junction. With ureteral tapering, muscle thickness and the ability of the ureteral fibers to contract remains unchanged. The decrease in radius resulting from tapering in itself, from the Laplace relationship, could account for higher intraluminal pressures which could improve urine transport. The tapered ureter can coapt its walls more readily and generate higher intraluminal pressure even though the muscle quality itself has not been changed. Figure 16–15 shows in diagrammatic fashion how with ureteral tapering, force or the number of blocks remains unchanged, but intraluminal pressure increases as the load is distributed over a smaller area. Thus, the height of the pile of blocks increases. Although the possibility of deleterious effects resulting from the wide "nonobstructed" ureter remains a controversial subject, these theoretical considerations should be considered in management and in the interpretation of our current modalities for accurately diagnosing obstruction.

BIBLIOGRAPHY

Backlund L, Grott G, Reuterskiold A: Functional stenosis as a cause of pelvi-ureteric obstruction and hydronephrosis. Arch Dis Child 40:203, 1965.

Backlund L, Reuterskiold AG: Activity in the dilated dog ureter. Scand J Urol Nephrol 3:99, 1969a.

Backlund L, Reuterskiold AG: The abnormal ureter in children. Scand J Urol Nephrol 3:219, 1969b.

Barr L, Berger W, Dewey MM: Electrical transmission at the nexus between smooth muscle cells. J Genet Physiol 51:347, 1968.

Biancani P, Hausman M, Weiss RM: Effect of obstruction on ureteral circumferential force-length relations. Am J Physiol 243:F204, 1982.

Biancani P, Zabinski MP, Weiss RM: Bidimensional deformation of acutely obstructed in vitro rabbit ureter. Am J Physiol 225:671, 1973.

Biancani P, Zabinski MP, Weiss RM: Time course of ureteral changes with acute and chronic obstruction. Am J Physiol 231:393, 1976.

Bozler E: The activity of the pacemaker previous to the discharge of a muscular impulse. Am J Physiol 136:543, 1942.

Bratt CG, Aurell M, Nilson A, et al: Diuretic urography and renography in the diagnosis of hydronephrosis. Contrib Nephrol 11:142, 1978.

Constantinou CE: Renal pelvic pacemaker control of ureteral peristaltic rate. Am J Physiol 226:1413, 1974.

Coolsaet BLRA, Griffiths DJ, Van Mastrigt R, et al: Urodynamic investigation of the wide ureter. J Urol 124:666, 1980.

Djurhuus JC, Constantinou CE: Chronic ureteric obstruction and its impact on the coordinating mechanisms of peristalsis (pyeloureteric pacemaker system). Urol Res 10:267, 1982.

Djurhuus JC, Stage P: Percutaneous intrapelvic pressure registration in hydronephrosis during diuresis. Acta Chir Scand 472:43, 1976.

Edmond P, Ross JA, Kirkland IS: Human ureteral peristalsis. J Urol 104:670, 1970.

Gosling JA, Dixon JS: Species variation in the location of upper urinary tract pacemaker cells. Invest Urol 11:418, 1974.

Gottschalk CW, Mylle M: Micropuncture study of pressures in proximal tubules and peritubular capillaries of the rat kidney and their relation to ureteral and renal venous pressures. Am J Physiol 185:430, 1956.

Griffiths DJ: The mechanics of urine transport in the upper urinary tract. II. The discharge of the bolus into the bladder and dynamics at high rates of flow. Neurourology, 2:167, 1983.

Hausman M, Biancani P, Weiss RM: Obstruction induced changes in longitudinal force-length relations of rabbit ureter. Invest Urol 17:223, 1979.

Hendren WH: A new aproach to infants with severe obstructive uropathy: early complete reconstruction. J Pediatr Surg 5:184, 1970.

Kinn AC, Nergardh A: Autonomic receptor functions in the normal and dilated renal pelvis: an in vitro study in man and rabbit. Urol Res 7:261, 1979.

Kobayachi M: Conduction velocity in various regions of the ureter. Tohoku J Exp Med 83:220, 1964.

Koff SA, Thrall JH: Diagnosis of obstruction in experimental hydroureteronephrosis. Urology 17:570, 1981a.

Koff SA, Thrall JH: The diagnosis of obstruction in experimental hydroureteronephrosis: mechanism for progressive urinary tract dilation. Invest Urol 19:85, 1981b.

Koff SA, Thrall JH, Keyes JW Jr: Diuretic radionuclide urography: a non-invasive method for evaluating nephroureteral dilatation. J Urol 122:451, 1979.

Koff SA, Thrall JH, Keyes JW Jr: Assessment of hydroureteronephrosis in children using diuretic radionuclide urography. J Urol 123:531, 1980.

Kuriyama H, Osa T, Toida N: Membrane properties of the smooth muscle of guinea-pig ureter. J Physiol (Lond) 191:225, 1967.

Libertino JA, Weiss RM: Ultrastructure of human ureter. J Urol 108:71, 1972.

McGuire EJ: Physiology of the lower urinary tract. Am J Kidney Dis 2:402, 1983.

McGuire EJ, Woodside JR, Borden TA, et al: Prognostic value of urodynamic testing in myelodysplastic patients. J Urol 126:205, 1981.

Nilson AE, Aurell M, Bratt CG, et al: Diuretic urography in the assessment of pelviureteric junction obstruction in patients with wide renal pelves. Acta Radiol Diagn 21:499, 1980.

Notley RG: The musculature of the human ureter. Br J Urol 42:724, 1970.

O'Reilly PH, Testa HJ, Lawson RS, et al: Diuresis renography in equivocal urinary tract obstruction. Br J Urol 50:76, 1978.

Reuterskiold AG: Ureteric pressure variations at different flow rates and varying bladder pressures in normal dogs. Acta Soc Med Upsal 74:94, 1969.

Reuterskiold AG: The abnormal ureter in children. II. Perfusion studies on the refluxing ureter. Scand J Urol Nephrol 4:99, 1970.

Rose JG, Gillenwater JY: Pathophysiology of ureteral obstruction. Am J Physiol 225:830, 1973.

Rose JG, Gillenwater JY: Effects of obstruction upon ureteral function. Urology 12:139, 1978.

Rose JG, Gillenwater JY, Wyker AT: The recovery of function of chronically obstructed and infected ureters. Invest Urol 13:125, 1975.

Schweitzer FAW: Intrapelvic pressure and renal function studies in experimental chronic partial ureteric obstruction. Br J Urol 45:2, 1973.

Stage KH, Lewis S: Use of the radionuclide washout test in evaluation of suspected upper urinary tract obstruction. J Urol 125:379, 1981.

Struthers NW: The role of manometry in the investigation of pelviureteral function. Br J Urol 41:129, 1969.

Thrall JH, Koff SA, Keyes JW Jr: Diuretic radionuclide renography and scintigraphy in the differential diagnosis of hydroureteronephrosis. Semin Nucl Med 11:89, 1981.

Toguri AG, Fournier G: Factors influencing the pressure-flow perfusion system. J Urol 127:1021, 1982.

Tsuchida S, Yamaguchi O: A constant electrical activity of the renal pelvis correlated to ureteral peristalsis. Tohoku J Exp Med 121:133, 1977.

Uehara Y, Burnstock G: Demonstration of "gap junctions" between smooth muscle cells. J Cell Biol 44:215, 1970.

Vaughan ED Jr, Shenasky JH II, Gillenwater JY: Mechanism of acute hemodynamic response to ureteral occlusion. Invest Urol 9:109, 1971.

Vaughan ED Jr, Sorenson EJ, Gillenwater JY: The renal hemodynamic response to chronic unilateral ureteral occlusion. Invest Urol 8:78, 1970.

Vela-Navarrete R: Percutaneous intrapelvic pressure determinations in the study of hydronephrosis. Invest Urol 8:526, 1971.

Vereecken RL, Derluyn J, Verduyn H: The viscoelastic behavior of the ureter during elongation. Urol Res 1:15, 1973.

Weiss RM: Clinical implications of ureteral physiology. J Urol 121:401, 1979.

Weiss RM: Clinical correlations of ureteral physiology. Am J Kidney Dis 2:409, 1983.

Weiss RM, Bassett AL, Hoffman BF: Dynamic length-tension curves of cat ureters. Am J Physiol 222:388, 1972.

Weiss RM, Biancani P: A rationale for ureteral tapering. Urology 20:482, 1982.

Weiss RM, Biancani P: Characteristics of normal and refluxing ureterovesical junctions. J Urol 129:858, 1983.

Weiss RM, Lytton B: Vesicoureteral reflux and distal ureteral obstruction. J Urol 111:245, 1974.

Weiss RM, Wagner ML, Hoffman BF: Localization of pacemaker for peristalsis in the intact canine ureter. Invest Urol 5:42, 1967.

Whitaker RH: Methods of assessing obstruction in dilated ureters. Br J Urol 45:15, 1973.

Whitaker RH: Some observations and theories on the wide ureter and hydronephrosis. Br J Urol 47:377, 1975.

Whitaker RH: Clinical assessment of pelvic and ureteral function. Urology 12:146, 1978.

Whitaker RH, Flower CSR: Ureters that show both reflux and obstruction. Br J Urol 51:471, 1979.

Whitfield HN, Britton KE, Fry IK, et al: The obstructed kidney: correlation between renal function and urodynamic assessment. Br J Urol 49:615, 1977.

Whitfield HN, Britton KE, Hendry WF, et al: The distinction between obstructive uropathy and nephropathy by radioisotope transit times. Br J Urol 50:433, 1978.

Whitfield HN, Harrison NW, Sherwood T, et al: Upper urinary tract obstruction: pressure flow studies in children. Br J Urol 48:427, 1976.

Witherow RO, Whitaker RH: The predictive accuracy of antegrade pressure flow studies in equivocal upper tract obstruction. Br J Urol 53:496, 1981.

Woodburne RT, Lapides J: The ureteral lumen during peristalsis. Am J Anat 133:255, 1972.

Detection and Management of Hydronephrosis in Utero

STEPHEN A. KRAMER

High-resolution, gray-scale, real-time ultrasonography permits accurate differentiation between cystic and solid renal masses. Prenatal ultrasonography is a safe and noninvasive technique that can detect a variety of congenital abnormalities in utero (Cass et al; Farrant; Fourcroy et al; Hately and Nicholls; Hobbins et al; Kay et al; Kurjak et al; Matturri et al; Nelson et al; Okulski; Sanders and Graham; Walzer and Koenigsberg). Antenatal sonography is of proven benefit in the detection and follow-up of patients with oligohydramnios. Advances in ultrasonographic techniques have permitted improved visual-

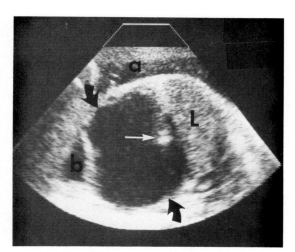

Figure 16-16. Real-time longitudinal sonogram shows large cystic mass in right renal fossa during percutaneous puncture. Needle tip *(small arrow)* is within 10 cm cystic mass *(curved arrows)* between liver (L) and urinary bladder (b). a, amniotic fluid. (From Kramer SA: Current status of fetal intervention for congenital hydronephrosis. J Urol *130*:641, 1983. © 1983, The Williams & Wilkins Company, Baltimore.)

Table 16-1. Errors in the Diagnosis of Obstructive Uropathy by Fetal Ultrasonography

Multicystic kidney	
Vesicoureteral reflux	
Megacalycosis	
Ureterocele	
Congenital, nonobstructive megaureter	Hydronephrosis
Prune-belly syndrome	
Simple renal cyst	
Duodenal atresia	
Bladder outlet obstruction	
"Physiologic hydronephrosis"	

ization of fetal anatomy, and the potential exists for detection of congenital anomalies as early as 12 to 15 weeks of gestation (Canty et al; Dubbins et al; Hadlock et al). Ultrasonography may identify accurately up to 90 per cent of fetal kidneys by 17 to 20 weeks of gestation and 95 per cent by 22 weeks of gestation. The widespread use of this study during pregnancy has led to an increased recognition of fetal hydronephrosis (Badlani et al; Garrett et al; Martin and Taylor; Pope et al) (Fig. 16-16).

Not all large sonolucent retroperitoneal masses in the fetal abdomen are the result of obstructive uropathy (Kramer; Mahan et al). The fetus with presumed hydronephrosis detected by prenatal ultrasonography must undergo repeated studies with real-time techniques for initial findings to be confirmed. Dilatation of the collection systems may be transient and may resolve before delivery. Overdistention of the bladder may produce intermittent hydronephrosis that disappears after the fetus voids (Sanders and Graham). Thus, it is important to obtain ultrasonograms at several phases of bladder filling.

CAUSES OF COLLECTING SYSTEM DILATATION

Multicystic kidney is probably the most common entity confused with congenital ure-teropelvic junction obstruction (Stuck et al) (Table 16-1). Ultrasonography in neonates and infants often can differentiate the classic multicystic kidney from obstruction at the ureteropelvic junction (Bearman et al). The morphologic appearance of ureteropelvic junction obstruction is readily discernible from the usual type of multicystic kidney secondary to pelvioinfundibular atresia (Griscom et al) (Fig. 16-17). Stuck et al recently outlined ultrasonographic criteria for identifying multicystic kidney: (1) presence of interfaces between cysts; (2) nonmedial location of largest cyst; (3) absence of an identifiable renal sinus; (4) multiplicity of oval or round cysts that do not communicate; and (5) absence of parenchymal tissue. It is noteworthy, however, that atresia of the ureter or pelvis during intrauterine development may produce the hydro-

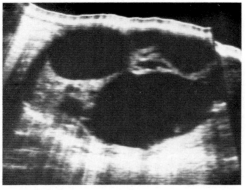

Figure 16-17. Parasagittal scan of left kidney demonstrates 8 cm mass composed of multiple cystic spaces of different sizes. This finding is consistent with multicystic dysplastic kidney. (From Kramer SA: Current status of fetal intervention for congenital hydronephrosis. J Urol *130*:641, 1983. © 1983, The Williams & Wilkins Company, Baltimore.)

nephrotic type of multicystic kidney that simulates ureteropelvic junction obstruction (Felson and Cussen). In these selected patients, the distinction between multicystic kidney and ureteropelvic junction obstruction in utero can be extremely difficult, and misdiagnosis may result in inappropriate fetal or obstetric intervention.

Several children with significant vesicoureteral reflux have been presumed to have obstructive uropathy on the basis of results of prenatal ultrasonography. Children with dilatation of the renal pelvis secondary to reflux usually have ureteral dilatation, which is not present in patients with congenital ureteropelvic junction obstruction (Fig. 16–18).

Prune-belly syndrome and nonobstructed dilatation of the collecting system have been diagnosed incorrectly as obstructive uropathy in utero (Oesch et al) (Fig. 16–19). Ultrasonographic findings in children with prune-belly syndrome include an enlarged bladder, bilateral ureteral dilatation, small kidneys, and oligohydramnios. Infrequently, these children have hydronephrotic kidneys; however, megaureters and megacystis should allow differentiation from ureteropelvic junction obstruction.

Duodenal atresia with an enlarged stomach has also led to a presumptive diagnosis of ureteropelvic junction obstruction (Hodgson NB, personal communication, 1982). Conversely, bilateral ureteropelvic junction obstruction and polyhydramnios may result in a misdiagnosis of duodenal atresia (Cass et al; Martin and Taylor; Sanders and Graham).

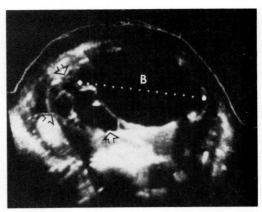

Figure 16–19. Transverse sonogram of fetus demonstrates 14.2 cm cystic mass consistent with urinary bladder (B). Adjacent cystic spaces represent dilated ureters *(arrows)*. (From Kramer SA: Current status of fetal intervention for congenital hydronephrosis. J Urol *130*:641, 1983. © 1983, The Williams & Wilkins Company, Baltimore.)

Patients with bladder outlet obstruction, such as those with posterior urethral valves or neuropathic disease, have dilatation of the bladder and one or both ureters. These findings should differentiate vesical outlet obstruction from obstruction at a higher level.

Furthermore, some observers have reported a 20 per cent incidence of "physiologic hydronephrosis" in the third trimester of pregnancy, which can be responsible for additional false positive findings.

ASSESSMENT OF RENAL FUNCTION

Currently, no reliable tests exist to accurately assess renal function or the potential for recoverability of fetal kidneys with obstructive uropathy. Furthermore, early in gestation, simple congenital hydronephrosis is extremely difficult to distinguish from cystic renal dysplasia secondary to obstructive uropathy (Felson and Cussen). Renal function in the fetus can be estimated by the volume of amniotic fluid detected by ultrasonography. Oligohydramnios is an accurate reflection of decreased urinary output and is the most important measure of renal impairment. A normal amniotic fluid volume indicates that at least one renal unit is functioning. It has been suggested that the intravenous administration of furosemide (Lasix) to the mother results in increased fetal urine output, which can be assessed by ultrasonic determination of blad-

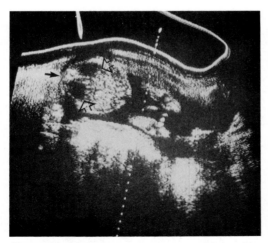

Figure 16–18. Transverse sonogram of fetus demonstrates dilated intrarenal collecting systems *(open arrows)* secondary to vesicoureteral reflux. Black arrow points to spine.

der volume (Wladimiroff). Failure to visualize the bladder after this stimulation test suggests that adequate functioning renal parenchyma is absent (Harrison et al, 1981). Although useful in bilateral renal agenesis or severe bilateral renal dysplasia, this technique has not been helpful in those with partial urinary obstruction (Harrison et al, 1982c).

The analysis of fetal urine by aspiration of the bladder or kidneys has not been of prognostic value. The ability of the bladder to refill after aspiration in utero similarly has not proved to be an effective predictor of renal function (Harrison et al, 1982a).

RENAL DYSPLASIA

The extent and timing of ureteral obstruction in utero correlate with the severity of renal dysplasia. Early obstruction of the developing kidney results in dysplastic changes (Beck; Fetterman et al; Harrison et al, 1982d; Tanagho, 1972a, 1972b, 1972c). Ureteral obstruction during the latter half of embryogenesis results in hydronephrosis without histologic changes of renal cystic dysplasia (Beck; Harrison et al., 1982d; Tanagho, 1972a, 1972b, 1972c). Clinical studies similarly have shown that the degree of obstructive uropathy and the time during which obstruction occurs are the two most important factors responsible for the severity of abnormal renal development (Osathanondh and Potter). There has been a recent report of death at 18 weeks of gestation in a fetus with posterior urethral valves (Bellinger et al). Histologic studies of the kidneys demonstrated significant renal dysplasia even at this early gestational age. Recent studies of chick embryos have shown that the primitive ducts associated with renal dysplasia may originate from branches of the ureteral bud that developed without condensed metanephrogenic mesenchyme (Maizels et al). These observations suggest that the most severe examples of renal dysplasia develop as a result of an abnormal location of the ureteral bud. These insults affect the kidney before nephrogenesis is complete.

TECHNIQUES FOR FETAL INTERVENTION

It has been postulated that unrelieved, high-grade urinary obstruction in utero may produce progressive renal damage. This supposition has resulted in the development of techniques for fetal intervention in attempts to correct obstructive uropathy and arrest renal dysplasia. The options currently available for the fetus with presumed hydronephrosis include the following.

Needle Aspiration of Bladder or Kidney

Percutaneous decompression of the bladder or renal pelvis by needle aspiration may avoid dystocia and cesarean section and allow for spontaneous vaginal delivery. However, repeat aspirations of the bladder or kidney have not been effective in the management of patients with congenital hydronephrosis. Antenatal decompression of the bladder has been performed in patients with prune-belly syndrome and megacystis (Oesch et al). Although technically successful, this technique has not produced resolution of hydronephrosis or arrested the development of renal dysplasia. Furthermore, the hydronephrotic kidney may be secondary to multicystic renal dysplasia and would not benefit from in utero decompression (Kramer).

Diversion of Urine into the Amniotic Fluid by Internal Shunt Drainage

Golbus et al developed a technique for percutaneous placement of a catheter shunt from the bladder to the amniotic cavity. This procedure has been successful in adequately decompressing the upper tracts but has not arrested the associated renal dysplasia or altered the course of abnormal renal development (Harrison et al, 1982c).

Open Surgical Diversion

The feasibility of open surgical diversion for the fetus with congenital hydronephrosis has been well documented (Harrison et al, 1982d). Harrison et al (1982a) performed extensive studies on the pathophysiology of congenital hydronephrosis in the fetal lamb model. These investigators developed successful anesthetic, surgical, and tocolytic techniques for fetal surgery in nonhuman primates and in the human fetus. Harrison et al (1982c) recently reported their cumulative experience in a group of 26 fetuses with dilated urinary tracts. This series included one fetus who underwent bilateral cutaneous ureterostomies at 21 weeks of gestation because of obstructive uropathy secondary to posterior urethral valves. Although surgery was technically successful, the infant died on the first day of life, and postmortem examination revealed renal dysplasia and pulmonary hypoplasia.

Early Delivery

Although the factors contributing to the development of pulmonary hypoplasia are poorly understood, a minimum volume of amniotic fluid appears to be critical to normal pulmonary embryogenesis. A deficiency in amniotic fluid prevents normal chest compliance and adversely affects normal lung development. The status of pulmonary maturity can be assessed through measurement of the lecithin-sphingomyelin ratio in the amniotic fluid or by the presence of phosphatidylglycerol. It is often possible to induce production of pulmonary surfactant by administration of steroids to the mother (Harrison et al, 1982c). However, pulmonary response to steroids in the presence of pulmonary dysplasia may not be predictable. This technique and recent advances in the respiratory care of premature infants have permitted early elective delivery with an excellent chance of survival in selected patients at 32 weeks of gestation.

RISKS VERSUS BENEFITS

Hemorrhage, sepsis, abortion, and premature labor (risk of respiratory distress syndrome) are significant risks to the fetus and mother subjected to in utero intervention (Table 16–2). The risks of hysterotomy for open surgical decompression have been enumerated by Harrison et al (1982a). These are that (1) the fetus or mother might die; (2) hemorrhage or sepsis, with resultant abortion, might occur; (3) cesarean section delivery would be required; (4) surgery might be unsuccessful; and (5) surgery might be successful but renal dysplasia and pulmonary hypoplasia might not be prevented. These risks must be weighed against the benefits of potential salvage of nephrogenesis and arrest of pulmonary hypoplasia.

TREATMENT GROUPS

Fetuses with congenital hydronephrosis may be separated into four treatment groups: (1) unilateral hydronephrosis; (2) bilateral hydronephrosis with good function; (3) bilateral hydronephrosis with poor function; and (4) bilateral hydronephrosis with equivocal function (Harrison et al, 1982c).

The fetus with unilateral hydronephrosis and a normal contralateral renal unit does not have oligohydramnios and will have normal renal function. Furthermore, there is no evidence to suggest that unilateral hydronephrosis causes pulmonary hypoplasia. These patients can be observed expectantly, and in utero intervention is not necessary except occasionally to permit vaginal delivery.

The fetus with bilateral hydronephrosis and adequate amniotic fluid volume has nearly normal renal and pulmonary function and does not need fetal intervention. These patients should be followed expectantly with serial ultrasound examinations and observation.

Bilateral hydronephrosis and oligohydramnios in the fetus have been associated uniformly with severe renal dysplasia and pulmonary hypoplasia (Harrison et al, 1982b, 1982c). Although successfully accomplished in these patients, early surgical intervention in utero has not yet altered the outcome beneficially.

The approach to the fetus with bilateral hydronephrosis and equivocal renal function was the subject of a recent review (Harrison et al, 1982c). This series included children with posterior urethral valves and prune-belly syndrome, all of whom had urethral obstruction, a thick-walled bladder, and bilateral hydronephrosis. Fetal intervention early in gestation in this group of patients similarly did not prevent renal dysplasia or pulmonary hypoplasia.

Table 16–2. Risks and Benefits of Fetal Intervention

Risks	Benefits
Hemorrhage	Potential salvage of nephrogenesis?
Sepsis	
Abortion	Potential prevention of pulmonary hypoplasia?
Premature labor (risk of respiratory distress syndrome)	
Fetal death	
Maternal death	

COMMENT

Currently there are no reliable tests to assess fetal renal function or the potential recoverability of kidneys with obstructive uropathy. Prenatal ultrasonography has been associated with a significant number of false results and cannot differentiate low-pressure, nonobstructed dilatation of the upper tracts from true obstructive uropathy at the ureteropelvic junction, ureterovesical junction, or bladder outlet. This is particularly true in attempts to distinguish the hydronephrotic type of multicystic kidney from ureteropelvic obstruction. It is important, therefore, to repeat the ultrasonogram after delivery to establish an accurate diagnosis and to evaluate the status of the contralateral kidney.

Functional tests after birth, such as renal scans and excretory urography, are mandatory to establish the proper diagnosis and assess the need for operative intervention. Prenatal ultrasonography is useful, however, for identification of the high-risk pregnancy and allows for early referral of these patients to medical centers where postnatal care can be instituted promptly.

Although in utero intervention for diagnosis or treatment of congenital hydronephrosis has been technically successful, little evidence exists to support the concept that early surgical decompression beneficially alters the outcome in children with congenital hydronephrosis. Experimental and clinical evidence strongly suggests that histologic changes of renal dysplasia occur early in gestation, long before in utero intervention is technically feasible.

In the fetus with obstructive uropathy, there is no evidence to suggest that relief of obstruction in utero will result in improvement in renal or pulmonary function beyond that achieved by pyeloplasty, vesicostomy, or ablation of posterior urethral valves in the neonate. Most fetuses with hydronephrosis have dilated low-pressure systems with adequate urinary output and amniotic fluid volume and can be followed safely to term delivery (Kramer; Lebowitz and Teele). The experience accumulated to date indicates that the fetus with congenital hydronephrosis detected in utero should be managed expectantly with serial ultrasound and observation. The natural history of congenital urinary tract dilatation in the fetus requires more extensive experimental study before fetal intervention by either radiography or in utero surgery can be recommended in the clinical setting.

BIBLIOGRAPHY

Badlani G, Abrams HJ, Kumari S: Diagnosis of fetal hydronephrosis in utero using ultrasound. Urology 16:315, 1980.

Bearman SB, Hine PL, Sanders RC: Multicystic kidney: a sonographic pattern. Radiology 118:685, 1976.

Beck AD: The effect of intra-uterine urinary obstruction upon the development of the fetal kidney. J Urol 105:784, 1971.

Bellinger MF, Comstock CH, Grosso D, et al: Fetal posterior urethral valves and renal dysplasia at 15 weeks gestational age. J Urol 129:1238, 1983.

Canty TG, Leopold GR, Wolf DA: Maternal ultrasonography for the antenatal diagnosis of surgically significant neonatal anomalies. Ann Surg 194:353, 1981.

Cass A, Smith S, Godec C, et al: Prenatal diagnosis of fetal urinary tract abnormalities by ultrasound. Urology 18:197, 1981.

Dubbins PA, Kurtz AB, Wapner RJ, et al: Renal agenesis: spectrum of in utero findings. JCU 9:189, 1981.

Farrant P: Early ultrasound diagnosis of fetal bladder neck obstruction. Br J Radiol 53:506, 1980.

Felson B, Cussen LJ: The hydronephrotic type of unilateral congenital multicystic disease of the kidney. Semin Roentgenol 10:113, 1975.

Fetterman GH, Ravitch MM, Sherman FE: Cystic changes in fetal kidneys following ureteral ligation: studies by microdissection. Kidney Int 5:111, 1974.

Fourcroy JL, Blei CL, Glassman LM, et al: Prenatal diagnosis by ultrasonography of genitourinary abnormalities. Urology 22:223, 1983.

Garrett WJ, Kossoff G, Osborn RA: The diagnosis of fetal hydronephrosis, megaureter and urethral obstruction by ultrasonic echography. Br J Obstet Gynaecol 82:115, 1975.

Golbus MS, Harrison MR, Filly RA, et al: In utero treatment of urinary tract obstruction. Am J Obstet Gynecol 142:383, 1982.

Griscom NT, Vawter GF, Fellers FX: Pelvoinfundibular atresia: the usual form of multicystic kidney: 44 unilateral and two bilateral cases. Semin Roentgenol 10:125, 1975.

Hadlock FP, Deter RL, Carpenter R, et al: Sonography of fetal urinary tract anomalies. AJR 137:261, 1981.

Harrison MR, Anderson J, Rosen MA, et al: Fetal surgery in the primate I. Anesthetic, surgical, and tocolytic management to maximize fetal-neonatal survival. J Pediatr Surg 17:115, 1982a.

Harrison MR, Golbus MS, Filly RA: Management of the fetus with a correctable congenital defect. JAMA 246:774, 1981.

Harrison MR, Golbus MS, Filly RA, et al: Fetal surgery for congenital hydronephrosis. N Engl J Med 306:591, 1982b.

Harrison MR, Golbus MS, Filly RA, et al: Management of the fetus with congenital hydronephrosis. J Pediatr Surg 17:728, 1982c.

Harrison MR, Nakayama DK, Noall R, et al: Correction of congenital hydronephrosis in utero. II. Decompression reverses the effects of obstruction on the fetal lung and urinary tract. J Pediatr Surg 17:965, 1982d.

Hately W, Nicholls B: The ultrasonic diagnosis of bilateral

hydronephrosis in twins during pregnancy. Br J Radiol 52:989, 1979.

Hobbins JC, Grannum PA, Berkowitz RL, et al: Ultrasound in the diagnosis of congenital anomalies. Am J Obstet Gynecol 134:331, 1979.

Kay R, Lee TG, Tank ES: Ultrasonographic diagnosis of fetal hydronephrosis in utero. Urology 13:286, 1979.

Kramer SA: Current status of fetal intervention for congenital hydronephrosis. J Urol 130:641, 1983.

Kurjak A, Kirkinen P, Latin V, et al: Ultrasonic assessment of fetal kidney function in normal and complicated pregnancies. Am J Obstet Gynecol 141:266, 1981.

Lebowitz RL, Teele RL: Fetal and neonatal hydronephrosis. Urol Radiol 5:185, 1983.

Mahan J, Gonzales R, Godec CJ, et al: Intrauterine obstructive uropathy: is early detection and intervention beneficial? Presented at the annual meeting of the Northwestern Pediatric Society, Chanhassen, Minnesota, September 24, 1982.

Maizels M, Simpson SB, Firlit CF: Understanding the morphogenesis of renal dysplasia. Presented at the meeting of the North Central Section of the American Urological Association, Marco Island, Florida, October 17–23, 1982.

Martin JJ, Taylor ES Jr: Diagnosis of bilateral hydronephrosis in utero by ultrasonography. Urology 17:272, 1981.

Matturri M, Peters BE, Kedziora JA: Prenatal and postnatal sonographic demonstration of bilateral ureteropelvic junction obstruction. Med Ultrasound 4:94, 1980.

Nelson LH, Resnick MI, Sumner TE: Sonolucencies in fetal and infant abdomen: implications for management. Urology 15:528, 1980.

Oesch I, Jann X, Bettex M: Ultrasonographic antenatal detection of obstructed bladder: diagnosis and management. Eur Urol 8:78, 1982.

Okulski TA: The prenatal diagnosis of lower urinary tract obstruction using B scan ultrasound: a case report. JCU 5:268, 1977.

Osathanondh V, Potter EL: Pathogenesis of polycystic kidneys: type 4 due to urethral obstruction. Arch Pathol 77:502, 1964.

Pope TL Jr, Alford BA, Buschi AJ, et al: Nuclear scintigraphy and ultrasound in the diagnosis of congenital ureteropelvic junction obstruction. J Urol 124:917, 1980.

Sanders R, Graham D: Twelve cases of hydronephrosis in utero diagnosed by ultrasonography. J Ultrasound Med 1:341, 1982.

Stuck KJ, Koff SA, Silver TM: Ultrasonic features of multicystic dysplastic kidney: expanded diagnostic criteria. Radiology 143:217, 1982.

Tanagho EA: Surgically induced partial urinary obstruction in the fetal lamb. I. Technique. Invest Urol 10:19, 1972a.

Tanagho EA: Surgically induced partial urinary obstruction in the fetal lamb. II. Urethral obstruction. Invest Urol 10:25, 1972b.

Tanagho EA: Surgically induced partial urinary obstruction in the fetal lamb. III. Ureteral obstruction. Invest Urol 10:35, 1972c.

Walzer A, Koenigsberg M: Prenatal evaluation of partial obstruction of the urinary tract. Radiology 135:93, 1980.

Wladimiroff JW: Effect of frusemide on fetal urine production. Br J Obstet Gynaecol 82:221, 1975.

Calyx

Reza S. Malek

Generalized calycectasis is undoubtedly one of the best recognized radiologic manifestations of obstructive uropathy. Poorly understood and ill classified, however, are a number of unusual conditions characterized by single or multiple dilated calyces in one or both kidneys. Synonymous use by some authors of such terms as hydrocalycosis, megacalycosis, calyceal diverticulm, pyelogenic cyst, and communicating cyst of the renal pelvis has further confused the issue (Williams et al).

The unusual forms of dilated calyces and their diverticula may be segregated into three distinct categories. A practical etiologic classification is provided in Table 16–3.

HYDROCALYCOSIS

The term hydrocalycosis simply denotes dilatation or "hydronephrosis" of one or more calyces. The cystic cavity is derived from the ureteral bud, and unless altered by prolonged infection and fibrosis, it is lined by transitional epithelium. Its stenotic infundibulum communicates directly with the renal pelvis (not with another calyx), and it may assume a size large enough to become clinically palpable (Williams and Mininberg).

Some children with hydrocalycosis present with urinary infection accompanied by pain that is directly referable to the renal lesion; occasionally, a loin mass is palpable. Other

Table 16-3. Unusual Calyceal Dilatation and Diverticulum

Lesion	Etiology
Hydrocalycosis	**Intrinsic obstruction**
	Congenital Infundibular stenosis Infundibulopelvic stenosis ?Achalasia
	Acquired Inflammation, perhaps with stone Localized obliterating pyelonephritis Tuberculosis Tumor (malignant or benign) Trauma
	Extrinsic obstruction
	Congenital Vascular compression
	Acquired Tumor (malignant or benign) Trauma
Megacalycosis	*Congenital* Faulty metanephric-ureteral bud embryogenesis Maldeveloped pelvicalyceal muscle Hypoplasia of juxtamedullary glomeruli
	Acquired? Intrauterine obstruction (fetal ureteral folds)
Calyceal diverticulum	*Congenital* Nondegeneration of third- and fourth-order divisions of ureteral bud

cases of the disease are diagnosed incidentally in the course of evaluating such urinary tract problems as urethral valves, reflux, ureteral ectopy, and meatal stenosis, and their usual sequelae.

Intrinsic Obstruction

CONGENITAL. Infundibular stenosis is a rare congenital form of hydrocalycosis. It is a lesser form of the disease, in which the renal pelvis is unaffected. The obstruction is clearly intrinsic, it produces one or more long stenotic (hypoplastic) infundibula with variably dilated calyces that may actually become extrarenal, and it may involve both kidneys (Fig. 16–20). The infundibulopelvic variety represents an extension of the stenotic process beyond the infundibula to the renal pelvis

(Fig. 16–21); the two varieties may coexist in the same child (Fig. 16–22). The stenotic (hypoplastic) infundibula, which are intrinsically obstructive, drain variably dilated calyces of cystic appearance, and these in turn communicate at their distal ends with a diminutive pelvis (Fig. 16–22). Attenuation of the parenchyma of the hydrocalyx may be so pronounced that differentiation from a renal cyst may become impossible (Figs. 16–20F and 16–23).

The basic defect is likely to be related to untimely budding of the ureter—too early or too late—during fetal life. This can lead to interruption or premature or delayed union of the ureter with the metanephric mass. Thus, the ureter enters the metanephric mass at a time when this tissue lacks potential for development. This may lead to anomalous divi-

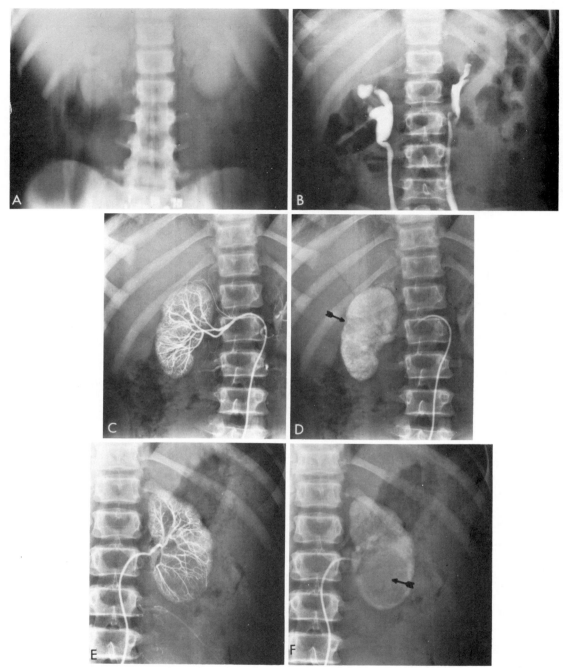

Figure 16–20. Hydrocalycosis of bilateral infundibular stenosis in 11-year-old boy who presented with polyuria, polydipsia (renal insufficiency), and poor stream. He was free of infection and reflux, but small urethral valves were found and resected, and symptoms improved. *A,* Excretory urogram. Poor opacification bilaterally. Note "extrarenal" calyx on right and masslike lesion in lower left renal pole. *B,* Retrograde ureteropyelogram (bilateral). Ureters and renal pelves are normal, but there are stenotic infundibula beyond which contrast medium has not passed except into middle "extrarenal" calyx on right. *C, D, E,* and *F,* Selective right (*C* and *D*) and left (*E* and *F*) renal angiograms. Note abnormal vascular pattern and diminished parenchymal thickness. Also note location of "extrarenal" calyx on right *(arrow)* and avascular cystic calyx on left *(arrow).*

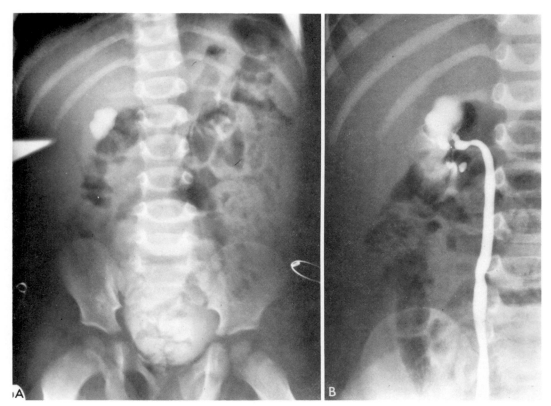

Figure 16–21. Hydrocalycosis in unilateral infundibulopelvic stenosis in 3-month-old boy who presented with urinary tract infection. Megacystis without reflux and meatal stenosis were found. Patient had remained trouble-free after urethral meatotomy. (Courtesy of Dr. Robert H. Halley.) *A*, Excretory urogram. Normal left kidney and a single dilated calyx in an otherwise unopacified right kidney. Note large bladder. *B*, Retrograde ureteropyelogram. Marked stenosis of right renal pelvis and infundibula with tubular backflow. Note essentially normal ureter.

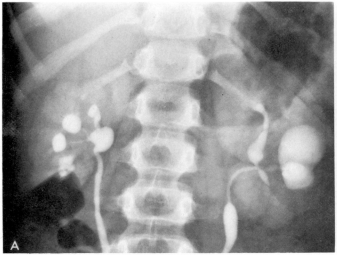

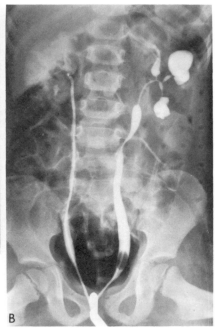

Figure 16–22. Hydrocalycosis of infundibulopelvic stenosis in 3-year-old boy with bilaterally ectopic ureteral orifices (at vesical neck) and other congenital anomalies, who presented with urinary infection. Reflux was not demonstrable, and patient has remained uninfected on chronic suppressive treatment. There has been no urographic change for 5 years. *A*, Excretory urogram. Right infundibular and left infundibulopelvic stenosis. *B*, Retrograde ureteropyelogram (bilateral). Mildly dilated left ureter. Note diffuse tubular backflow on right.

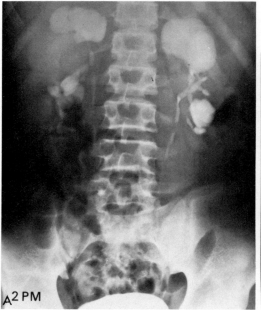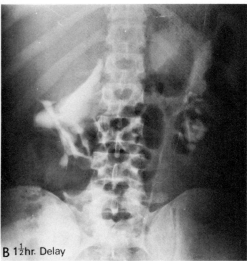

A 2 PM B 1½hr. Delay

Figure 16–23. *A* and *B*, Excretory urograms in a 15-year-old boy. (From Kelalis PP, Malek RS: Infundibulopelvic stenosis. J Urol *125*:568–571, 1981. © 1981, The Williams & Wilkins Company, Baltimore.)

sion or cystic dilatation of the tubules derived from the ureteral bud. Anomalies of the ureterovesical junction in four of eight children (five boys and three girls) with infundibulopelvic stenosis seen at the Mayo Clinic (Table 16–4) are another manifestation of such faulty embryogenesis and further substantiate this point (Kelalis and Malek; Mackie).

Clearly, there is a spectrum of obstructive renal disease, the degree of which depends on the extent of obstruction of the ureter and its intrarenal derivatives and on its relationship to the developing kidney. Its mildest form is represented by generalized pyelocalycectasis due to stenosis at the ureteropelvic junction (Fig. 16–24A). Its most severe form is the hydrocalycosis of the functionless multicystic dysplastic kidney, usually with atresia of the infundibula, pelvis, and variable lengths of the ureter. More aptly, this extreme end of the spectrum has been described as "congenital cystic hydrocalycosis" (Fink et al). The contention that this multicystic dysplastic kidney is an end-stage hydronephrosis is supported, at least in some instances, by the presence of luminal (pelvicalyceal) continuity during specimen radiography (Fig. 16–24E), by percutaneous antegrade pyelocalyceography (Fig. 16–25), and by calyceal crescents seen on excretory urography.

The type of renal dysmorphism that is characterized by various degrees of infundibular or infundibulopelvic narrowing is a central link in the obstructive hydronephrotic spectrum (Fig. 16–24B, C, and D). The clinical, radiographic, and pathologic features of these entities, together with their frequent association with other urinary tract anomalies (Table 16–4), point to a spectrum of advancing congenital malformations. It can be easily discerned that, had such malformation progressed to the extreme, the typical atretic ureter and associated bunch-of-grapes–like

Table 16–4. Findings in Eight Cases of Infundibulopelvic Stenosis

Bilateral	4
Unilateral	4
Contralateral multicystic kidney, 2	
Contralateral ureteropelvic junction, 1	
Megaureter	1
Vesicoureteral reflux	2
Ureteral ectopy	1
Urethral valves	1
Cryptorchidism	3
Anomalies of other systems	4

From Kelalis PP, Malek RS: Infundibulopelvic stenosis. J Urol *125*:568, 1981. © 1981, The Williams & Wilkins Company, Baltimore.

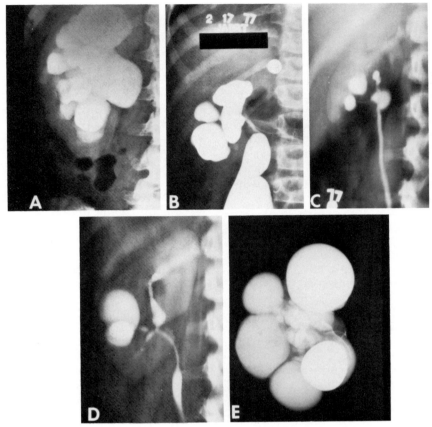

Figure 16–24. Spectrum of hydronephrosis: due to ureteropelvic stenosis (A), pelvic stenosis (B), infundibular stenosis (C), infundibulopelvic stenosis (D), and cystic dysplastic kidney (E). In cystic hydrocalycosis injected with radiopaque medium, note intraluminal communication suggesting extreme degree of hydronephrosis as in Figure 16–25. (A, B, and E from Kelalis PP, Malek RS: Infundibulopelvic stenosis. J Urol 125:568–571, 1981. © 1981, The Williams & Wilkins Company, Baltimore.)

Figure 16–25. Newborn infant with right hydronephrosis and functionless left kidney. Percutaneous puncture of the left renal pelvis followed by injection of contrast medium shows a left hydropelvis (P) and multiple cysts (C) in the left kidney. Multicystic kidney disease with hydropelvis was found on the left at surgery. (Reproduced with permission from Friedland GW: Hydronephrosis in infants and children, Part I. In Moseley RD Jr, et al (eds): Current Problems in Diagnostic Radiology. Copyright © 1978 by Year Book Medical Publishers, Inc., Chicago.)

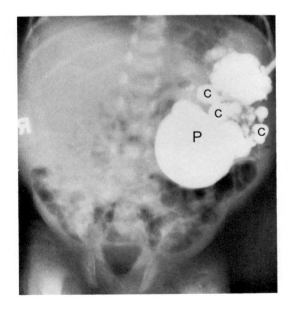

multicystic dysplastic kidney would have been the end result (Fig. 16–24). As a corollary, regression or perhaps "skipping" of these lesions through the pelvic variety leads to stenosis at the ureteropelvic junction, the most common form of hydronephrosis. The involvement of the contralateral kidney by ureteropelvic junction obstruction or multicystic renal dysplasia when unilateral infundibulopelvic stenosis is present further substantiates this concept (Table 16–4). Infundibular achalasia, although theoretically an attractive postulate, has never been demonstrated.

The clinical significance of these lesions lies in the need to differentiate them from renal malignancy and the more usual and correctable forms of hydronephrosis, and in taking into consideration their effects on renal function, superimposed infection, occasional stone formation, and poor intrarenal drainage. All forms of diagnostic urographic and angiographic techniques thus may have to be used to achieve accurate diagnosis of the more extensive lesions (see Fig. 16–20). Antibacterial chemotherapy and correction of lower urinary tract anomalies are the treatments of choice.

In the absence of infection, the renal lesions

may be only slowly progressive. Intubated infundibulotomy may improve the intrarenal transport of urine and may help to eradicate urosepsis; it is seldom justified, and it usually does not bring about urographic improvement (Williams). Partial nephrectomy to relieve the compression effect of a symptomatic poorly draining or totally obstructed and expanding calyceal cavity is rarely necessary. The "cavity" into which urine is actively excreted (in contrast to a true calyceal diverticulum) must be totally excised and its infundibular communication carefully obliterated. Simple unroofing of the cystic cavity without recognition of the underlying problem will lead to urinary extravasation. Occasionally, ureterocalycostomy may be helpful (Fig. 16–26).

ACQUIRED. Infundibular cicatrization with hydrocalycosis and stone formation may follow specific and nonspecific infections, urothelial tumors, and trauma. Hydrocalycosis of localized obliterating pyelonephritis develops gradually. The infected calyceal lining is rough and irregular, and it is fibrotic; in addition, other calyces usually appear pyelonephritic, with cortical scarring (Williams and Mininberg).

These conditions are all unusual during in-

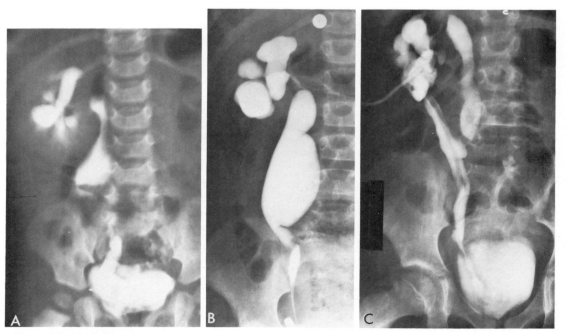

Figure 16–26. *A,* Excretory urogram shows stenotic pelvis and megaureter. *B,* Confirmation by retrograde pyeloureterogram. *C,* Nephrostogram postoperatively reveals creation of incomplete duplication and ureterocalycostomy. (From Kelalis PP, Malek RS: Infundibulopelvic stenosis. J Urol *125:*568–571, 1981. © 1981, The Williams & Wilkins Company, Baltimore.)

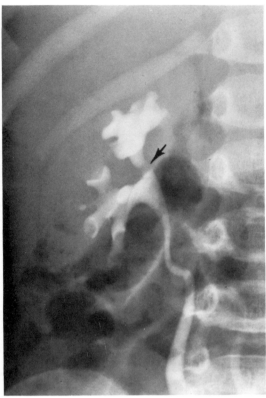

Figure 16–27. Hydrocalycosis due to vascular compression in asymptomatic 2-year-old boy whose bladder was ruptured in car accident. Excretory urogram shows dilatation of right upper calyx and infundibular compression by renal vessels (arrow).

fancy and childhood. Correction of the underlying disorder is the treatment of choice.

Extrinsic Obstruction

CONGENITAL. Dilatation of the upper pole calyceal group as a result of intrarenal vascular compression of its infundibulum is the most common form of hydrocalycosis (Fig. 16–27). This phenomenon has been observed in 27.5 per 1000 pediatric excretory urograms. It affects the two sexes equally, occurs almost 11 times more commonly on the right side, and is rarely bilateral (Rusiewicz and Reilly).

The arterial branch is usually anterior to the infundibulum. Together with a posteriorly running vein, or (rarely) another artery, it embraces the infundibulum in a "scissors grip" fashion (Johnston and Sandomirsky; Malek et al). Despite its relatively frequent occurrence, this form of hydrocalycosis is very rarely of clinical significance. Nephralgia with or without loin tenderness, and occasionally with other urinary tract symptoms, may be associated with significant hydrocalycosis, delayed emptying, and, on rare occasions, thinness of the upper pole renal cortex. Limited experience with Fraley's "dismembered infundibulopyelostomy" indicates that relief of pain, but little urographic improvement, can be achieved with this procedure in bona fide cases (Johnston and Sandomirsky).

ACQUIRED. Calyceal dilatation can occur as a result of the compression effect of mass lesions or various forms of trauma. Therapy is aimed at the underlying cause.

MEGACALYCOSIS

Megacalycosis was first described by Puigvert (Fig. 16–28). It is usually unilateral and has the following characteristics:

1. The involved kidney may be larger than its normal mate or equal in size.

2. The calyces, which are generally dilated and malformed (polygonal, faceted, mosaic), may be normal in number or may be increased to as many as 20 or 25.

3. The renal pelvis, which contracts infrequently (one to three times per minute), and pelviureteral confluence are of normal funnel-shaped configuration.

4. The appearance time of contrast medium is the same on both sides; however, complete opacification of the pelvicalyceal system, which shows very little variation in size, is delayed for 15 to 30 minutes because of the larger volume of urine that must be displaced.

5. The renal parenchyma, although unscarred, is generally and uniformly thinner than that of the normal kidney. The thickness of the renal cortex is normal (0.5 to 0.8 mm); however, the medulla is uniformly thin, possibly owing to hypoplasia, so that the ratio of the cortex to the medulla is changed from the normal $1:2$ to $1:1$ or more. Selective renal angiography demonstrates these changes and discloses an entirely normal arterial system (interlobular arteries are attenuated in post-obstructive atrophy).

6. Scintiphotography with a proximal tubular agent (technetium-99m penicillamine) discloses a normal amount of functioning cortical tissue on either side. This is corroborated

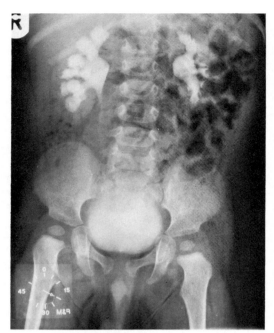

Figure 16–28. Megacalycosis of right kidney in 1-year-old boy. (From Johnston JH: Megacalicosis: a burnt-out obstruction? J Urol *110*:344–346, 1973. © 1973, The Williams & Wilkins Company, Baltimore.)

by normal overall creatinine clearance. Occasionally, in keeping with the underdevelopment of the medulla, renal concentrating ability may be moderately diminished (Talner and Gittes).

Megacalycosis is most likely a congenital defect. Faulty embryogenesis at the time of division of the ureteral bud and its junction with the metanephros, maldevelopment of the pelvicalyceal musculature, and primary hypoplasia of juxtamedullary glomeruli have all been described (Galian et al; Puigvert; Talner and Gittes).

Johnston has proposed that the condition is a "burnt-out obstruction" acquired during intrauterine life from fetal ureteral folds that later involute.

Megacalycosis is not hereditary and does not result in any impairment of overall renal function. Calyceal urinary stasis can predispose to urinary infection during childhood, and in later life stone formation may complicate the picture. A recent review of nearly 60 cases reported in the literature indicates that the condition is diagnosed usually because of the above-mentioned complications and occasionally in the course of urographic evaluation for unrelated conditions such as hypertension (Kimche and Lask).

Megacalycosis is not associated with reflux, and it must be carefully distinguished from obstructive disease, because pyeloplasty is of no value in treating megacalycosis.

CALYCEAL DIVERTICULUM

Calyceal diverticulum is a renal parenchymal cavity, lined with transitional epithelium, that originates with a narrow isthmus from the fornix of an otherwise normal minor calyx

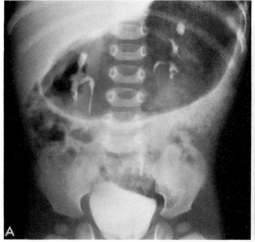
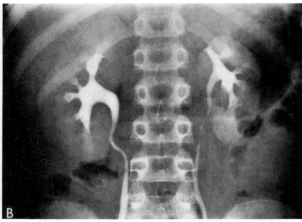

Figure 16–29. Calyceal diverticulum in 1-year-old boy who presented with fever of unknown origin. *A,* Excretory urogram. Normal kidneys and calyceal diverticulum arising with narrow isthmus from normal left upper pole calyx. *B,* Excretory urogram. Normal right kidney and appearance of left kidney 9 years after excision of its upper diverticulum-bearing pole.

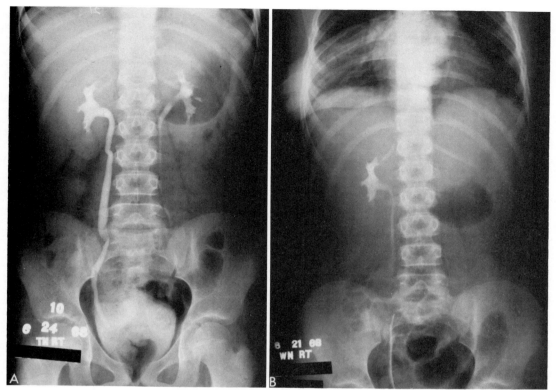

Figure 16–30. Calyceal diverticulum in 10-year-old girl who presented with right flank pain. *A*, Excretory urogram. Normal kidneys with faintly opacified calyceal diverticulum arising from normal right upper pole calyx. *B*, Retrograde ureteropyelogram. Normal right collecting system that fails to demonstrate the diverticulum, whose isthmus is now obstructed as a result of active inflammation.

(Fig. 16–29). It is usually noted incidentally in 3.3 of 1000 pediatric excretory urograms (Timmons et al). The similarity of the incidence rate of this lesion in children and adults, its occurrence in the newborn, and its frequent coexistence with genitourinary and other anomalies in children support the theory of an embryologic origin: the third- and fourth-order divisions of the ureteral bud at the 5-mm stage of embryonic development fail to degenerate, persisting as calyceal diverticula (Lister and Singh; Timmons et al).

There is no side of predilection. The diverticulum is usually found in the upper renal pole. Approximately one third of the children with this disorder may become symptomatic, with loin pain or urinary infection, or both. Rarely, gross hematuria may develop, and in later life as many as 40 per cent of such patients may have diverticular calculi (Lister and Singh; Timmons et al). The diverticular cavity is usually filled by "retrograde" flow during excretory urography; contrast medium pools in it, and emptying is delayed. Retrograde pyelography still may fail to demonstrate the

diverticulum, however, because of active inflammation combined with an edematous, self-obstructing isthmus (Fig. 16–30).

Excision of the diverticulum and obliteration of its isthmus or partial nephrectomy are indicated only when there is persistent pain referable to the diverticulum (with or without calculi), intractable urosepsis or gross hematuria, or evidence of progressive renal damage. However, medical management should be given an adequate trial before the child is subjected to an operation.

BIBLIOGRAPHY

Fink AJ, Garlick WB, Stein A: Congenital cystic hydrocalicosis (unilateral multicystic disease). J Urol 78:22, 1957.

Fraley EE: Dismembered infundibulopyelostomy: improved technique for correcting vascular obstruction of the superior infundibulum. J Urol 101:144, 1969.

Friedland GW: Hydronephrosis in infants and children, Part 1. Curr Probl Diagn Radiol 7:1, 1978.

Galian P, Forest M, Aboulker P: La mégacalicose. Presse Med 78:1663, 1970.

Johnston JH: Megacalicosis: a burnt-out obstruction? J Urol *110*:344, 1973.

Johnston JH, Sandomirsky SK: Intrarenal vascular obstruction of the superior infundibulum in children. J Pediatr Surg 7:318, 1972.

Kelalis PP, Malek RS: Infundibulopelvic stenosis. J Urol *125*:568, 1981.

Kimche D, Lask D: Megacalycosis. Urology *19*:478, 1982.

Lister J, Singh H: Pelvicalyceal cysts in children. J Pediatr Surg *8*:901, 1973.

Mackie GG: Abnormalities of the ureteral bud. Urol Clin North Am *5*:161, 1978.

Malek RS, Aguilo JJ, Hattery RR: Radiolucent filling defects of the renal pelvis: classification and report of unusual cases. J Urol *114*:508, 1975.

Puigvert A: Mégacalicose—diagnostic différentiel avec l'hydrocaliectasie. Helv Chir Acta *31*:414, 1964.

Rusiewicz E, Reilly BJ: The significance of isolated upper pole calyceal dilatation. J Can Assoc Radiol *19*:179, 1968.

Talner LB, Gittes RF: Megacalyces: further observations and differentiation from obstructive renal disease. Am J Roentgenol Radium Ther Nucl Med *121*:473, 1974.

Timmons JW Jr, Malek RS, Hattery RR, et al: Caliceal diverticulum. J Urol *114*:6, 1975.

Williams DI: Urology in childhood. Encyclopedia of Urology. Vol 15 Suppl. New York, Springer-Verlag, 1974, pp 175–177.

Williams DI, Mininberg DT: Hydrocalycosis: report of three cases in children. Br J Urol *40*:541, 1968.

Williams G, Blandy JP, Tresidder GC: Communicating cysts and diverticula of the renal pelvis. Br J Urol *41*:163, 1969.

Ureteropelvic Junction

PANAYOTIS P. KELALIS

The most common site of obstruction in the upper urinary tract is the ureteropelvic junction. The causes of such obstruction are quite variable and complex and often are disputed, but basically the end result is the same—namely, various degrees of hydronephrosis.

Obstruction of the ureteropelvic junction occurs in utero and becomes apparent throughout infancy and childhood. In some of the published series, the incidence was highest in the first year or even the first 6 months of life (Uson et al, 1968, 1969; Williams and Karlaftis), but this may be due to samplings taken from highly specialized pediatric urologic practice. In larger series, the peak incidence is after age 5 years. A definite but unexplained predilection for the left side exists, but the condition is often bilateral (Kelalis et al). In boys, and especially in the first year of life, there is a tendency toward bilaterality; in later years, the obstruction tends to be unilateral, with approximately equal distribution between the two sides. A familial occurrence has been reported (Cohen et al).

PATHOGENESIS

Nearly all obstructions of the ureteropelvic junction are congenital in origin, being produced by mechanical narrowing that is caused by intrinsic stenosis or mechanical compression, as from a band or vessel. Such obstruction also may be functional, resulting from ureteropelvic incoordination secondary to abnormal development of, or injury to, the muscle fibers in this region.

Intrinsic Abnormalities

Intrinsic abnormalities are the most common cause of obstruction. The basic obstructive lesion is caused by abnormality of the muscle bundles—which is usually congenital, but also may be acquired (Allen)—leading to impaired conduction of urine across the ureteropelvic junction. According to Murnaghan, this narrow aperistaltic segment results from replacement of the normal spirals of muscle by longitudinal fibers. Increased distention merely elongates the longitudinal bundles without increasing their girth, producing narrowing instead of the widening that occurs with the normal circular fibers. Others have studied excised segments of ureteropelvic junction, and, despite variation in the histologic interpretation, all report various abnormalities of muscle fibers or their replacement by fibrous tissue, perhaps as a result of developmental arrest of indeterminate cause (Allen; Foote et al).

Perhaps the most appealing explanation to date is that suggested by Ruano-Gil et al, who have clearly shown that the embryonic ureter goes through a solid phase with subsequent recanalization. Thus, ureteropelvic junction obstruction may result from a failure of the upper ureter to completely recanalize.

Physiologically, the end result is the failure of the peristaltic wave to propagate from the pelvis to the ureter. Instead, there are multiple ineffective pelvic peristaltic waves that eventually cause hydronephrosis by incompletely emptying the pelvic contents. This model is corroborated by fluoroscopic observations on the diseased ureteropelvic junctions.

Furthermore, according to Hanna, in a moderately dilated pelvis, a progressive improvement of muscle cell quality is seen by electron microscopy as sections are examined in a more cephalad direction from the ureteropelvic junction. However, in gross hydronephrosis, severe muscle damage and increased collagen and ground substance are found over a wider area of the pelvis, so that the pelves must be excised in such cases. In general, the condition of the pelvis on biopsy correlates well with postpyeloplasty urographic improvement.

Kinks, Bands, and Adhesions

Kinks, bands, and adhesions are frequently found around the ureteropelvic junction, even in the absence of inflammation. They may produce a sharp angulation of the ureter against the lower margin of the pelvis, causing obstruction. As the pelvis dilates, the ureter may be carried proximally in such a way that the most dependent portion of the pelvis is not drained. Such high insertions of the ureter into the pelvis are most often secondary phenomena related to the directions in which the hydronephrotic pelvis enlarges—anteriorly as well as inferiorly. Johnston has reported that lysis of such external adhesions

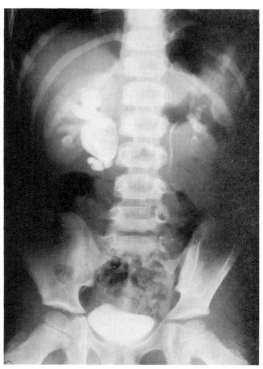

Figure 16–31. Ureteroureteral angulation below ureteropelvic obstruction. Hydronephrosis with massive hematuria also was present.

frequently re-establishes a free flow in the ureteropelvic junction without formal pyeloplasty.

Ureteroureteral angulations just below the ureteropelvic junction are produced by infoldings of the ureteral mucosa and musculature and may lead to acute kinking and obstruction. In such instances, the adventitia of the ureter bridges these defects and obliterates them, so that they are difficult to recognize macroscopically until the pelvis is opened and the upper ureter is calibrated. They probably represent persistence of an exaggerated form of the folds found in the fetal ureter (Fig. 16–31).

Aberrant Vessels

Aberrant vessels are present in at least one third of patients with ureteropelvic obstruction, an incidence that is much higher than that in the normal population. True aberrant vessels cross the ureter posteriorly, but anterior accessory and polar vessels are often referred to collectively as "aberrant" in nature (Fig. 16–32). This intimate relationship of aberrant vessels with the upper ureter or ure-

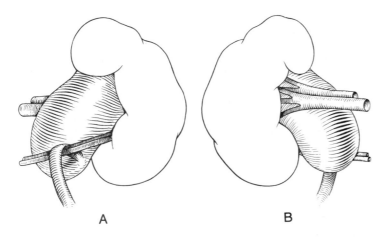

Figure 16–32. *A*, Aberrant vessels. *B*, Accessory or polar vessels.

teropelvic junction has led many to believe that accessory vessels are commonly the cause of the obstruction. More likely, they usually aggravate rather than initiate such an obstruction, because intrinsic pathologic changes are nearly always found in the ureter. The fact that aberrant vessels often are associated with ureteropelvic obstruction can hardly be considered entirely coincidental, however. It has led some researchers to suggest that the close proximity of vessels to the ureteropelvic junction creates mechanical pressure in the region, possibly causing intrinsic abnormalities in the ureteral wall itself, in the form of developmental arrest (Allen).

Polyps and Valves

Valvular mucosal infoldings or minute polypoid lesions have been described as obstructing the ureteropelvic junction, but they are exceedingly rare. That they do occur,

Figure 16–33. Total left vesicoureteral reflux simulating ureteropelvic obstruction. *A*, Excretory urogram. *B*, Cystogram.

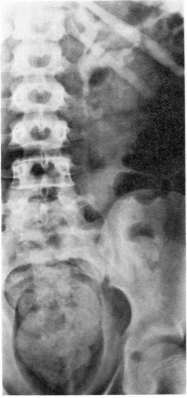
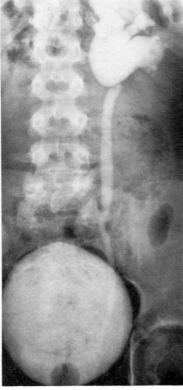

A   B

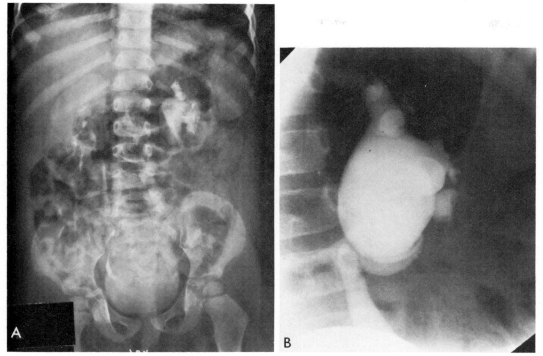

Figure 16-34. *A,* Excretory urogram. Pyelectasis on left. *B,* Cystogram. Vesicoureteral reflux with early ureteropelvic obstruction on left.

however, emphasizes the need to explore the ureteropelvic junction by opening the pelvis in all cases, even when lysis of external adhesions seems to allow the ureter to straighten (Dajani et al; Gup; Maizels and Stephens).

Vesicoureteral Reflux

The most common entity that mimics primary ureteropelvic junction obstruction is vesicoureteral reflux. Complete vesicoureteral reflux can increase the urine load, and therefore the flow rate, beyond the emptying capacity of the pelvis. As a result, the pelvis may dilate. This dilatation may appear on retrograde cystography, simulating ureteropelvic obstruction (Figs. 16-33 and 16-34). As the ureter dilates further, elongates, and becomes tortuous, kinking appears at the ureteropelvic junction. Periureteritis from infection may then result in stenosis and adhesions between adjacent and parallel segments of the ureter. In such circumstances, ureteral dilatation beyond the point of obstruction and vesicoureteral reflux should be regarded as signs that the stasis and dilatation are secondary to infection and reflux (Jimenez-Mariscal and Moussali Flah).

In a closed type of renal pelvis, reflux can induce hydronephrosis that remains or even becomes symptomatic long after the reflux has spontaneously disappeared (Figs. 16-35 and 16-36). At operation, secondary kinking at the ureteropelvic junction is seen (Hutch et al). In this group, the pelvis balloons out during micturition and remains full, but this phenomenon disappears after correction of the reflux. If reflux and pelvic dilatation are noted during voiding cystourethrography, observing how long the pelvis remains full is particularly important, since even the most grossly distended pelves during reflux empty readily after voiding. True secondary ureteropelvic obstruction is clinically demonstrated by significant reflux filling the ureter only to the ureteropelvic junction in association with an excretory urogram that demonstrates hydronephrosis. Occasionally, concomitant reflux of a minor degree is present in addition to the ureteropelvic problem. This should be considered an incidental finding that is irrelevant to the cause of hydronephrosis and that usually will cease spontaneously (Whitaker).

Intrapelvic Pressures

The basic pressure of the normal pelvis depends on the urine flow rate; it ranges be-

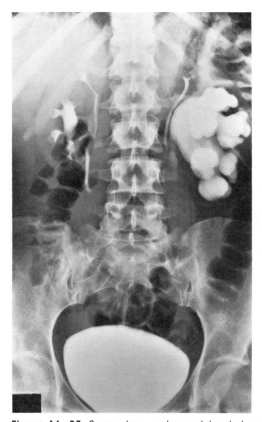

Figure 16–35. Secondary ureteropelvic obstruction of lower segment of complete duplication on left. Old vesicoureteral reflux, same segment.

tween 5 and 25 cm H_2O. Contrary to expectation, low intrapelvic pressures are the rule rather than the exception in hydronephrotic kidneys. Johnston found increased pressures (greater than 25 cm H_2O) in only 7 of 36 kidneys made hydronephrotic by ureteropelvic obstruction. Low pressures suggest a state of equilibrium between the dilated pelvis and its obstructed outlet, at least at the rate of urine flow present when the normal pressure is recorded. Increases in intrapelvic pressure conceivably take place during diuresis, when the flow rate may exceed the emptying capacity of the obstructed pelvis. This probably explains the observation that untreated hydronephrotic kidneys may remain anatomically and functionally stable over prolonged periods.

Intermittent Hydronephrosis

The syndrome known as intermittent hydronephrosis was first described by Nesbit, who studied patients with intermittent attacks of colicky flank pain. Between such attacks, the excretory urograms were normal; during attacks, pyelectasis was demonstrated on the painful side. In such patients, the pelvis is likely to be full and extrarenal on examinations between attacks. Roentgenographically, it can be demonstrated that hydronephrosis

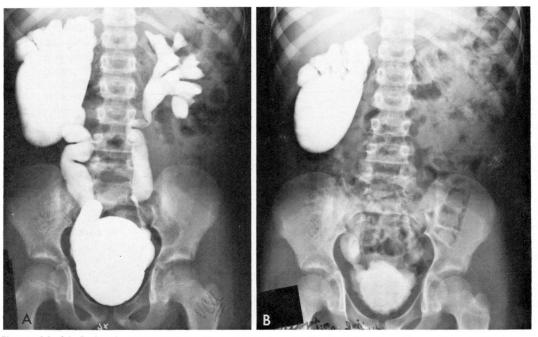

Figure 16–36. Reflux in megaureter with secondary ureteropelvic junction obstruction. *A*, Cystogram. Bilateral reflux in megaureters. *B*, Plain film several hours later, showing retention of dye in renal pelvis from secondary obstruction at ureteropelvic junction on right.

results when the urine flow rate has increased beyond the ability of the pelvis to empty, because the urine flow is limited in such instances by the relatively nondistensible ureteropelvic junction (Genereux and Monks). Cinepyelographic studies made during increasing diuresis have shown that this type of pelvis has difficulty handling an increased flow of urine (Hanley). Limitation of the rate of flow through the ureteropelvic junction has also been demonstrated at the time of surgical exposure. Such studies tend to complement and indeed confirm the existence of physiologic abnormalities of the ureteropelvic junction. The cause of the pain in intermittent hydronephrosis is renal pelvic distention, and at times pain can be reproduced by the diuretic urogram.

CLINICAL FEATURES

In infants, there may be more than one presenting sign. A palpable renal mass is the most frequent sign in bilateral cases. Vomiting and failure to thrive, with consequent increases in blood urea and creatinine concentrations, may occur as a result of renal impairment; in others, screaming suggests attacks of abdominal pain. Mild anemia and even polycythemia have been noted as uncommon presentations of the disease.

In older children, ureteropelvic obstruction may simulate gastrointestinal disease, obscuring the renal origin, which may not be discovered for many years. In approximately one third of patients, the abdominal pain is vague and paraumbilical and is often associated with nausea or vomiting. This combination of symptoms often leads to a misdiagnosis of appendicitis, gastroenteritis, or spastic colon. The next most common symptom is recurrent attacks of pain localized to the flank and usually colicky in nature. Such pain may be accentuated by an unusually large fluid intake. The most common urologic complaint is varying degrees of gross hematuria that at times may be excessive even in the absence of trauma; this is probably the result of fluctuating intrapelvic pressures or of episodes of acute obstruction, both of which can lead to sudden distention of the renal pelvis and to rupture of a dilated vessel. Contrary to the classic theory that obstruction leads to residual urine that predisposes to infection, symptoms of urinary infection are relatively uncommon. When found, infection should arouse suspicion that vesicoureteral reflux or lower urinary tract disease is also present. If infection is present, fever may be noted. In some instances, there has been sudden onset of hypertension, which appears to result from activation of the renal pressor system (Grossman et al; Munoz et al). Urine extravasation secondary to obstruction at the ureteropelvic junction has also been reported (Levitt and Lutzker).

Investigation of refractory urinary abnormalities may uncover ureteropelvic obstruction. Routine urographic investigation of other abnormalities, such as hypospadias or Hirschsprung's disease, has occasionally led to the diagnosis of ureteropelvic obstruction. Infection accompanying this disease is de-

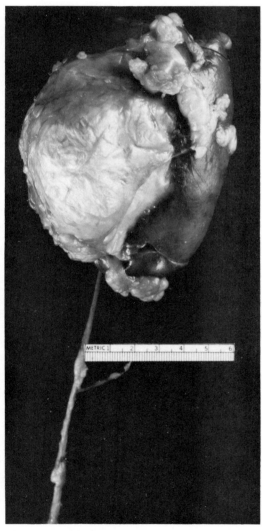

Figure 16–37. Gross specimen: ureteropelvic obstruction.

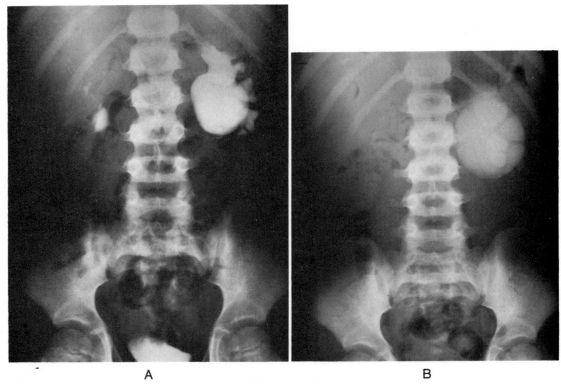

A   B

Figure 16–38. Excretory urograms, showing left ureteropelvic obstruction. *A*, At 20 minutes. *B*, At 2 hours, delayed film shows accentuation of hydronephrosis and obstruction.

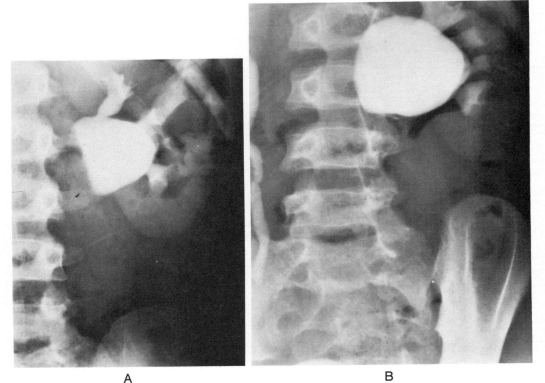

A   B

Figure 16–39. Films during infusion urography under fluoroscopic control; films 10 minutes apart show rapid progression of pyelectasis with no medium in ureter because of ureteropelvic obstruction.

tected by urine culture in only 15 to 20 per cent of cases. The presence of moderate to severe azotemia is confined, of course, to patients with bilateral ureteropelvic obstruction, solitary kidney, or ureteropelvic obstruction associated with contralateral renal disease.

On physical examination, the finding of a mass with the characteristics of a renal enlargement raises the possibility of neoplasm or polycystic disease, especially when the mass is quite firm. One is likely to feel the distended, greatly enlarged pelvis, whereas the renal cortex may be palpable on its surface as a firmer protuberance in the form of a cup (Fig. 16–37). Transillumination by the use of fiberoptic light should be tried, but it is unlikely that this will be successful.

DIAGNOSTIC STUDIES

Excretory Urography

The diagnosis of ureteropelvic obstruction is established when excretory urography demonstrates the typically dilated renal pelvis. Nonvisualization of the ipsilateral ure-

ter below the dilated pelvis tends to confirm the diagnosis. Delayed films are most informative because they tend to document the continuing obstruction and confirm the diagnosis (Fig. 16–38). Urographic examinations, however, are not always totally dependable, especially if the study has been done under conditions of severe dehydration. The same pelvis under stress during a diuretic phase may exhibit spectacular differences (Fig. 16–39). Infusion urography obviates these difficulties, and its value is greatly enhanced if it is carried out under simultaneous fluoroscopic control, with spot films (Fig. 16–40). The obstructing segment is identified by its failure to propagate the contrast medium—that is, a persistent "hang-up" of medium will be noted at this point.

High degrees of pelvic dilatation may occur while the calyces look delicate and normal, but in instances of severe obstruction, dilated calyces are often all that can be seen in early films. Infants in general have a more advanced degree of hydronephrosis (Fig. 16–41). In severe cases of hydronephrosis, a crescentic collection of contrast medium is

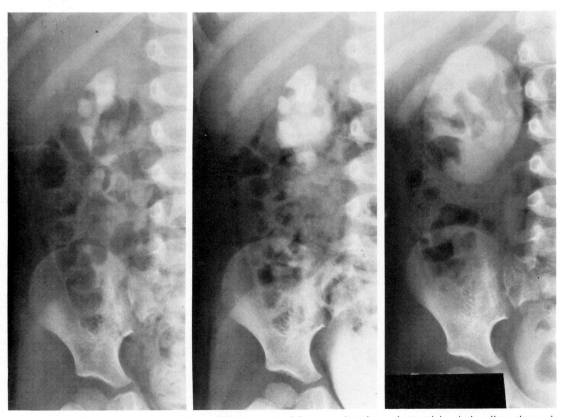

Figure 16–40. Progressive distention of right renal pelvis secondary to ureteropelvic obstruction, shown in films taken over a 5-hour period during infusion urography.

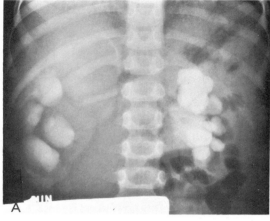
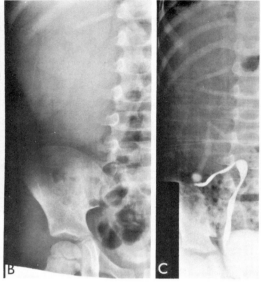

Figure 16–41. Ureteropelvic obstruction on right. A, Excretory urogram, early film. B, Same, late film. C, Retrograde ureterogram.

occasionally observed in the renal parenchyma, overlying nonopacified calyces. Referred to as the "crescent sign," this phenomenon is caused by contrast medium appearing first in the stretched collecting duct and is usually demonstrable in the early films of excretory urography (Fig. 16–42). The crescent sign gradually disappears as the calyces are opacified. The appearance of calyceal crescents requires dilated calyces and collecting ducts as well as preservation of renal concentrating ability. This crescent sign should be considered a reliable sign not only of upper urinary tract obstruction but also of recoverable renal function.

Evidence of fluid levels in the hydronephrotic kidney signifies that gas or air is present (Fig. 16–43). Urographic visualization may be delayed or totally absent. In such instances, ultrasound examination may lead to the correct diagnosis. Every attempt should be made to obtain a satisfactory profile of the ureter and thereby to obviate retrograde ureterography. If azotemia is present, double-dose excretory urography or infusion urography is likely to outline the details satisfactorily.

In the child with intermittent pain and only mild pelvic dilatation, a study should be sought during an episode of pain, when in-

Figure 16–42. Crescent sign of hydronephrosis.

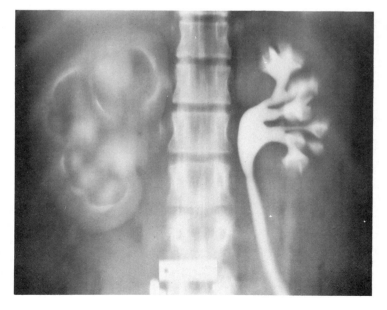

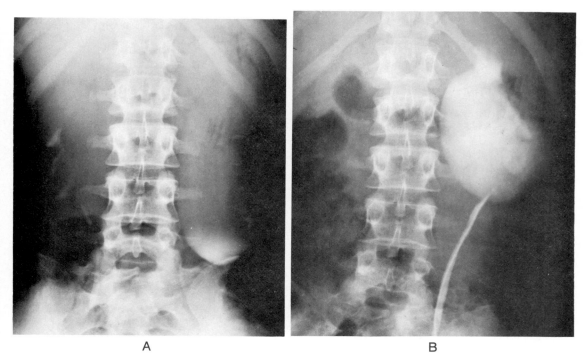

Figure 16–43. *A*, Excretory urogram, showing fluid level on left side. *B*, Retrograde pyelogram, showing left ureteropelvic obstruction.

creased hydronephrosis will confirm the renal origin of the pain. Otherwise, administration of a diuretic at the time of excretory urography will stress the ureteropelvic junction with an increase of urine flow. Increase in hydronephrosis, especially in association with pain, is positive proof of significant obstruction at the ureteropelvic junction (Fig. 16–44).

Cystourethrography

As mentioned, complete vesicoureteral reflux may simulate ureteropelvic obstruction, because the reflux at times increases the contents of the renal pelvis beyond its emptying capacity (Fig. 16–45). Certainly, in refluxing ureters, considerable dilatation of the pelvis

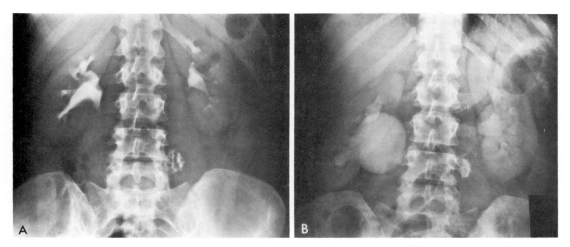

Figure 16–44. *A*, Conventional excretory urogram. *B*, Same, with furosemide. Classic ureteropelvic obstruction on right.

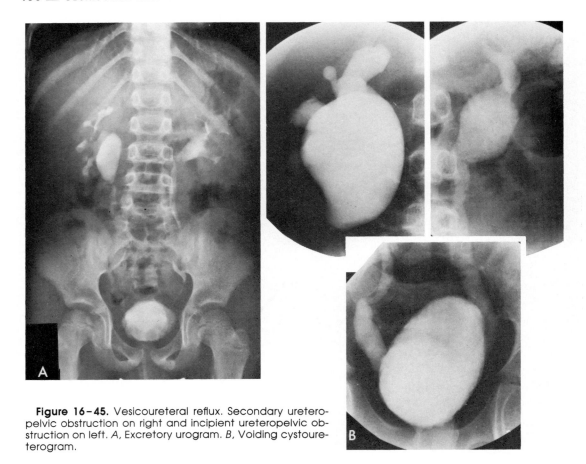

Figure 16–45. Vesicoureteral reflux. Secondary ureteropelvic obstruction on right and incipient ureteropelvic obstruction on left. *A,* Excretory urogram. *B,* Voiding cystoureterogram.

can occur during micturition, and evacuation of the pelvis may be delayed for prolonged periods. In such instances, suggestive ureteral dilatation will be noted, especially in the pelvic portion of the ureter, although such dilatation may be minimal. But it probably is wise to exclude vesicoureteral reflux in all cases of suspected ureteropelvic obstruction. Sometimes, of course, a minor degree of reflux can be present on the same side as a typical ureteropelvic junction obstruction, and in such cases one can safely assume that the association is merely coincidental.

Retrograde Ureterography

Improvement in urographic techniques and the use of ultrasonography have considerably diminished the need for retrograde ureterography. Such an examination may still be necessary when a urographically functionless kidney is found or when the profile of the ureter is not completely outlined (Fig. 16–46). Retrograde ureterography should be done when the patient is anesthetized for the surgical exploration. This way, the risk of iatrogenic infection is diminished and the hazards of a second episode of anesthesia are avoided.

Antegrade Pyelography

Antegrade pyelography has almost completely eliminated the need for retrograde studies. Percutaneous pyelography does not require anesthesia and can be helpful in a hydronephrotic functionless kidney not only in assisting in the correct diagnosis but also in assessing renal function. The procedure is preferable to use of ureteral catheters, because even the smallest one can cause appreciable edema of an infant's ureteral orifice and delayed emptying—an important point if tubeless pyeloplasties are to be used.

Ultrasonography and Computed Tomography

Ultrasound examination usually confirms the diagnosis. It is particularly useful in functionless renal masses (Fig. 16–47) and for detection of a dilated ureter to differentiate between ureteropelvic and ureterovesical obstruction. In exceptional instances, computed tomography scans may be of help, especially when the diagnosis in huge functionless renal masses continues to be elusive (Fig. 16–48).

Arteriography

Rarely, there may be doubt as to the true diagnosis; in such cases, arteriography is used. This examination has been suggested for elucidation of the relationship of the collecting system to the aberrant vessels; however, because these vessels must be defined at the time of operation, arteriography for this purpose appears superfluous.

Radioisotope Studies

Radioisotope studies have great potential for the assessment of total and individual renal function in hydronephrosis. They are also useful in assessing obstruction in the dilated system and in monitoring progress after surgical correction with less radiation than conventional urography.

Technetium-99m dimercaptosuccinic acid (DMSA) scan, a valuable recent addition, helps establish the percentage contribution of

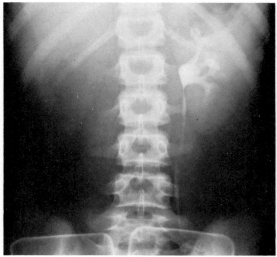

A

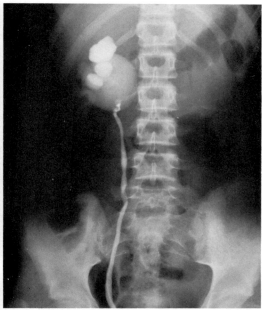

B

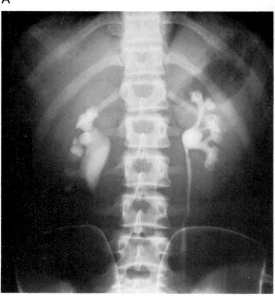

C

Figure 16–46. A 12-year-old girl had pain and vomiting and recent onset of hypertension. *A*, Excretory urogram shows functionless right kidney. *B*, Retrograde pyelogram shows right ureteropelvic obstruction. *C*, Excretory urogram taken 6 months after operation shows return of function in right kidney. Patient is asymptomatic and normotensive.

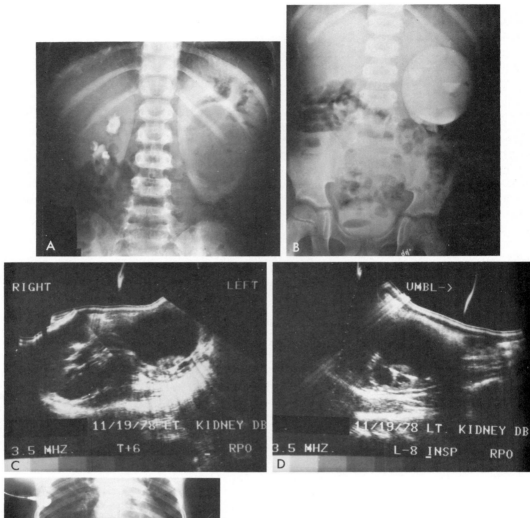

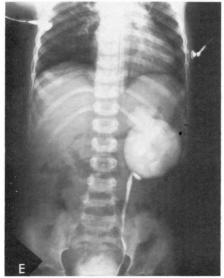

Figure 16–47. Example of ureteropelvic obstruction on left. *A* and *B*, Excretory urogram. *C* and *D*, Ultrasonography. *E*, Retrograde ureterogram.

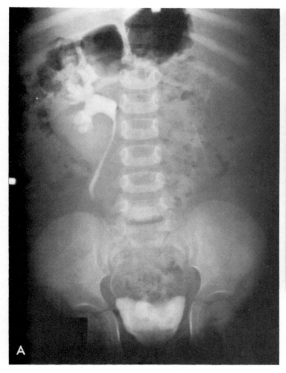

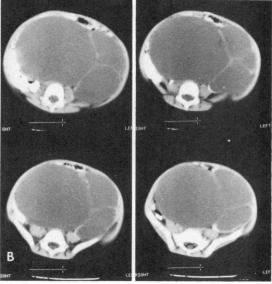

Figure 16–48. *A,* Functionless kidney on left. *B,* Computed tomography scan shows huge hydronephrosis filling entire abdomen. Ureteropelvic obstruction.

each kidney to renal function (Parker et al). Isotope transit times through the parenchyma of the kidney offer a means of determining whether obstructive uropathy is affecting nephron function (Whitfield et al). Diuretic radionuclide urography is a noninvasive method for accurately and reliably assessing urinary tract dilatation. Even though such studies do not measure the factors responsible for progression of the hydronephrosis or renal damage, a good correlation exists between the functional diuretic renogram and morphohistologic patterns of the renal pelvis (Lupton et al; Koff et al). Obstruction impedes the urine flow at either low or high rates, and, provided that adequate renal function exists, impedance is reflected in the renogram curve. Isotope renography can also be used in evaluating the postoperative results of pyeloplasty, because it gives greater detail of function and emptying rate of individual kidneys than the conventional urogram (O'Reilly et al). However, false positive results simulating obstruction can be obtained because of acute tubular necrosis, infection, reflux, and, of course, clinical error (Krueger et al). If much redundant pelvis remains even though the obstruction has been eliminated, the obstructive pattern is likely to remain on the standard renogram; a diuretic should then be given to assess the ability to drain.

Pressure-Flow Studies

From time to time in truly equivocal obstructions, neither urographic nor isotopic techniques can settle the issue. In such instances, perfusion (pressure-flow) studies are used to assess more accurately the degree of obstruction. Such studies, although well documented and valuable, are nonetheless invasive, because percutaneous puncture of the dilated pelvis under fluoroscopic or sonographic control is necessary unless a nephrostomy tube is already in place (Whitaker). The upper limit of normal differential (pelvis minus bladder) pressure with a perfusion rate of 10 ml/min is up to 14 cm of water with the bladder empty and 10 cm with the bladder full (Newhouse et al). Equivocal obstruction after pyeloplasty, according to Odiase and Whitaker, can be settled by this study, but a questionable area between 15 and 20 cm of water pressure is found in a small percentage of cases.

Equivocal Ureteropelvic Obstruction

Less frequently in children than in adults, it is necessary to establish the pressure or degree of obstruction in patients with large renal pelves. Diuresis urography in this situation is

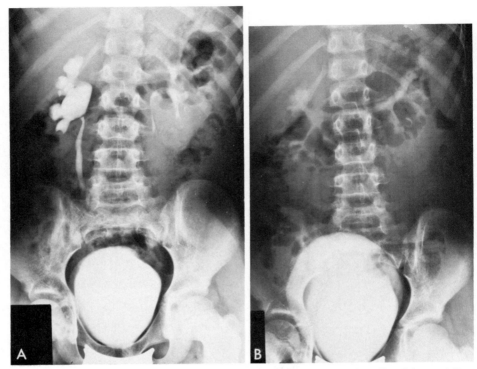

Figure 16–49. *A*, Excretory urogram. Postoperative pyeloplasty on right. Questionable persisting obstruction. *B*, Synchronous furosemide study shows prompt elimination of dye that is confirmed by isotopic study. No obstruction.

useful. In most patients with equivocal obstruction on routine urography, dilution and drainage of the contrast medium occur promptly without further dilatation after furosemide (Lasix) stimulation (Fig. 16–49). The demonstration of the ability of the ureteropelvic junction to transfer a full diuretic load is convincing evidence of the absence of obstruction (Whitaker).

TREATMENT

The indications for surgical intervention and the choice between nephrectomy and pyeloplasty are the two cardinal considerations in the treatment of ureteropelvic obstruction. Minimal degrees of pyelectasis, with well-preserved calyces that are delicate and normal in appearance, usually remain unchanged for many years and, provided that the patient is asymptomatic, should be left undisturbed (Alton) (Figs. 16–50 and 16–51). If there is doubt about the need for treatment, re-evaluation is preferable to immediate surgical intervention. However, if calycectasis is present, if the obstruction is symptomatic, if

renal infection is found, or, especially, if progressive pyelocalycectasis is demonstrated, surgical intervention becomes mandatory.

Nephrectomy versus Pyeloplasty

The choice between pyeloplasty and nephrectomy is difficult at times. Extreme conservatism is justified, because the recovery potential of the kidney is greater in children than in adults and is totally unpredictable. It is a good rule to assume that almost all ureteropelvic obstructions are salvageable. Furthermore, the fact that bilaterality can appear later in life must be taken into consideration. When nephrectomy is performed, the added load on the remaining kidney, especially during growth, may precipitate ureteropelvic obstruction on the other side (Fig. 16–52). If parenchymal infection is present or cystic changes are noted, nephrectomy usually is preferable. With utmost conservatism, fewer than 5 per cent of kidneys with ureteropelvic obstruction require nephrectomy.

Probably, more recoverable kidneys are encountered in childhood, especially in the neonatal period. Technetium-99m DMSA study

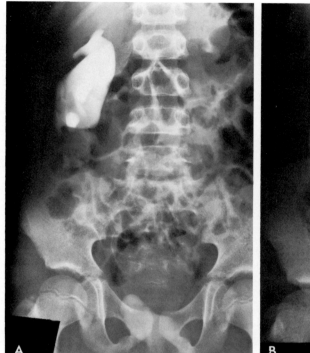 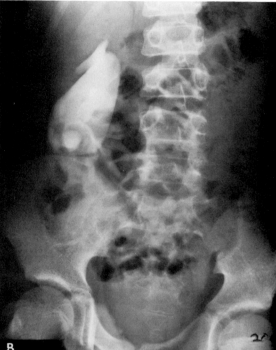

Figure 16–50. Excretory urogram. *A* and *B*, Same patient, 6 years apart; no change. Apparent pyelectasis. Negative furosemide radionuclide study.

allows evaluation of the relative function present in an obstructed kidney and is superior to the urogram in evaluating residual renal function—a fact particularly important in the newborn, in whom urographic studies are of poor quality. Such imaging does not always correlate well with urographic function (Parker et al).

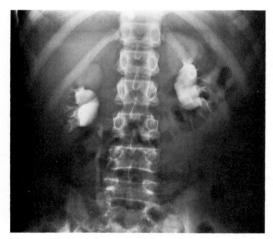

Figure 16–51. Pyelectasis with delicate calyces bilaterally. Furosemide study negative. Excretory urogram.

Bilateral Ureteropelvic Obstruction

Approximately one fifth of ureteropelvic obstructions are bilateral. The incidence is much higher in infants and young children (Figs. 16–53 and 16–54). Furthermore, in infants the contralateral kidney frequently is involved with multicystic dysplastic changes, a probable finding in patients whose contralateral kidney cannot be visualized urographically. Such kidneys often represent an extreme degree of hydronephrosis, and the term *hydrocalycosis* is probably preferable (Kelalis and Malek).

Surgical correction of the symptomatic side should take precedence. If a decision to proceed with unilateral nephrectomy has been made, the pyeloplasty should precede this. A transabdominal, transperitoneal approach obviates the difficult choice of side and, in the infant, allows mobilization of the pelvis without disturbing the kidney, but this advantage must be weighed against the incidence of subsequent intestinal obstruction due to adhesions in about 3 per cent of cases (Drake et al). Separate transverse flank extraperitoneal incisions during the same period of

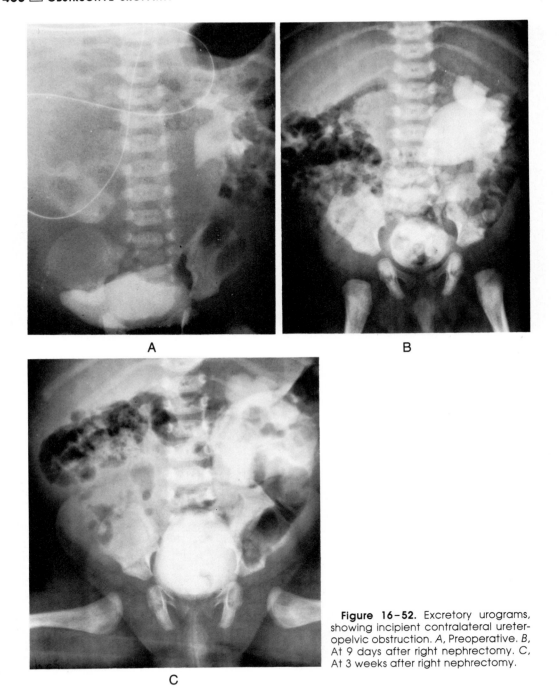

A

B

C

Figure 16–52. Excretory urograms, showing incipient contralateral ureteropelvic obstruction. *A*, Preoperative. *B*, At 9 days after right nephrectomy. *C*, At 3 weeks after right nephrectomy.

anesthesia for simultaneous correction of the obstruction in both sides appears now to be the approach preferred by most in bilateral ureteropelvic obstruction.

Preliminary Urinary Diversion

Percutaneous insertion of a nephrostomy tube under fluoroscopic control or, in the functionless kidney, ultrasonic guidance is a useful procedure in patients who require temporary drainage. Because of the large size of the renal pelvis, it can usually be accomplished without difficulty (Saxton). Little or no reaction occurs, and the procedure is unlikely to interfere with the subsequent definitive treatment.

At present, the legitimate role of formal

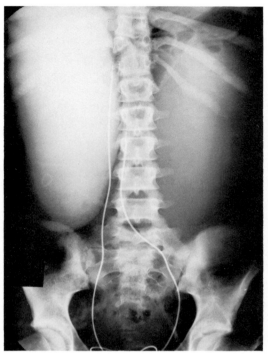

Figure 16–53. Massive bilateral pyelocalycectasis in a 13-year-old girl, caused by obstruction at the ureteropelvic junction. This patient had vague abdominal complaints for many years.

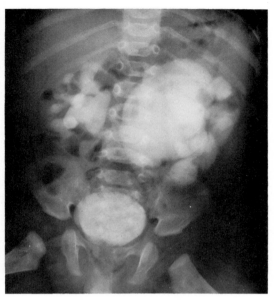

Figure 16–54. Excretory urogram, showing bilateral ureteropelvic obstruction, more advanced on the left, in a 4-month-old boy.

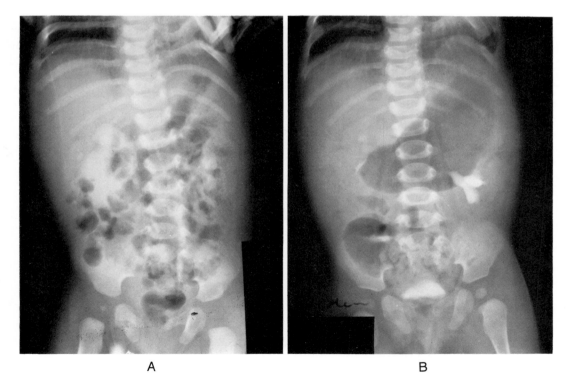

A   B

Figure 16–55. Excretory urograms in infant with right ureteropelvic obstruction. *A*, Preoperative. *B*, After cutaneous pyelostomy.

nephrostomy is extremely limited. In special situations, temporary cutaneous pyelostomy appears an attractive alternative (Fig. 16–55). The large, dilated pelvis makes the procedure easy to perform, and it may be used occasionally to control infection (Marshall et al). Repair of the ureteropelvic junction may then be accomplished several months later, when the renal pelvis has regressed in size and the technical difficulties are less formidable.

Pyeloplasty

Anatomic variations in ureteropelvic obstruction cause dissimilarities in therapeutic problems, so that no single type of pyeloplasty is sufficient for all situations (Culp). Any type of pyeloplasty should create a ureteropelvic junction that is dependent in position, funnel-shaped, and of adequate caliber. The transition from pelvis to ureter is not readily distinguishable in normal patients, but this transition can be identified when ureteropelvic dysfunction or obstruction is present. Further definition of such an obstructing segment (functional or anatomic) is aided by distending the pelvis with saline injected through a 20-gauge needle mounted on a syringe. Subjecting the emptying capability of the pelvis to further stress in this way usually leads to clear identification of the dysfunctioning segment of upper ureter (Fig. 16–56).

Regardless of the method of pyeloplasty used, the pelvis should always be opened and the ureteropelvic junction inspected. Calibration of the ureter distally should be carried out routinely to detect concomitant ureteral strictures; if such strictures are not found and treated, they may compromise the repair at the ureteropelvic junction. The incision in the pelvis and ureter should be closed with interrupted fine 5-0 and 6-0 catgut sutures, with the knots tied outside and closely placed to achieve as tight a closure as possible. Particular care should be taken in the placement of the apical sutures. If the size of the pelvis must be reduced, the edges are closed with continuous interlocking sutures. Finally, it should be constantly borne in mind that more than one factor may be responsible for obstruction at the ureteropelvic junction.

The extraperitoneal approach via transverse flank incision is preferred. In bilateral cases, two separate incisions are used. In some, the ureteropelvic junction can be exposed more easily by retraction of the lower

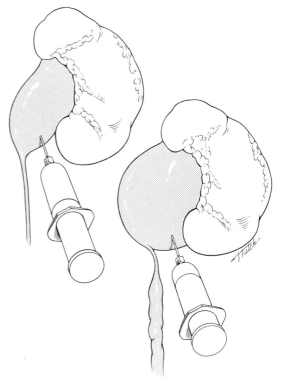

Figure 16–56. Distention of pelvis by injection of saline for identification of dysfunctioning segment of ureter.

pole of the kidney upward and laterally; in others, rotation of the kidney will reveal the ureteropelvic region posteriorly. To reduce the chances of twisting, angulation, or interference with blood supply, one should leave the kidney and upper ureter relatively undisturbed. Ureteral and pelvic traction sutures facilitate the anastomosis. Flap or plastic operations for the repair of ureteropelvic junction obstruction have been almost totally replaced by ureteropyelostomy, particularly in children, in whom the situations in which these techniques are applicable are extremely rare. They are mentioned for the sake of completeness.

THE Y-PLASTY (FOLEY). The principle of the Foley operation is the conversion of a Y-shaped pyeloureterotomy incision into a V closure. The Y-plasty is particularly suitable when the ureter inserts high on the pelvis and when the inferior portion of the pelvis between the ureter and hilus of the kidney is generous in size. The incisions on the pelvis must be on the anterior and posterior surfaces; they should be long enough to create a dependent juncture and to enlarge the caliber

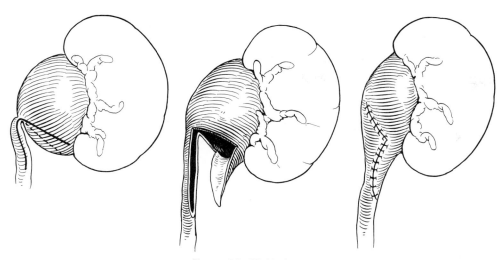

Figure 16–57. Y-plasty.

of the defective ureter. The tail of the Y must be on the lateral aspect of the ureter and must be carried to a point well below the obstruction (Fig. 16–57).

THE SPIRAL FLAP (CULP). The spiral flap is suitable for the relatively long stenotic but dependent ureteropelvic obstruction. A pelvic flap is outlined by converging incisions that start with a broad base and follow the spherical contour of the pelvis to avoid angulation after the flap has been rotated (Fig. 16–58). The vertical flap (Scardino) is a similar technique, but the spiral method affords longer flaps to bridge longer narrowings, admittedly a rare occurrence in children.

INTUBATED URETEROTOMY. For long constrictions (miniureter), for multiple strictures not amenable to any type of revision using existing tissues, or for strictures too low to reach with a spiral flap without putting tension on existing tissues, the Davis intubated ureterotomy should be used in combination with one of the flap operations. The narrow ureter is left open to heal over a ureteral stent of appropriate size, preferably a soft rubber catheter large enough to fit comfortably into the lumen of the ureter. The catheter is brought out through the lower calyx with a nephrostomy tube; both catheter and tube are left indwelling for 10 days to 3

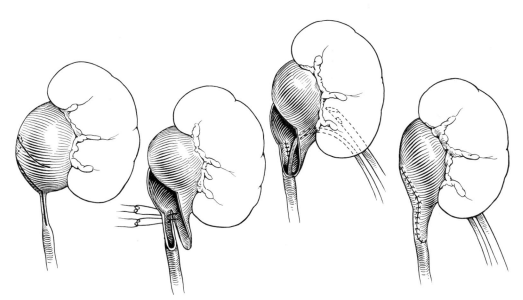

Figure 16–58. Spiral flap.

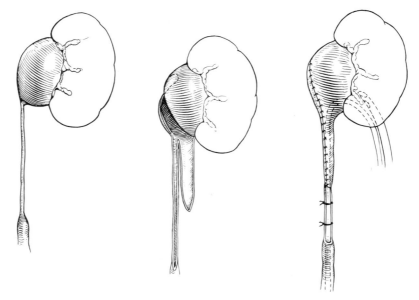

Figure 16–59. Intubated ureterotomy.

weeks (Fig. 16–59). For such situations, admittedly very rare in children, a ureterocalycostomy is preferable when the ureter is long enough to reach the transected lower pole.

ABERRANT VESSELS. There are few well-documented cases in which the ureteropelvic junction has been obstructed solely because of aberrant vessels. More commonly, these vessels aggravate the obstruction; correcting the anatomic relationship of the vessel to the pelvis relieves the hydronephrosis considerably but rarely obliterates it completely. Every attempt should be made to preserve the arteries running to the lower pole, because division will lead to segmental renal ischemia and possibly to persistent hypertension. A procedure of tagging the vessel into a pelvic sleeve has been described by Hellstrom et al, but, because ureteropelvic obstruction or dysfunction is usually coexistent, it is preferable to excise the abnormal ureteral segment, transpose the ureter anteriorly, and subsequently anastomose it to the pelvis.

Ureteropyelostomy

The existence of a defective obstructive segment of ureter at the ureteropelvic junction has been convincingly established both functionally and histologically; excision of the defective segment is therefore a sound surgical principle. In the past, interrupting the continuity of the ureteropelvic junction was viewed with trepidation. Because the propagation of peristalsis is now thought to be mainly myogenic, such fears appear to have no physiologic foundation, a realization that has led to the increasing acceptance of this technique. In pelvic flap operations, sutures are closely placed on the longitudinally opened, narrowed strip of ureter; this may lead to postoperative strictures caused by interruption of the blood supply.

Now that the pathophysiology and the histopathology of the problem of ureteropelvic obstruction have been elucidated, dismembered pyeloplasty appears to be the only technique satisfying all the criteria for successful repair. Nonetheless, routine excision of the pelvis—reductive pyeloplasty—should not be necessary unless gross hydronephrosis exists. There is little support for the notion that excision of the pelvis improves renal function and calyceal details to a greater degree than ureteropyelostomy alone. So-called urographic improvement after such a procedure reflects the extent of surgery and is simply a reduction of the pelvic size in the postoperative urogram.

The abnormal segment of ureter is excised by oblique incisions in the pelvis and in the ureter. The ureter is next spatulated liberally for 1 or 2 cm laterally to avoid the blood supply that lies on the medial ureter and to enlarge the area of the anastomosis to prevent a constricting stenosis at that level (Fig. 16–60). Modifications, such as varying the pattern of the incision to produce pelvic flaps to fit the spatulated ureter, have been described. These maneuvers are probably super-

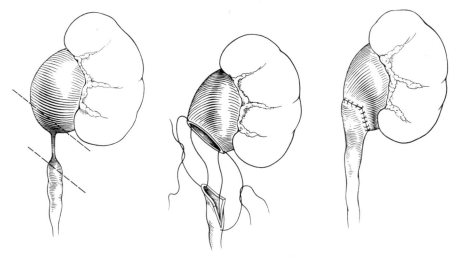

Figure 16–60. Ureteropyelostomy.

fluous, because the pelvis has sufficient elasticity to conform to the shape of the anastomosis. Functional ureteropelvic continuity is established within 1 month, as evidenced by the transmission of normal peristalsis seen fluoroscopically during excretory urography (Caine and Hermann).

Dismembered ureteropyelostomy is the most versatile of all operations for obstruction, its only limitation being that excision of an unusually long ureteral stricture would put the anastomosis of the ureter to the pelvis under tension.

Reductive Pyeloplasty

Unless the redundant pelvis is decompensated and fibrotic or grossly enlarged, partial pelvectomy should not be necessary; the size of the pelvis will regress dramatically once the obstruction is relieved. For partial pelvectomy, the redundant pelvis is excised longitudinally, and the spatulated ureter is anastomosed to the pelvic flap in the most inferior portion of the pelvis. The pelvic incisions are closed with either interrupted or continuous interlocking fine chromic catgut. A common error is to resect too much pelvis; when the obstruction is relieved, there will be spontaneous reduction in the renal pelvic size (Fig. 16–61).

Adjuncts to Reconstructive Procedures

NEPHROPEXY. One of the advantages of the transperitoneal approach is that the repair of the ureteropelvic obstruction can be accomplished without mobilization of the kidney. In the flank approach, a limited amount of mobilization is necessary but does not in itself interfere with subsequent drainage of the newly created junction. Rarely, mobilization is so extensive that nephropexy is necessary. Nephropexy, however, is often necessary after pyeloplasty in horseshoe kidney when the isthmus has been divided. Several interrupted figure-of-eight heavy chromic catgut sutures are placed between the posterior capsule of the kidney and the psoas fascia.

STENTS AND NEPHROSTOMY TUBES. In the past, the use of the ureteral stents (ureteral intubation) and nephrostomy drainage (diversion) was considered an integral part of ureteropelvic reconstructive proce-

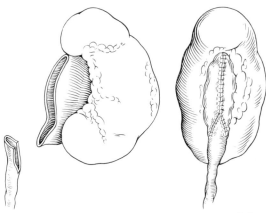

Figure 16–61. Ureteropyelostomy and partial resection of pelvis.

dures. Use of these techniques is still mandatory if a Davis ureterotomy must be performed or if the patient has an infected kidney. Also, in secondary operative procedures, when a difficult dissection may somewhat compromise the wall of the ureter, intubation and diversion may be used to add a measure of safety. Nephrostomy protects against renal damage from recurrent obstruction and prevents flank drainage of urine at the anastomotic site. The purpose of an indwelling stent is to ensure patency of the anastomosis and to carry the urine past the anastomotic site without leakage and subsequent fibrosis. Conversely, the stent can block the lumen of the ureter and promote a urine leak.

The major disadvantage of the stent is that the presence of a foreign body at the site of healing impairs local vascularity and may delay healing. When the anastomosis is wide and surgically satisfactory, there is no need for a stent; when the anastomosis is narrow and the ureteral end is of doubtful viability, the stent may be harmful. It is best, therefore, to fashion the anastomosis over a stent and then to remove the stent at the conclusion of the procedure. No proximal urinary diversion, nephrostomy, or vent is necessary. A suction Hemovac tube with multiple openings is used to drain the anastomotic site.

However, opinions about the use of stents, usually Silastic tubing of appropriate size, or nephrostomy vary. Certainly for acute (intermittent) obstruction in which the pelvis is minimally dilated and possesses good musculature and tone, the use of either stent or nephrostomy would appear to be superfluous. Nephrostomy may be used for only a few days postoperatively to protect the kidney from obstruction of the ureteropelvic anastomosis caused by edema (Hendren et al). It also

allows for the performance of a nephrostogram and, if necessary, a pressure flow study to assess the patency of the anastomosis objectively before removal of the nephrostomy tube. Others have suggested the use of both nephrostomy and stent in the very young to avoid the risk of adhesions across the anastomosis resulting from apposition of the walls (Persky et al; Snyder et al). An alternative to nephrostomy coming into fairly common use of present is the double-J stent, which provides adequate internal drainage.

It would appear, however, that in general the results of pyeloplasty with and without the use of tubes are generally comparable. The tubeless technique does reduce hospitalization significantly (Rickwood and Phadke). It is likely that this argument will never be resolved completely, even though the tendency clearly is toward tubeless pyeloplasty.

Chemotherapy. If infection is found, an attempt should be made to sterilize the urine before the operation with appropriate antibiotic treatment. When nephrostomy tubes are used, either preliminarily or adjuvant to the surgical procedure, suppressive chemotherapy should be given. Once all tubes have been removed, the patient should be initially treated with specific antibiotics chosen on the basis of culture and sensitivity test results and should be given suppressive chemotherapy for several weeks until healing is complete and the urine is sterile.

Ureteropelvic Obstruction in Neonates and Infants

The use of prenatal ultrasonography (Figs. 16–62 and 16–63) and contrast studies for other anomalies, primarily cardiac, early in life is responsible for the increasing number of neonates seen for repair of ureteropelvic ob-

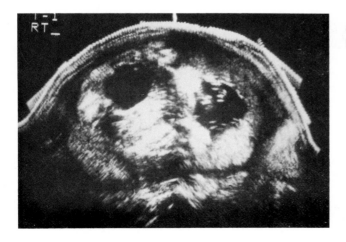

Figure 16–62. Maternal ultrasound. Bilateral hydronephrosis and bilateral ureteropelvic obstruction.

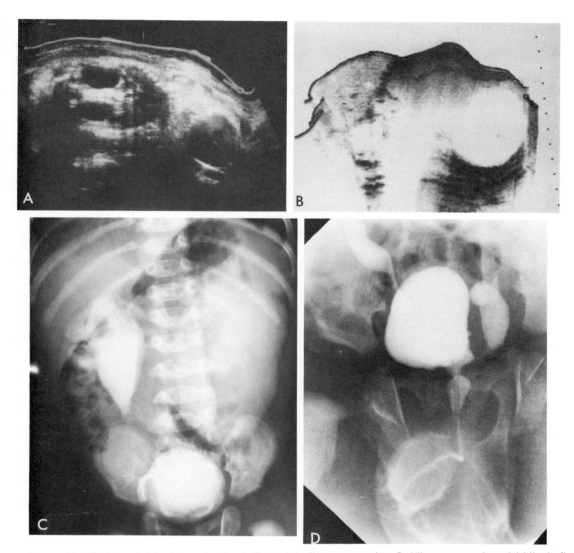

Figure 16–63. Prenatal hydronephrosis. *A,* Prenatal ultrasonography. *B,* Ultrasonography at birth. Left hydronephrosis. *C,* Excretory urogram. Massive left hydronephrosis secondary to ureteropelvic obstruction. *D,* Voiding cystourethrogram. Also, bilateral vesicoureteral reflux.

struction (Roth and Gonzales). The early recognition and correction of such obstruction is extremely important, because evidence accumulated to date suggests that relief of obstruction in the first few months of life is associated with greater return of renal function than is relief in older children or adults, apparently because of the possibility of nephron maturation in the cortical zone (McCrory; Beck; Mayor et al).

A mass, generally large, and urinary infection are the main presenting symptoms in obstruction not discovered prenatally. Bilaterality in the neonatal and infant group is characteristic, occurring in up to 50 per cent of males (Robson et al). The possible presence of severe contralateral disease, particularly mul-

ticystic kidney and absence of function, deserves emphasis.

The urographic findings have already been referred to under the section on diagnostic studies (Figs. 16–64 and 16–65). Despite the poorly functioning kidneys and advanced degree of hydronephrosis, retrograde pyelography is rarely necessary to determine the lesion (Perlmutter et al). When additional information is considered essential, percutaneous antegrade pyelography, especially before exploration, is a safe and effective method of defining the level of obstruction in the poorly opacified system (Fowler and Jensen). Furthermore, careful ultrasonographic examination of the involved side for identification of a dilated ureter suggesting ureterovesical ob-

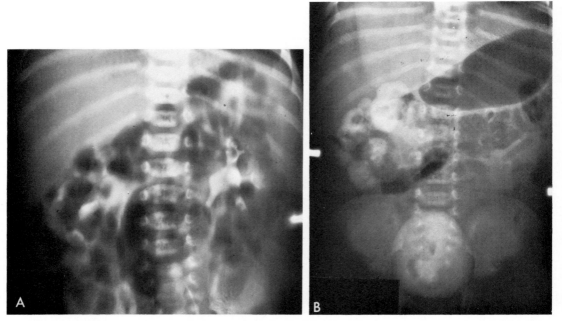

Figure 16–64. Neonatal hydronephrosis from ureteropelvic obstruction on right. *A*, Conventional excretory urogram. *B*, Same, with furosemide.

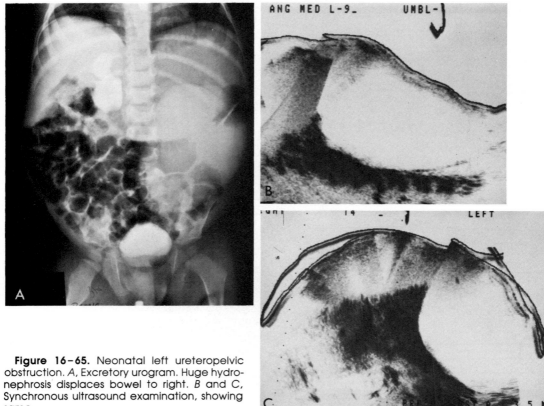

Figure 16–65. Neonatal left ureteropelvic obstruction. *A*, Excretory urogram. Huge hydronephrosis displaces bowel to right. *B* and *C*, Synchronous ultrasound examination, showing same.

struction can be of additional help in determining the correct diagnosis. Nephrectomy, except in patients with multicystic dysplastic kidney, is almost never justified. The incidence of bilaterality, especially contralateral disease appearing later in life, and the marked recuperative power of the infant kidney, which is totally unpredictable by any measures available at present, clearly suggest the need for utmost conservatism.

The pyeloplasty should be performed by extraperitoneal anterior flank or subcostal incision and, if the condition is bilateral, on both sides during the same period of anesthesia. Because of the usually severe degree of hydronephrosis, reduction of the size of the pelvis in addition to ureteropyelostomy is the rule rather than the exception. The same considerations in the use of nephrostomy and stents as those already discussed are applicable for neonatal pyeloplasty (Bejjani and Belman). Improvement in hydronephrosis is generally dramatic, and recovery of parenchymal architecture is impressive (Fig. 16–66).

Postoperative Complications and Follow-Up

The usual complications common to all reconstructive procedures are encountered here. Transitory obstruction at the anastomosis due to edema, at times lasting several weeks and leading to excessive urine leakage in the tubeless technique, occurs occasionally, especially in the very young. Interestingly, the use of stents does not prevent this complication (Snyder et al). It should be corrected by early placement of indwelling ureteral catheters or a double-J stent of appropriate size that is left in for a few days. Results are better in kidneys that are free of infection at the time of operation. Intrarenal bleeding may fill the pelvis with clots that will be evident on a postoperative urogram. Most failures are the result of postoperative stricture at the anastomotic site. Such failures are usually evident soon after operation. Balloon dilatation of the postoperatively obstructed anastomosis has been accomplished with success (Kadir et al).

A limited urographic examination in the early postoperative period will assure proper function and drainage in the reconstructed ureteropelvic obstruction, but conventional urography generally is deferred for 3 to 6 months after the operation, the time in which the maximum urographic improvement will become evident (Fig. 16–67). Rarely, asymptomatic obstruction of the kidney occurs despite initial improvement after pyeloplasty (McAlister et al).

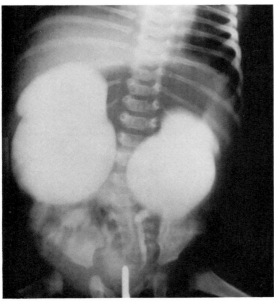
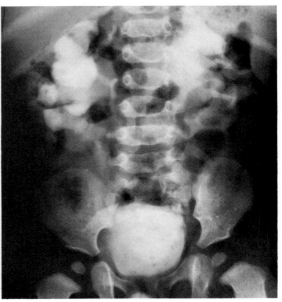

A

B

Figure 16–66. *A,* Preoperative bilateral retrograde pyelogram in 8-week-old infant with advanced bilateral hydronephrosis. Excretory urogram showed nearly functionless kidneys. *B,* Excretory urogram at 8 months after pyeloplasty.

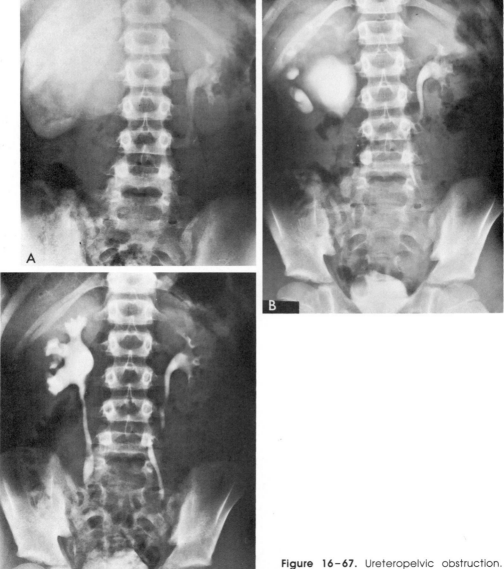

Figure 16–67. Ureteropelvic obstruction. Right ureteropyelostomy. *A,* Preoperative excretory urogram. *B,* Spot excretory urogram on fifth postoperative day. *C,* Excretory urogram 3 months later.

Evaluation of Postoperative Results

All formulas for evaluating postoperative results are inadequate, because none can take all factors into account simultaneously. Renal function is likely to improve postoperatively, especially in bilateral obstruction with compromised renal function initially, as shown by improved glomerular filtration rates (Williams and Kenawai). The functional result is difficult to assess in unilateral cases, although renography may be of value. The method readily available and universally used is, of course, comparison of the urograms before and after surgery — a method concerned with anatomic rather than functional assessment and at best quite subjective. If a preoperative isotope renal scan is carried out, differential renal functions can be compared postoperatively. Additionally, the half-times of the diuretic renal scans can also be used for comparison, although 6 months should elapse before any definitive conclusion is made about residual obstruction.

It is therefore reasonable to classify results

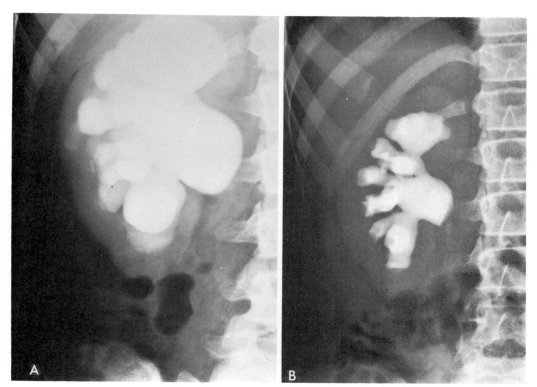

Figure 16–68. Ureteropelvic obstruction. *A,* Excretory urogram, preoperative. *B,* Excretory urogram, 3 months after ureteropyelostomy. Elimination of symptoms and regression but incomplete resolution of hydronephrosis. Dye enters right ureter.

as either successes or failures. Pyeloplasty gives excellent results in more than 90 per cent of cases, even though only a small number of kidneys return to normal urographically. As a rule, the greatest improvement is seen in cases in which the excretory urogram was made preoperatively during a phase of acute obstruction. In kidneys with severe calycectasis, even though some shrinkage might be expected after removal of the obstruction, there is seldom any noteworthy improvement in the shape of the calyces (Fig. 16–68). It is important, however, that pyelographic assessment of the calyces be made, because improvement in the appearance of the pelvis is simply the result of operative excision rather than relief of obstruction (Figs. 16–66, 16–69, and 16–70).

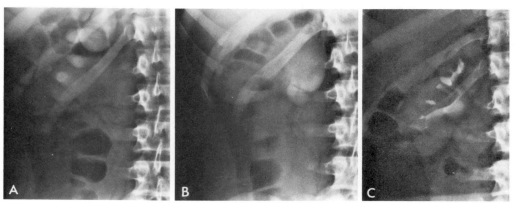

Figure 16–69. Ureteropelvic obstruction. Reductive pyeloplasty. *A* and *B,* Excretory urogram. *C,* Same, postoperative.

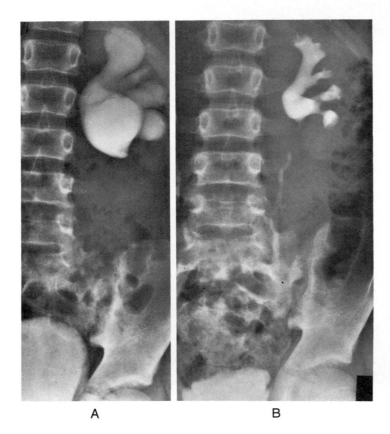

A   B

Figure 16–70. Excretory urograms. *A*, Preoperative showing left ureteropelvic obstruction. *B*, At 3 months after ureteropyelostomy.

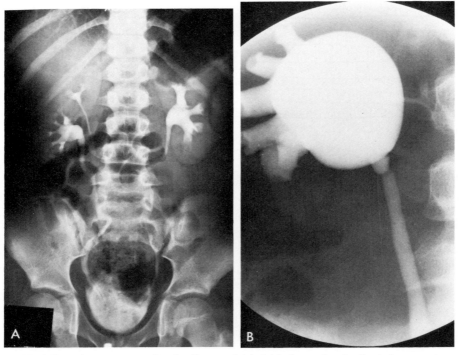

Figure 16–71. *A*, Excretory urogram. Duplication on right. *B*, Vesicoureteral reflux in lower segment on left. Early ureteropelvic obstruction?

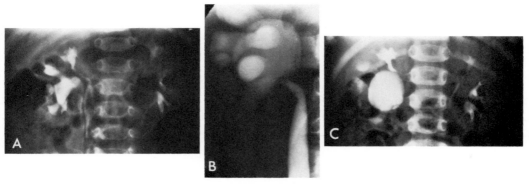

Figure 16–72. Bilateral duplication with vesicoureteral reflux in right lower segment. *A*, Excretory urogram. *B*, Voiding cystourethrogram. *C*, Secondary ureteropelvic obstruction in right lower segment (3 years later).

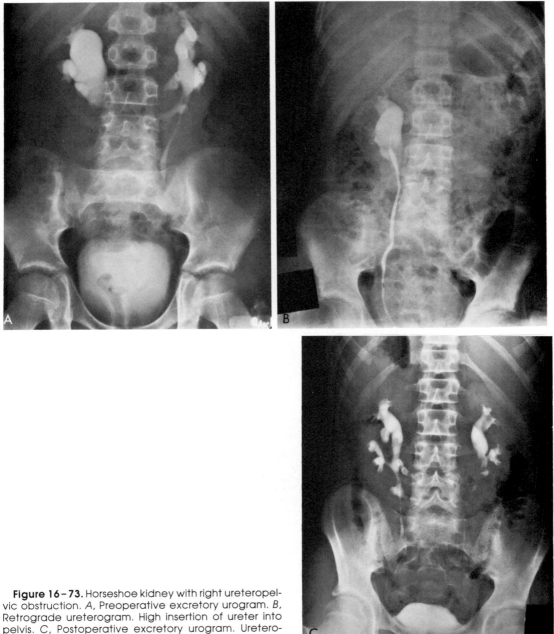

Figure 16–73. Horseshoe kidney with right ureteropelvic obstruction. *A*, Preoperative excretory urogram. *B*, Retrograde ureterogram. High insertion of ureter into pelvis. *C*, Postoperative excretory urogram. Ureterocalycostomy.

Special Situations

URETEROPELVIC JUNCTION OB-STRUCTION IN THE LOWER SEGMENT OF THE DUPLEX SYSTEM. Most often, ureteropelvic obstruction in the lower segment of the completely duplicated system is secondary to vesicoureteral reflux. Clearly, unless significant obstruction can be demonstrated at the renal level, ureteroneocystostomy should be the initial procedure and is, in fact, the only one usually necessary (Fig. 16–71). If significant obstruction is demonstrated, pyeloplasty should be the initial procedure (Fig. 16–72). Should anatomic variations in the region prevent conventional pyeloplasty, pyeloureterostomy should be done, either by anastomosis of the distal end of the pelvis to the upper segment ureter (end-to-side) or simply by joining of the two by adjacent vertical incisions (side-to-side). In incomplete duplication, a short connecting ureteral segment below the ureteropelvic junction and an adjacent narrow upper segment of ureter may further complicate correction (Ossandon et al).

URETEROPELVIC OBSTRUCTION IN THE HORSESHOE KIDNEY. The time-honored view that hydronephrosis in the horseshoe kidney is caused by obstruction at the isthmus and that the isthmus should therefore be routinely divided is no longer tenable. In general, the results of pyeloplasty in the horseshoe kidney are equally satisfactory without division of the isthmus (Pitts and Muecke). Because of the high insertion of the ureter into the pelvis, a long side-to-side anastomosis between the pelvis and the ureter is often preferable to ureteropyelostomy (Hendren), although both procedures have worked well. However, an option that has gained increasingly wide use, especially when the pyelocalycectasis is severe, is ureterocalycostomy (Mollard and Braun) (Fig. 16–73).

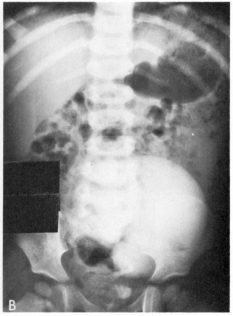

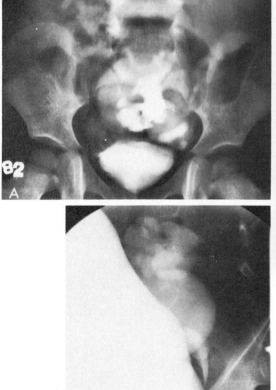

Figure 16–74. Solitary pelvic kidney. *A*, Excretory urogram. Dilated pelvis anterior to kidney is faintly visualized. *B*, Excretory urogram, late film. Pyelectasis is clearly shown. *C*, Cystogram. Vesicoureteral reflux.

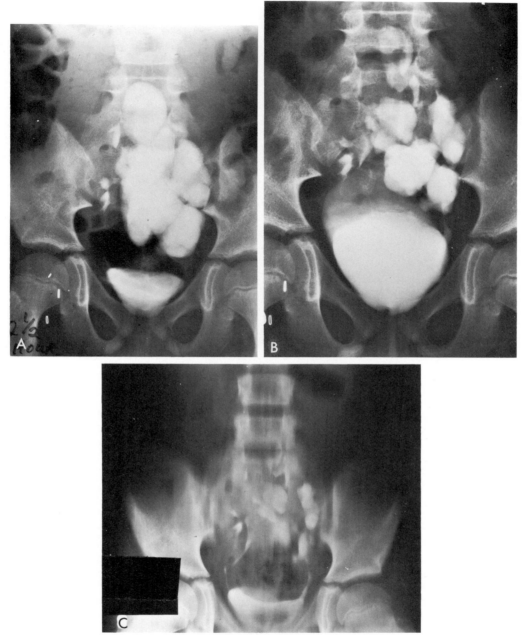

Figure 16–75. Pelvic fused kidney with left ureteropelvic obstruction. *A*, Preoperative excretory urogram. *B*, Ureterocalycostomy. Early postoperative urogram. *C*, Final result at 1 year. Postoperative excretory urogram.

URETEROPELVIC OBSTRUCTION IN THE PELVIC KIDNEY. High insertion of the ureter into the pelvis is a frequent cause of hydronephrosis in the pelvic kidney. It is of the utmost importance that both reflux and apparent but nonobstructive pyelectasis, both known to mimic ureteropelvic obstruction, be adequately excluded by suitable drainage studies, cystourethrography, and a diuretic-assisted renogram (Fig. 16–74).

A transabdominal approach offers the best exposure. Kinking of the ureteropyelostomy should be carefully avoided, a difficult undertaking because of the anomalous blood supply of the kidney and the resulting relative immobility, which can also prevent a freely

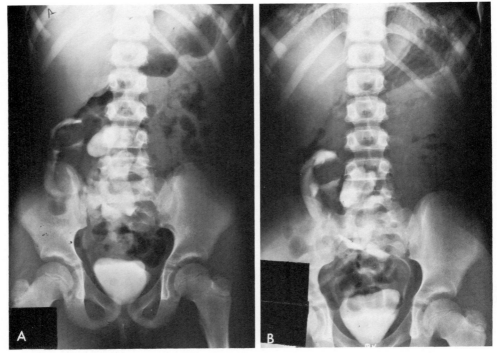

Figure 16–76. *A,* Ureteropelvic obstruction in crossed segment of fused kidney. *B,* After ureterocalycostomy.

dependent ureteropelvic junction repair. For these reasons, ureterocalycostomy may be a superior procedure in some cases of ureteropelvic obstruction in renal ectopy, both in the pelvic variety and crossed ectopy with or without fusion (Figs. 16–75 and 16–76).

Ureterocalycostomy

Ureterocalycostomy is generally considered an exceptional procedure rarely used in clinical situations in which normal renal drainage cannot be established by the conventional techniques. It is particularly suited after unsuccessful pyeloplasty with destruction of the renal pelvis (Fig. 16–77), avulsion or long stricture of the proximal ureter, congenital pelvic stenosis, or intrarenal pelvis (Couvelaire et al; Wesolowski). As already discussed, specific problems encountered in anomalies of renal fusion or ectopy make ureteropelvic repair by conventional pyeloplasty at times unsatisfactory. In all these situations, ureterocalycostomy deserves special consideration. In the horseshoe kidney, ureterocalycostomy also eliminates the need for division of the isthmus.

Neuwirk performed the first ureterocalycostomy by pulling the splayed ureter into the cortex and suturing the ureter to the renal capsule. Later experience showed that ureterocalycostomy without amputation of the lower pole of the kidney leads to scarring and contracture of the intrarenal ureteral segment owing to fibrosis of the cortex (Jameson et al).

According to Hawthorne, cardinal features of a successful ureterocalycostomy should include amputation of enough lower pole cortex to free the ureter from entrapment by contracting fibrosis of the renal cortex (Fig. 16–78A), tangential sectioning of the calyx and spatulation of the ureter to create a maximally patent anastomosis and a noncircumferential suture line (Fig. 16–78B), and cystoscopic placement of a retrograde catheter to ease identification of the ureter in instances of reoperation, subsequent removal, and creation of anastomoses over ureteral stent and nephrostomy drainage. (Fig. 16–78C).

The likelihood of success is comparable with that in other secondary operations on the ureteropelvic junction (Fig. 16–79) and is quite favorable in unusual clinical situations in which it is a primary procedure.

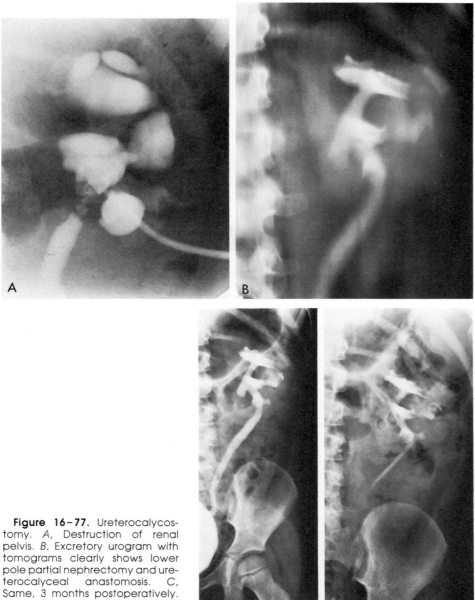

Figure 16-77. Ureterocalycostomy. *A*, Destruction of renal pelvis. *B*, Excretory urogram with tomograms clearly shows lower pole partial nephrectomy and ureterocalyceal anastomosis. *C*, Same, 3 months postoperatively. *D*, Same, 9 months postoperatively.

Figure 16-78. Ureterocalycostomy (see text).

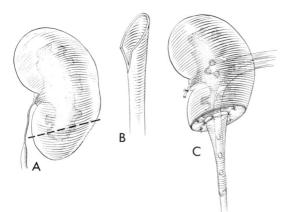

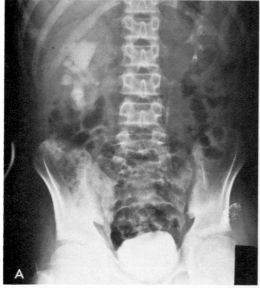

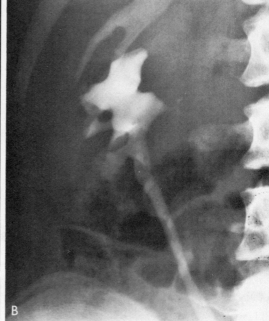

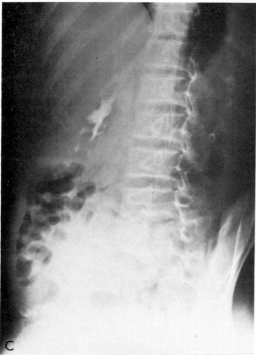

Figure 16–79. *A*, Unsuccessful right pyeloplasty (three attempts). Persisting obstruction at uretero-pelvic junction. Right ureterocalycostomy. *B* and *C*, Postoperative excretory urogram, showing free drainage through ureterocalycostomy and regression of hydronephrosis.

BIBLIOGRAPHY

Allen TD: Congenital ureteral strictures. J Urol *104*:196, 1970.

Alton DJ: Pelviureteric obstruction in childhood. Radiol Clin North Am *15*:61, 1977.

Anderson JC: Hydronephrosis: a fourteen years' survey of results. Proc R Soc Med *55*:93, 1962.

Beck AD: The effect of intra-uterine urinary obstruction upon the development of the fetal kidney. J Urol *105*:504, 1971.

Bejjani B, Belman AB: Ureteropelvic junction obstruction in newborns and infants. J Urol *128*:770, 1982.

Butcher HR Jr, Sleator W Jr: The effect of ureteral anastomosis upon conduction of peristaltic waves: an electroureterographic study. J Urol *75*:650, 1956.

Caine M, Hermann G: The return of peristalsis in the anastomosed ureter. Br J Urol *42*:164, 1970.

Carella JA, Silber I: Hyperreninemic hypertension in an infant secondary to pelviureteric obstruction treated successfully by surgery. J Pediatrics *89*:987, 1976.

Cohen B, Goldman SM, Kopilnick M, et al: Ureteropelvic junction obstruction: its occurrence in 3 members of a single family. J Urol *120*:361, 1978.

Couvelaire R, Auvert J, Moulonguet A, et al: Implantations et anastomoses urétéro-calicielles: techniques et indications. J Urol Neprhol *70*:437, 1964.

Culp OS: Management of ureteropelvic obstruction. Bull NY Acad Med 43:355, 1967.

Culp OS, DeWeerd JH: A pelvic flap operation for certain types of ureteropelvic obstruction: preliminary report. Proc Staff Meet Mayo Clin 26:483, 1951.

Culp OS, Rusche CF, Johnson SH III, et al: Hydronephrosis and hydroureter in infancy and childhood: a panel discussion. J Urol 88:443, 1962.

Dajani AM, Dajani YF, Dahbrah S: Congenital ureteric valves—a cause of urinary obstruction: a report of 5 cases. Br J Urol 54:98, 1982.

Drake DP, Stevens PS, Eckstein HB: Hydronephrosis secondary to ureteropelvic obstruction in children: a review of 14 years of experience. J Urol 119:649, 1978.

Dunn DH, Williams RD, Gonzalez R: Intermittent hydronephrosis: a cause of abdominal pain. Arch Surg 113:329, 1978.

Eckstein HB, Kamal I: Hydronephrosis due to pelvi-ureteric obstruction in children: an assessment of the anterior transperitoneal approach. Br J Surg 58:663, 1971.

Foley FEB: A new plastic operation for stricture at the uretero-pelvic junction: report of 20 operations. J Urol 38:643, 1937.

Foote JW, Blennerhassett JB, Wiglesworth FW, et al: Observations on the ureteropelvic junction. J Urol 104:252, 1970.

Fowler R, Jensen F: Percutaneous antegrade pyelography in small infants and neonates. Br J Radiol 48:987, 1975.

Garrett J, Polse SL, Morrow JW: Ureteral obstruction and hypertension. Am J Med 49:171, 1970.

Genereux GP, Monks JH: Intermittent ureteropelvic junction obstruction: pathophysiologic-radiologic features. J Can Assoc Radiol 23:75, 1972.

Grossman IC, Cromie WJ, Wein AJ, et al. Renal hypertension secondary to ureteropelvic junction obstruction: unusual presentation and new therapeutic modality. Urology 17:69, 1981.

Gup A: Benign mesodermal polyp in childhood. J Urol 114:619, 1975.

Hanley HG: The pelvi-ureteric junction: a cine-pyelography study. Br J Urol 31:377, 1959.

Hanna MK: Some observations on congenital ureteropelvic junction obstruction. Urology 12:151, 1978.

Hawthorne NJ, Zincke H, Kelalis PP: Ureterocalicostomy: an alternative to nephrectomy. J Urol 115:583, 1976.

Hellstrom J, Giertz G, Lindblom K: Pathogenesis and treatment of hydronephrosis. In VIII Congreso de la Sociedad International de Urologia, Paris, 1949.

Hendren WH: Abdominal masses in newborn infants. Am J Surg 107:502, 1964.

Hendren WH, Donahoe PK: Renal fusions and ectopia. In Pediatric Surgery. Third ed. Edited by Ravitch MM, Welch KJ, Benson DC, et al. Chicago, Year Book Medical Publishers, 1978, p 1166.

Hendren WH, Radharkrishnan J, Middleton AW Jr: Pediatric pyeloplasty. J Pediatr Surg 15:133, 1980.

Hinman F Jr, Oppenheimer R: Ureteral regeneration. VI. Delayed urinary flow in the healing of unsplinted ureteral defects. J Urol 78:138, 1957.

Hjort EF, Boe OW: Partial resection of the renal pelvis and lower pole of the kidney for hydronephrosis. Br J Urol 43:406, 1971.

Homsy Y, Simard J, Debs C, et al: Pyeloplasty: to divert or not to divert? Urology 16:577, 1980.

Hutch JA, Hinman F, Miller ER: Reflux as a cause of hydronephrosis and chronic pyelonephritis. J Urol 88:169, 1962.

Hutch JA, Tanagho EA: Etiology of non-occlusive ureteral dilatation. J Urol 93:177, 184, 1965.

Jameson SG, McKinney JS, Rushton JF: Ureterocalyostomy: a new surgical procedure for correction of ureteropelvic stricture associated with an intrarenal pelvis. J Urol 77:135, 1957.

Jimenez-Mariscal JL, Moussali Flah L: Ureteropelvic junction obstruction secondary to vesicoureteral reflux: later complication after successful vesicoureteral reimplant. Urology 18:203, 1981.

Johnston JH: The pathogenesis of hydronephrosis in children. Br J Urol 41:724, 1969.

Kadir S, White RI Jr, Engel R: Balloon dilatation of a ureteropelvic junction obstruction. Radiology 143:263, 1982.

Kelalis PP, Culp OS, Stickler GB, et al: Ureteropelvic obstruction in children: experiences with 109 cases. J Urol 106:418, 1971.

Kelalis PP, Malek RS: Infundibulopelvic stenosis. J Urol 125:568, 1981.

Kendall AR, Karafin L: Intermittent hydronephrosis: hydration pyelography. J Urol 98:653, 1967.

Koff SA, Thrall JH, Keyes JW Jr: Diuretic radionuclide urography: a non-invasive method for evaluating nephroureteral dilatation. J Urol 121:153, 1979.

Krueger RP, Ash JM, Silver MM, et al: Primary hydronephrosis: assessment of diuretic renography, pelvic operative findings and renal and ureteral histology. Urol Clin North Am 7:231, 1980.

Leadbetter GW Jr, Monaco AP, Russell PS: A technique for reconstruction of the urinary tract in renal transplantation. Surg Gynecol Obstet 123:839, 1966.

Levitt SB, Lutzker LG: Urine extravasation secondary to upper urinary tract obstruction. J Pediatr Surg 11:575, 1976.

Lich R Jr: The obstructed ureteropelvic junction. Radiology 68:337, 1957.

Lupton EW, Testa HJ, O'Reilly PH, et al: Diuresis renography and morphology in upper urinary tract obstruction. Br J Urol 51:10, 1979.

Maizels M, Stephens FD: Valves of the ureter as a cause of primary obstruction of the ureter: anatomic, embryologic and clinical aspects. J Urol 123:742, 1980.

Marshall FF, Jeffs RD, Smolev JK: Neonatal bilateral ureteropelvic junction obstruction. J Urol 123:107, 1980.

Mayor G, Genton N, Torrado A, et al: Renal function in obstructive nephropathy: long-term effect of reconstructive surgery. Pediatrics 56:740, 1975.

McAlister WH, Manley CB, Siegel MJ: Asymptomatic progression of partial ureteropelvic obstruction in children. J Urol 123:267, 1980.

McCrory WW: Regulation of renal functional development. Urol Clin North Am 7:243, 1980.

McCrory WW, Shibuya M, Leumann E, et al: Studies of renal function in children with chronic hydronephrosis. Pediatr Clin North Am 18:445, 1971.

Melick WF, Karellos D, Naryka JJ: Pressure studies of hydronephrosis in children by means of the strain gauge. J Urol 85:703, 1961.

Michalowski E, Modelski W, Kmak A: Die End-zu-End-Anastomose zwischen dem unteren Nierenkelch und Harnleiter (Ureterocalicostomie). Z Urol Nephrol 63:1, 1970.

Mollard P, Braun P: Primary ureterocalycostomy for severe hydronephrosis in children. J Pediatr Surg 15:87, 1980.

Munoz A, Pascual Y Baralt JF, Melendez MT: Arterial hypertension in infants with hydronephrosis: report of six cases. Am J Dis Child 131:38, 1977.

Murnaghan GF: The dynamics of the renal pelvis and ureter with reference to congenital hydronephrosis. Br J Urol 30:321, 1958a.

Murnaghan GF: The mechanism of congenital hydronephrosis with reference to the factors influencing surgical treatment. Ann R Coll Surg Engl 23:25, 1958b.

Murnaghan GF: Experimental aspects of hydronephrosis. Br J Urol 31:370, 1959.

Nesbit RM: Diagnoses of intermittent hydronephrosis: importance of pyelography during episodes of pain. J Urol 75:767, 1956.

Neuwirk K: Implantation of the ureter into the lower calyx of the renal pelvis. In VII Congrès de la Société Internationale d'Urologie, part 2, pp 253–255, 1947.

Newhouse JH, Pfister RC, Hendren WH, et al: Whitaker test after pyeloplasty: establishment of normal ureteral perfusion pressures. AJR 137:223, 1981.

Nixon HH: Hydronephrosis in children: a clinical study of seventy-eight cases with special reference to the role of aberrant renal vessels and the results of conservative operations. Br J Surg 40:601, 1953.

Odiase V, Whitaker RH: Dynamic evaluation of the results of pyeloplasty using pressure-flow studies. Eur Urol 7:324, 1981.

O'Reilly PH, Lawson RS, Shields RA, et al: Idiopathic hydronephrosis–the diuresis renogram: a new non-invasive method of assessing equivocal pelviureteral junction obstruction. J Urol 121:153, 1979.

Ossandon F, Androulakakis P, Ransley PG: Surgical problems in pelviureteral junction obstruction of the lower moiety in incomplete duplex systems. J Urol 125:871, 1981.

Parker RM, Perlmutter AD: Upper urinary tract obstruction in infants. J Urol 102:355, 1969.

Parker RM, Rudd RG, Wonderly RK, et al: Ureteropelvic junction obstruction in infants and children: functional evaluation of the obstructed kidney preoperative and postoperatively. J Urol 126:509, 1981.

Pathak IG, Williams DI: Multicystic and cystic dysplastic kidneys. Br J Urol 36:318, 1964.

Perlmutter AD, Kroovand RL, Lai Y-W: Management of ureteropelvic obstruction in the first year of life. J Urol 123:535, 1980.

Persky L, McDougal WS, Kedia K: Management of initial pyeloplasty failure. J Urol 125:695, 1981.

Pitts WR Jr, Muecke EC: Horseshoe kidneys: a 40-year experience. J Urol 113:743, 1975.

Rattner WH, Fink S, Murphy JJ: Pressure studies in the human ureter and renal pelvis. J Urol 78:359, 1957.

Rickwood AM, Phadke D: Pyeloplasty in infants and children with particular reference to the method of drainage post-operatively. Br J Urol 50:217, 1978.

Robson WJ, Rudy SM, Johnston JH: Pelviureteric obstruction in infancy. J Pediatr Surg 11:57, 1976.

Roth DR, Gonzales ET Jr: Management of ureteropelvic junction obstruction in infants. J Urol 129:108, 1983.

Ruano-Gil D, Coca-Payeras A, Tejedo-Maten A: Obstruction and normal recanalization of the ureter in the human embryo: its relation to congenital ureteric obstruction. Eur Urol 1:287, 1975.

Saxton HM: Percutaneous nephrostomy: technique. Urol Radiol 2:131, 1981.

Shopfner CE: Ureteropelvic junction obstruction. Am J Roentgenol Radium Ther Nucl Med 98:148, 1966.

Snyder HM III, Lebowitz RL, Colodny AH, et al: Ureteropelvic junction obstruction in children. Urol Clin North Am 7:273, 1980.

Squitiera AP, Ceccarelli FE, Bobka JC: Hypertension in an infant secondary to pelviureteric obstruction treated successfully by surgery. J Pediatr 88:987, 1976.

Uson AC, Cox LA, Lattimer JK: Hydronephrosis in infants and children. II. Surgical management and results. JAMA 205:327, 1968.

Uson AC, Levitt SB, Lattimer JK: Giant hydronephrosis in children. Pediatrics 44:209, 1969.

Wesolowski S: Corrective operative procedure after unsuccessful pelvi-ureteric plastic surgery. Br J Urol 43:679, 1971.

Wesolowski S: Uretero-calicostomy. Eur Urol 1:18, 1975.

Whitaker RH: Reflux induced pelvi-ureteric obstruction. Br J Urol 48:555, 1976.

Whitfield HN, Britton KE, Hendry WF, et al: The distinction between obstructive uropathy and nephropathy by radioisotope transit times. Br J Urol 50:433, 1978.

Williams DI, Kenawai MM: The prognosis of pelviureteric obstruction in childhood: a review of 190 cases. Eur Urol 2:57, 1976.

Williams DI, Karlaftis CM: Hydronephrosis due to pelvi-ureteric obstruction in the newborn. Br J Urol 38:138, 1966.

Ureter and Ureterovesical Junction

LOWELL R. KING

RETROCAVAL URETER

In the condition known as retrocaval ureter, the upper third of the ureter makes an abrupt turn medially, passes behind the vena cava, continues forward between the vena cava and the aorta, and then courses laterally, anterior to the vena cava to reach its normal position (Fig. 16–80). This anomaly originates from a developmental error in the formation of the vena cava, not the ureter. Normally, the infrarenal segment of the inferior vena cava is formed from the supracardinal vein, a venous channel that lies dorsal to the ureter. If the subcardinal vein, which lies ventral to the ureter, persists instead as the infrarenal segment of the vena cava, the ureter passes behind the definitive vein but in front of the

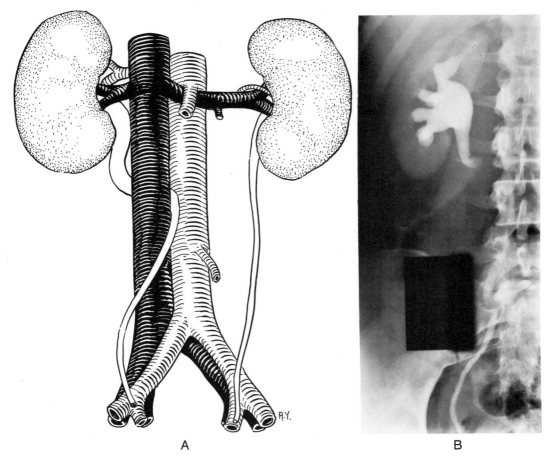

Figure 16–80. Retrocaval ureter. *A*, Drawing. (From Hollinshead WH: Anatomy for Surgeons. Vol 2. Second ed. © 1971 by Harper and Row, Inc. Reproduced by permission.) *B*, Excretory urogram.

dorsally formed iliac vein and necessarily hooks around the anomalously formed vena cava (Fig. 16–81). Thus, the majority of retrocaval ureters result from the persistance of a ventral embryologic venous element with disappearance of a dorsal element. Occasionally, both elements persist; the ureter then passes between the duplicated venae cavae.

Since the condition was originally described in 1940, cases have been recorded with increasing frequency (Considine). The association of this anomaly with gonadal dysgenesis and with Turner's syndrome has been described (Uson et al). Retrocaval ureter is the only anomaly of the genitourinary system that is essentially limited to the right side, although a single case of a left-sided retrocaval ureter has been recorded in association with situs inversus (Brooks).

Retrocaval ureter is of clinical significance only when hydronephrosis results from obstruction of the ureter where it passes behind the vena cava. In any patient with pyelectasis and ureterectasis of the upper third of the right ureter, retrocaval ureter should be suspected. Urographic confirmation is easily achieved by inserting a catheter into the ureter. The ureteral catheter passes toward the midline, overlying the vertebral column in the region of L3 and L4. Performing simultaneous inferior venacavography is superfluous, but an ultrasound examination alone may be misinterpreted as ureteropelvic junction obstruction.

Treatment, if necessary, consists of dividing the distal portion of the dilated upper ureter and moving the distal limb of the ureter, transposing it to a position in front of the vena cava, and re-establishing ureteral continuity (Fig. 16–82). A procedure combining resection of the vena cava with anatomically correct repositioning of the ureter and reanastomosis of the vessel has also been reported (Goodwin et al, 1957). This seems more ardu-

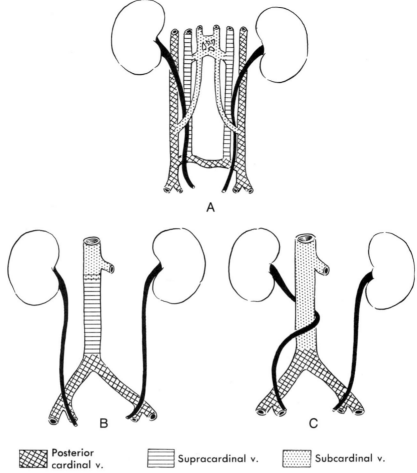

Posterior cardinal v.   Supracardinal v.   Subcardinal v.

Figure 16-81. Relationship between development of infrarenal portion of the inferior vena cava and retrocaval ureter. *A,* Primitive condition with ureter winding among three cardinal veins. *B,* Usual method of formation of vena cava from right supracardinal vein (dorsal to ureter). *C,* Main portion of vena cava formed from subcardinal vein. (From Hollinshead WH: Anatomy for Surgeons. Vol 2. Second ed. © 1971 by Harper and Row, Inc. Reproduced by permission.)

ous than the technique just described, because some lumbar veins must be identified and carefully divided to permit adequate mobilization of the transected vena cava.

URETERAL STRICTURES

Congenital ureteral strictures at the ureteropelvic and ureterovesical junctions are described elsewhere in this chapter. Until recently, strictures of the ureter itself were diagnosed with extreme rarity. In a 1971 study of the morphology of a large number of ureteral strictures in children with hydronephrosis, Cussen found at least one third of the strictures to be in the midureter. Most were composed of what he terms *segmental* or *serpig-*

inous stenosis. As evidence of obstruction, Cussen cites the finding that the muscle above the obstruction was both hypertrophic and hyperplastic.

Others report such strictures in the midureter in the region of the pelvic brim as it crosses the common iliac vessel. These investigators suggest that such strictures are the result of impaired muscularization consequent to compression by the vessel during embryogenesis (Allen). Such strictures must be differentiated from ureteral atresia. Retroperitoneal fibrosis or lymphoma also may be considered in the differential diagnosis, but the former is exceedingly rare in children, and the latter is identified by other signs.

Treatment depends on the condition of the kidney. Nephrectomy is elected when the re-

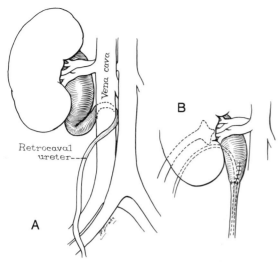

Figure 16-82. Surgical correction of retrocaval ureter. (From Goyanna R, Cook EN, Counseller VS: Circumcaval ureter: report of case in which diagnosis was made preoperatively. Proc Staff Meet Mayo Clin 21:356–360, 1946. Reproduced by permission.)

sultant hydronephrosis is extreme. Otherwise, excision of the strictured segment with ureteroureterostomy is the preferred mode of treatment.

Ureteroureterostomy is done by anastomosing the cut ends of the sectioned ureter with fine interrupted sutures of catgut or Dexon, the knots being placed on the outside. For small-caliber ureters, spatulating the cut ends of the ureter enlarges the anastomotic area and helps to prevent subsequent stenosis. Often, however, the disparity between the diameters of the upper and lower segments of the ureter is great. In such instances, Z-plasty ureterostomy is preferable. The Z-plasty technique is particularly applicable because varying the angle of the incisions mitigates the difference in the diameter of the two segments, the greater angle being in the normal segment and the lesser angle in the dilated one (Fig. 16–83).

Conduction of the peristaltic waves across

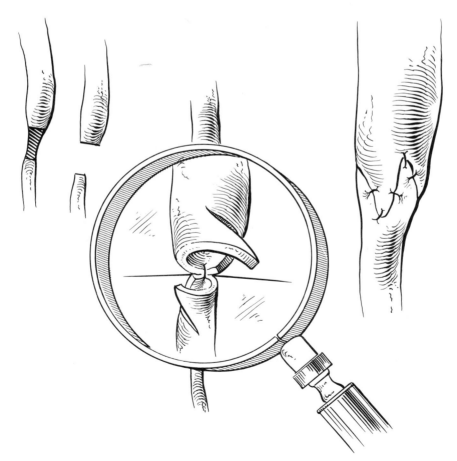

Figure 16-83. Z-plasty ureterostomy for ureteral stricture. (From DeWeerd JH, Henry JD: Z-plastic ureteroureterostomy. J Urol 93:690–692, 1965. © 1965, The Williams & Wilkins Company, Baltimore.)

the anastomotic site, as judged by cineradiographic investigation, returns by the fourth postoperative week, when coordinated contraction of the ureter across the anastomosis becomes normal (Caine and Hermann).

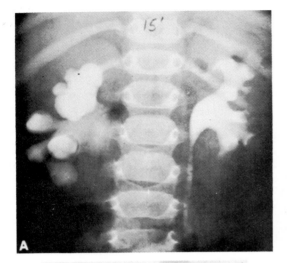

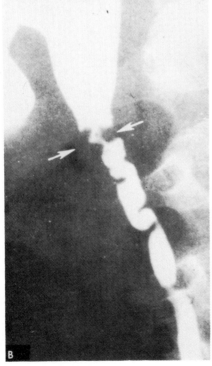

Figure 16–84. Ureteral valves. *A*, Fifteen-minute excretory urogram in 3-year-old boy, demonstrating right hydronephrosis and corkscrew appearance of left ureter. *B*, Partially obstructive valves *(arrows)* are clearly shown on the right retrograde ureterogram. Below this level the ureter has the same corkscrew appearance as on the left side. (From Albertson KW, Tainer LB: Valves of the ureter. Radiology *103:*91–94, 1972. Reproduced by permission of The Radiological Society of North America, Inc.)

URETERAL VALVES

Ureteral valves are rare. About a dozen cases, several of them in infants and children, have been reported (Passaro and Smith). The distinguishing characteristic necessary to substantiate a diagnosis of ureteral valves is an anatomically demonstrable transverse fold of ureteral mucosa that contains smooth muscle fibers with obstructive changes above but not below the valve. Ureteral valves are thought to represent the persistence of the exaggerated physiologic folds often seen in the ureters of the fetus and the neonate. They are usually close to the ureteropelvic junction (Albertson and Talner).

Ureteral valves have also been found in the juxtavesical ureter, prompting the suggestion that the valves result from persistence of Chwalla's membrane. However, this theory does not account for the formation of valves in the upper ureter nor for multiple valve formations. Ureters involved by these folds usually become more normal in function and appearance with growth.

The symptoms of ureteral valves are those of ureteral obstruction. The valve may be cuplike or iridiform; it may produce various degrees of hydronephrosis; and it may be palpable at the time of surgical exploration. Preoperative diagnosis is infrequent unless hydronephrosis is present, even though the excretory urogram may raise suspicion that a valve exists (Fig. 16–84). Resection of the portion of the ureter bearing the valve is required. If the valve is close to the ureteropelvic junction, ureteropyelostomy is elected. For lower ureteral valves, ureteroneocystostomy is used; otherwise ureteroureterostomy is necessary.

DIVERTICULUM OF THE URETER

True ureteral diverticula, a few cases of which have been reported in children, contain all the ureteral layers and communicate with the ureter by way of a distinct stoma. A diverticulum may be round or globular, and it can occur at any level from the renal pelvis to the bladder (Culp). Diverticula of the renal pelvis reported in infants and children most likely represent pseudodiverticula or a blind-ending duplication or triplication of the pelvis, with concomitant dilatation. Ureteral diverticula must be differentiated from blind-ending ure-

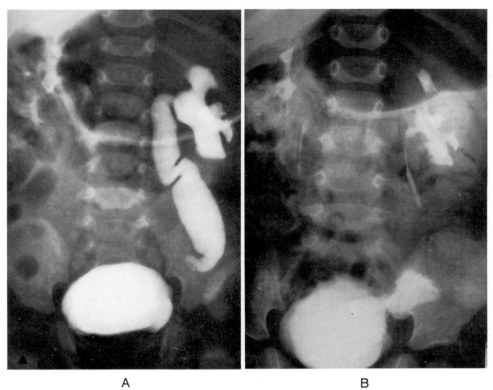

A   B

Figure 16–85. Vascular obstruction to ureter. Obstruction of lower ureter by distal hypogastric artery. *A*, Excretory urogram at age 1 month, showing partial obstruction of distal left ureter. Vessel was resected. *B*, Postoperative excretory urogram at age 14 months, showing decreased ureteropyelocalycectasis. Distal colon and rectum are filled with contrast medium from earlier demonstration of a rectourethral fistula. (From Trackler RT, McAlister WH: Obstruction of the lower ureter by the distal hypogastric (umbilical) artery. Am J Roentgenol Radium Ther Nucl Med 98:160–162, 1966. Reproduced by permission of the American Roentgen Ray Society.)

ters and have been confused with hydronephrosis, ureterocele, and vesical diverticula (Culp). Nevertheless, they probably represent a rudimentary blind branch of the ureteral bud that has become dilated. Symptoms are those of ureteral obstruction and infection. The choice of surgical procedure depends on the location of the diverticulum and the state of the associated kidney.

Diverticula in the pelviureteric region have also been reported in children (Williams and Goodwin). They are possibly caused when some collecting tubules fail to be absorbed into the main calyces.

VASCULAR OBSTRUCTION TO URETER

The relation of aberrant or accessory vessels to ureteropelvic obstruction has been discussed above. The lower ureter also may be obstructed by blood vessels, but, as with the ureteropelvic junction, the role that such vessels play in the production of hydronephrosis must always be questioned. In most cases, concomitant pathologic changes such as reflux or obstruction at the ureterovesical junction are sufficient to account for the ureteral dilatation, suggesting that anomalous vessels aggravate, rather than produce, the hydronephrosis. Nonetheless, division of a vessel alone has occasionally produced regression of the ureteral dilatation (Fig. 16–85). Obstruction in such instances most often occurs at the juxtavesical ureter and is produced by persistence of the umbilical branch of the hypogastric artery. This condition is apt to be confused with ureterovesical obstruction and congenital nonobstructed megaureter.

The ovarian vein syndrome should be considered when a postpubertal girl presents with right-sided flank pain and right hydronephrosis, even though this syndrome tends to occur in women only after multiple pregnancies, and its very existence has been questioned by some.

Abnormal passage of the ureter behind the

common iliac artery and vein, or between the two, occurs rarely. Bilateral retroiliac ureter in a 2-year-old boy whose multiple congenital anomalies included horseshoe kidney and vesicoureteral reflux is reported by Hanna. The ureteral dilatation was probably caused by the reflux. There were also associated abnormalities of both vasa deferentia.

DISTAL URETERAL ATRESIA

Despite its name, the condition called distal ureteral atresia simply represents a failure of the distal ureter to communicate with the bladder or with any other normal structures. Instead, it terminates as a cul-de-sac. If a functioning renal segment is present, it tends to enlarge gradually. Thus, the clinical problem becomes one of the differential diagnosis of abdominal tumors. The cystic mass may be associated with infection and sepsis. On physical examination, the protuberant abdomen will be evident. The mass can also be palpated on rectal examination. Urographically, the mass exhibits additional features of retroperitoneal lesions. The colon is displaced anteriorly or medially, and the bladder shows extrinsic pressure deformity. The obstructed kidney is functionless unless duplication is present. On lateral films, an increase in the space between the bladder and rectum is noted (Fig. 16–86).

A ureteral cyst must be differentiated from other retroperitoneal tumors, cysts, hydronephrosis, teratoma, and neuroblastoma. The treatment is excision of the dilated ureter and the obstructed renal segment.

MEGAURETER

Much of the debate surrounding the diagnosis and treatment of "megaureter" stems from confusion in nomenclature; the term means a single specific disease to some, while it carries a more general connotation to others. Caulk first used the term to denote the condi-

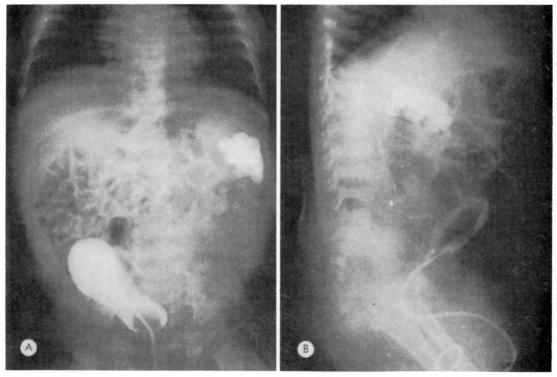

Figure 16–86. Distal ureteral atresia. Four-month-old infant with abdominal mass. *A,* Excretory urogram shows left pyelocalycectasis (upper pole of duplication) with renal, ureteral, and bladder displacement and distortion by extensive mass. *B,* Lateral pyelogram shows the mass to be retroperitoneal and demonstrates increase in the space between the bladder and rectum. (From Gordon M, Reed JO: Distal ureteral atresia. Am J Roentgenol Radium Ther Nucl Med 88:579–584, 1962. Reproduced by permission of Charles C Thomas, Publisher.)

Table 16−5. Dimensions of the Normal Ureter in Infancy and Childhood

Age	30 wk gestation	3 month	3 year	6 year	12 year
Height	40 cm	60 cm	90 cm	120 cm	150 cm
Weight	2 kg	5 kg	13 kg	20 kg	35 kg
Length:					
Ureter	5	10	15	20	25
Intravesical ureter	0.4	0.6	0.8	1.0	1.2
Submucosal ureter	0.2	0.3	0.4	0.5	0.6
Diameter and French gauge:					
Ureteropelvic junction	0.05 (2)	0.15 (4)	0.20 (8)	0.25 (8)	0.30 (10)
Middle spindle	0.15 (4)	0.35 (10)	0.40 (12)	0.45 (14)	0.50 (16)
Distal end of extravesical ureter	0.05 (2)	0.10 (3)	0.15 (4)	0.18 (5)	0.20 (6)

These normal dimensions of the child's ureter at various stages of growth are taken from cadaver measurements (Cussen). All measurements are given in centimeters. French (Charriere) catheter gauge is indicated in brackets.

tion of a 32-year-old woman with distal ureterectasis without pyelectasis or calycectasis. The word itself is simply a combination of *mega,* meaning "big," and *ureter.* Thus, it may be argued that the term can be applied to any dilated ureter.

Cussen has established normal measurements of ureteral diameter in infants and children from 30 weeks gestation to 12 years of age (Table 16−5). It can be argued that any ureter exceeding these norms, at most 7 mm at age 12, is abnormal and should be considered a "megaureter." However, in the clinical setting megaureter usually denotes more than minimal ureterectasis. The term has been expanded to include dilated ureters with or without pyelocalycectasis, which may or may not be associated with demonstrable obstruction. Debate centers on precise differentiation of the obstructed from the nonobstructed megaureter. The practical reason for differentiating these causes is that obstructed ureters require surgical correction, whereas dilated ureters that neither reflux nor are obstructed can generally be successfully managed with a modicum of surveillance only or, at most, antibacterial prophylaxis. In addition, nonobstructed but dilated ureters do not improve after successful reimplantation, but seem prone to surgical complications that may result in increased hydronephrosis. Recent emphasis on the furosemide-assisted excretory urogram and renogram and the Whitaker test in differentiating the obstructed from the nonobstructed state has advanced our understanding of the causes of ureterectasis. However, significant problems may occur in the interpretation of these tests.

One purpose of this section is to define megaureter in a reasonable way, and to establish guidelines for differential diagnosis in ways that are of practical use to the clinician. Emphasis is placed on the classification of megaureter so that the various causes will leap to mind when one is confronted with such a case. The various anatomic causes of obstructed megaureter are described, but once this diagnosis is made techniques of successful surgical correction become much more important than considerations of etiology, which may remain, in any case, somewhat unclear.

All dilated ureters have characteristics in common, especially lack of effective peristalsis caused by inability of the walls of the dilated ureter to coapt. However, lack of peristalsis does not itself result in renal damage or failure of the kidney to grow. Therefore, to stop the evaluation at the diagnosis of "big ureter" or to advise ureteral tailoring and reimplantation in all such cases is to do the patient a disservice. Furthermore, the congenital nonobstructed megaureter is often associated with megacalycosis, which is calyceal dilatation without obstruction. Thus, the presence of ureteral dilatation with calycectasis is not in itself absolutely indicative of ureterovesical junction (UVJ) obstruction. It is safest initially to consider megaureter a radiographic finding and to train oneself to proceed systematically from there to exclude reflux or UVJ obstruction as causes.

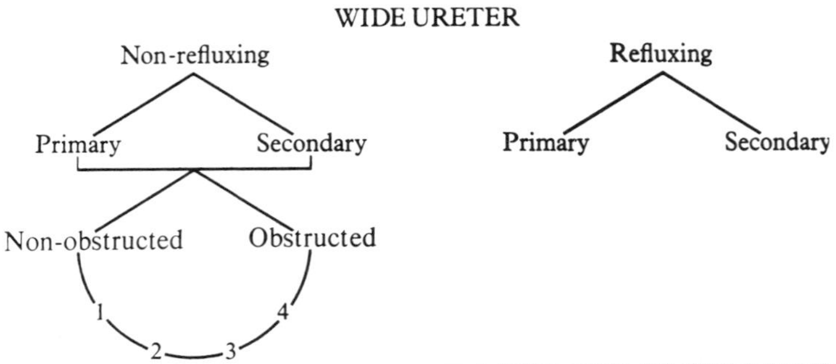

WIDE URETER

Figure 16–87. Whitaker's classification of "wide" ureters. The nonrefluxing megaureter may be obstructed or nonobstructed, with room for an intermediate group as well.

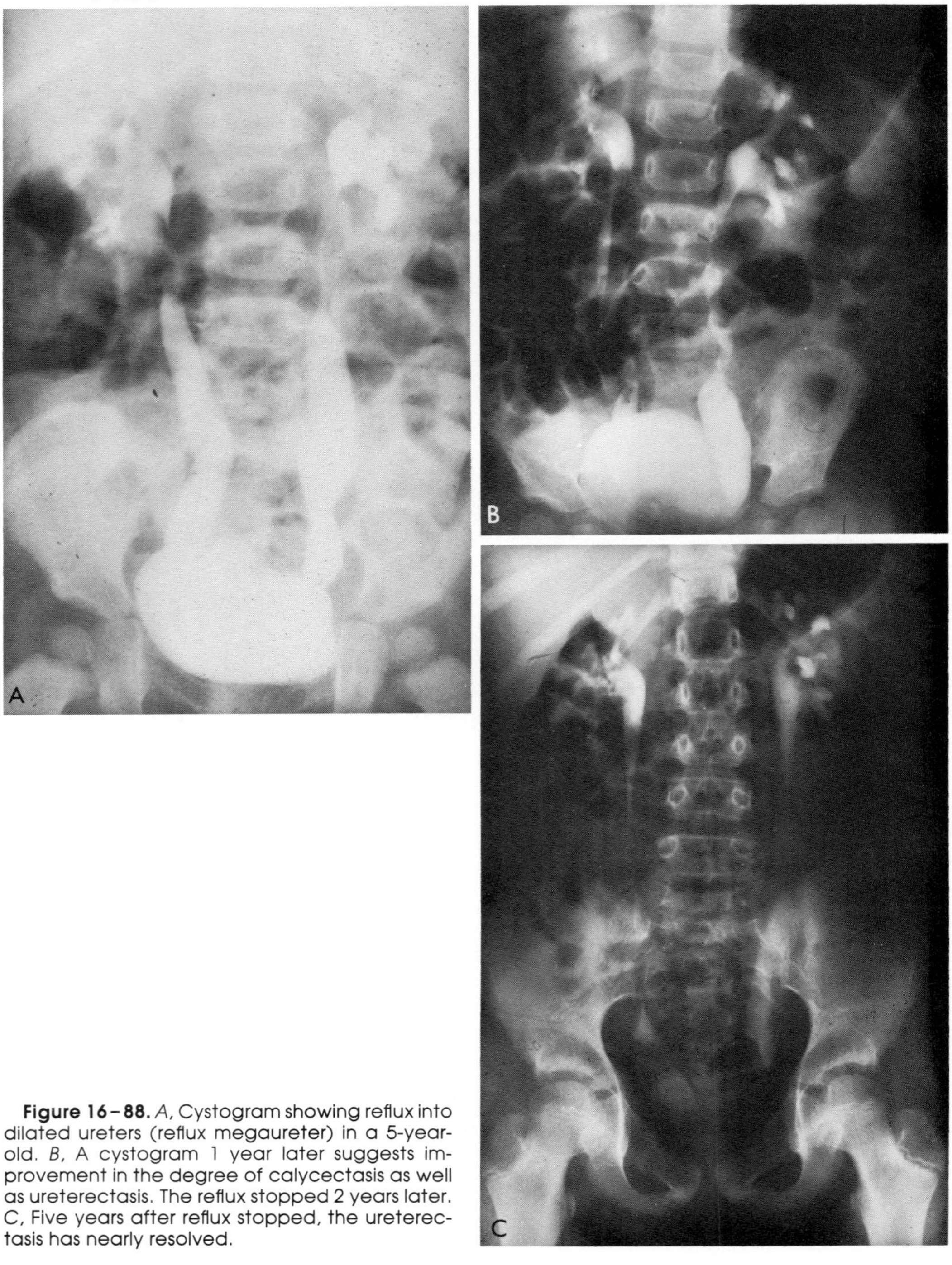

Figure 16–88. *A,* Cystogram showing reflux into dilated ureters (reflux megaureter) in a 5-year-old. *B,* A cystogram 1 year later suggests improvement in the degree of calycectasis as well as ureterectasis. The reflux stopped 2 years later. *C,* Five years after reflux stopped, the ureterectasis has nearly resolved.

Classification

All the modern attempts to classify mega-ureter have been in response to the practical need to differentiate the obstructed from un-obstructed varieties. Whitaker and others have pointed out that relatively severe reflux may result in the appearance of megaureter on excretory urography (Figs. 16–87 and 16–88). More recent classifications have at-tempted to start with ureterectasis, with or without calycectasis, and include all possible causes. The international classification of Smith et al is the most comprehensive (Table 16–6). In this scheme, megaureter may be due to obstruction or reflux, or may be idio-pathic—that is, developmental, and not as-sociated with either reflux or obstruction. Each of these major categories may then be subdivided into a primary and a secondary group. Thus, the cause of primary obstructive megaureter is obstruction at or just above the ureterovesical junction. In secondary obstruc-tive megaureter the ureterectasis is due to infravesical obstruction from valves, prolaps-ing ureterocele, calculi, granulomatous dis-ease, or other causes.

Primary refluxing megaureter is due to a short or absent intravesical ureter, congenital paraureteral diverticulum, or other derange-ment of the ureterovesical junction. In sec-ondary refluxing megaureter, reflux is present together with another anomaly such as neu-ropathic bladder, infravesical obstruction, or other bladder anomalies.

In primary nonobstructive, nonrefluxing megaureter there is no juxtavesical obstruc-tion, reflux, bladder anomaly, or outlet ob-struction. The ureterectasis is isolated or asso-ciated with calycectasis, but upper tract drainage is good by all functional parameters. In children, such systems tend to improve in radiographic appearance with growth, though some ureterectasis usually persists (Fig. 16–89). In secondary nonrefluxing, non-obstructive megaureter the dilatation of the upper tract is due to urinary infection, dia-betes insipidus, or other rare causes of very high rates of urine formation.

This is an exhaustive and useful classifica-tion. The main advantage is that all patients with ureterectasis can be classified within the system. Glassberg and others have found its use cumbersome, however, when dealing with what most consider typical megaureter. They argue that in general use the term megaureter is not applied to hydroureter caused by overt neuropathic bladder or typi-cal bladder outlet obstruction with bladder trabeculation and residual urine. The term megaureter is usually reserved for more mys-tifying conditions in which the bladder and bladder outlet are normal but the ureter is dilated to some extent (Figure 16–90).

Dilated ureters of the prune-belly syn-drome are given a category of their own. However, it must be recognized that in the Eagle-Barrett syndrome the ureterectasis commonly associated may be due to reflux or to ureterovesical junction obstruction, or may be of the nonobstructive variety. Glassberg has also addressed the cause of residual ure-terectasis commonly seen after successful re-section of urethral valves (Table 16–7) (see the section on the posterior urethra later in this chapter).

One drawback in the minds of some au-thors has been that none of these systems include a category specifically for iatrogenic ureterectasis that begins or worsens after ure-teral reimplantation. Postoperative patients can be studied and categorized within either system, however.

Our own practical classification of mega-ureter is given in Table 16–8. We tend to agree that the international classification is more complex than necessary, and that to most physicians megaureter means ureteral dilatation in the absence of another overt dis-ease. The prune-belly and iatrogenic mega-ureters can be categorized, after evaluation, into one of the four groups, as appropriate diagnostic studies need to be done in nearly every case to rule out obstruction. We added

Table 16–6. International Classification of Megaureter

	Primary	Secondary
Obstructed	Intrinsic ureteral obstruction	To urethral obstruction or extrinsic lesions
Reflux	Reflux is only abnormality	Associated with bladder outlet obstruction or neurogenic bladder
Nonrefluxing, nonobstructed	Idiopathic ureteral dilation	To polyuria (diabetes insipidus) or infection (?)

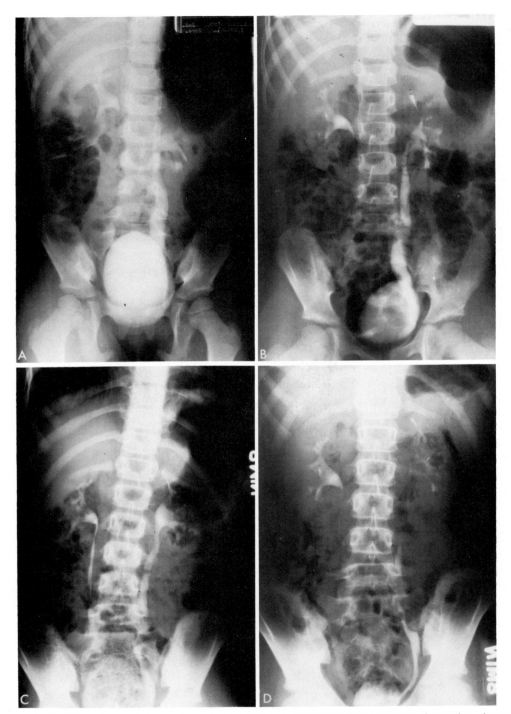

Figure 16–89. Idiopathic variety of primary megaureter. *A,* Initial excretory urogram, done when 4-year-old child presented with a urinary infection. No obstruction at ureteral orifice. No hydronephrotic drip. No reflux on cystogram. *B,* Same girl, 2 years later. Little intercurrent problem with urinary infections. No reflux. *C,* Same girl, aged 8. *D,* Same girl, aged 10 and completely well for 4 years.

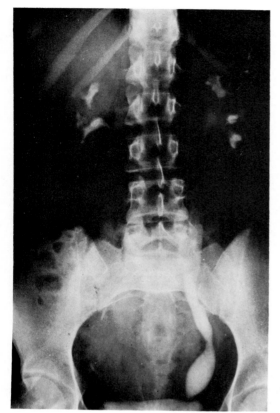

Figure 16-90. Excretory urogram typical of megaureter. Note the fusiform distal ureteral dilatation with normal renal collecting system and proximal ureter.

the category of reflux with UVJ obstruction to call attention to the fact that reflux and obstruction can coexist in a small proportion of patients. In these instances, the reflux is often the most obvious finding, and concomitant obstruction may not be considered unless the possibility of dual lesions is kept in mind. If

Table 16-7. Johnson-Glassberg Classification of Megaureter

I. Primary megaureter
  A. With functional obstruction
  B. With congenital stricture (anatomic obstruction)
II. Refluxing megaureter
III. Dysmorphic ureter (prune-belly ureter)
IV. Hydroureter—includes ureterectasis due to trauma, stone, neurogenic bladder or bladder outlet obstruction.

Iatrogenic (obstructed) megaureter and ectopic ureters are not included in this classification.
From Glassberg KI: Dilated ureter. Classification and approach. Urology 9:1, 1977.

Table 16-8. Simplified Classification of Primary Megaureter

1. Nonobstructing, nonrefluxing megaureter—without obstruction or reflux
2. Obstructive megaureter—due to ureterovesical obstruction
3. Refluxing megaureter
4. Megaureter due to ureterovesical obstruction masked by reflux

This simplified system is useful when there is no infravesical obstruction, reflux, or overt abnormality of the urinary tract except for hydroureteronephrosis. Megaureter can then be due to UVJ obstruction or reflux, and category 4 is included to remind the clinician that these lesions can coexist. Ureterectasis not associated with obstruction or reflux is also a variety of primary megaureter (category 1).

a delayed film is obtained after the cystogram, poor drainage of one or both upper tracts may suggest associated UVJ obstruction (Fig. 16-91). This can then be confirmed or excluded by further evaluation. In a series of over 400 refluxing renal units, Weiss et al found concomitant UVJ obstruction in nine. This can be an important observation, since proven obstruction generally requires early surgical correction, whereas reflux is often treated by surveillance, at least for a time.

The reader should employ the system of megaureter classification that seems most useful. The main thing to be kept in mind is that ureterectasis does not always mean obstruction, even when calycectasis is also present. Primary megaureter is an inherently compound term and usually includes both primary obstructed megaureter and primary nonobstructive megaureter, as shown in Figure 16-92.

Etiology

Nonobstructive, Nonrefluxing Megaureter

The cause of isolated nonobstructed megaureter is not clear. There is no stenosis of the juxtavesicular ureter, but the ureter is usually dilated beginning at a point just above the bladder. The dilatation may involve the entire ureter or may be segmental. The lowermost ureter is usually the widest, and bulbous in appearance with a sharp cutoff and little tortuosity (Fig. 16-93). Rarely, only the midportion of the ureter may be dilated.

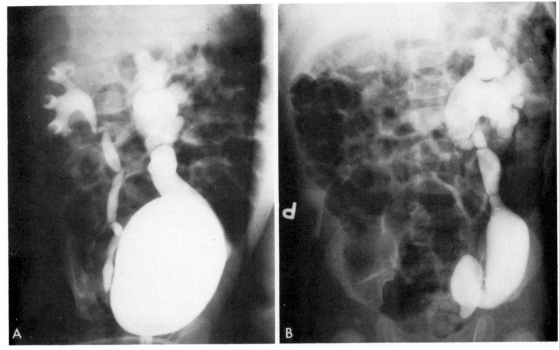

Figure 16-91. *A,* Child with bilateral reflux and dilated collecting system with significant calycectatic changes. *B,* Six-hour drainage film of same patient. Note that the right side is completely empty; note also the sharp cutoff on the left at ureterovesical junction. This left side combines the worst features of two problems, reflux and obstruction.

This configuration is sometimes reminiscent of the dilated ureters often seen in boys with the prune-belly syndrome, so a primary abnormality of the ureteral musculature or absence of normal intra-abdominal pressure are suspected causes.

Refluxing Megaureter

This term implies that the appearance of megaureter on excretory urography, minimally some ureterectasis, is due to reflux. The presence of reflux is usually noted on cystography. Any of the various causes of reflux may be at fault. The reflux can be managed according to the etiology, that is, by surveillance or by early operative correction. The choice of therapy in such instances is discussed extensively in Chapter 15.

Obstructed Megaureter

The presence of a narrowed juxtavesicular ureteral segment that will not convey the peristaltic wave nor dilate enough to permit free passage of urine is the most important cause of primary obstructive megaureter. The narrow segment measures from 0.5 to 4 cm in

length. Grégoir and Debled described four histologic types, the majority (60 per cent) exhibiting increased collagenous tissue in the terminal 3 to 4 cm of the ureter. A band of circumferential tissue devoid of muscle in the most distal portion of the narrowed segment is another cause (MacKinnon et al). At times a band of thickened muscle is arranged in a nearly circular pattern and seems to be the site of obstruction. It is postulated that such obstruction is initially caused by focal congenital absence of the spiral musculature of the lowermost ureter and that consequent local secondary muscular hypertrophy then compounds the problem.

McLaughlin et al (1973) reviewed the histopathology of 32 typical primary megaureters (obstructed and nonobstructed). Four anatomic varieties could be distinguished. Five ureters were normal histologically in the narrowed portion and contained longitudinal as well as spiral muscle fibers (Fig. 16-94). These were presumably patients with nonobstructive megaureter, but physiologic studies to rule out obstruction were not performed, as the furosemide renogram and Whitaker test were not then in use. The smooth muscle in two segments was predominantly circular in

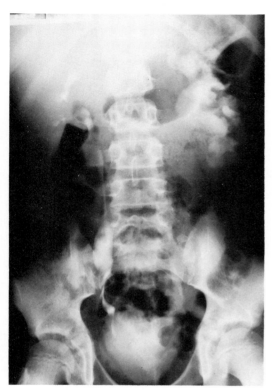

Figure 16-92. Excretory urogram of a brother of the girl whose urograms are reproduced in Figure 16-89. Of seven siblings, all but these two had normal studies. One parent proved to have ureteral duplication. On the right, this boy exhibits a spindle-shaped deformity of the midureter, a variety of idiopathic primary megaureter not associated with obstruction. On the left, there is primary obstructive megaureter, with a hydronephrotic drip of 20 ml. Left ureteral reimplantation was done to relieve obstruction with a good result—the degree of calycectasis subsequently improved somewhat.

orientation, and three showed mural fibrosis with little or no musculature. The fourth and most common type, found in 69 per cent (22 of 32), was pronounced muscular hypoplasia and atrophy of the muscle fibers, which were separated by sheets of fibrotic tissue (Fig. 16-95). McLaughlin et al (1973) concluded that obstruction had two causes: (1) absence of muscle fibers, which prevents transmission of peristalsis, and (2) fibrotic rigidity of the ureteral wall, which prevents expansion and free passive urine egress.

Also in 1973, Tanagho presented an embryologic explanation of these changes, based on studies in the fetal lamb. He noted that the distal ureter is the last portion to develop its muscular coat and that early muscular differentiation is primarily of muscle with circular orientation. This observation suggests that arrest late in development results in absence of the longitudinally oriented musculature that conducts the peristaltic wave, and that this then results in obstruction by the circular muscle fibers, which often then undergo hypertrophy.

When conveying a bolus of urine, each muscular component of a ureteral segment or spindle contracts to force the fluid into the adjacent spindle (Murnaghan). Obstruction at the terminal ureter causes partial retrograde emptying. Ureteral dilatation is potentially dependent upon the rate of urine flow in that all ureters become dilated if their volume capacity is exceeded (Hutch and Tanagho, diabetes insipidus model). The retrograde flow of urine from the most distal ureter combined with urine newly excreted produces an exces-

Figure 16-93. Artist's conception of megaureter. Ureteral dilatation begins above the ureterovesical junction, usually a few millimeters or more above the bladder. (Courtesy of Dr. AP McLaughlin, III.)

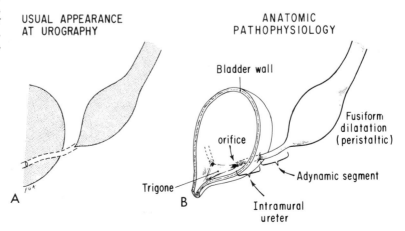

APERISTALTIC DISTAL URETERAL SEGMENT
(PRIMARY MEGALOURETER)

USUAL APPEARANCE
AT UROGRAPHY

ANATOMIC
PATHOPHYSIOLOGY

Bladder wall

orifice

Trigone

Fusiform
dilatation
(peristaltic)

Adynamic segment

Intramural
ureter

Normal

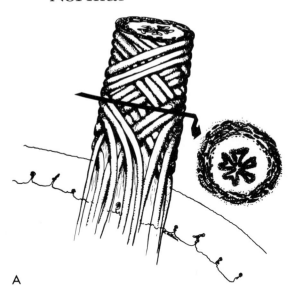

A

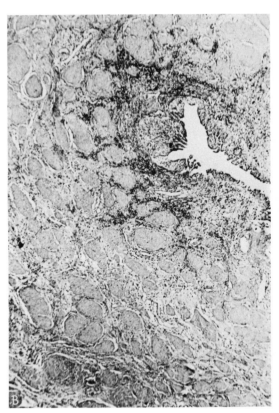

B

Figure 16-94. *A,* Normal ureteral muscular orientation seen in five ureters in McLaughlin's series. *B,* Photomicrograph from section of ureter noted in *A.* (From McLaughlin AP III, Pfister RC, Leadbetter WF, et al: The pathophysiology of primary megaloureter. J Urol *109*:805–811, 1973. © 1973, The Williams & Wilkins Company, Baltimore.)

Hypoplasia

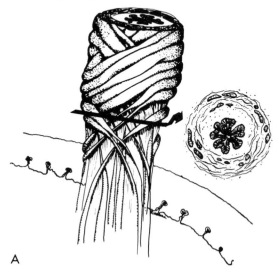

A

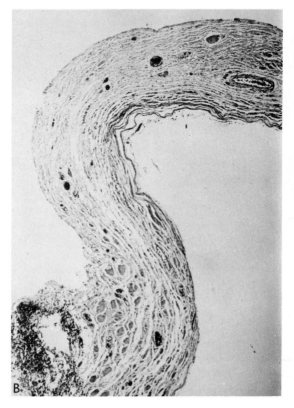

B

Figure 16-95. *A,* Hypoplasia and atrophy of ureteral muscle as seen in 22 patients in McLaughlin's series. *B,* Photomicrograph from section of ureter noted in *A.* (From McLaughlin AP III, Pfister RC, Leadbetter WF, et al: The pathophysiology of primary megaloureter. J Urol *109*:805–811, 1973. © 1973, The Williams & Wilkins Company, Baltimore.)

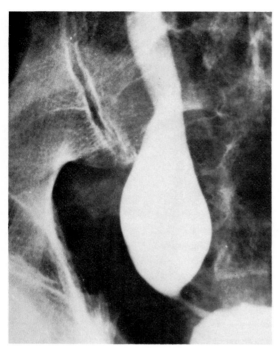

Figure 16–96. Narrowed ureteral segment at the juxtavesical level. Only rarely is this configuration visualized on excretory urogram. (From McLaughlin AP III, Pfister RC, Leadbetter WF, et al: The pathophysiology of primary megaloureter. J Urol 109:805–811, 1973. © 1973, The Williams & Wilkins Company, Baltimore.)

lief that 50 per cent of children with megacolon also had enlarged bladders. A parasympathetic lesion producing independent or combined lower bowel and bladder dysfunction was postulated. Absence of ureteral parasympathetic ganglia, as found in Hirschsprung's disease, has not been noted in children with ureterectasis, however (Grégoir and Debled; Leibowitz and Bodian; Notley).

Radiographic Appearance

In obstructive megaureter the distalmost segment is so close to the bladder wall that the narrow segment is usually obscured by the overlying contrast filled bladder; it was visualized on the initial excretory urogram in only 3 of 38 megaureters reviewed by Pfister et al (Fig. 16–96 and 16–97). The chances of visualizing the obstructing segment are improved by getting oblique views or postvoiding films. Distal ureteral dilatation may be so severe that the bulbous lower ureter prolapses below the proximal portion of the narrowed segment so that the distal dilated portion and the narrow lowermost ureter appear side by

sive load, which results in dilatation of the normal ureter proximal to the stenotic segment. Vesicoureteral reflux, in quantity, evokes a similar response, and ureterectasis occurs when refluxed bladder urine exceeds the ureter's normal carrying capacity.

Several electron microscopic studies of the lower ureter in nonrefluxing megaureter confirm the variable nature of the lesion (Tokunaka and Koyanagi; Tokunaka et al, 1980a, 1980b, 1982; Hanna et al; Pagano and Passerini). However, pathologic studies of the narrow ureteral segment have not yet been correlated with the findings and diagnosis arrived at by diuretic renogram or Whitaker test in adequate numbers of patients.

Ureterectasis without obstruction must occur by a different mechanism, or obstruction might be present during early development that results in residual ureterectasis even though the obstruction itself somehow resolves. At the time of his original description Caulk equated megaureter and Hirschsprung's disease, a concept supported by Swenson and Fisher and by Swenson et al. In their reviews, these authors expressed the be-

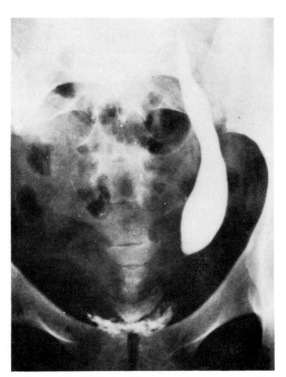

Figure 16–97. Postvoiding excretory urogram. Delayed emptying of distal ureter is obvious along with abrupt cutoff proximal to the distal narrowed segment. The narrowed segment itself is not visualized.

Table 16–9. Clinical Findings Associated with Megaureter

Study	Infection (%)	Hematuria (%)	Pain (%)	Uremia (%)
Williams and Hulme-Moir, 1970	73	13	29	11
Flatmark et al, 1970	86	—	—	14
Pfister et al, 1971	32	52	42	0
Pagano and Passerini, 1977	90	—	10	—
Pfister and Hendren, 1978	70	7	5	7
Rabinowitz et al, 1979b	78	17	10	10

side. This has given birth to the term "ureteral valve," which, used in this context, is quite descriptive but sometimes misleading. First, the term ureteral valve is too easily confused with urethral valve phonetically. More importantly, the septum or valve between the dilated portion of the ureter and the narrow part is seldom, if ever, the primary cause of such obstruction, which seems clearly to be due to intrinsic stenosis of the distalmost segment. The valvelike flap may compound the obstruction, but rarely occurs alone without a very narrow and more distal justavesical segment, which is the hallmark of obstructed megaureter.

Almost regardless of the severity of upper ureteral dilatation, active movement of the ureteral wall is seen on cineradiographic studies in almost all cases. Effective peristalsis is absent when the walls of the ureter cannot coapt, and, like ureteral peristalsis, this movement is reduced by bacterial exotoxins during some infections. Usually the ureteral movements convey contrast media to the narrowed segment, where most of the bolus simply floods back up the ureter. If the upper ureter is of normal or near normal caliber, this "refluxed" urine will initiate a wave of retrograde peristalsis. It seems likely that such peristalsis damps the pressure and prevents dilatation of

the pelvis. When only the lower ureter is dilated, the pelvis is usually normal in size. When the entire ureter is dilated, some pelvic dilatation is commonly present also.

Mode of Presentation

Most children with megaureter with or without calycectasis present with urinary infection, which may be cystitis and urelated to the upper tract anomaly, with hematuria, or with otherwise unexplained abdominal pain. It is not unusual for the dilated ureter to be noted at the time of appendectomy or other abdominal surgery. Uremia, anemia, renal rickets, failure to thrive, or other signs of renal failure are fortunately rare presenting complaints (Table 16–9). Megaureter is bilateral in about 25 per cent of patients. Children presenting prior to 1 year of age are more apt to have bilateral megaureter than older patients (Williams and Hulme-Moir). The incidence in males is 1.5 to 4.8 times greater than in females. The left ureter is involved 1.6 to 4.5 times more than the right. The incidence of contralateral renal agenesis is about 9 per cent (Table 16–10). The condition is not known to be hereditary, but families with more than one member with megaureter have been described.

Table 16–10. Incidence of Megaureter

Study	Bilateral Lesions (%)	Left/Right Ratio	Male/Female Ratio	Contralateral Agenesis
Johnston, 1967	14.8	3.3 to 1	4.8 to 1	5 of 35
Williams and Hulme-Moir, 1970	25.7	—	3.5 to 1	—
Flatmark et al, 1970	50.0	4.5 to 1	2.0 to 1	9 of 100
Pfister et al, 1971	22.6	1.7 to 1	4.8 to 1	2 of 31
Pagano and Passerini, 1977	17.2	1.4 to 1	1.6 to 1	3 of 46 2/duplication
Pfister and Hendren, 1978	38.6	4.4 to 1	2 to 1	6 of 57
Rabinowitz et al, 1979b	19.6	1.6 to 1	3.1 to 1	1 of 41

Differential Diagnosis of Obstructive versus Nonobstructive Megaureter

Since reflux of moderate or severe degree is usually diagnosed without difficulty on cystogram, further discussion will center on differentiating obstructed from nonobstructed megaureter. Many tests are clinically useful in this regard, and these are summarized below. Since the child with megaureter usually presents with urinary tract infection, hematuria, or a flank mass, we assume that a cystogram and an excretory urogram are performed and that the x-rays show the ureteral dilatation without reflux or intravesical obstruction as an obvious cause (Fig. 16–98). Renal scans are preferred to excretory urography in the neonate, performed as described below.

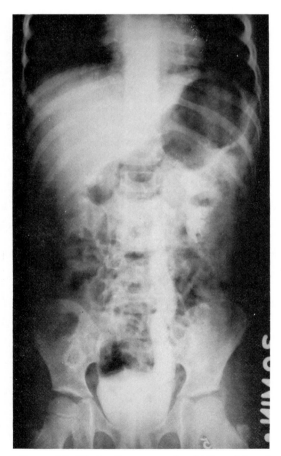

Figure 16–98. Another example of idiopathic primary megaureter. This girl was followed for 10 years with gradual improvement in urographic appearance. The ureter remains wider than normal. An excretory urogram was performed after a first urinary infection; she never had another infection.

The next evaluation can be cystoscopy, but a renogram using furosemide is now commonly employed to stimulate washout of the dilated collecting system if the renogram curve appears obstructive (see Chapter 8 and the beginning of this chapter). This test is in wide use, but normal parameters that rule out obstruction have not yet been clearly established. One reason for this difficulty in interpretation is that if the hydronephrosis is very severe, even a relatively well-functioning kidney may not be able to diurese fast enough to clearly demonstrate good drainage after the administration of furosemide. Also, a poorly functioning kidney may not be able to excrete enough urine under any conditions to clear the radioactivity at a "normal" rate. Furthermore, variations in the degree of hydroureteronephrosis mean that varying degrees of diuresis will dilute the radioactive isotope already excreted by varying amounts, so a spectrum of unobstructed drainage patterns is to be expected (see Chapter 8). Therefore, the furosemide renogram allows various interpretations, severely and unequivocally obstructed, unobstructed, and one or two groups of variable size in which the diagnosis is not clear. This latter group needs further evaluation. However, some guidelines for the test can be summarized.

The child should have no prior dehydration or enemas. Technetium-99m diethylenetriaminepentaacetic acid (DTPA) is used to estimate renal blood flow. Alternately, iodine-131 hippuran is given and images of the kidney and ureter are made at 2, 5, 10, 15, 20, 25, and 30 minutes. The counting crystals should be centered over the area where the isotope is pooled, and a catheter should be indwelling to keep the bladder empty. The hippuran renogram is a sensitive test, so the initial renogram curve will often look obstructed in most cases of megaureter of any etiology. If a catheter is not in place, the child is asked to void, or is catheterized, to determine the effect of bladder emptying on the curve. If it remains obstructed, furosemide, 1 mg/kg, is administered. If the amount of radioactivity is reduced by half in less than 10 minutes, the study is normal and there is no UVJ obstruction. When the half-time clearance is 10 to 20 minutes, the study is equivocal and further tests are needed. A half-time clearance of radioactivity requiring longer than 20 minutes is indicative of obstruction unless renal function is very poor or hydronephrosis extreme as noted above.

Some potential pitfalls in the use of the

furosemide renogram can be avoided by careful attention to test conditions. Accidental dehydration may minimize the diuresis effect. The technician may accidently alter the Y axis of the renogram curve. The furosemide dose must be standardized and weight-related, as the diuretic effect increases with larger doses. Hippuran must be used to gauge the furosemide response, not DTPA. Furosemide affects tubular function; hippuran is secreted by the tubules, and hippuran is cleared faster than DTPA. Furosemide administration less than 30 minutes after DTPA may result in the collecting system being washed out by "hot" (i.e., radioactive) urine, which would yield a false positive result. The child's position during the test should be standardized, as posture may affect drainage of the dilated collecting system. If only the ureter is dilated, the counting crystal should be placed over the area of ureterectasis, not the kidney.

In spite of these qualifications, mainly difficulties in interpretation, the furosemide renogram is a useful test. In fact, Kass has recently compared the furosemide renogram with the more invasive Whitaker test and found diuretic renography to be as accurate (Table 16–11). Those with hydroureter without obstruction are then spared more invasive investigations. Also, even though some furosemide renograms are equivocal in patients with megaureter, such tests are quite reproducible in the same patient when performed in exactly the same manner. Therefore, if the results fall into the equivocal range, a follow-up

study several months after the first may demonstrate improved drainage and exclude obstruction.

In children who continue to appear to have possible ureteral obstruction an equivocal or obstructed furosemide renogram is often an indication for further diagnostic studies. These include cystoscopy with ureteral catheterization to see if a "hydronephrotic drip" is present and measurement of the renal pelvic pressure at which fluid flows into the bladder across the site of possible obstruction (Whitaker test). It is difficult to make a firm rule as to which of these examinations should be performed first. Many children with megaureter have had previous cystoscopic examinations to rule out urethral obstruction, so a Whitaker test often seems most pertinent. If cystoscopy has not been done, I usually choose to do that first. The anterior urethra is calibrated with bougies, and inspected to look for an anterior or posterior valve. More than mild bladder trabeculation suggests outflow obstruction. Since the voiding cystogram was normal in these children, the urethra will usually in fact be normal but outlet obstruction may still be caused by sphincter dyssynergia, and the hydroureter may be the result of the neurogenic non-neurogenic bladder syndrome. Urodynamic studies are then indicated. Attention is next turned to the ureteral orifices. Are they normal, or does their size and position suggest reflux, which is occasionally not detected on cystogram? Is there a small ureterocele? If the orifice is normal, the next step is to pass a 4 or 5 F ureteral catheter, the caliber depending on the size of the child. A diameter of at least 4 F is preferable so that a hydronephrotic drip can be detected. Occasionally, the ureteral catheter will not pass. This may be due to technical factors — a difficult angle — or to ureteral meatal stenosis, which is an uncommon cause of ureterectasis that is usually susceptible to transurethral or percutaneous meatotomy. Usually in primary obstructive megaureter the point of obstruction is above the ureteral hiatus, about 5 to 15 mm from the bladder. The ureteral catheter may stop at that point, but it will usually pass. If a large volume of urine then comes out of the ureteral catheter in a steady drip, a so-called hydronephrotic drip, obstruction is deemed likely to be present.

Contrast material is then introduced and drainage films are made. The normal rate of drainage from a dilated collecting system in a dehydrated child has not been quantified, but

Table 16–11. Comparison of the Diuretic Renogram and Whitaker Test in the Diagnosis or Exclusion of Obstruction in 33 Kidneys

Results	Furosemide Renal Scan	Pressure Perfusion
Unequivocally positive	18/19 (95%)	18/19 (95%)
Unequivocally negative	11/13 (85%)	10/11 (91%)
Indeterminant	1/33 (3%)	3/33 (9%)
Definitely positive or negative	29/33 (88%)	28/33 (85%)
True positive	18	18
True negative	11	10
False positive	2	1
False negative	1	1
Indeterminant	1	3

Data courtesy of Dr. Evan Kass.

persistence of contrast material in the ureter for 6 hours is usually indicative of obstruction. Conversely, complete drainage within 1 or 2 hours is usually most compatible with the diagnosis of nonobstructed, nonrefluxing megaureter. If obstruction is absent, the total volume of the continuous hydronephrotic drip is also apt to be less than one would expect from the size of the dilated collecting system as seen on excretory urography. These cystoscopic tests to differentiate obstructed from nonobstructed megaureter are all subjective, and yet it seems that the results are in fact fairly accurate. It is hard to conceive that a dilated ureter that produces 20 ml immediately after catheterization and retains contrast material for several hours after filling is not an obstructed ureter.

Whitaker Test

The other way to evaluate the dilated ureter more completely is to measure the renal pelvic pressure at which a high volume of fluid, 10 ml/min, passes the site of possible obstruction. This is a well thought out and physiologic test and has a great advantage in that it is quantitative. A number, the maximum renal pressure during sustained flow minus the bladder pressure, is produced. The drawbacks are that the test is relatively invasive and usually requires a general anesthetic in children, and that, like the furosemide renogram, it is at times difficult to interpret with certainty. Nonetheless, it has come into wide use to differentiate hydroureteronephrosis due to obstruction from the nonobstructive causes of ureterectasis or calycectasis.

The test requires a nephrostomy or pyelostomy, or most commonly, insertion of long percutaneous needles, using fluoroscopic control. Needles of gauge 20 or 22 are commonly employed, although some prefer a larger bore. The needle resistance is subtracted from the renal pressure. An urethral catheter is inserted. A pump capable of delivering a constant flow then perfuses the renal pelvis at 10 ml/min. Manometers or strain gauges are attached to the perfusion catheter and bladder outflow tubing. Perfusion is maintained until the collecting system is filled and the renal pressure reaches a plateau, or is obviously increasing and far above the physiologic range, indicating obstruction. Maximum renal relative pressures (renal pelvis pressure minus needle resistance minus blad-

der pressure) below 15 cm of H_2O are considered to indicate an absence of obstruction. Conversely, higher pressures are regarded as indicative of obstruction, although some cases with marginal elevation may remain equivocal, as discussed below. In typical ureteropelvic junction (UPJ) obstructions, the relative renal pressure may be very elevated during the test, but most UPJ obstructions are readily diagnosed by the typical appearance of the dilated pelvis and calyces on excretory urography or ultrasound. Megacalycosis, defined as underdevelopment of the renal pyramids in the absence of obstruction, may occur with ipsilateral nonobstructed megaureter (Von Niederhäusern and Tuchschmid; Talner and Gittes; Whitaker and Flower) as noted above. In this situation, further evaluation is generally needed, as it is when moderate pyelocalycectasis is combined with typical megaureter. When the volume of the collecting system is extreme, drainage on the diuretic renogram is often equivocal, as noted above. A Whitaker test is usually diagnostic in this situation and will yield relative renal pressures in the normal — usually low normal — or unequivocally obstructed range. Patients with obstruction are then operated upon, while those without obstruction are followed with an occasional excretory urogram or diuretic renogram to make absolutely certain that the upper tracts do not deteriorate.

When the test is normal there does not appear to be much risk of misdiagnosis. Witherow and Whitaker reported on 21 of the patients — all but 4 children — evaluated by Whitaker test in 1973. They were divided into four groups. Nine of 11 with elevated pressures that underwent corrective surgery exhibited improved pyelograms and/or clearances more than 5 years later. In 5 children with an elevated relative renal pressure no operation was performed. Four of these patients were boys with valves in whom the hydroureteronephrosis persisted after valve resection and reimplantation was deferred. In two, the bladder pressures indicated a noncompliant bladder, and this elevated pressure was reflected in the kidney although the relative renal pressure (renal pressure minus bladder pressure) was not elevated. Renal function deteriorated with time in both these boys. One of the patients with valves was studied soon after valve resection. The relative renal pressures were elevated. This boy improved. It is surmised that the ureters were obstructed by the hypertrophied detrusor and that as the hypertrophy subsided the obstruction was relieved.

In seven patients the pressure flow study was normal and no operation was performed. After 5 to 9 years all upper tracts are stable in appearance and function. In four patients a low relative pressure was found, but operation was performed on clinical grounds. The Whitaker test was introduced in 1973, but its accuracy was then uncertain, so these four patients were treated surgically. Two had bilateral and two unilateral megaureter. A good surgical result was obtained in each instance. However, after 5 to 8 years, the pyelographic appearance of the kidneys had not changed, except that the tailored lowermost ureter looked less dilated, and renal function was stable. One must conclude that these were patients with nonobstructed megaureter, and that ureteral tailoring and reimplantation could not improve them even though an optimal surgical result was achieved.

The false positive test in the boy with valves, described above, is illustrative of problems in interpretation that are not uncommon. Two groups of children, particularly, seem prone to misleading or uninterpretable test results. Some are boys with residual hydroureteronephrosis after relief of bladder outlet obstruction, usually due to urethral valves, while others are children of either sex with persistent or worsened ureterectasis after ureteral reimplantation. The vagaries of the Whitaker test in boys with residual hydronephrosis after valve resection is so great that Glassberg et al use the test results to define four different types of megaureter encountered in such patients. They consider relative renal pressures between 15 and 20 cm H_2O to be an inherently equivocal test, and 3 of 14 renal units studied fell into this marginal category. Only 4 of the kidneys had low pressures with the bladder both full and empty and were clearly unobstructed. No evaluated patients had unequivocally high relative renal pressures, but in 7 of 14 renal units the test was difficult to interpret. The reason was that renal pressures were normal with the bladder empty but rose quickly into the pathologic range when the bladder began to fill. Thus, strictly speaking, the Whitaker test was normal if done as originally described with a catheter draining the bladder, but since some boys with noncompliant bladders after valve ablation develop progressive renal damage, it seems that this observation is important. Also, it seems futile to reimplant such ureters into

the bladder with expectation that drainage will be improved or that the bladder will then function more normally. Glassberg et al advise following such patients for at least 6 months. If the upper tracts do not improve and renal pressures remain elevated when the bladder fills, they advocate augmentation cystoplasty to reduce the bladder pressure (also favored by Mitchell) or ileocecocystoplasty using the plicated or reinforced ileocecal valve as the antireflux mechanism, moving the ureters into the terminal ileum above the valve. This is also my usual preference. I think the success of either operation depends upon removal of the bulk of the noncompliant bladder, retaining only the disk around the urethra or trigone to which the bowel segment is anastomosed. However, we find that only a small proportion of boys with residual hydronephrosis and no reflux after valve resection need further intervention, and that loss of bladder compliance, rather than ureteral obstruction, is the major indication for such surgery.

Other common problems with interpretation of the Whitaker test and results falsely negative for obstruction are seen in children who have persistent or worsening hydronephrosis after ureteral reimplantation, commonly antireflux surgery. Such children may also exhibit noncompliant bladders, with renal pressures rising sharply as the bladder begins to fill. Most such children have normal relative renal pressures with the bladder empty. The bladder seems usually to recover with time, and the child then does well long-term, although interval vesicostomy may be required if ureterectasis increases. Occasionally, specific children will have a completely normal test with a compliant bladder and a low relative renal pressure. In spite of this, hydronephrosis may occasionally increase dramatically, even over only a few months. The reason for this appears to be that as scar matures the once unobstructed ureter becomes obstructed, usually at the new hiatus as it passes through the detrusor. This is not a common sequence, but occurs often enough to warn that the Whitaker test must be interpreted with caution in postoperative patients. A negative test does not necessarily mean that obstruction will not occur in the future.

Even with all these provisos, renal pressure-flow measurements have become our most accurate test to differentiate obstructed from nonobstructed megaureter. The test is quite accurate in patients who have not been operated upon in whom the bladder is compliant. Alternately, it may be performed intraoperatively to document obstruction, although at that point it is a little late if obstruction is not found. The dilated ureters in the prune-belly syndrome may be obstructed or nonobstructed, just as in other types of megaureter, and can be accurately categorized using the Whitaker test.

The only potential problem caused by nonobstructed megaureter is due to stasis caused by the inability of the walls of the ureter to coapt. This loss of effective peristalsis seems clearly not to prevent renal growth, either in children or animal models, but such ureterectasis seems occasionally the predisposing cause of urinary infection.

Management of Primary Obstructed Megaureter

History of Surgical Treatment

Caulk treated his initial patient with transurethral endoscopic meatotomy in 1923. The patient did well clinically, but of course it is not certain whether this was a case of obstructed or nonobstructed megaureter. Lewis and Kimbrough performed ureteral meatotomy after ureteral dialatations and nephroureterolysis failed to result in improvement, but reflux resulted. In 1954, in view of the poor surgical results up to that time, Nesbit and Withycombe concluded that megaureter should not be treated surgically. In retrospect, it seems that ureteral meatotomy was doomed to fail, since the obstruction, when present, is extravesical. In fact, the intravesical ureter is seldom involved, though an occasional child will have severe stenosis at the ureteral meatus without a ureterocele.

The use of a tapered isolated portion of small bowel to replace the ureter in patients with extreme hydronephrosis was reported by Swenson et al (1956). No attempt was made to form an antireflux anastomosis with the bladder. Also in 1956, Lewis and Cletsoway reported using a ureteral nipple similar to that fashioned in a Paquin ureteral reimplantation for reflux. The ureter was not tapered, but the lower extremely dilated portion was excised. Good surgical results were achieved, and reflux was not demonstrable postoperatively in any of 12 ureters so treated.

Goodwin et al (1959) also replaced the dilated ureter with isolated ileal segments. Partial extravesical intussusception of the upper

ileum into the lower for a distance of 1 to 2 inches was the antireflux mechanism employed. Good long-term results have been achieved. Politano (personal communication, 1984) also used small bowel to replace megaureters with success. He incorporated a long everted nipple of the distalmost ileal segment into the bladder anastomosis as the antireflux mechanism. All authors have emphasized the need to remove a disk of bladder equal in size to the lumen of the bowel to prevent obstruction when an ileal segment is employed to replace the ureter, and the orientation of the bowel loop must always be isoperistaltic. Hirschhorn and Politano have sought to restore ureteral peristalsis in patients with megaureter by wrapping the dilated ureter with an isolated segment of small bowel from which the mucosa had been removed. The bowel segment must always run the full length of the ureter, preferably from the pelvis to the bladder.

Creevy, in 1967, was the first to report extensive ureteral tailoring combined with a Politano type antireflux reimplantation. He clearly defined the radiographic characteristics of the different types of megaureter and felt that ureteral reimplantation was generally indicated when calycectasis was present. Thus, some of his patients probably had nonobstructed megaureter with megacalycosis. Bischoff (1972) advocated tapering of the lowermost ureter only in most instances in order to achieve an antireflux reimplantation.

Current Therapy

The majority of patients with primary megaureter, particularly those presenting as older children or adults, prove to have the nonobstructed variety of megaureter and do not require surgical intervention (Figure 16–99). In pediatric cases, the ureter generally becomes less dilated as the child grows. In a review of their experience with primary megaureter, Williams and Hulme-Moir presented in detail many cases in children followed for more than 5 years. Those with terminal ureterectasis only always remained stable or improved.

Surgery should be reserved for patients with progressive ureterectasis or extreme generalized hydroureteronephrosis with parenchymal loss, and patients with lesser degrees of dilatation in whom the diuretic renogram and/or the Whitaker test is unequivocally positive for obstruction.

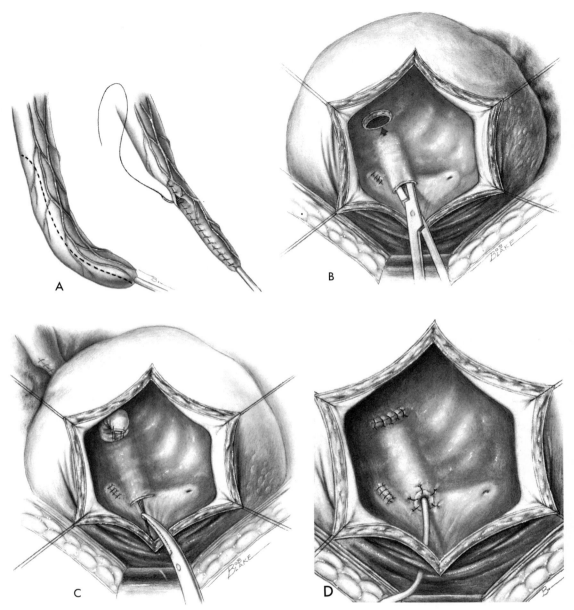

Figure 16–99. Surgical correction of megaureter. *A*, The dilated ureter is detached from the bladder extravesically. After limited mobilization to straighten very severe kinks, excess ureteral length is trimmed away. About 5 cm of the distalmost remaining ureter is then tapered around a 10 or 12 F stent. A second suture is employed to close the adventitia to reduce the risk of an extravesical or intravesical leak or fistula. Usually the best blood supply is on the medial aspect of the ureter, and this is preserved. *B*, A new hiatus site is selected well cephalad and medial to the original hiatus, which is closed. A generous submucosal tunnel, about 4 cm in length, is fashioned. *C*, The tailored ureter is then led into the bladder through the new hiatus and the new tunnel. *D*, The orifice is sutured in place, and mucosal rents are closed where possible. The stent is maintained for 7 to 10 days.

Another indication for surgery in children with megaureter is recurrent or persistent infection that can be localized to the hydronephrotic upper tract by culturing samples taken from the collecting system. The urine can be obtained by ureteral catheterization or by percutaneous aspiration. This group may include some with nonobstructed megaureter but severe stasis. As noted earlier, nonobstructed upper tracts seldom improve in function or appearance after surgery, but the infection may be eliminated. It is in this group with persistent infection that the strongest case can be made for tailoring the dilated ureter above the bladder, wrapping the ureter with denuded bowel, or replacing the ureter with a bowel segment to restore peristalsis.

Surgical Correction of Megaureter

The standard surgical therapy for primary obstructive megaureter descends from the work of Paquin, Creevy, and Hendren. Paquin and Bischoff advocated tapering only that portion of the wide ureter which would become the new intravesical ureter after reimplantation, but would then permit a reliable type of antireflux anastomosis. Hendren showed that with care more of the lower ureter could be narrowed without devascularizing the most distal portion. The key to success is atraumatic manipulation of the ureter and preservation of the blood vessels that enter the wall of the dilated ureter on its medial aspect. If dilatation of the upper ureter persists or infection persists, the upper ureter is occasionally similarly narrowed 6 to 8 weeks later (Fig. 16–99). Hanna has devised a technique to permit narrowing the entire length of the ureter in a single operation. In this procedure the ureteral adventitia with its rich blood supply is preserved intact. Above the bladder stepwise windows are made in the adventitia to permit exposure of the dilated ureter. A strip of the medial and posterior aspect of the ureter 12 to 14 mm in width is left attached to the adventitia. This strip is tubularized with two layers of absorbable suture to narrow the ureter to a uniform caliber of approximately

12 F. Stents are left in place for a week or more after ureteral reimplantation with extravesical tailoring.

A simpler, limited approach has proved to be adequate in most children with obstructed megaureter. If obstruction is relieved and reflux prevented, the dilated ureter above the bladder will narrow and straighten as the child grows. This means that tailoring long ureteral segments, with an increased risk of distal ureteral ischemia and stenosis even when care is taken to preserve the blood supply, is unnecessary. In practice, we find that tailoring the lowermost 5 cm of ureter that is to be retained and serve mainly as the new intravesical ureter after reimplantation is adequate. This tapered segment, about 12 F in diameter, is reimplanted into the bladder rostral and medial to the original hiatus so that a 4 cm intravesical course can be achieved, taking care that the medial blood supply of the juxtavesical ureter is not disrupted (Fig. 16–99) (Hendren, 1978). Alternately, a cross-trigonal method of implantation can be employed. This also permits a relatively long intravesical course, and Ahmed and Cohen, as well as Hensle et al, believe that intravesical tailoring and preservation of the original hiatus reduces the risk of distal ureteral ischemia or of obstruction due to angulation outside the bladder.

In 1977, Kalicinski et al introduced an alternative to ureteral tailoring that still permits narrowing the lower ureter enough to facilitate an antireflux reimplantation while possibly better preserving the blood supply. Instead of excision of the lateral wall of the dilated ureter, this portion is excluded from

Table 16–12. Results of Surgical Correction of Megaureter

Study	Patients Treated	Evaluated Postop	Failures No.	%	Unchanged No.	%	Improved No.	%
Johnston, 1967	41	32	4	12	8	24	20	62
Williams and Hulme-Moir, 1970 Without antireflux reimplantation	10	10	3	30	6	60	1	10
With antireflux reimplantation	45	45	7	16	7	16	31	69
McLaughlin et al, 1971	31	31	2	6	6	19	23	74
Pagano and Passerini, 1977	40	40	4	10	5	12	31	78
Pfister and Hendren, 1978	57		5					
Rabinowitz et al, 1979b	49	46	3	7	6	14	37	84

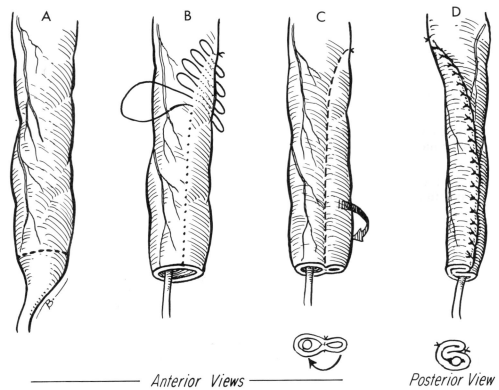

Figure 16–100. Diagram of Kalicinsky's technique of ureteral tailoring. The excess lateral aspect of the ureter is simply excluded from the lumen with a running absorbable suture. This excluded portion is then turned under the medial aspect of the ureter. Surprisingly, there is little excess bulk, and the maneuver facilitates the achievement of adequate tunnel length to prevent reflux.

the lumen with a running absorbable suture, effectively narrowing the lower ureter. The lateral excluded lumen is then folded underneath the intact lumen and held in position by absorbable tacking sutures along the medial wall (Fig. 16–100). This procedure is also described in Chapter 15 and has been discussed in detail by Starr. Ehrlich observes that the fold underneath does not result in unmanageable bulk, and that reimplantation is easily performed thereafter using Cohen's transverse technique, usually retaining the original ureteral hiatus. In 12 patients (17 ureters) Ehrlich experienced no failures from either obstruction or reflux, and cites 6 more successful cases. The procedure has proved reliable in our hands also.

Whether excision or folding is elected, it seems clear that only that portion of the megaureter which will serve as the new intravesical ureter need be narrowed in treating a large majority of children with obstructive megaureter successfully. Such limited tailoring reduces the risk of subsequent obstruction.

BIBLIOGRAPHY

Ahmed S: Transverse advancement ureteral reimplantation: pull-through alternative in megaloureter. J Urol 123:218, 1980.

Ahmed S, Tan H: Complications of transverse advancement ureteral reimplantation: Diverticulum formation. J Urol 127:970, 1982.

Albertson KW, Talner LB: Valves of the ureter. Radiology 103:91, 1972.

Allen TD: Congenital ureteral strictures. J Urol 104:196, 1970.

Belman AB: Megaureter: classification, etiology, and management. Urol Clin North Am 1:497, 1974.

Bjordal RI, Stake G, Knutrud O: Surgical treatment of megaureter in the first few months of life. Ann Chir Gynaecol 69:10, 1980.

Bischoff P: Betrachtungen zur Genese des Megaureters. Urol Int 11:257, 1961.

Bischoff PF: Problems in treatment of vesicoureteral reflux. J Urol 107:133, 1972.

Bishop MC, Askew AR, Smith JC: Reimplantation of the wide ureter. Br J Urol 50:383, 1978.

Boxer RJ, Fritsche P, Skinner DG, et al: Replacement of the ureter by small intestine: clinical application and results of the ileal ureter in 89 patients. J Urol 121:728, 1979.

Brooks RE Jr: Left retrocaval ureter associated with sinus inversus. J Urol 88:484, 1962.

Burkowski A: Operative treatment of megaureter in adults. Int Urol Nephrol 9:105, 1977.

Caine M, Hermann G: The return of peristalsis in the anastomosed ureter: a cine-radiographic study. Br J Urol 42:164, 1970.

Carlson HE: The intrapsoas transplant of megalo-ureter. J Urol 72:172, 1954.

Caulk JR: Megaloureter: the importance of the uretero-vesical valve. J Urol 9:315, 1923.

Cohen SJ: Ureterozystoneostomie. Eine Neue Antireflux-technik. Akt Urol 6:1, 1975.

Considine J: Retrocaval ureter: a review of the literature with a report on two new cases followed for fifteen years and two years respectively. Br J Urol 38:412, 1966.

Creevy CD: The atonic distal ureteral segment (ureteral achalasia). J Urol 97:457, 1967.

Culp OS: Ureteral diverticulum: classification of the literature and report of an authentic case. J Urol 58:309, 1947.

Cussen LJ: The morphology of congenital dilatation of the ureter: intrinsic ureteral lesions. Aust NZ J Surg 41:185, 1971.

Derrick FC Jr: Management of the large, tortuous, ady-namic ureter with reflux. J Urol 108:153, 1972.

Deter RL, Hadlock FP, Gonzales ET, et al: Prenatal detection of primary megaureter using dynamic image ultra-sonography. Obstet Gynecol 56:759, 1980.

Ehrlich RM: Ureteral folding technique for megaureter surgery. Soc for Ped Urol Newsletter, May 5, 1982.

Fitzer PM: Congenital ureteral valve. Pedatr Radiol 8:54, 1979.

Flatmark AL, Maurseth K. Knutrud O: Lower ureteric obstruction in children. Br J Urol 42:431, 1970.

Garrett WJ, Kossoff G, Osborn RA: The diagnosis of fetal hydronephrosis, megaureter and urethral obstruction by ultrasonic echography. Br J Obstet Gynaecol 82:115, 1975.

Gearhart JP, Woolfenden KA: The vesico-psoas hitch as an adjunct to megaureter repair in childhood. J Urol 127:505, 1982.

Glassberg KI: Dilated ureter. Classification and approach. Urology 9:1, 1977.

Glassberg KI: Schneider M, Haller JD, et al: Observations on persistently dilated ureter after posterior urethral valve ablation. Urology 20:20, 1982.

Goodwin WE, Burke DE, Muller WH: Retrocaval ureter. Surg Gynecol Obstet 104:337, 1957.

Goodwin WE, Winter CC, Turner RD: Replacement of the ureter by small intestine: clinical application and results of the "ileal ureter." J Urol 81:406, 1959.

Gosling JA, Dixon JS: Functional obstruction of the ureter and renal pelvis. A histological and electron micro-scopic study. Br J Urol 50:145, 1978.

Grana L, Kidd J, Idriss F, et al: Effect of chronic urinary tract infection on ureteral peristalsis. J Urol 94:652, 1965.

Grana L, Swenson O: A new surgical procedure for the treatment of aperistaltic megaloureter. Am J Surg 109:532, 1965.

Grégoir W, Debled G: L'etiologie du reflux congénital et du méga-uretère primaire. Urol Int 24:119, 1969.

Hanna MK: Early surgical correction of massive refluxing megaureter in babies by total ureteral reconstruction and reimplantation. Urology 18:562, 1981.

Hanna MK, Jeffs RD: Primary obstructive megaureter in children. Urology 6:419, 1975.

Hanna MK, Jeffs RD, Sturgess JM, et al: Ureteral structure and ultrastructure. Part II. Congenital ureteropelvic junction obstruction and primary obstructive mega-ureter. J Urol 116:725, 1976.

Heal MR: Primary obstructive megaureter in adults. Br J Urol 45:490, 1973.

Hendren WH: Operative repair of megaureter in children. J Urol 101:491, 1969.

Hendren WH: Restoration of function in the severely decompensated ureter. In Problems in Paediatric Urol-ogy. Edited by JH Johnston, RJ Scholtmeijjer. Amsterdam, Excerpta Medica, 1972.

Hendren WH: Complications of megaureter repair in children. J Urol 113:238, 1975.

Hendren WH: Tapered bowel segment for ureteral re-placement. Urol Clin North Am 5:607, 1978.

Hensle TW, Berdon WE, Baker DH, et al: The ureteral "J" sign: radiographic demonstration of iatrogenic distal ureteral obstruction after ureteral reimplantation. J Urol 127:766, 1982.

Hirschhorn RC: The ileal sleeve. II. Surgical technique in clinical application. J Urol 92:120, 1964.

Hodgson NB, Thompson LW: Technique of reductive ureteroplasty in the management of megaureter. J Urol 113:118, 1975.

Hurst AF, Gaymer-Jones J: A case of megalo-ureter due to achalasia of the uretero vesical sphincter. Br J Urol 3:43, 1931.

Hutch JA: Non obstructive dilatation of the upper urinary tract. J Urol 71:412, 1954.

Hutch JA, Tanagho EA: Etiology of non-occlusive ure-teral dilatation. J Urol 93:177, 1965.

Johnston JH: Reconstructive surgery of mega-ureter in childhood. Br J Urol 39:17, 1967.

Johnston JH: Hydro-ureter and mega-ureter. In Paedi-atric Urology. Edited by DI Williams. London, Butter-worth and Co., 1968, pp. 160–174.

Johnston JH, Farkas A: The congenital refluxing mega-ureter: experiences with surgical reconstruction. Br J Urol 47:153, 1975.

Kalicinski ZH, Kansy J, Kotarbinska B, et al: Surgery of megaureters—modification of Hendren's operation. J Pediatr Surg 12:183, 1977.

King LR: Megaloureter: definition, diagnosis and man-agement (editorial). J Urol 123:222, 1980.

King LR, Kazmi SO, Campbell JA, et al: Vesicoureteral reflux: the case for non-surgical management. In Cur-rent Controversies in Urologic Management. Edited by R Scott Jr. Philadelphia, WB Saunders Co., 1972.

Leibowitz S, Bodian M: A study of the vesical ganglia in children and the relationship to the megaureter mega-cystis syndrome and Hirschsprung's disease. J Clin Pathol 16:342, 1963.

Lewis EL, Cletsoway RW: Megaloureter. J Urol 75:643, 1956.

Lewis EL, Kimbrough JC: Megalo-ureter: new concept in treatment. South Med J 45:171, 1952.

Lockhart JL, Singer AM, Glenn JF: Congenital mega-ureter. J Urol 122:310, 1979.

Mackie GG, Stephens FD: Duplex kidneys: a correction of renal dysplasia with position of the ureteral orifice. J Urol 114:274, 1975.

MacKinnon KJ: Primary megaureter. Birth Defects 13:15, 1977.

MacKinnon KJ, Foote JW, Wiglesworth FW, et al: The pathology of the adynamic distal ureteral segment. Trans Am Assoc Genitourin Surg 61:63, 1969.

McLaughlin AP III, Leadbetter WF, Pfister RC: Recon-structive surgery of primary megalo-ureter. J Urol 106:186, 1971.

McLaughlin AP III, Pfister RC, Leadbetter WF, et al: The pathophysiology of primary megaloureter. J Urol 109:805, 1973.

Mitchell ME: The role of bladder augmentation in undiversion. J Ped Surg 16:790, 1981.

Mollard P, Paillot JM: Primary megaureter (pathogenesis and treatment 104 patients—131 ureters). Prog Pediatr Surg 5:113, 1973.

Murnaghan GF: Experimental investigation of the dynamics of the normal and dilated ureter. Br J Urol 29:403, 1957.

Nanninga J, King LR, Downing J, et al: Factors affecting the outcome of 100 ureteral reimplantations done for vesicoureteral reflux. J Urol 102:772, 1969.

Nesbit RM, Withycombe JF: The problem of primary megaloureter. J Urol 72:162, 1954.

Notley RG: Electron microscopy of the primary obstructive megaureter. Br J Urol 44:229, 1972.

Pagano P, Passerini G: Primary obstructed megaureter. Br J Urol 49:469, 1977.

Paquin AJ Jr: Surgery of the ureterovesical junction. In Urologic Surgery. Edited by JF Glenn, WH Boyce. New York, Hoeber Medical Division, Harper & Row, 1969, pp 191–252.

Passaro E Jr, Smith JP: Congenital ureteral valve in children: a case report. J Urol 84:290, 1960.

Pfister RC, Hendren WH: Primary megaureter in children and adults. Clinical and pathophysiologic features of 150 ureters. Urology 12:160, 1978.

Pfister RC, McLaughlin AP III, Leadbetter WF: Radiological evaluation of primary megaloureter: the aperistaltic distal ureteral segment. Radiology 99:503, 1971.

Pitts WR Jr, Muecke EC: Congenital megaloureter: a review of 80 patients. J Urol 111:468, 1974.

Rabinowitz R, Barkin M, Schillinger JF, et al: Salvaging the iatrogenic megaureter. J Urol 121:330, 1979a.

Rabinowitz R, Barkin M, Schillinger JF, et al: Surgical treatment of the massively dilated primary megaureter in children. Br J Urol 51:19, 1979b.

Retik AB, McEvoy JP, Bauer SB: Megaureters in children. Urology 11:231, 1978.

Skinner DG, Goodwin WE: Indications for the use of intestinal segments in management of nephrocalcinosis. Trans Am Assoc Genitourin Surg 66:158, 1974.

Sommer JT, Stephens FD: Morphogenesis of nephropathy with partial ureteral obstruction and vesicoureteral reflux. J Urol 125:67, 1981.

Starr A: Ureteral plication: a new concept in ureteral tailoring for megaureter. Invest Urol 17:153, 1979.

Stephens FD: Treatment of megaureters by multiple micturition. Aust NZ J Surg 27:130, 1957.

Swenson O, Fisher JH: The relation of megacolon and megaloureter. N Engl J Med 253:1147, 1955.

Swenson O, Fisher JH, Cendron J: Megaloureter: investigation as to the cause and report on the results of newer forms of treatment. Surgery 40:223, 1956.

Swenson O, MacMahon HE, Jaques WE, et al: A new concept of the etiology of megaloureters. N Engl J Med 246:41, 1952.

Swenson O, Smyth BT: Aperistaltic megaloureter: treatment by bilateral cutaneous ureterostomy using a new technique: preliminary communication. J Urol 82:62, 1959.

Talner LB, Gittes RF: Megacalyces: further observation

and differentiation from obstructive renal disease. Am J Roentgenol Radium Ther Nucl Med 121:473, 1974.

Tanagho EA: Ureteral tailoring. J Urol 106:194, 1971.

Tanagho EA: Intrauterine fetal ureteral obstruction. J Urol 109:196, 1973.

Tanagho, EA: A case against incorporation of bowel segments into the closed urinary system. J Urol 113:196, 1975.

Tatu W, Brennan RE: Primary megaureter in a mother and daughter. Urol Radiol 3:185, 1981.

Tokunaka S, Koyanagi T: Morphologic study of primary nonreflux megaureters with particular emphasis on the role of ureteral sheath and ureteral dysplasia. J Urol 128:399, 1982.

Tokunaka S, Koyanagi T, Matsuno T, et al: Paraureteral diverticula: clinical experience with 17 cases with associated renal dysmorphism. J Urol 124:791, 1980a.

Tokunaka S, Koyanagi T, Tsuji I: Two infantile cases of primary megaloureter with uncommon pathological findings: ultrastructural study and its clinical implication. J Urol 123:1214, 1980b.

Tokunaka S, Koyanagi T, Tsuji I, et al: Histopathology of the nonrefluxing megaloureter: a clue to its pathogenesis. J Urol 17:238, 1982.

Tscholl R, Tettamatti F, Zingg E: Ileal substitute of ureter with reflux-plasty by terminal intussusception of bowel. Urology 9:385, 1977.

Turner RD, Goodwin WE: Experiments with intussuscepted ileal valve in ureteral substitution. J Urol 81:526, 1959.

Tveter KJ, Goodwin WE: The use of ileum as substitute for the ureter. In Current Trends In Urology. Vol 2. Edited by MI Resnick. Baltimore, Williams and Wilkins, 1982, pp 1–15.

Udall DA, Hodges CV, Pearse HM, et al: Transureterostomy: experience in pediatric patient. Urology 2:401, 1973.

Uson AC, Braham SB, Abrams CAL, et al: Retrocaval ureter in a child with Turner's syndrome. Am J Dis Child 119:267, 1970.

Von Niederhäusern W, Tuchschmid D: Une association mal connue: le méga-uretère congénital primarie et le rein a méga-calices, Ann Urol (Paris) 5:225, 1971.

Weber AL, Pfister RC, James AE Jr, et al: Megaureter in infants and children: roentgenologic, clinical, and surgical aspects. Am J Roentgenol Radium Ther Nucl Med 112:170, 1971.

Weiss RM, Biancani P: Rationale for ureteral tapering. Urology 20:482, 1982.

Whitaker RH: Methods of assessing obstruction in dilated ureter. Br J Urol 45:15, 1973a.

Whitaker RH: Diagnosis of obstruction in dilated ureters. Ann R Coll Surg Engl 53:153, 1973b.

Whitaker RH, Flower CDR: Megacalices—how broad a spectrum? Br J Urol 53:1, 1981.

Williams DI, Eckstein HB: Surgical treatment of reflux in children. Br J Urol 37:13, 1965.

Williams DI, Hulme-Moir I: Primary obstructive megaureter. Br J Urol 42:140, 1970.

Williams JL, Goodwin WE: Congenital multiple diverticula of the ureter. Br J Urol 37:299, 1965.

Witherow RO, Whitaker RH: The predictive accuracy of antegrade pressure flow studies in equivocal upper tract obstruction. Br J Urol 53:496, 1981.

Bladder and Bladder Neck

R. DIXON WALKER, III

BLADDER DIVERTICULA

Many diverticula seen in children are associated with reflux, obstructed urethras, or neurogenic bladders and are discussed in those respective chapters. Congenital diverticula do occur, however, unassociated with these diseases (Johnston). The diagnosis of congenital diverticulum is made after first ruling out obstruction and neurogenic bladder.

Classification, Definitions, and Pathology

A *diverticulum* is a protrusion of bladder mucosa through bundles of the detrusor muscle. This can occur in areas where the muscle is inadequately formed, typically at the ureterovesical junction, or between bundles of hypertrophied muscle. A true diverticulum should contain only two layers, mucosal and adventitial, although some diverticula may have small amounts of muscle below the mucosa. A *herniation* represents a protrusion of all layers of the bladder into or toward a portion of the muscular pelvis (Bell and Witherington). Most of these are encountered in adults within an inguinal hernia, but the bladder "ears" seen predominantly in male infants also represent physiologic bladder hernias (Fig. 16–101).

Diverticula that occur with obstruction, particularly in association with posterior valves (Fig. 16–102), are very similar to those that occur with neurogenic bladder (Fig. 16–103). Such diverticula tend to be multiple and associated with cellules, saccules, and severe trabeculation. The cause of diverticula in both diseases is related to the hypertrophy of the detrusor muscle and increased intravesical pressure. The detrusor hypertrophy results in muscular bridges with interposed weak areas that progress from cellules to saccules to diverticula. The point at which a saccule becomes a diverticulum cannot be clearly defined. Kelalis and McLean have suggested that a saccule larger than 2 cm seen on cystography should be considered a diverticulum. Although diverticula associated with obstructed or neurogenic bladders may become large, most saccules are less than 1 cm in diameter. The pathology in these diverticula is varied; those that are newly evolved from saccules may still have a muscular layer, whereas those that are larger may have only mucosa and adventitia. One problem with diverticula, along with their associated saccules and trabeculations, is that they increase the difficulty of bladder surgery. Diseased bladders are less satisfactory than normal bladders for ureteral reimplantation, urinary undiversion, and renal transplantation.

The paraureteral diverticula associated with reflux are commonly termed "Hutch" diverticula, although Hutch initially described these in neuropathic bladders (Hutch). Stephens has indicated that the disorder needs to be clarified since some are associated with reflux and some are not (Stephens). Anatomically, these diverticula occur through the muscular hiatus. Reflux will not occur if the orifice remains in the bladder with a tunnel of sufficient intramural length, but will occur if the intramural tunnel is short or if the ureter enters the diverticulum (Figs. 16–104 to 16–106).

Congenital diverticula unassociated with obstruction or neuropathic bladder are un-

Figure 16–101. Physiologic bladder "ears" in male infant.

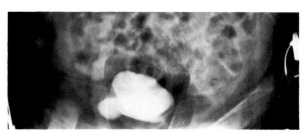

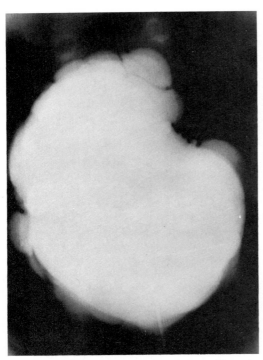

Figure 16–102. Diverticula associated with posterior urethral valves.

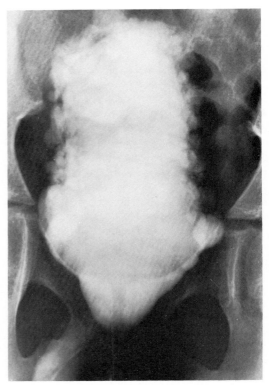

Figure 16–103. Small diverticula and saccules in patient with neurogenic bladder.

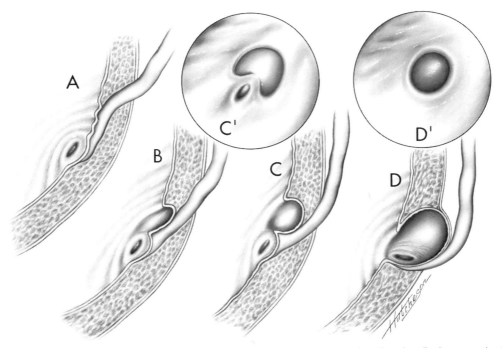

Figure 16–104. Development of paraureteral saccule or diverticulum leading to displacement of the submucosal and intramural ureter with subsequent loss of its muscular support and resultant incompetence of the ureterovesical angle. The ureteral orifice can be displaced within the diverticulum and lost to cystoscopic view.

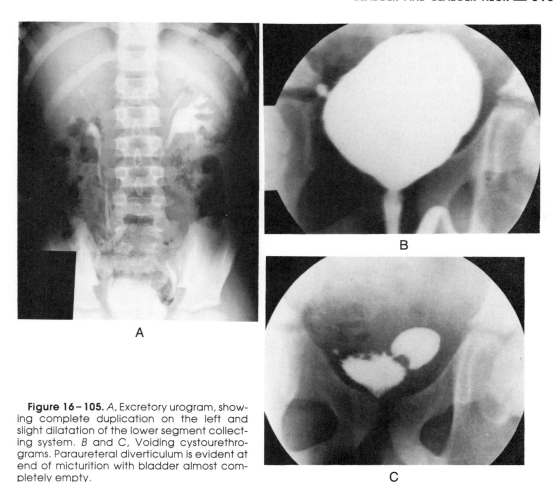

Figure 16–105. *A*, Excretory urogram, showing complete duplication on the left and slight dilatation of the lower segment collecting system. *B* and *C*, Voiding cystourethrograms. Paraureteral diverticulum is evident at end of micturition with bladder almost completely empty.

usual but not rare, and almost always occur in boys (Fig. 16–107). Although these diverticula are not necessarily paraureteral diverticula as described above, they may be located in close proximity to the ureteral hiatus and may be associated with reflux. Johnston states that these diverticula probably start near the ureteral orifice but not in the hiatal area. As the diverticulum enlarges, it may incorporate the intramural tunnel so that the orifice empties into the diverticulum and reflux ensues. Congenital diverticula are often larger than those caused by neurogenic bladder or by obstruction. They may have some muscle fibers in their walls. The remainder of the bladder is usually smooth, but on occasion may have

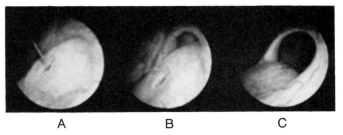

Figure 16–106. Endoscopic views, showing development of paraureteral diverticulum with progressive distention of the bladder. *A*, Heaped-up mucosa around ureteral orifice simulates ureterocele. *B*, Early development of paraureteral diverticulum. *C*, With bladder full or slightly overdistended, the ureteral orifice has been displaced by the diverticulum.

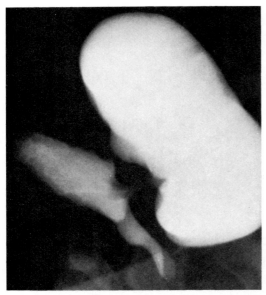

Figure 16-107. Solitary congenital diverticulum in male infant. No urethral obstruction is present. In this postvoiding film the bladder, on the left, is nearly empty while the diverticulum remains full.

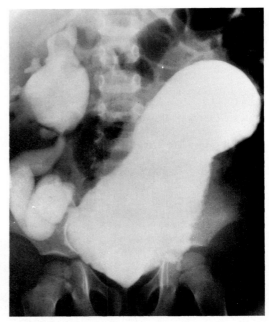

Figure 16-109. Prune-belly bladder with urachal diverticulum.

associated mild trabeculation probably related to the inefficiency of bladder emptying caused by the diverticulum. Congenital diverticula have been found associated with Menkes' syndrome, an abnormality of copper metabolism (Daly and Rabinovitch).

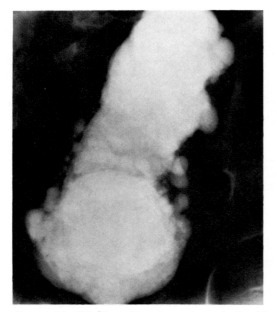

Figure 16-108. Hourglass shape in patient with neurogenic bladder.

Abnormal bladder shapes may be reminiscent of diverticula but do not necessarily represent true diverticula. The hourglass bladder (Fig. 16-108) is associated with a neuropathic bladder and is probably caused by high intravesical pressure and ineffective emptying. The upper part of the hourglass bladder is not a diverticulum but a thick, fully formed portion of the bladder. Similarly, the bladder in the prune-belly patient (Fig. 16-109) is commonly said to have a urachal diverticulum. This is also not a true diverticulum but rather an abnormally developed bladder with that portion of the bladder adjacent to the urachus undergoing segmentalization. This segment has all layers and, indeed, hypertrophied muscle, and its cause is not related to obstruction, but to the maldevelopment of all the muscular layers of the ureter, bladder, and posterior urethra.

Clinical Presentation

A diverticulum rarely produces any specific symptomatology that suggests its presence. It is most often diagnosed radiographically during an evaluation for urinary tract infection, incontinence, or obstruction. Therefore, a discussion of the clinical presentation of bladder diverticula must include signs and symptoms referable to the disease processes associated with diverticula.

An occasional diverticulum may be of sufficient size that it is palpable or visualized on inspection of the abdomen. These diverticula are often larger than the bladders from which they arise. Nevertheless, the precise diagnosis is still radiologic rather than clinical.

Bladder diverticula may reach sufficient size that they obstruct the urethra and result in obstructive voiding symptoms (Fig. 16–110) (Taylor et al). Obstruction of one or both ureters may result in hydronephrosis. This diagnosis is usually not suspected until the radiologic study discloses the presence of a large diverticulum.

Diverticula may not empty adequately and effectively and thus cause a significant retention of urine. This situation increases the possibility of urinary tract infection and may also be associated with incontinence. It has been suggested that urine retention is related to development of carcinoma of the bladder in the diverticulum in later life, but recent evidence indicates that this is not so (Fellows). Whether or not the incidence of carcinoma is increased, the prognosis for cure of a tumor is probably made worse because of the decreased thickness of the diverticulum wall. These patients are also prone to stone formation as adults.

Both an excretory urogram and a voiding cystourethrogram should be obtained in evaluating a diverticulum. Smaller diverticula may be obscured by the heavy contrast on a voiding cystourethrogram and show more clearly on the bladder phase of an excretory urogram. The voiding cystourethrogram may also indicate a diverticulum with high-pressure reflux that on the urogram actually proves to be a ureterocele. The voiding cystourethrogram should include films made during voiding with oblique and lateral views. A diverticulum is one of the few lesions that will shift the course of the lower ureter. Cystoscopy is usually unnecessary, but may be needed to evaluate the relationship of a refluxing ureteral orifice to the diverticulum, or to exclude bladder outlet obstruction definitely. The diverticulum should then be located, the size of the neck measured, and the proximity to the ureteral orifices noted. Further studies should include a thorough neurologic evaluation, cystometrogram, and electromyography of the urethral sphincter if obstruction is suspected. The diagnosis and cause of the diverticula can be determined by evaluating the results of the aforementioned data.

Treatment

Most bladder diverticula do not require excision. Small diverticula (less than 1 to 2 cm) associated with neurogenic bladder and posterior urethral valves cannot be easily removed, and treatment should be directed toward relieving the obstruction and stabilizing the bladder. Bladder "ears" are physiologic and will disappear as the child matures. The abnormally shaped bladder, such as the hourglass bladder, will usually not require operative therapy but rather treatment directed toward improving voiding or emptying patterns.

The prune-belly child with the large urachal "diverticulum" may have repeated episodes of urinary infection or retention, and the urachal segment of the bladder may need to be excised if it fails to empty. This is discussed in Chapter 20. The patient with an everting ureterocele forming a diverticulum will require heminephroureterectomy, and probably resection of the ureterocele with reconstruction of the bladder base.

Paraureteral diverticula may or may not require surgical management (Allen and Atwell). If reflux is severe and surgical management is required, then the muscular hiatus will be repaired at the same operation. Lower-grade reflux associated with small diverticula often stops with growth and does not require surgical intervention.

The treatment for symptomatic congenital

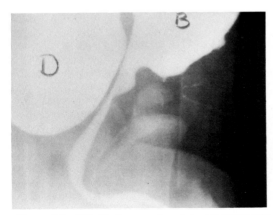

Figure 16–110. Cystogram in a boy presenting in urinary retention. The bladder (B) and the urethra are compressed by the diverticulum (D).

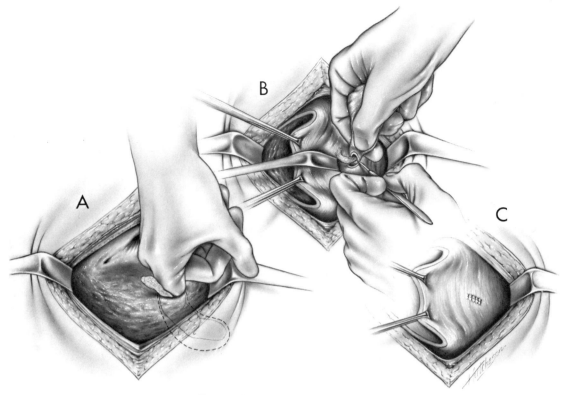

Figure 16–111. Diverticulectomy.

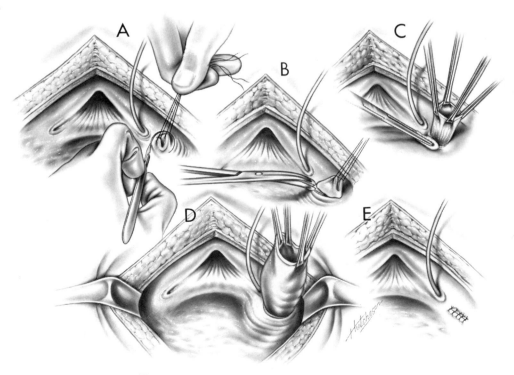

Figure 16–112. Transvesical diverticulectomy.

diverticula of the bladder, which are not due to obstruction, is surgical removal. Occasionally, larger diverticula associated with posterior urethral valves or neurogenic bladder may also require surgical management. After the appropriate diagnostic studies have been performed, the bladder is approached through a transverse suprapubic incision. It is opened and the proximity of the diverticulum to the ureteral orifice is identified. Both ureteral orifices may be catheterized with infant feeding tubes. The diverticulum can be filled with moist surgical gauze and then dissected extravesically (Fig. 16–111), separating the diverticulum with a combination of blunt and sharp dissection from all of the adjacent structures. Since almost all of these patients are male children, particular attention needs to be given to preservation of the vas deferens and the ureter on the ipsilateral side. The neck of the diverticulum is incised, and the bladder is closed in layers using fine catgut for the mucosal layer and stronger catgut for the muscular layers (Fig. 16–110C). Diverticula may be resected entirely intravesically, although the relationship of the diverticulum to vital structures is sometimes harder to determine precisely using this approach (Fig. 16–112). A Fogarty catheter may be placed within the diverticulum to aid in the dissection (Colodny). The mouth of the diverticulum is incised and the diverticulum itself is dissected free by a combination of blunt and sharp dissection. After removal of the diverticulum, the muscular defect in the bladder is closed in layers using absorbable sutures.

BLADDER NECK OBSTRUCTION

What has been termed *primary* bladder neck obstruction actually represents two different diseases: the bladder neck obstruction that historically was associated with urinary tract infection or reflux, and the current concept of bladder neck obstruction as a rare but real entity whose diagnosis is primarily one of exclusion. *Secondary* bladder neck obstruction is less confusing in both concept and management. This article will try to place bladder neck obstruction in proper historical perspective and will present the objective data necessary to assign bladder neck obstruction its true place with the other obstructive uropathies in children.

Historical Perspective

Primary bladder neck obstruction was first described by Marion, who examined postmortem specimens from children who died of obstructive uropathy. With the advent of the voiding cystourethrogram, radiologic techniques allowed visualization of the urethra. Normal and abnormal anatomy could then be defined based on the observation that the bladder neck should open during voiding (Fig. 16–113); if it did not, this unopened bladder neck might have been obstructed. We know now that this was a tremendous oversimplification of voiding dynamics. There is a wide range of normal appearances of the urethra on voiding cystourethrogram.

Figure 16–113. Normal bladder neck in boy as seen on voiding cystourethrogram.

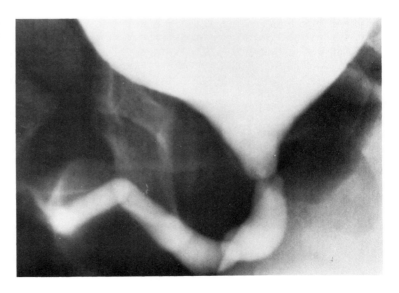

In 1953, Young advocated a Y-V plasty for children with recurrent urinary tract infection and believed that bladder neck obstruction was an important etiologic factor. McDonald et al surveyed 368 children with recurrent urinary tract infection and thought that 85 per cent had either urethral or bladder neck obstruction. In panel discussions of the relation of bladder neck obstruction to urinary tract infection, a wide range of opinion was expressed. Some experienced urologists believed that it was present in almost all children with urinary tract infection. In one such discussion (Spence et al), bladder neck obstruction was described in 41 of 140 children with urinary tract infection. Schoenberg et al found bladder neck obstruction in 10 of 24 children with urinary tract infection, almost all of whom improved after Y-V plasty of the bladder neck. Similar data were generated by Grieve, who performed Y-V plasties on 37 of 38 children with urinary tract infection and noted that all but 4 children were cured.

In none of these groups were randomized studies performed, and patients were concurrently treated with antibiotics. Thus, the reports of good results were often quite subjective. Because bladder neck obstruction and reflux were strongly believed by many to be related and because often these patients were undergoing operative treatment for their reflux, a Y-V plasty of the bladder neck was often performed at the same time. Leadbetter and Leadbetter reviewed their early data from refluxing patients and thought that 40 per cent had associated bladder neck obstruction. Baker et al found that of 555 patients with bladder neck or urethral obstruction, 24 per cent had vesicoureteral reflux. Harrow et al criticized the frequent diagnosis of bladder neck obstruction and found that in 217 patients with recurrent urinary tract infections, 90 of whom had vesicoureteral reflux, only 3 had cystoscopic and radiologic evidence of bladder neck obstruction. The popularity of bladder neck revision continued into the 1970's, however, in some medical centers, even though accumulating data indicated that whether or not a bladder neck revision was performed made little difference in the success rate of ureteral reimplantation. Many believed that patients who had bladder neck revisions were generally improved and had fewer postoperative urinary tract infections, but most of these data were not subjected to critical analysis.

Pathogenesis

Marion described fibrous tissue causing a circular contraction of the bladder neck in autopsy specimens. Bodian subsequently examined patients in whom elastic tissue was identified by appropriate histologic staining and then described similar pathology as fibroelastosis. Young (1965) suggested that the fibroelastosis may be a reaction to recurrent infection. Presman et al thought that the tissue resected was typical of fibromuscular hyperplasia. Kaplan and King found a range of pathologic tissue explaining the apparent variability in the degree of obstruction. Their patients had various amounts of normal smooth muscle, hypertrophied smooth muscle, fibrosis, and elastic tissue.

Outlet obstruction in some young adult males has been theorized to be functional. Bates et al believed that tightening of the bladder neck as the detrusor contracts causes obstruction in patients without evidence of increased fibrosis.

More recently, Woodside demonstrated that the obstruction could be due to a dyssynergic bladder neck or failure of bladder neck relaxation, and this has remained the modern explanation of most cases. Anderson et al, however, think that the pathogenesis is obscure and may be associated with the previously described pathologic findings, while Yalla et al have stated that since some bladder neck obstructions do not respond well to alpha adrenergic blockage, this is indicative of anatomic pathology.

Primary bladder neck obstruction probably represents a spectrum between the pathologic entities described by Kaplan and King and the functional abnormality described by Bates et al and by Woodside.

Table 16–13. Classification of Bladder Neck Obstruction

Primary
Obstructive
Functional
Secondary
Urethral obstruction (valves, stricture)
Neurogenic bladder
Ureterocele
Trigonal curtain
Polyp, tumor
Trigonal cyst
Iatrogenic

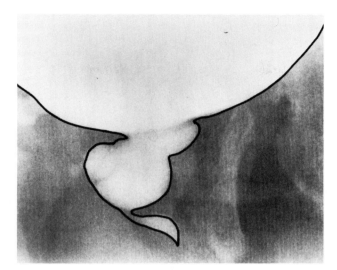

Figure 16–114. Bladder neck obstruction secondary to posterior urethral valve. (Enhanced photograph.)

Classification and Incidence

Primary bladder neck obstruction may be either functional or obstructive (Table 16–13). The functional classification has been introduced for those bladder neck obstructions diagnosed by urodynamics that may or may not have the *pathologic* features of an obstructive bladder neck disorder. Secondary bladder neck obstruction can occur from muscular hypertrophy of the internal sphincter, and is most often secondary to distal obstruction caused by anterior or posterior urethral valves (Fig. 16–114). The secondary form may also be related to hypertrophy associated with

neuropathic bladder dysfunction (Fig. 16–115). In addition, secondary bladder neck obstruction can occur owing to a prolapsing ureterocele (Fig. 16–116), bladder neck polyp, prostatic sarcoma (Fig. 16–117), or trigonal cyst or curtain, or iatrogenically as a result of an operative procedure such as imperforate anus repair.

Primary bladder neck obstruction is rare. Gierup reported that although he and his associates have an interest in bladder neck obstruction, they see only two cases per year. Kaplan and King indicated they found only

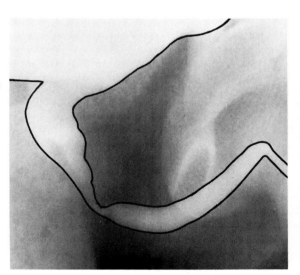

Figure 16–115. Bladder neck obstruction secondary to neurogenic bladder. (Enhanced photograph.)

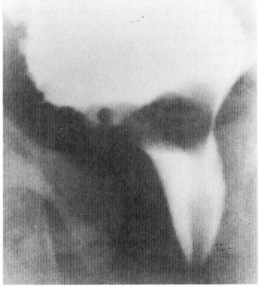

Figure 16–116. Bladder neck obstruction in male infant secondary to ureterocele.

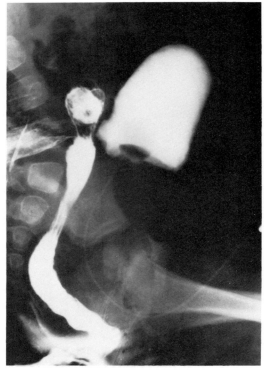

Figure 16–117. Bladder neck obstruction secondary to prostatic sarcoma. Barium in rectum allows appreciation of the marked elevation of the bladder base.

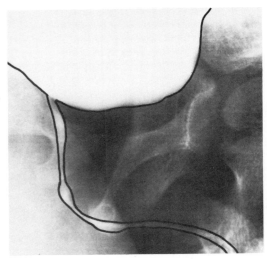

Figure 16–118. Primary bladder neck obstruction on voiding cystourethrogram. (Enhanced photograph.)

six cases per year in a busy pediatric practice. In retrospect, some of their patients probably had functional obstruction due to internal sphincter dyssynergia. In a round-table discussion on urethral obstruction, prominent European urologists were interviewed regarding their thoughts about bladder neck obstruction (Cukier and Gosalbez). Hohen-

fellner believed that primary bladder neck obstruction was nonexistent. Whitaker thought that it was rare but could occur in both sexes. Cukier stated that he had seen five cases of bladder neck obstruction; two were mild and three required surgery. Melchior thought that there was no primary structural bladder neck disease, but only a dyssynergic imbalance between the urethra and bladder. In my pediatric urologic practice in the past 10 years, I have twice made the diagnosis of primary bladder neck obstruction (Figs. 16–118 and 16–119). During this same decade, I have seen 44 patients with posterior urethral valves, 15 with Eagle-Barrett syndrome, and 18 with exstrophy of the bladder, so the lesion is clearly rare.

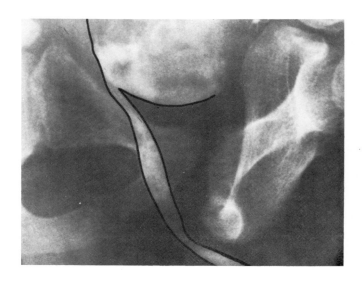

Figure 16–119. Primary bladder neck obstruction on retrograde urethrography. (Enhanced photograph.)

Most data indicate that primary bladder neck obstruction occurs almost exclusively in males. The argument advanced by Kaplan and King is that bladder neck obstruction is not known to occur in adult women, and one would have to presuppose that if the lesion was congenital and not diagnosed in childhood, it would be found in later life. This argument is refuted by Barnes, who has reportedly found bladder neck obstruction characterized by urinary retention in young women. Racial predilection does not appear to be a factor in primary bladder neck obstruction because there have been reports in white, black, and Oriental children.

Our current concept is that primary bladder neck obstruction is an extremely rare disease that occurs primarily in male children, adolescents, and young adults. The obstruction may be structural or functional and, if structural, may have a varied pathologic picture with admixtures of muscular hypertrophy, elastic tissue, and fibrosis.

Clinical Presentation

One would presume that primary bladder neck obstruction would always be accompanied by obstructive symptoms, although historically that is not true. Most cases were believed to be associated with reflux or urinary tract infection. Reports of bladder neck obstruction associated with reflux or urinary tract infection generally gave little attention to objective evidence of outlet obstruction. The diagnosis was a radiologic one or derived from the empiric observation that children with reflux or urinary tract infections who had bladder neck revision seemed to improve. Unfortunately, most of these observations proved misleading in that improvement was due to concomitant use of antibacterials, and the majority of those who believed that bladder neck obstruction was common now agree that it is rare.

Kaplan and King observed that patients with supposed bladder neck obstruction associated with reflux or urinary tract infection were almost always girls and that bladder neck surgery was unlikely to be effective in reducing voiding pressure. In a group of predominantly male patients in whom obstructive signs were present, 88 per cent improved with bladder neck surgery. In retrospect, many of these boys probably had sphincter dyssynergia, as mentioned above. Gierup et al indicated that 14 of 18 boys with bladder neck obstruction had obstructive symptoms characterized by difficulty in starting the urinary stream, by straining to void, and by poor or inadequate stream, all of which are also symptoms of dyssynergia. All of these boys also had urinary tract infection.

Urinary retention secondary to bladder neck obstruction has been reported in 239 young women and girls (Barnes). In addition to symptoms of retention, they had difficulty in initiating voiding and painful urination. This entity in girls and in young women has not been confirmed by other observers, and a portion of these cases are undoubtedly manifestations of psychologic problems.

Urologic Evaluation

Since the diagnosis of primary bladder neck obstruction is exclusionary, made after other obstructive diseases are considered, radiologic, urodynamic, and endoscopic evaluation are the most important tests in establishing the diagnosis.

Radiologic findings vary considerably. The traditional radiologic description was that by Rudhe and Ericsson, who described a distinct narrowing of the bladder neck with failure to funnel on voiding cystourethrogram. In patients described by Gierup et al, none had hydronephrosis, dilated ureter, or bladder diverticulum, although five boys had a trabeculated bladder and four had vesicoureteral reflux. The patient presented by Wacksman et al had severe bilateral hydronephrosis with renal failure. Kaplan and King indicated that 50 per cent of the patients in their series had azotemia and some radiologic evidence of obstructive uropathy.

Urodynamic studies in children should include urethral pressure profile and urinary flow studies. Because of discomfort, however, urethral pressure profiles are often inaccurate, at least on the initial study. Gierup et al found that results of urinary flow studies were abnormal in 14 of 18 boys in whom such abnormalities were suspected. They also reported that cystometrograms were normal in all patients. Of the 14 with abnormal flow studies, there was no consistent pattern but rather a wide variety of abnormalities. These abnormal flow patterns included variations in outflow resistance and intermittency of flow (Fig. 16–120).

The cystoscopic findings are usually of a firm ridge of tissue which is circumferential but appears to protrude into the bladder from

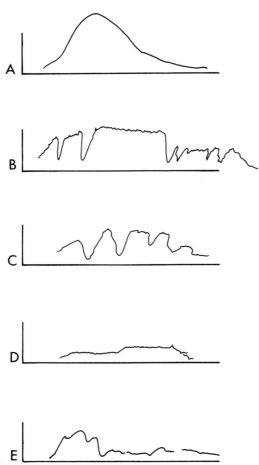

Figure 16–120. Examples of flow patterns in boys with primary bladder neck obstruction. (From Gierup J, Ericsson N, Hedenberg C: Urodynamic studies in boys with disorders of the lower urinary tract. Scand J Urol Nephrol 12:195, 1978.)

the floor of the urethra. This tissue appears to be either fibrous or muscular. In these patients, there is no cystoscopic or radiographic evidence of distal obstruction. The bladder may show trabeculation, cellules, or diverticula, and minimally will show otherwise unexplained trabeculation.

Treatment

The treatment of primary bladder neck obstruction is straightforward, with a choice between open (Fig. 16–121) and endoscopic (Fig. 16–122) surgery. Andreassen described Y-V plasty of the bladder neck. This procedure and its variations are all based on widening the anterior bladder neck by placing a flap or normal bladder tissue across the stenotic area.

The procedure is performed through a transverse suprapubic incision, the bladder is exposed, and the perivesical fat is dissected from the anterior bladder wall and bladder neck. After adequate mobilization of the bladder neck and urethra, the appropriate incision is made and carried through the obstructed bladder neck into the normal urethra. The wound margins are closed with absorbable sutures and the urine is diverted by suprapubic cystotomy for 1 week.

Andreassen's procedure adequately accomplishes the desired result, but Young and Goebel also found resecting a posterior wedge of bladder neck to be advantageous. Kaplan and King use a "T" incision converted to a "V" and believe that this causes less buckling of tissue.

Endoscopic surgery is favored by Cukier, who suggested incision of the posterior bladder neck rather than circular resection (Fig. 16–122A). Zade described resection of the posterior bladder neck and removal of the dome of the associated large bladder (Cukier and Gosalbez). Anderson et al described an endoscopic incision with electrocautery at the 5 o'clock and 7 o'clock positions of the bladder neck (Fig. 16–122B).

All of these procedures in boys carry some risk of retrograde ejaculation after maturation. This is less likely after anterior widening only than after a posterior wedge resection. The treatment of functional bladder neck obstruction is less direct. Limited experience indicates that treatment with pharmacologic agents, mainly phenoxybenzamine, may be disappointing, in which case either open or endoscopic surgery may become appropriate (Yalla et al). However, clean intermittent catheterization is another effective means of managing this problem in a manner that does not result in retrograde ejaculation in males.

Surgery for secondary bladder neck obstruction is related to the primary disease. It is contraindicated in most children with neurogenic bladder, since a principal form of therapy now is clean intermittent catheterization. With posterior urethral valves, some element of bladder neck hypertrophy almost always exists initially, but the intact bladder neck may be important in maintaining continence and in most patients should not be resected. Hendren has indicated that in unusual instances the prominent bladder neck may be obstructive and endoscopic incisions may be necessary.

Management of a bladder neck obstructed by ureterocele is determined by the quality of

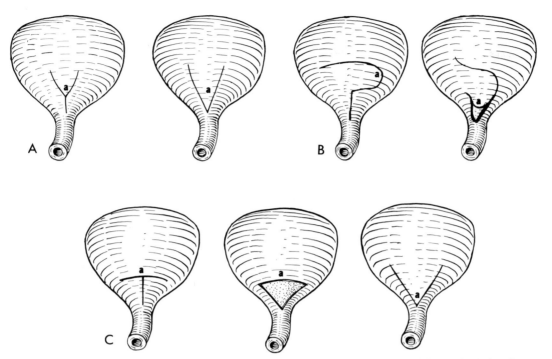

Figure 16–121. Open bladder neck plasty with modifications for primary bladder neck obstruction.

the kidney that the ureterocele drains. Often both heminephrectomy and reconstruction of the bladder floor will be required, although in many cases excision of the obstructed ureter and renal segment will result in collapse of the ureterocele and resolution of the problem. Occasionally a ureterocele remnant, especially from a cecoureterocele, may be left behind at the bladder neck and become obstructive. This remnant, which acts like a valve, can be resected endoscopically. Lesions such as bladder veils (valves) or polyps may also be endoscopically resected.

RESULTS OF SURGERY. The results of bladder neck surgery are difficult to measure by today's standards because the number of

patients currently undergoing such surgery are so few. The measure of success used to be decreased recurrences of infection or ablation of reflux, but these criteria alone no longer seem appropriate. Improvement in urinary flow and decreased residual urine are more objective signs of relief of obstruction. Gierup et al showed that five of seven boys with an abnormal flow study had improvement or were normal after bladder neck surgery. Yalla et al also showed improvement in urinary flow after bladder neck surgery in boys who had not improved after alpha adrenergic blockade.

COMPLICATIONS. Some children who have had extensive bladder neck surgery may

Figure 16–122. Methods of transurethral management of primary bladder neck obstruction.

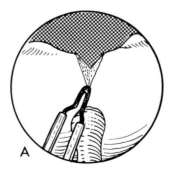
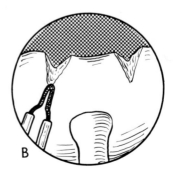

be made incontinent. This is particularly true of patients with posterior urethral valves in whom the intact bladder neck may be necessary to maintain continence. Cukier has reported that recurrent iatrogenic bladder neck obstruction can be a complication of extensive endoscopic resection of the entire bladder neck. Retrograde ejaculation and reflux of urine into the vas deferens are other complications seen following bladder neck revision.

RARE BLADDER LESIONS

In some children, bladder outlet obstruction appears to be the result of loose mucosal folds or valves. In many instances the mucosal fold involves the trigone, and sometimes, in girls, the folds may prolapse through the urethral meatus (Espinosa et al). This situation has been referred to as trigonal curtains, bladder neck valve, or mucosal redundancy. The most common presenting complaint is difficulty in micturition, in the form of intermittent obstruction, although in some cases the diagnosis was established at autopsy. It is important to remember that these signs may represent unusual types of ectopic ureterocele, or ureterocele remnants after rupture. A search for a double urinary system should be made. The treatment is excision of the fold, often suprapubically, because this approach affords a better opportunity to establish the exact diagnosis.

Another rare anomaly in the trigonal area is the trigonal cyst, which may cause obstruction to bladder outflow. This may be the result of cystic transformation of glands (Brunner's glands) in the trigone. The symptoms are sometimes similar to those of an ectopic ureterocele, and, in fact, a diagnosis of trigonal cyst should not be made until the possibility of a ureterocele has been thoroughly excluded.

BIBLIOGRAPHY

BLADDER DIVERTICULA

Allen NH, Atwell JD: The paraureteric diverticulum in childhood. Br J Urol 52:264, 1980.
Bell ED, Witherington R: Bladder hernias. Urology 15:127, 1980.
Colodny AH: An improved surgical technique for intravesicle resection of bladder diverticuli. Br J Urol 47:399, 1975.

Daly WJ, Rabinovitch HH: Urologic abnormality in Menkes' syndrome. J Urol 126:262, 1981.
Fellows GJ: The association between vesicle carcinoma and diverticulum of the bladder. Eur Urol 4:185, 1978.
Hutch JA: Saccule formation at the ureterovesical junction in smooth walled bladders. J Urol 86:390, 1961.
Johnston JH: Vesical diverticula without urinary obstruction in childhood. J Urol 84:535, 1960.
Kelalis PP, McLean P: The treatment of diverticulum of the bladder. J Urol 98:349, 1967.
Mackellar A, Stephens FD: Vesical diverticula in children. In Congenital Malformations of the Rectum, Anus, and Genitourinary Tracts. Edited by R Webster. Edinburgh, E & S Livingstone, 1963, pp 246–259.
Stephens FD: The vesicoureteral hiatus and paraureteral diverticula. J Urol 121:786, 1979.
Taylor WN, Alton D, Toguri A, et al: Bladder diverticula causing posterior urethral obstruction in children. J Urol 122:415, 1979.
Williams DI, Eckstein HB: Bladder disorders: diverticula. In Paediatric Urology. Edited by DI Williams. London, Butterworth & Co., 1968, pp 213–227.

BLADDER NECK OBSTRUCTION

Anderson JT, Nordling J, Meyhoff HH, et al: Functional bladder neck obstruction. Scand J Urol Nephrol 14:17, 1980.
Andreassen M: Vesicle neck obstruction in children. Acta Chir Scand 105:378, 1953.
Ashcraft KW, Hendren WH: Bladder outlet obstruction after operation for ureterocele. J Pediatr Surg 14:819, 1979.
Baker R, Maxted W, McCrystal H, et al: Unpredictable results associated with treatment of 133 children with ureterorenal reflux. J Urol 94:362, 1965.
Barnes RW: Vesicle neck obstruction: rare cause of female urinary retention. Urol Times 11:3, November, 1981.
Bates CP, Arnold EP, Griffiths DJ: The nature of the abnormality in bladder neck obstruction. Br J Urol 47:651, 1975.
Bodian M: Some observations on the pathology of congenital "idiopathic bladder neck obstruction" (Marion's disease). Br J Urol 29:393, 1957.
Boissonnat P, Bouteau P: Volumineux kyste du trigone chez un garçon de 3 ans. J Urol (Paris) 60:688, 1954.
Cukier J, Gosalbez R: Congenital cervicourethral obstruction in children. Eur Urol 6:1, 1980.
Gierup J, Ericsson N, Hedenberg C: Urodynamic studies in boys with disorders of the lower urinary tract. Scand J Urol Nephrol 12:195, 1978.
Grieve J: Bladder neck stenosis in children—is it important? Br J Urol 39:13, 1967.
Harrow BR, Sloan JA, Witus WS: A critical examination of bladder neck obstruction in children. J Urol 98:613, 1967.
Hendren WH: Urethral valves. Birth Defects 13:5, 1977.
Kaplan GW, King LR: An evaluation of Y-V vesicourethroplasty in children. Surg Gynecol Obstet 130:1059, 1970.
Leadbetter GW, Leadbetter WF: Ureteral reimplantation and bladder neck reconstruction—four and one-half years experience. JAMA 175:349, 1961.
Learmonth JR, Watkins KH: A rare type of valvular obstruction of the neck of the bladder: report of two cases. Br J Urol 22:879, 1935.
Marion G: Surgery of the neck of the bladder. Br J Urol 5:351, 1933.
McDonald HP, Upchurch WE, Celaya CL: Vesicle neck obstruction in children. Amer Surg 27:603, 1961.

Michon L, Boyet C, Cammenos A: Kyste du trigone chez une fillette de 3 ans. J Urol (Paris) 59:529, 1953.

Poole-Wilson DS: Congenital valvular obstruction of the neck of the bladder. Br J Urol 15:11, 1943.

Presman D, Ross LS, Nicosia SV: Fibromuscular hyperplasia of the posterior urethra: a cause of lower urinary tract obstruction in male children. J Urol 107:149, 1972.

Rudhe U, Ericsson NO: Roentgen evaluation of primary bladder neck obstruction in children. Acta Radiol (Diagn) (Stockh) 3:237, 1968.

Schoenberg HW, Tristan TA, Murphy JJ: The effect of urethral meatotomy in girls with bladder neck dysfunction. J Urol 96:921, 1966.

Spence HM, Murphy JJ, McGovern JH, et al: Urinary tract infections in infants and children. J Urol 91:623, 1964.

Wacksman J, Lalli AF, Kallen RJ, et al: Bladder neck contracture: primary vs secondary disease. Am J Dis Child 135:561, 1981.

Woodside JR: Urodynamic evaluation of dysfunctional bladder neck obstruction in men. J Urol 124:673, 1980.

Yalla SB, Blute RD, Snyder H, et al: Isolated bladder neck obstruction of undetermined etiology (primary) in adult male. Urology 17:99, 1981.

Young BW: The retropubic approach to vesicle neck obstruction in children. Surg Gynecol Obstet 96:150, 1953.

Young BW: Elastic components of the vesicle neck and urethra in childhood. Invest Urol 3:20, 1965.

Young BW, Goebel JL: Retropubic wedge excision in congenital vesicle neck obstruction. Stanford Med Bull 12:106, 1954.

RARE BLADDER LESIONS

Espinosa RR, Blanco RL, Picornell BV: Prolapsing trigonal mucosa in infant. J Pediatr 54:446, 1958.

Posterior Urethra

LOWELL R. KING

POSTERIOR URETHRAL VALVES

The precise diagnosis and management of posterior urethral valves has posed one of the great challenges in pediatric urology, and even now the optimum modes of treatment remain controversial in many areas. On the surface, the problem and therapy seem straightforward; in practice there are many variables — different degrees of obstruction, reflux, superimposed infection, and/or renal dysgenesis. Technical problems in surgical removal, especially in infants, also dictate indirect treatment, which is more complex than simple resection, in many instances.

The purpose of this article is to formulate criteria for exact diagnosis and to put forth a safe and workable scheme of therapy that will minimize the risk of further renal damage. A consensus in managing children with valves is emerging that is based on the clear need to conserve renal function and to retain any ability that the damaged kidneys may have to grow with the child. In general, this means that obstruction should be relieved as soon as the diagnosis is made, and renal infection should be prevented or treated aggressively with antibiotics or with temporary urinary diversion — whichever is needed to quickly eradicate the infection and prevent further renal damage. There are also many continuing controversies regarding embryology, diagnosis, and nuances in management that continue to stimulate the urologist and repay the study of this interesting disease.

Most credit Largenbeck with the first description of valves in his treatise on lithotomy in 1802. Budd (1840), Pickard (1855), and Tolmatschew (1870) reported autopsy dissections of patients with valves; the latter is credited with the first systematic study of the lesion. In 1912, Knox and Sprunt published the first American report of a case discovered at autopsy. Young, also in 1912, was the first to make the diagnosis of posterior urethral valves endoscopically. He then fulgurated the valves from above through a cystostomy. Subsequently, Young used his perineal approach with forcible rupture of the valves with sounds. This may have worked in treating an obstructing mucosal diaphragm (type III valve), but the more common type I leaflet valves are not often susceptible to rupture by dilatation. Young probably recognized the limitations of dilatation, because in 1915 he performed the first successful transurethral treatment in an adult using an endoscopic punch of his own design. In 1920 he employed the same technique in a child. In 1921, Randall recognized valves in a patient that he treated with transurethral fulguration, a technique that has stood the test of time and has evolved into standard modern therapy.

After these initial cases were reported, many urologists became skeptical of the existence of valves because they were unable to identify these lesions in their own patients. For example, between 1942 and 1953 Lattimer and Hubbard found only 3 cases of urethral valves in over 2000 pediatric urologic admissions. However, Campbell, working among the same population, made the diagnosis frequently, and in 1949 McCrea reviewed a total of 207 cases that had been reported up to that time. In retrospect the reason for the discrepancy in diagnosis seems clear—voiding cystourethrography had not yet come into clinical use. When urethroscopy and bougienage were the only tools available to evaluate the urethra, precise diagnosis was even more difficult than it is today.

Embryology

There is no question that posterior urethral valves are congenital. Young (1972) found typical type I valves at autopsy in a 6 month fetus. Campbell (1931) discovered valves at autopsy in an infant who died 5 hours after birth. In many institutions nearly half of all the children treated for valves are now diagnosed within the first month of life, and many are diagnosed antenatally by fetal ultrasound.

Valves have no known genetic basis, and are very rarely encountered in the same family. Familial cases have been reported by Campbell, Counseller and Menville, and Kjellberg et al. Valves have been discovered in twins, but even in identical twins often only one twin is affected (Gonzales, 1983).

A high incidence of congenital anomalies in other organ systems is occasionally reported in conjunction with urethral valves. In most series, however, this is not a prominent feature, and most boys with valves do not have serious lesions beyond the urinary tract. There is an obstructive lesion of the distal portion of the dilated posterior urethra that telescopes during voiding in some boys with the prune-belly syndrome and mimics a posterior urethral valve; this is often termed a type IV valve (Stephens, FD, personal communication, 1983), but in this situation the "valve" is composed of hypoplastic prostatic tissue (Moerman et al).

In male fetuses with a severe degree of obstruction from valves or other causes, renal development may become abnormal as a consequence of the obstruction. In extreme instances this may result in renal dysplasia or dysgenesis, microcystic disease, and an inability of the kidney to grow, which eventually results in renal failure. Marked impairment of urine formation in utero is associated with oligohydramnios. The fetal lungs then develop poorly, and fetal respiratory distress syndrome is likely after delivery, especially if the birth is premature. Lack of amniotic fluid probably also results in skeletal molding and the Potter facies so typical of babies born with severe congenital renal disease.

We must now consider the formation of the lower urinary tract in an attempt to elucidate the abnormal pathoembryology that may result in a urethral valve. (Figs. 16–123 to 16–126). Normally, the urorectal or cloacal septum, a tongue of tissue formed from entoderm, grows caudally to fuse with the cloacal membrane, dividing the primitive cloaca into an anterior urogenital sinus and a posterior rectum. The anterior portion of the cloacal membrane then becomes the urogenital membrane, which perforates at the 12 to 16 mm stage of development.

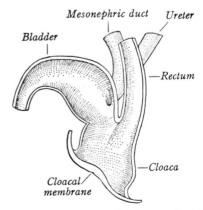

Figure 16–123. Partial division of the human cloaca: 8 mm stage. (From Arey LB, Developmental Anatomy, Revised seventh ed. Philadelphia, WB Saunders Co., 1974.)

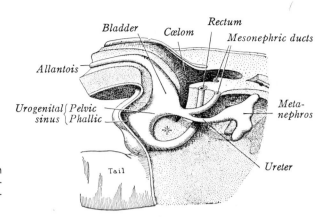

Figure 16–124. Further division of the human cloaca: 11 mm stage. (From Arey LB, Developmental Anatomy, Revised seventh ed. Philadelphia, WB Saunders Co., 1974.)

The wolffian ducts—originally the pronephric and mesonephric ducts—open into the primitive cloaca. As the urorectal septum grows caudally the wolffian ducts are incorporated into the ventral wall of the urorectal septum, forming Müller's tubercle. The ureteral buds arise from the wolffian ducts in the 5 to 6 mm embryo; the distal ends eventually migrate cephalad to form the borders of the trigone. The portion of the urogenital sinus proximal to Müller's tubercle becomes the entire urethra in the female or the prostatic urethra in the male.

The remaining urogenital sinus, extending caudally from the tubercle, can be further divided into two portions. The more proximal portion, directly below Müller's tubercle, is larger and develops longitudinal ridges, the urethrovaginal folds, in its lateral walls. These ridges run from the tubercle to the point of origin of Cowper's or Bartholin's glands, which, at this stage, are located in the anterior urethral wall. Williams has observed urethrovaginal folds in 60 to 100 mm fetuses. Stephens (1963) believes that these folds are related to the wolffian ducts and mark their course of regression as they become more cephalad in position. In the male the cranial vestiges of these urethrovaginal folds remain as the plicae colliculi, migrating laterally by lateral growth and by fusion of the bulbous and cavernous portions of the urethra. Similar growth probably accounts for the final position of Cowper's glands.

How then do valves develop, and why is there a predilection for this region? Many theories have been proposed. Tolmatschew suggested that valves represent extreme development of the normal folds, described above. As distention of the exaggerated fold

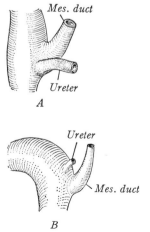

Figure 16–125. *A, B,* Cephalad migration of ureteral buds at 6 and 7 weeks gestation, respectively. (From Arey LB, Developmental Anatomy, Revised seventh ed. Philadelphia, WB Saunders Co., 1974.)

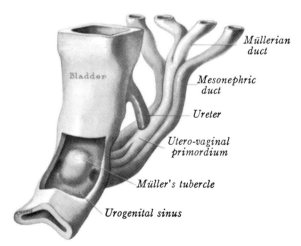

Figure 16–126. Differentiation of urogenital sinus at 9 weeks. (From Arey LB, Developmental Anatomy, Revised seventh ed. Philadelphia, WB Saunders Co., 1974.)

occurs the membranes become thinner but greater in area, eventually compromising the urethral lumen and causing obstruction. This theory, however, doesn't really account for the circumferential nature of valves that have anterior attachments, since normal plicae insert posterolaterally on the urethral wall. However, the typical type I valve does seem an exaggeration of the normal plicae in the sense that the plicae are replaced by the valve. However, Tolmatschew's theory does not account at all for type III valves, which are circumferential narrowings below, or occasionally above, the level of the embryonic folds.

Bazy suggested that valves are remnants of the urogenital membrane in that they occur at a site close to the junction of the anterior and posterior urethra. Lowsley believed that valves were the result of an abnormal junction of the ejaculatory (wolffian) duct and the prostatic utricle (müllerian duct); he described fibers from this area passing around the entire circumference of the urethra in an autopsy specimen. Watson deduced that valves represent the fusion of epithelium of the seminal colliculus with the roof of the urethra, the posterior urethral groove. Stephens, in an eloquent discussion (1963), argued that type I valves result from an abnormal insertion and persistence of the distalmost extremity of the wolffian ducts (Fig. 16–127), whereas type III valves represent persistence of the urogenital membrane. Stephens also described some extraordinary urethral membranes that may be

quite long and pedunculated, with only a tiny perforation to provide some continuity in the lumen of the urethra. These extreme anomalies are seldom encountered in surviving babies (Fig. 16–128).

Classification

No simple system really encompasses all the lesions that have been described as urethral valves. Young (1919) devised his classification primarily on the basis of autopsy findings. His system is still in general use. According to Young, type I valves are sails, or exaggerated plicae colliculi, which extend distally from either side of the verumontanum to attach to the anterolateral walls of the urethra. Type II valves are folds that arise from the verumontanum and pass proximally toward the bladder neck, where they divide into finlike membranes. Type III valves are diaphragms with a small central perforation located distal or proximal to the verumontanum, but not attached to it (Fig. 16–129).

This system of classification is clear and has never been seriously challenged. However, there is a real question whether the type II "valves" cause obstruction. Both obstructing cusps and diaphragms are found in the anterior urethra but are unrelated to posterior urethral valves, at least in etiology.

Before continuing, it is also pertinent to review the normal topographic anatomy of the male posterior urethra as described by

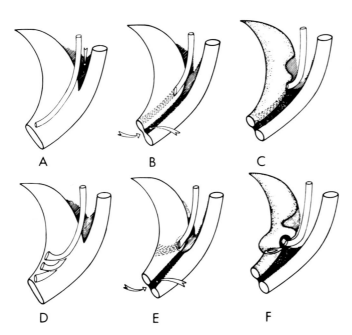

Figure 16–127. Development of type I valves. (These previously unpublished drawings are supplied through the courtesy of Dr. F. D. Stevens.) A–C. Development of the normal urethral crest. Migration of the orifice of the wolffian duct from its anterolateral position in the cloaca to the site of Müller's tubercle on the posterior wall of the urorectal septum, occurring synchronously with cloacal division. (Dots denote pathway of migration.) This pathway is swept laterally and posteriorly and remains as the normal inferior crest and the plicae colliculi. D–F, Abnormal anterior positions of the wolffian duct orifices and consequent abnormal migration of the terminal ends of the ducts, resulting in circumferential obliquely oriented ridges that comprise the value.

A   B   C

D   E   F

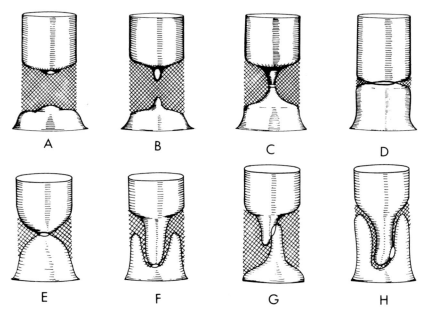

Figure 16–128. Development of type III valves. *A–D*, Normal canalization of the urogenital membrane. *D* shows normal slight constriction at the level of the perineal membrane. *E*, Stricture formation. *F*, Canalization by central downgrowth and circumferential ingrowth resulting in a bulging membrane with a central stenotic orifice. *G* and *H*, Side openings creating valvular "wind-sock" membranes. (Drawings and descriptions supplied through the courtesy of Dr. F. D. Stephens.)

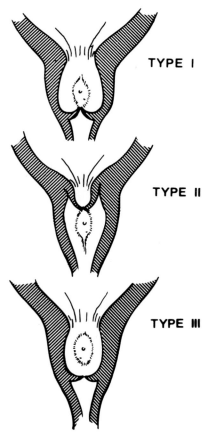

Figure 16–129. H. H. Young's classification of valves into three types.

Stephens (1963). The urethral crest is a straight tapering ridge that arises in the posterior midline at the verumontanum and ends distally, dividing into two to four fins, the plicae colliculi (Fig. 16–130). These fins diverge laterally and distally into the membranous urethra, disappearing at approximately the level of the embryonic perineal

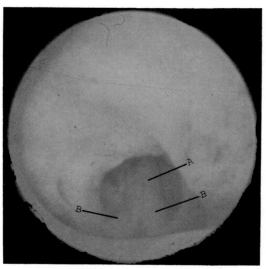

Figure 16–130. Endoscopic photograph of normal urethra in a 4-year-old male. *A* indicates the urethral crest and *B* the plicae colliculi.

membrane. The plicae represent the embryonic urethrovaginal folds. In some patients one can identify fins cephalad to the verumontanum. These may be traces of the course taken by the embryonic ureteral buds in their migration to form the trigone, as proposed by Young (1972), or they may be unrelated longitudinal bands of fibroelastic tissue in the prostatic wall, as suggested by Robertson and Hayes.

We must now reconsider Young's classification on the basis of the embryology and anatomy of the posterior urethra. Type II valves have no obvious embryologic precursor. The fins that run from the verumontanum toward the bladder neck on the floor of the posterior urethra are almost longitudinally oriented. It does not seem possible that they could obstruct urinary outflow. Some authors have proposed that valves in females might be the type II variety. If this were so, however, they should insert at the external meatus, but they are always described in the midportion of the female urethra. Campbell (1931), Graham et - al, Hendren (1971), Lowsley, and McCrea have reported type II valves in boys, so they are not easily dismissed. However, most series do not include type II valves. In the case reported by Graham et al there was a more distal obstruction as well. It does seem possible that the type II folds might be the longitudinal bands of fibroelastic tissue described vividly by Robertson and Hayes, which may stand out prominently when the rest of the posterior urethra becomes dilated. In any case, type II valves are a rarity.

Robertson and Hayes studied type I valves at autopsy in 17 patients. Specimens were prepared by distending the bladder and urethra with formalin and allowing the tissue to fix before opening the urethra. After fixation the anterior urethras were unroofed tangentially instead of by the usual technique of cutting open the urethra longitudinally. The valve was then better preserved and better visualized (Figs. 16 – 131 and 16 – 132). In all 17 specimens a slitlike opening in a tilted, obliquely placed diaphragm was found. This anatomic study clearly demonstrated that type I valves are also really diaphragms, with anterior fusion of the cusps that were originally described and that are so much more obvious endoscopically than the circumferential nature of the obstruction. This also raises the question of whether type I and type III valves might really be variations in the same lesion, differing mainly in location.

On balance, however, it seems best that

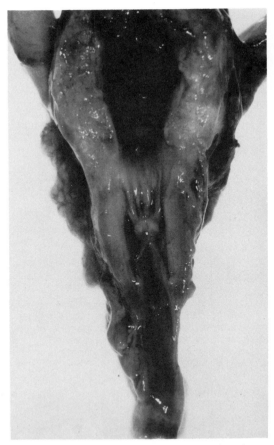

Figure 16 – 131. Specimen of valves at autopsy opened in conventional manner so that it appears that there are two folds. (From Robertson WB, Hayes JA, Br J Urol 41:592 – 598, 1969. Reproduced by permission.)

posterior urethral valves be characterized as two distinct lesions that have a different embryogenesis and slightly different anatomy. The first, and most common, corresponds to Young's type I. This lesion is probably caused by anterior fusion of the urethrovaginal folds, perhaps with an abnormal insertion into the verumontanum. It is also possible that failure of Cowper's glands to migrate is the causative factor. Anatomically this lesion consists of an obliquely placed diaphragm formed by paired cusps that arise from the verumontanum and pass distally and laterally to fuse dorsally. The folds may be thin and diaphanous, composed mainly of their epithelial surfaces, or may be fleshy with a definite stromal component. The cusps are usually somewhat rigid compared with the normal plicae, which are pliable and thin and insert on the lateral walls of the urethra without an anterior circumferential extension. The Vest straight-ahead lens system enables one to appreciate the slitlike

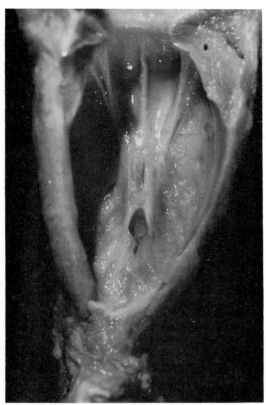

Figure 16–132. Autopsy specimen of valves opened by unroofing rather than incising anterior urethral wall. The folds in Figure 16–131 are now clearly seen to be an oblique diaphragm. Note also the type II "valves" cephalad to the verumontanum. (From Robertson WB, Hayes JA, Br J Urol 41:592–598, 1969. Reproduced by permission.)

opening in the type I valve and the true diaphragmatic nature of the lesion at endoscopy.

The other type of valve that commonly occurs in the posterior urethra corresponds to Young's type III. In the view of both Bazy and Stephens, this type is a consequence of persistence of the urogenital membrane. The anatomic result is a diaphragm with a small, more or less central perforation. This valve is a diaphragm that is perpendicular to the long axis of the urethra and is usually located just distal to the verumontanum and proximal to the junction of the bulbous and membranous portions of the urethra. Young also describes such lesions above the verumontanum, and similar lesions are occasionally found in the bulbous and pendulous urethra. The supramontane position must be very unusual, and is not considered a possible site for a type III valve by some authors (Kaplan, Stephens), mainly on embryologic grounds. The orifice

of the type III valve is occasionally eccentric, or there may be multiple perforations. The type III valve may occasionally balloon into the more distal urethra, resulting in the "windsock" configuration described by Field and Stephens.

Incidence

It is difficult to estimate the true incidence of posterior urethral valves, in part because many insist that only those with the typical appearance on voiding cystourethrogram should be counted. Mahony and Hendren, however, encounter valves not infrequently in older boys with few radiographic signs of obstruction who usually present with wetting. I concur that such a population exists, but believe that subtle obstruction from valves is an infrequent cause of diurnal enuresis overall.

Rattner et al identified 21 cases of valves in 2569 autopsies over a 12 year period. Although most valves are identified in childhood, 20 per cent of those reported by Landes and Rall were in patients over 20 years old at the time of diagnosis. Their oldest patient was 89. Williams et al (1973) reported 206 cases diagnosed in the previous 22 years and pointed out that valves are the most common cause of severe urethral obstruction in male infants. Over half of these patients were diagnosed before they were 1 year of age. Other pediatric urologists report an accrual rate of two to eight cases a year in busy pediatric urologic practices.

When first using the voiding cystourethrogram systematically to investigate children with urologic problems, Kjellberg et al found valves in 52 of 1461 patients studied by cystourethrography. They established the modern radiographic criteria for the diagnosis with this study. As cystourethrography came into clinical use, the diagnosis of valves was made more frequently and on more objective grounds than had been possible using urethroscopy alone.

In general, valves seem about as common as multicystic kidney, and have a probable incidence of 1 in 5000 to 8000 boys. Anterior urethral valves are about eight times less common, with a probable incidence of 1 in 40,000.

Pathophysiology

Histologically, both type I and type III valves are thick or thin membranes covered

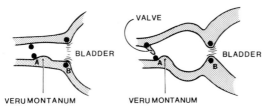

Figure 16–133. The pathophysiology of valvular obstruction. See text for description. *A* represents the valve and *B* the vesical neck. The left figure depicts the normal condition and the right depicts valvular obstruction.

on both sides with transitional epithelium. The epithelial lining may be ulcerated by inflammation or infection. The valves are probably thick folds or diaphragms of mucous membrane initially that become stretched and thinner as they obstruct urinary flow (Fig. 16–133). The intervening stroma consists of fibrous tissue combined with some elastic tissue and fibers of smooth or striated muscle. The stroma is often edematous and infiltrated with round cells. Several observers have noted increased amounts of elastic tissue in the urethral wall adjacent to the valves.

All pathologic consequences follow from the location and severity of the obstruction. When severe, the valves can be thought of as a rigid membrane obstructing urine egress. The proximal urethra dilates and elongates. The detrusor must perform extra work, resulting in bladder thickening, manifested by trabeculation, cellules, and eventually diverticula. The bladder neck, a part of the detrusor, also hypertrophies and shifts the internal urethral meatus ventrally, producing the characteristic posterior lip and the appearance of a "bladder neck contracture" (Fig. 16–134). In some instances the vesical neck will dilate and become incompetent, however. The thickened bladder also produces hydroureteronephrosis. If primary reflux is present owing to short intravesical ureters, the degree of reflux is worsened by the obstruction. Paraureteral diverticula may also result in reflux, even when the intravesical ureters were potentially normal from a developmental viewpoint.

Severe obstruction causing intrauterine hydronephrosis may be associated with renal parenchymal damage during development of the metanephros — the permanent kidney — and result in renal dysplasia, microcystic disease, and/or interstitial nephritis.

Dysplasia is most common in conjunction with reflux. Osathanondh and Potter believe that dysplasia is usually a consequence of urinary obstruction. However, in most experi-

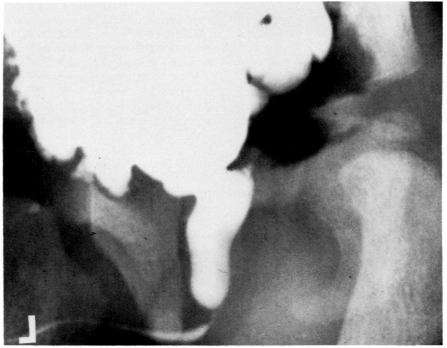

Figure 16–134. Voiding cystourethrogram of 4-month-old infant, showing type I posterior urethral valves. Note the indentations at the bladder neck, which are caused by secondary hypertrophy.

mental animals fetal urethral obstruction early in gestation leads to a patent urachus, without hydronephrosis or dysplasia, which does not seem to correspond to the picture in obstructed human newborns. Later in gestation, experimental ureteral obstruction results in hydronephrosis but not dysplasia. In addition, dysplasia is often unilateral, rather than bilateral as one would expect if it resulted from fetal urethral obstruction. Kaplan cited a newborn with valves and massive bilateral hydronephrosis. There was unilateral reflux only. The kidney on the refluxing side was dysplastic, whereas the nonrefluxing side, on biopsy, showed changes compatible with hydronephrosis but without dysplasia. This combination is frequent enough to be considered one of the syndromes seen with urethral valves. Stephens (1983) believes that dysgenesis is the result of a primary ureteral bud anomaly. The bud arising from the wolffian duct medial to the usual site reaches the metanephric blastema only tangentially, and fails to induce a normal kidney. The abnormal bud site also results in a lateral ureteral orifice, with reflux, but this is a coincident though related abnormality. The reflux of urine is not thought itself to cause the dysgenesis, which has occurred before urine formation and possible reflux begins. Kaplan also reported a child with exstrophy, with a dilated ureteral orifice and a dysplastic kidney above. Obviously, there was no obstructive component that might have been responsible for the renal dysgenesis in this instance.

Boys with valves with the most severe degrees of obstruction are diagnosed in early infancy because of inability to void at all, or, more commonly, because of a palpable bladder or kidneys. Rattner et al found histologic evidence of renal dysplasia in 10 of 21 such infants. Cendron et al, on the other hand, rarely encountered dysgenesis in valve patients. Bernstein's was an autopsy series (Rattner et al), whereas Cendron reviewed clinical cases, which probably accounts for the difference. Duckett found dysplasia, eventually, in 5 of 27 neonates with valves treated initially by vesicostomy. Thus, the incidence of renal dysplasia in boys with severe valvular obstruction, diagnosed in early infancy, would seem to be about 15 to 20 per cent. Such patients rapidly outgrow their fixed renal function and are not helped for long by any therapy except dialysis and transplantation.

On balance it seems most likely that dys-plasia results from a primary anomaly of the ureteral bud and metanephros that is sometimes associated with urethral valves but not actually caused by the urethral obstruction per se. Harrison, particularly, is putting this theory to the test by decompressing some fetuses with valvular obstruction in utero, hoping to prevent dysgenesis or extreme renal damage from hydronephrosis.

In Utero Diagnosis and Treatment

With the advent of ultrasonography it has become quite feasible to make the presumptive diagnosis of obstructive uropathies in the fetus. Since the fetus with a severly obstructed bladder makes less urine than normal, the indication for the examination is often oligohydramnios—a uterus that is small for gestational age. When the baby's bladder is seen to be distended the sonogram is repeated to see if the bladder will empty. If the bladder is always distended, urethral valves become the presumptive diagnosis.

Harrison and coworkers have done pioneering research on the means to prevent abortion after fetal surgery. Nonetheless, at this writing, fetal surgery is still definitely best regarded as experimental. It seems, however that some role will be found for in utero intervention in the treatment of valves, since methods have been worked out for successful surgical intervention. A compelling reason for such decompression is also to prevent the pulmonary hypoplasia and respiratory distress syndrome, which is often encountered even in babies born at term when there is associated oligohydramnios. Harrison has reported bilateral ureterostomies draining the urine into the amniotic sac in a 20 week fetus. Since the metanephros does not excrete urine until about the fourteenth or fifteenth week of gestation, it seems unlikely that the diagnosis of valves will be made much earlier. The ureterostomies drained well and the fetus was carried nearly to term, but the baby's renal function was inadequate to sustain life.

Another method of decompression of the fetal urinary tract is to place a sort of miniature double J catheter in the bladder, or the dilated kidneys, by percutaneous puncture. The other end of the stent is left to drain into the amniotic fluid. This is a much simpler procedure, and is therefore an attractive alternative to open fetal ureterostomy or vesicostomy. At present, the prognosis seems poorest when oligohydramnios is profound. In a few treated cases only, poor renal function has resulted even after in utero relief of obstruction.

All fetuses with constantly dilated bladders may not, however, have extreme degrees of obstruction. There is a spectrum in severity even when the valves cause residual urine and in utero hydronephrosis just as there is after birth. Early delivery to treat such babies has not been a success because of the severity of the associated pulmonary hypoplasia. The degree of oligohydramnios may be an index of the degree of obstruction. Thus, when valves are discovered by serendipity — that is, when oligohydramnios is not the reason for the maternal ultrasound — fetal renal function is probably potentially better. These fetuses are probably best managed by prompt treatment — valve resection, vesicostomy, or supravesical tubeless diversion — at birth, or by the percutaneous insertion of fetal catheters, as described above. A minority of obstructed fetuses have associated moderate oligohydramnios, and these may potentially benefit the most from in utero decompression, since the kidneys make some urine and are presumably less severely damaged than when oligohydramnios is profound. This group constituted only 3 of 28 fetuses evaluated by Harrison with the presumptive diagnosis of valves. In 15, the degree of oligohydramnios was severe, and renal function remained markedly impaired even after relief of obstruction in utero or immediately after birth.

Tests are being developed to estimate the renal function of the fetus. These include percutaneous aspiration of the fetal bladder to permit the rate of refilling to be estimated, the response of the fetal kidney to furosemide, and fetal cystography. Reflux is common in premature infants, and cystography will often therefore permit visualization of the kidneys. Since renal dysplasia is unusual in the absence of reflux even in babies with severe congenital obstruction, lack of reflux should be a good prognostic sign.

Today fetal intervention is limited to a few centers where the obstetric, sonographic, surgical, and neonatal services have made a commitment to study and evaluate the risks and benefits of fetal intervention. This approach is reasonable since, for one thing, all fetal anomalies that can be diagnosed do not necessarily need to be treated, especially before birth. Urethral valves, however, do represent a lesion that is not infrequently lethal in the neonate, and intrauterine decompression of the urinary tract offers an attractive potential method for limiting the degree of renal damage. Increasing the volume of amniotic fluid also should reduce the problems resulting from pulmonary immaturity.

Mode of Presentation

Ultrasonic examination of the fetus near term is becoming widespread, and this is resulting in earlier diagnosis and reducing the age at which valves are diagnosed. In general, after birth, boys with the worst degrees of obstruction present the earliest, occasionally with inability to void at all. Voiding normally occurs the first day after birth, but about 3 per cent of babies wait for 48 hours to initiate urination. Other young infants present because of a thickened palpable bladder that remains firm and hard even after voiding, or with flank masses that are hydronephrotic kidneys. Both multicystic kidney and ureteropelvic junction obstruction are more common causes of flank masses in the newborn, but hydroureteronephrosis is a close third.

Urinary ascites is not an infrequent mode of presentation in the neonatal period. A healthy-appearing baby becomes progressively obtunded in the first few days of life, and fails to eat well. The diagnosis is sometimes confusing unless frank ascites is suspected, because the urinary ascites seems to decompress the kidneys, and not much hydronephrosis may be detected by ultrasound or seen on an excretory urogram. Such decompression often seems to protect kidney function somewhat; the degree of renal damage is often less than one would expect given the severity of the bladder changes. Reflux is usually present also.

The site of the urinary leak is often difficult to localize. A few cases in which a bladder diverticulum ruptured intraperitoneally have been reported. More commonly, the urine reaches the peritoneum as a transudate through the posterior parietal peritoneum. The site of the urinary extravasation is from the renal fornices in most cases, but the leak may be diffuse and like a transudate in that no frank rupture of the collecting system may be demonstrable.

The diagnosis of ascites is usually made on clinical grounds and is confirmed by a plain x-ray of the abdomen that shows the bowel

Table 16–14. Rate of Incidence of Presenting Symptoms at Various Ages in Patients with Posterior Urethral Valves

Presenting Symptom	Rate of Incidence (Per Cent)*		
	Infants	*Toddlers*	*Children or Adults*
Urinary Symptoms			
Decreased stream	0 to 12	10 to 23	4 to 32
Distended bladder	47 to 70	42 to 64	9 to 43
Dribbling	0 to 20	3 to 23	2 to 48
Enuresis	—	3	23
Hematuria	0 to 8	3 to 14	2 to 10
Hesitancy	13	23	32
Infection	13 to 18	13 to 70	15 to 39
Palpable kidney	54	—	—
Renal failure	33	—	—
Retention	3 to 27	5 to 36	5 to 7
Urinary extravasation	1	—	—
Nonurinary Symptoms			
Abdominal distention	40	19 to 30	4
Abdominal pain	—	9	—
Anemia	—	1	—
Constipation	—	—	5
Diarrhea	2 to 3	—	—
Dystocia	3	—	—
Edema	—	1 to 2	—
Failure to thrive	35	50	5
Fever of unknown origin	—	26	—
Hypertension	—	8	—
Irritability	—	6	—
Jaundice	1	—	—
Microcephaly	33	—	—
Rectal prolapse	—	1	—
Respiratory distress	4	—	—
Seizures	6	—	—
Vomiting	33	20 to 54	4

* These figures are gleaned from several series in the literature and consequently represent approximations, at best.

"floating" in the central abdomen. Urinary ascites is confirmed by finding that an aspirate of the peritoneal fluid has a higher creatinine level than the serum, or by doing a voiding cystourethrogram that demonstrates the valves. Occasionally, the urine is confined in the retroperitoneum as a localized "spontaneous" urinoma. Also, a minority of infants with urinary ascites will have a sympathetic pleural effusion, or urine may be transported into the pleural cavity by transudation or a direct leak.

The mechanism of urinary ascites in infants with valves is not well understood. When the ureter is obstructed, some urine formation continues. If the urine can find no egress, this urine is ordinarily absorbed by the renal lymphatics, and in general nontraumatic rupture of the obstructed renal segment does not occur unless the lymphatics are also blocked, as by a diffuse retroperitoneal malignancy. Immaturity of the renal lymphatics is therefore an obvious, but unproven, mechanism that may lead to the sort of diffuse urinary leaking from the thinnest portion of the collecting system, observed in most cases of urinary ascites.

When these obvious and suggestive physical findings are absent, the infant may present with fever (urinary tract infection), anemia, failure to thrive, or even weight loss, seizures, jaundice, or hemorrhagic diathesis, as detailed in Table 16–14, resulting from superimposed infection or renal failure. Vomiting and diarrhea may be symptoms of renal failure alone or of infection. Respiratory distress, sometimes with spontaneous pneumothorax or mediastinal air, is an occasional symptom of otherwise unsuspected valves in newborn infants. One should be suspicious of valves or other severe renal anomalies in any full-term boy with respiratory distress syndrome.

As azotemia and renal failure progress, dehydration and electrolyte imbalances occur. Infants may develop dysphagia secondary to a dry and fissured tongue. Hypertension may be present, and indeed may be the cause of seizures, but these symptoms are otherwise nonspecific.

Valves account for a little over one third of the infants who present with azotemia. One must remember that a normal serum creatinine in a term infant is on the order of 0.1 to 0.4 mg/dl. A serum creatinine over 0.8 mg/dl is definitely elevated, and a cause should be sought.

Urethral valves may also present as neonatal hematuria, because the trauma of delivery may cause bleeding from the hydronephrotic upper tracts. This is a somewhat more common mode of presentation in older boys, who may bleed from a hypertrophied bladder and may not even exhibit hydronephrosis. As a general rule, the older the boy with valves at the time of presentation, the less severe the obstruction is likely to be. Though boys over age 6 may present with infection, many are diagnosed during the evaluation of diurnal enuresis. The stream may be diminished, but since this is "normal" for the patient he will not remark it. These patients have, as a rule, little or no hydronephrosis, no reflux, and good renal function, so that the prognosis is far different from the prototype case we have discussed in which significant renal damage has occurred in utero. As Hendren has emphasized, most diseases have a spectrum of severity. Valves are an excellent example of this dictum, having been discovered in octogenarians without renal damage.

Older infants and toddlers with valves do not present with urinary ascites, and are much less apt to have palpable kidneys. They commonly present with urinary infection, a palpable bladder, poor stream, or, occasionally, renal rickets. However, young boys with valves may exhibit a reasonably good urinary stream as long as the bladder is compensated, so this sign is inconsistent. Many children with hydronephrosis present with hematuria, and this is a common presenting complaint in valve patients also. Straining to void may be noticed by the parents, and may also result in rectal prolapse. Campbell, particularly, thought this a common mode of presentation and noted that the children strain so hard to void that their faces turned purple. Severe straining may also be associated with inguinal hernias.

Any child with a fever of unknown origin needs a urinalysis, and almost all authors seem agreed that boys merit radiologic investigation of the urinary tract after a first infection.

The older child with valves usually manifests fewer signs and symptoms, and presents chiefly with urinary infection or diurnal enuresis. Valves in these older boys may not produce much obstruction, and they may lack the characteristic configuration of the posterior urethra that is the hallmark of urethral valves in younger patients.

Laboratory Studies

No laboratory study is specifically indicative of urethral valves, but many findings of routine studies may direct attention to the severely damaged or obstructed urinary tract. Chief among these are elevation of the blood or serum urea nitrogen and serum creatinine, anemia, proteinurea, hematuria, and urinary tract infection.

Since the fetus is dialyzed through the placenta, urea and creatinine levels are normal at birth. They may rise quickly after delivery, calling attention to abnormal kidney function, but most babies with valves who are diagnosed as neonates have palpable flank masses — the kidneys — or a thickened palpable bladder and are already suspect. Older children, with lesser degrees of obstruction, occasionally present because of the laboratory detection of azotemia, however. Kaplan states that 8 to 10 per cent of boys with valves have anemia, but, again, this is an unusual mode of presentation.

In the infant blood gases may be useful in assessment of the exact metabolic status. Sullivan et al have pointed out that in infants the usual serum urea/creatinine ratio is about 10.8 to 1. In two cases of urinary ascites the urea/creatinine ratio was 31 to 1. This finding is associated with hyperchloremic acidosis and abdominal distention. The high urea/creatinine ratio then suggests urinary ascites as the immediate cause of the distention.

Many have suggested that a presumptive diagnosis of urinary ascites can be confirmed by chemical examination of the ascitic fluid and comparison with serum and urine. Although urea and creatinine levels in the ascitic fluid are usually higher than serum concentrations, they are usually much lower than those in the urine. The reason is that the peritoneum acts as a dializing membrane and there is near equilibrium of urea and creatinine between the serum and peritoneal cavity. The peritoneum may secrete a proteinaceous exudate, so the protein content of the ascitic

POSTERIOR URETHRA ☐ 539

fluid is often higher than that in the urine with peritonitis of almost any cause. Furthermore, in boys with severe obstruction, urea and creatinine concentration in the urine is impaired. The urinary ascitic fluid may therefore come into equilibrium with the serum quickly, and the resulting differences in the levels of these waste products are sometimes minimal.

Urinary ascites must therefore be a diagnostic consideration in any obtunded young infant, particularly any male with frank ascites that lacks another obvious cause. Recovery of vital dyes that are excreted in the urine, such as indigo carmine, from the ascitic fluid cannot be assumed, as impaired renal function may prevent enough concentration in the urine for easy detection after further dilution with peritoneal transudate.

Once the possibility of urinary ascites comes to mind, the presence of severe obstruction of the urinary tract is most easily established by a voiding cystourethrogram, which will demonstrate valves in most such infants, or by a renal scan, which will reveal impaired function, hydronephrosis, and gradual accumulation of radioactivity in the ascitic fluid.

Excretory urography is of limited value in the neonate. The kidneys at birth are immature, and contrast material may not be concentrated well enough to image the collecting system adequately. This is especially likely when renal function is further impaired by obstruction. However, if reflux is present, as it is in about 50 per cent of neonatal kidneys obstructed by valves, the upper tracts are visualized on the cystogram.

Overall, urinalysis is abnormal in about 60 per cent of boys with valves. Proteinurea alone is uncommon, but does occur. Most, at least 40 per cent, present with urinary infection or fever of unknown origin that is eventually traced to urinary infection. Half of these patients are chemically azotemic at the time of diagnosis, and renal damage may be severe enough that metabolic acidosis is a prominent feature of their illness.

Voiding Cystourethrogram

As noted earlier in this article, urethral valves were reported relatively infrequently for a long time after Young's initial description. In retrospect, the reason for this omission seems clear. Endoscopically the most striking finding in children with valves is usually bladder thickening and trabeculation with hypertrophy of the posterior bladder neck. The appearance of the detrusor in the absence of an overt neurologic problem indicates that obstruction is present. The elevation of the bladder neck is usually much more striking and easily appreciated than the valve itself, which indeed may not be clearly seen until the resectoscope loop is used to elevate the valve leaflets, or the filled bladder is forcibly expressed. Mainly for this reason, the primary obstruction was often mistakenly placed at the bladder neck on endoscopic grounds. To compound this problem, in an era when reflux was also thought usually to be secondary to bladder outlet obstruction, was the possibility that the valves would be accidentally disrupted at endoscopy, or eroded by an indwelling urethral catheter, often inserted at the time of bladder neck enlargement. The resulting confusion, and the occasional dramatic improvement after bladder neck revision, retarded the detection of valves even in most pediatric centers.

This unsatisfactory state of affairs persisted until voiding cystourethrography was reintroduced on a widespread clinical basis to detect and study reflux. Kjellberg et al emphasized the importance of voiding films in the detection of valves as well as reflux. They reported 52 boys with valves, including three sets of twins, and one other pair of brothers. Twenty-seven had hydronephrosis and 16 exhibited reflux. Nineteen of the children were over age 8 at the time of diagnosis, but the more severe cases of obstruction were found in those who presented earlier. Most importantly, Kjellberg et al illustrated the typical radiographic appearance of valves very convincingly, and made the point that the "bladder neck contracture," appearing as a posterior lip on the lateral voiding films, was secondary to more distal obstruction. The prostatic urethra was also dilated and elongated, which makes the bladder neck appear narrower than it really is. As cystourethrography has come into general use, the mystique involving the diagnosis of valves has largely disappeared, and treatment has come to be directed primarily to the valve rather than the bladder neck.

Cystourethrography should be performed in male infants and children with low abdominal or flank masses or after a first infection, because valves are a likely cause of obstruction. Older boys presenting with diurnal enuresis or even bedwetting alone will occasionally be found to have valves, and deciding who among this older and larger group should be selected for radiographic and cystoscopic evaluation is truly one of the arts that the urologist must master.

Before describing interpretation of the voiding cystourethrogram, it is helpful to review the normal radiologic appearance of the male urethra in boys seen in an oblique or lateral view. The bladder neck is usually clearly defined. There is often a posterior "lip" that persists through most of voiding, though this is not the rule. This seems usually the result of incomplete relaxation of the internal sphincter due to apprehension and the anomalous circumstances of voiding on the x-ray table, and is seldom in itself significant. The verumontanum is usually readily apparent as an oval filling defect less than 1 cm in length just below the bladder neck. The utricle may be visualized in the center of the verumontanum, and the plicae colliculi may occasionally be seen running from the verumontanum to the lateral urethral walls somewhat more distally.

The muscle of the urogenital diaphragm may indent the urethra distal to the verumontanum, often giving the appearance of a double concentric narrowing. Contraction of the external sphincter will cause some relative dilatation of the more proximal urethra.

Typical posterior urethral valves present quite a different appearance. The valve—type I or type III—may itself be seen as a filling defect in the contrast column in the urethra (Fig. 16–135).

The posterior urethra is dilated, and also elongated (Fig. 16–136). The stream is usually diminished distal to the valve, but this is not always the case. The dilated urethra undermines the bladder neck and the resulting "posterior lip" is very prominent. The bladder is trabeculated and is often elongated also. Cellules, if not frank diverticula, are the rule. About 45 to 50 per cent of all valve patients reflux (Fig. 16–137), and hydronephrosis and hydroureter are often severe in degree. When severe obstruction is present, this appearance is consistent throughout voiding. Dilatation of the posterior urethra can normally occur to some extent when the external sphincter closes during voiding. The key differential point is the elongation of the posterior urethra behind a valve—the verumontanum is much more distal in position when a valve is present.

Cystourethrography is usually safely and easily carried out by passing a urethral cath-

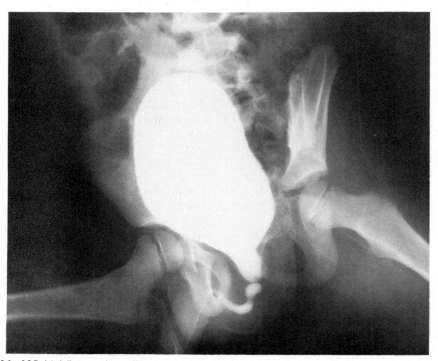

Figure 16–135. Voiding cystourethrogram, showing type III posterior urethral valves in a 4-year-old.

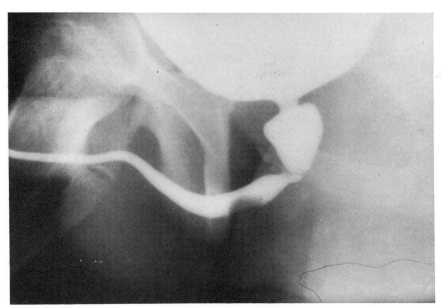

Figure 16–136. Voiding cystourethrogram in a boy with mild obstruction due to type I valves. The urethrogram also reveals a Cowper's duct cyst, seen as the filling defect on the floor of the bulbous urethra.

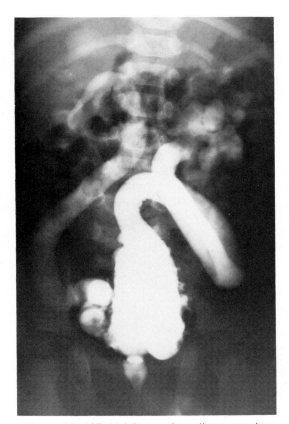

Figure 16–137. Voiding cystourethrogram demonstrating severe vesicoureteral reflux associated with type I valves. Half of valve patients reflux; the incidence is about 80 per cent in infants.

eter, measuring the volume present, obtaining a urine specimen, and filling the bladder with contrast material by gravity drip. The catheter is quickly removed when voiding begins, and films are made in a lateral or steep oblique position. Anteroposterior films may be difficult to interpret. Alternately, the bladder can be filled with contrast material by suprapubic puncture.

The cusps of type I valves lie more or less flat against the walls of the urethra except during voiding, and do not resist passage of a catheter. Type III valves have a more central opening that is fixed and may be difficult to enter or too small, in absolute terms, for the catheter. Thus, inability to pass a catheter suggests a type III valve or a stricture. In this situation a retrograde urethrogram may be helpful, particularly if the obstruction is distal to the urogenital diaphragm. The posterior urethra usually does not fill well enough for diagnostic purposes on a retrograde study, however, and an antegrade cystogram then becomes necessary. Alternately, if renal function is good, contrast material may fill the bladder well enough after an excretory urogram to permit a voiding film at the end of that study. Such studies are often not clear and sharp, but they may be adequate to exclude a valve from diagnostic consideration. The excretory urogram may, of course, itself suggest the presence of a valve when hydrouptereronephrosis is present or concentration of the contrast material is very poor.

Differential Diagnosis

The chief causes of dilatation of the posterior urethra on voiding cystourethrogram, aside from valves, are external sphincter dyssynergia, abnormal prostatic stroma as in the prune-belly syndrome, polyp of the verumontanum, and neurogenic bladder in some boys in whom the bladder neck is incompetent and widely dilated. The typical appearances of the urethra on voiding films in these conditions are illustrated in the appropriate chapters. One must emphasize, however, that external sphincter dyssynergia, a failure of the external sphincter to relax during voiding, is a urodynamic and not an x-ray diagnosis. The external sphincter may contract consistently during voiding without causing much dilatation of the prostatic urethra. More commonly,

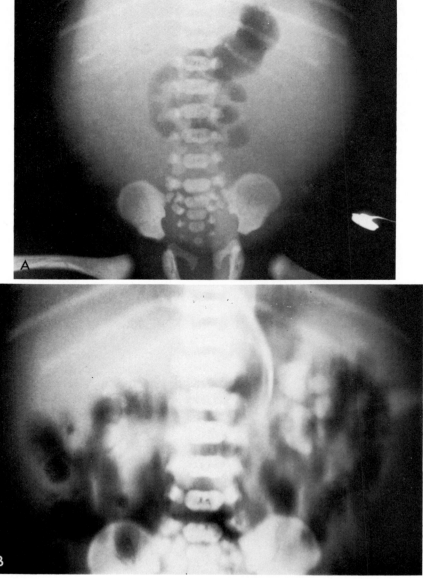

Figure 16–138. *A,* Urinary ascites at birth in a boy who had been found to have this condition in utero. Note the characteristic bulging of the flanks. The air-filled bowel is ''floating'' and is shifted toward the midline by the ascitic fluid. *B,* Infants with neonatal urinary ascites often retain better kidney function than would be expected, considering the severity of the obstruction. The collecting system leak may decompress the kidney sufficiently to protect renal function to some degree.

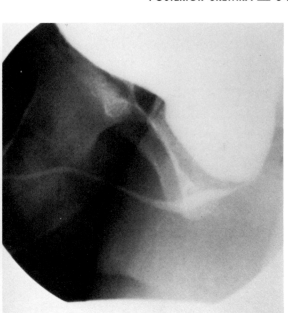

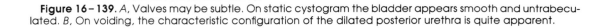

Figure 16–139. *A,* Valves may be subtle. On static cystogram the bladder appears smooth and untrabecu-lated. *B,* On voiding, the characteristic configuration of the dilated posterior urethra is quite apparent.

the appearance of a dilated posterior urethra is probably due to anxiety provoked by the test situation, and incomplete sphincter relaxation is therefore not necessarily a sign of clinically significant dyssynergia.

In the prune-belly syndrome, the musculature of the prostate is deficient, and the muscle fibers that are present are more widely separated than normal. The posterior urethra is also wide. On voiding films, the prostatic urethra is dilated, though the posterior urethra usually appears globular or spherical and not as elongated as when severe valvular obstruction is present. The redundancy of the posterior urethra in these patients may cause obstruction, but the syndrome is only rarely associated with valves of the type discussed in this chapter. Occasionally, one will encounter a boy without any other stigmata of the prune-belly syndrome in whom the urinary tract and posterior urethra suggest this diagnosis (Fig. 16–138). Idiopathic dilatation of the posterior urethra may also be seen in boys without any other urologic anomaly. In these cases the posterior urethra usually appears more globular than elongated, but cystoscopy is often warranted in these instances to be certain that a valve is not present.

Alternately, there are boys with real valves —type I or type III—in whom the radiographic appearance of the urethra on the voiding cystourethrogram is frankly misleading (Fig. 16–139). These present after attempted toilet training is unsuccessful or as late as adolescence. The usual symptom is daytime wetting, but urinary infection or nocturnal enuresis alone may be the only complaint. A trial of therapy for wetting is unsuccessful, leading to cystographic evaluation. Even then, the urethra may appear normal or nearly so, and the valve is discovered only at cystoscopy that is done because all other therapeutic manuevers have failed. These valves may be quite striking at urethroscopy even though they are not apparent, even in retrospect, in good quality voiding films (Fig. 16–140).

This produces a dilemma. Valves are certainly a rare cause of enuresis alone, and an unusual cause of diurnal enuresis (Fig. 16–141), which is much more likely to be due to inappropriate bladder contractures and/or sphincter dyssynergia. Yet a careful cystoscopy may eventually become warranted when these conditions do not respond to medical therapy.

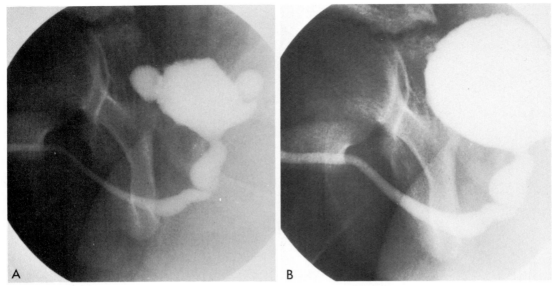

Figure 16-140. Valves may be atypical in their appearance on voiding cystourethrogram (VCUG). *A,* VCUG in a 10-year-old presenting with diurnal enuresis. The posterior urethra is somewhat dilated, but the appearance is not typical. *B,* The VCUG following valve resection shows resolution of the bladder diverticula, but some dilatation of the posterior persists, as it does in 20 to 25 per cent of patients. The wetting stopped promptly.

Management of Urethral Valves

Once the diagnosis is made, further management is determined by the overall condition of the patient. In older boys who are healthy and uninfected and have good renal

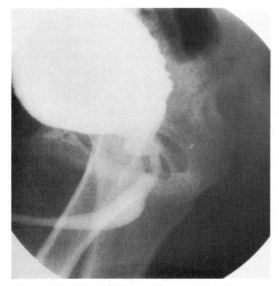

Figure 16-141. VCUG in a 12-year-old with persistent diurnal enuresis. The picture is not diagnostic, but the valve was an absolutely typical type I valve. The boy became dry for the first time 2 days after resection.

function, simple resection of the valves is the preferred method of treatment, and the only therapy necessary.

All patients should eventually have a postoperative cystogram, usually 6 to 12 weeks after surgery, to prove that the valve has been adequately resected.

At the other extreme is the infant with severe obstruction, increasing azotemia, and acidosis. Infection may be superimposed. In this situation, the first consideration is resuscitation. A feeding tube is placed in the bladder through the urethra to serve as a catheter, and correction of dehydration and acidosis is begun. During this period the infant should be carefully monitored in an intensive care setting, or transferred to a pediatric tertiary care facility by helicopter or mobile intensive care van.

Dehydration is reflected in sunken fontanelles, dry mucous membranes, and reduced skin elasticity. By the time these signs are apparent, there is a 6 to 10 per cent loss of body weight. Further dehydration results in a pale, apathetic, inert infant with poor muscle tone, abdominal distention, and slight cyanosis. The skin becomes wrinkled, and after loss of 15 per cent of body water shock may supervene, with hypotension, stupor, and cyanotic blotchy skin.

When infection is also present, sepsis may

further compound these diagnostic and therapeutic problems.

Azotemia may or may not be significant and depends upon the age of the infant since the waste products begin to accumulate only after placental separation. The hematocrit may be of some value in assessing the level of dehydration, but since infants have high hematocrit levels clinical evaluation is usually more accurate.

Fluid Management

If the infant is in shock, colloidal volume expanders should be given rapidly in a dose of 20 ml/kg body weight. If dehydration is less severe, fluid replacement can be more gradual, usually over a 24 hour period. In addition, maintenance fluid should be given using 100 ml/kg per day of 0.2 per cent normal saline in 5 per cent dextrose. If the dehydration is hypotonic, as determined by serum osmolality, fluid replacement can be more rapid. If dehydration has resulted in hyperosmolality, one might consider dialysis for replacement since the rapid administration of relatively hypotonic solutions may cause convulsions and brain damage.

Electrolyte Replacement

If electrolyte imbalances are present, one should correct sodium, chloride, and bicarbonate deficits while rehydrating the infant. The amount of replacement is calculated on the basis of the child's weight, assuming that these electrolytes are evenly distributed in total body water, which accounts for about 70 per cent of body weight. One half to two thirds of the calculated electrolyte deficit is given over about 12 hours, and the electrolyte status is then rechecked. Hyperkalemia is often a threat, although infants tolerate higher levels of serum potassium than adults without electrocardiographic changes. Infants with normal potassium levels need some potassium with their maintenance fluids. Dosages should be guided principally by the electrocardiographic findings. Hyperkalemia will often improve as hyponatremia is corrected. If elevated potassium levels persist, 1 to 3 g of Kayexalate may be administered by nasogastric tube or enema every 6 to 8 hours.

Drainage

A child who is not infected but azotemic and not in electrolyte imbalance needs no preoperative drainage. An indwelling catheter may introduce infection and necessitate catheter drainage in the postoperative period to avoid sepsis.

On the other hand, infected children and those with dehydration and acidosis require careful preoperative stabilization, as discussed above. This usually necessitates a period of catheter drainage while the appropriate intravenous therapy and antibiotics are administered. A urethral catheter will usually suffice for a few days, using a 5 F feeding tube in infants, and positioning the catheter carefully to optimize bladder emptying.

Suprapubic catheters may be employed if the urethral catheter falls out or cannot be maintained in optimal position. In this situation, a percutaneous suprapubic tube, such as the Stamey or Cystocath system, is usually preferable to formal cystostomy and obviates the need for an extra anesthetic in a sick infant. The presence of the suprapubic tube makes it difficult or impossible to eradicate infection, and the suprapubic tube should be seen as a tenuous solution employed until the child can be stabilized and the valve resected. Long-term catheter drainage or tubed cystostomy may lead to contracture of the hypertrophied bladder as well as continued infection.

There are several other considerations appropriate in infants who are already septic or who respond slowly or poorly to bladder level drainage. Chief among these is the possibility that the dilated ureters, often aperistaltic because of their width and the consequent inability of the walls to coapt, are producing functional obstruction. Additionally, bacterial exotoxins may paralyze the ureteral musculature, or the ureters may be partially obstructed as they pass through the thickened bladder wall. In this situation, renal level diversion becomes attractive, as this will optimize urinary drainage, minimize residual, and allow infection to be more effectively treated if residual urine is the factor permitting the infection to persist. Also, upper tract drainage, by removing any downstream impediment to urinary flow and neutralizing any effect of reflux, will allow the kidneys to recover to a maximal degree.

Percutaneous nephrostomies or pyelostomies can often be inserted using fluoroscopic or ultrasonic guidance with minimal difficulty. However, since such catheters are tenuous at best, they can usually be maintained for only a few days to a few weeks. They create a risk of infection, but they can provide a margin of safety over the short period needed for valve ablation, and are finding a place in the management of sick infants.

Cutaneous pyelostomy or high loop ureterostomy, or one of its variations, is usually a more attractive option when the infant is sick or remains septic. These operations are described in Chapter 17. Kidney biopsies may be obtained at the time of surgery for prognostic guidance. Kruger et al have reviewed the growth and eventual renal function achieved by young infants who were treated by primary valve resection and primary high diversion, usually by loop ureterostomy. The infants with better renal function at the time of presentation tended to be treated by valve resection alone, while those with more severe degrees of azotemia, sepsis, or frank uremia generally underwent high diversion. Two to 20 years later, these groups had reversed themselves in terms of renal function and somatic growth. Those treated primarily with loop ureterostomies had to undergo subsequent valve resection and reconstruction, or permanent diversion, yet exhibited better growth and renal function, as a group, than those in whom only resection of the valve was performed.

This experience establishes the safety of high diversion, but should not be as generalized to conclude that primary valve resection is unduly hazardous in all infants. The study was retrospective, and truly miniaturized fiberoptic equipment was available only in the last 5 years covered by the review. Some valves were surely not resected at the first attempt. Also, even after successful resection urinary infection would have been much more likely in those who underwent resection than in those who underwent diversion. No data are available on these points, but primary resection appears safe in a stable infant without sepsis. If infection supervenes, however, high diversion should be strongly considered as an immediate means of protecting the capacity for potential renal growth.

Other alternatives to loop ureterostomy — the Sober pelviureterostomy, William's ring, and ureteral chimney — are all designed to prevent bladder contracture in that the urinary tract remains intact, vented at the level of the upper ureter, but with some urine passing to the bladder. These procedures have the disadvantage of lengthening the primary operation, which is carried out in a sick infant, and usually need to be bilateral. The use of these variants of loop ureterostomy has declined with the realization that the defunc-

tionalized bladder will almost always re-expand promptly when the upper tract is reconstituted. Lome et al, however, reported on 30 boys treated with loop ureterostomies. After valve resection and reconstruction, half exhibited a normal bladder capacity, 27 per cent showed a temporary reduction only, and 23 per cent exhibited a permanent reduction in expected capacity. Defunctionalization alone cannot account for the reduction in capacity, for as Dahl and others have shown, the normal bladder can be defunctionalized for years yet recover fully and rapidly when the urinary tract is reconstituted. Those with small capacity after refunctionalization have residual bladder wall thickening and fibrosis, and such bladders are generally noncompliant. These bladders may not have functioned well even if temporary diversion were not employed. Be that as it may, a small minority of infants who undergo high diversion will need some type of cystoplasty before their reconstructed urinary tract becomes completely functional.

Duckett and others have shown that cutaneous vesicostomy is useful in babies with valves deemed too ill or too small for primary resection. Twenty-two of 27 infants survived, and the deaths were attributable, at least in part, to associated renal dysgenesis. My own preference is for cutaneous pyelostomy when the pelves are large enough to reach the skin easily. If they are not, high loop ureterostomy, as popularized by Johnson, will also optimalize drainage and reduce residual urine to nil. Reconstruction by ureteropyelostomy is quite reliable and can be carried out on a totally elective basis.

Put another way, if temporary diversion is deemed desirable because of sepsis, urinary ascites, or poor renal function, high diversion is optimal and safest. If diversion is elected because of prematurity, severe concurrent disease in other organ systems, a urethra that is too small to accommodate the required endoscopic equipment, or fear of causing urethral stricture by resection of the valve in an infant, vesicostomy drainage will usually suffice.

Valve Ablation

Removal of the valve, either primarily or after temporary diversion, may pose special problems in infants. The widespread availability of miniature fiberoptic cystoscopes and resectoscopes has mitigated these problems substantially in recent years. However, one should not ever stretch the infant's urethra, because the tissues are very delicate and even slight overdilatation may result in stricture. For this reason, it is still important to review therapeutic alternatives to endoscopic valve resection even though these are no longer often employed in medically sophisticated communities. There is a nonoperative approach that sometimes works. A catheter is simply inserted into the bladder through the urethra and left in place for several weeks. Either the catheter erodes the valve leaflets or mild bacterial activity, induced by the catheter, may destroy the valve. The author has seen two boys who were treated in this way by Michie in the early 1960's. Each had typical type I valves on cystourethrogram, and in each the obstruction was completely and permanently relieved after 3 weeks of catheter drainage. It seems likely that this "erosion treatment" may work when the valve is filmy and thin, but is likely to fail when the valvular tissues are more substantial in consistency. The obvious drawback to this form of treatment is that the long duration of catheter drainage usually results in infection, and the results are inconsistent. However, the observation is interesting, and before the advent of miniature fiberoptic equipment Brandesky, Bischoff, and Singer each individually advocated this approach as less apt to result in stricture or incontinence than valve resection.

Type III valves are occasionally definitively treated and ablated by dilatation. Again, the anterior urethra must first be calibrated with bougies to avoid passing a sound that would traumatize the urethra and result in stricture. A filiform is passed through the obstruction. It must be ascertained that the filiform is coiling in the bladder, not the urethra. Then a tapered LeFort following sound of the largest size that will pass without overdilating the distal urethra — this may be only 10 F — is inserted. An expression urethrogram may be made just afterward, before the child awakens, which will usually indicate whether the obstruction has been successfully dilated or ruptured. If it has not, the chances are that the child has a type I valve, and the operator should then proceed with endoscopy to confirm this assumption. If dilatation is achieved, the obstruction may be relieved temporarily but may still recur. Follow-up cystourethrography is necessary to make certain that this minimal form of therapy has been adequate.

Valves have been treated by excision after open exposure of the posterior urethra, usually employing a symphysiotomy to obtain the exposure needed. This approach is really much too cumbersome and may result in excessive bleeding, poor visualization, and incomplete valve excision or sphincter damage. However, one can visualize the valves directly by inserting an otoscope into the posterior urethra through a perineal urethrostomy. They may then be engaged by a hook electrode, or a bent ureteral catheter stylet protruding slightly from the ureteral catheter. The valve cusps may then be elevated and fulgurated much as one would do if working endoscopically.

In general, even in infants, endoscopic fulguration or resection of the valves is safer and simpler. The urethra is carefully calibrated to ascertain that passage of the cystoscope or resectoscope sheath will not be traumatic. A meatotomy may be performed. If the available instruments are too large, a perineal urethrostomy should be employed. Noe has found that even when the surgeon is conscious of the risk of overdilatation, transurethral valve resection in infants results in stricture in as many as 25 per cent of cases. This emphasizes the need to insert the instrument through the wider posterior urethra by perineal urethrostomy whenever a question of adequate urethral caliber arises. Walker has described strictures after resection via perineal urethrostomy, but these were usually radiographic narrowings of the posterior urethra at the site of the urethrostomy, and not clinically significant strictures. Unstinting use of perineal urethrostomy minimizes the risk of urethral stricture subsequent to valve resection. Occasionally, a stricture may occur at the level of the valve, possibly because of thermal injury to the surrounding tissues, irrespective of the technique employed.

Valves are best visualized through the straight-ahead lens that now accompanies most pediatric resectoscopes and cystoscopes. The valve may be engaged with the loop electrode, a hook electrode, or the angled tip of a ureteral catheter stylet that protrudes slightly from the ureteral catheter that serves to insulate the metal stylet. The ureteral catheter may be passed through the operating channel of a cystoscope, making a miniature resectoscope unnecessary. Alternately, a miniature Bugbee electrode (3 F) may be used to fulgurate the valve cusps.

Whichever instrument is chosen, the next step is to visualize the valve unequivocally. This requires a little practice. Valves must be distinguished from the plicae colliculi, which are normal nonobstructive structures (Fig.

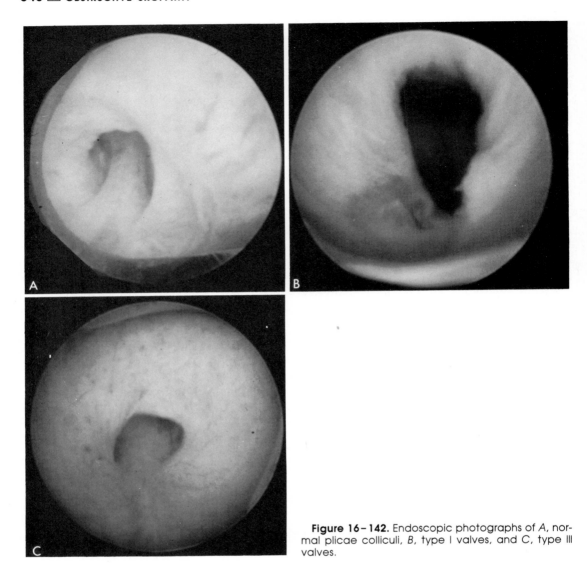

Figure 16–142. Endoscopic photographs of *A*, normal plicae colliculi, *B*, type I valves, and *C*, type III valves.

16–142). The operator must remember that many voiding cystourethrograms may be somewhat misleading when the x-rays are not absolutely typical. Valves will occasionally be encountered in patients with only minimal dilatation of the posterior urethra, and valves may be absent in boys with even marked dilatation, as discussed above. It is necessary to demonstrate the valve endoscopically to confirm its presence. This is usually best done by inspecting the posterior urethra and bladder and looking for objective evidence of obstruction at the outset. The bladder should be trabeculated. Cellules and diverticula are often present. If reflux is also occurring, this is the best time to inspect the orifices to judge whether the reflux may stop after the obstruction is relieved. Virtually all males with severe

obstruction from valves have marked secondary hypertrophy of the bladder neck (Fig. 16–143). This results in an elevated bladder neck, which is readily seen looking into the bladder from the level of the verumontanum. In occasional cases with mild obstruction, however, this secondary bladder neck elevation is absent.

The posterior urethra is also elongated in boys with valves. In normal males prior to puberty, the verumontanum seems to pop up into the urethra just below the bladder neck. In boys with valves, the verumontanum is more distal. When all these secondary signs are present, one is dealing with a valve. The valve itself may still be hard to visualize, however.

The resectoscope should be withdrawn to a

point below the verumontanum, with the utricle kept in view. The unactivated loop or hook electrode is extended and a sweep is made on either side of the verumontanum. In type I valves, the loop will engage the cusps of the valve that lie flat against the wall of the urethra when the water is running into the bladder from the fluid reservoir. Alternatively, one may express the filled bladder to elevate the valve cusps.

After the cusps are visualized, they are elevated with the extended electrode and drawn away from the urethral wall. The cutting current is then activated and the valve cusps are incised or excised. The depth of the cut should extend to, but not into, the urethral wall. In dealing with type I valves the same procedure is repeated on the other side of the verumontanum. Alternately, one can engage the valve at 12 o'clock and resect only in that quadrant. All valves are circumferential, and incision to the depth of the urethral wall at any point is sufficient to relieve obstruction. However, when one is dealing with type I valves it is usually easier to see the posterior cusps near their attachment to the verumontanum, and adequate resection of these structures is more easily ascertained.

Type III valves, which appear more nearly circular, are usually fulgurated or incised at three points to make as certain as possible that the obstruction is relieved.

Bleeding points are lightly fulgurated. If bleeding is minimal and the urine is uninfected, no catheter need be used postopera-

tively. If infection is present, a day or two of catheter drainage is desirable. Similarly, if the resection site remains bloody, a few days of postoperative catheter drainage is preferable to extensive fulguration in the region of the external sphincter.

Postoperatively, the child should be watched closely for postobstructive diuresis, which is rare, and electrolyte imbalance, which is common in infants with severe obstruction. Electrolyte replacement should include maintenance doses of potassium, which can usually be given orally if desired in doses of 0.25 to 0.5 g per day. Antibiotic coverage should be continued for 3 to 5 days and the child should be given an antibacterial, usually a urinary antiseptic like nitrofurantoin, sulfa, or a sulfa-trimethoprim combination for several weeks. Sulfas should not be given to premature infants or to term infants less than 1 month of age.

A postoperative cystogram should be obtained if any complications ensue, or in 8 to 12 weeks to make absolutely certain that the obstruction has been relieved.

A few valves of the female urethra have been reported (Everett and Brack; Nesbit et al; Stephens, 1983). In one of Nesbit's patients the lesion was diagnosed by voiding cystourethrography. He then used a button hook to engage and avulse the valve, or fold, which ran from side to side on the floor of the urethra approximately 1 cm above the meatus. In two of Everett's patients the folds were in the mid-urethra also.

These lesions are rare, and not much is known about them. They are not explained by conventional embryologic theory, and treatment must clearly be individualized. I can recall seeing only one such patient, a female infant, who was diagnosed in utero as probably having valves because the fetal bladder was always distended. It was a great surprise when a female child was born. However, she had a single cusp which looked just like a single leaflet of a type I valve without the verumontanum. The valve was mainly to the left of the midline and was easily resected. Matheson and Ward reported a very masculinized genetic female with adrenogenital syndrome who, at autopsy, was found to have definite prostatic tissue and type I urethral valves. One suspects that some of the "valves" occuring in females are the unrecognized urethral extension of a cecoureterocele left over after incision or perforation of the vesical portion of the ureterocele, or after

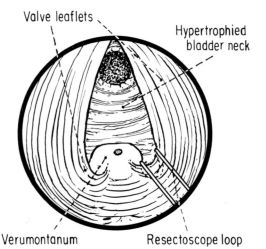

Valve leaflets

Hypertrophied bladder neck

Verumontanum

Resectoscope loop

Figure 16–143. Diagram representing engagement of valve leaflet with resectoscope loop. Note the secondary bladder neck hypertrophy, which is so prominent endoscopically.

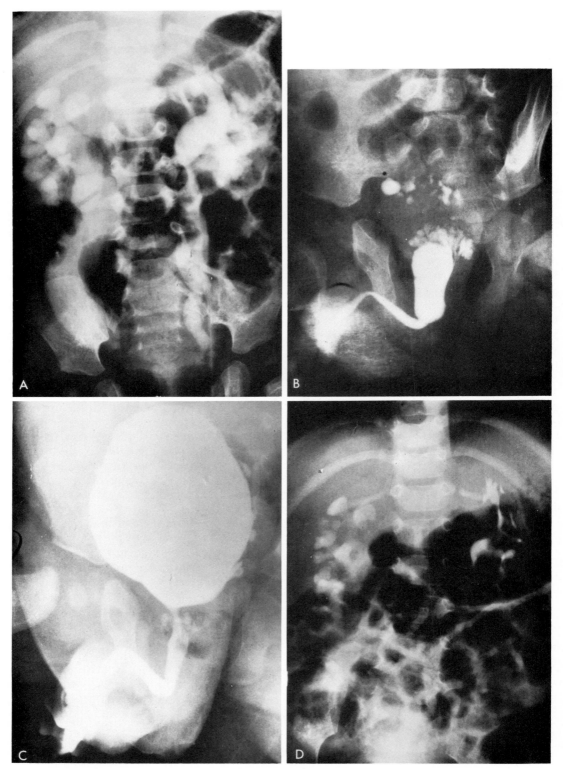

Figure 16–144. Excretory urogram *(A)* and voiding cystourethrogram *(B)* of a 5-month-old azotemic male with recurrent fever and failure to thrive. Posterior urethral valves were destroyed transurethrally. No other surgical treatment was employed. Voiding cystourethrogram at 5 weeks *(C)* and excretory urograms at 6 weeks *(D)*.

Illustration continued on opposite page

spontaneous rupture. The blind urethral extension of a ruptured cecoureterocele fills with urine during voiding and encroaches on the urethra just like a type I valve. Transurethral resection is usually the simplest form of therapy.

Other Problems in the Management of Infants with Severe Valvular Obstruction

The incidence of reflux with valves in boys that present in infancy because of a severe degree of urethral obstruction approaches 80 per cent. When reflux is present, renal dysplasia often limits the renal recovery seen after decompression. This in itself is an argument to treat such patients by high temporary diversion and renal biopsy when renal function is severely impaired or azotemia increases rapidly after birth. Some kidneys never demonstrate measurable function even if cutaneous pyelostomies are performed at 3 or 4 days of age and urinary drainage is optimized after that time. Until a few years ago the survival rate in babies with valves diagnosed in the first month after birth was only 29 to 61 per cent (Ellis et al; Johnson and Kulatilake; Waldbaum and Marshall; Williams). Survival rates are better now, partly because of the antenatal diagnosis of severely obstructing lesions, but mainly because of improvements in neonatal intensive care. Nonetheless, it is estimated that 15 to 30 per cent of boys diagnosed in infancy eventually outgrow their limited and somewhat fixed renal reserve,

and dialysis and transplantation become necessary in childhood or early adolescence.

Using data derived from 30 personal cases, followed as long as 30 years, Lyon has been able to predict with some certainty whether renal failure will occur before full growth is achieved. He has observed that if the serum creatinine falls below 1.0 mg/dl or the BUN below 15 mg/dl after valve resection or diversion, renal function will improve enough to support life even though azotemia may worsen as the boy grows. Conversely, if the creatinine level remains more elevated after successful relief of obstruction, renal failure will occur, usually within a few years, but occasionally not until the patient is fully grown. The usual inability to assess the potential of even the refluxing, obstructed, and often somewhat dysgenetic kidney in even the short term makes it necessary to try to salvage all renal tissue initially. Kidneys that never function significantly may be removed at the time of reconstruction of the urinary tract after high diversion, if reflux persists, or if they became a cause of hypertension.

In boys with reflux that did not require diversion, Williams found that 25 per cent stopped refluxing within a few years after valve ablation. In our own valve patients with reflux, 47 per cent ceased to reflux with time, and presumably with growth of the intravesical ureter (Fig. 16–144).

The results of antireflux surgery are usually better when relatively normal ureters can be reimplanted into a relatively normal bladder than when dilated ureters are reimplanted

Figure 16–144. *Continued. E,* Excretory urogram 18 years postoperatively demonstrates complete recovery anatomically and functionally. Valve resection will often suffice even when the upper tracts are quite dilated, unless infection supervenes. (Courtesy of Professor N. O. Ericsson.)

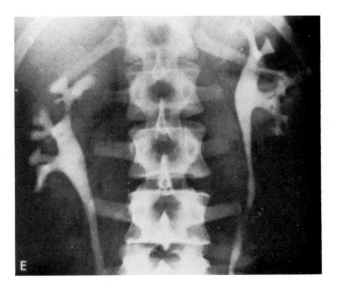

into a thickened trabeculated bladder that has only recently been obstructed. Thus, it is usually preferable to defer operative correction of reflux until the bladder returns to normal, or nearly normal, after valve resection. This may take a year or two. Ureterectasis usually lessens in degree with relief of obstruction, even though reflux may persist. In such circumstances the success rate of the antireflux surgery needed because of persistent reflux can be expected to be about 90 per cent, and perhaps even higher. Conversely, in a relatively small number of boys who underwent valve resection and immediate reimplantation, usually with ureteral tailoring, a 57 per cent initial success rate was the best that we could achieve. We feel therefore that the status of the bladder at the time of the antireflux surgery is the main determinant of success, and that such surgery should be deferred until the bladder becomes more thin-walled and compliant. If persistent or recurrent infection mandates earlier therapy, temporary diversion should be strongly considered in such patients.

Hendren, Knutrud, and others do not share this view. Hendren's successful technique of lower ureteral tailoring was devised to permit the treatment of just such patients in a single comprehensive operation. Faced with this situation, an infant with hydronephrosis and reflux, he stabilizes the infant preoperatively and then proceeds with valve ablation, bilateral ureteral tailoring with reimplantation, and often a limited anterior Y-V plasty. He emphasizes several important points in such surgery. Most importantly, the ureteral tailoring must be carried out without impairing the blood supply of the remaining strip of ureter. This is achieved by leaving the medial ureteral adventitia, with its relatively rich blood supply, intact. Only the lateral portion of the straightened lower ureter is removed. The ureteral edges are reapproximated in two layers (see Figs. 15–52, 16–99, and 16–100). A watertight closure is needed to prevent a fistula between the bladder and the ureter above the new meatus from resulting in reflux. The detached ureter is drawn into the bladder through a new hiatus cephalad and medial to the original point of entry. The suture line in the ureter is rotated against the bladder musculature to minimize the risk of the fistula. Alternately, the dilated ureter can be reduced in caliber by "modeling," which is described in Chapter 15 and in the article on the Ureter and Ureterovesical Junction in this chapter.

Only the portion of the lower ureter that becomes the new intravesical portion needs to be tapered. The extravesical ureter will straighten and narrow as the child grows if reflux is corrected and obstruction does not occur. This usually means that only about 5 cm of the lower ureter needs to be narrowed, and less in the infant, minimizing the risk of impairing the blood supply of the distalmost segment. Hendren has achieved consistently good results using this technique, and estimates that only 15 to 25 per cent of his infant patients with valves come to renal failure, and transplantation, before fully grown. This is about the same incidence of eventual renal failure encountered in this group of infants with valves even when more conservative staged treatment is elected.

Hendren emphasizes the diminished morbidity inherent in his single-stage approach when compared with temporary diversion, valve resection, restoration of the continuity of the urinary tract, and subsequent antireflux surgery, each usually performed as a separate operation. This is certainly a valid point when the total reconstruction is an unqualified success. However, implanting dilated ureters into an obstructed bladder has resulted in a complication rate of 30 to 60 per cent in the hands of many experienced urologists. Hendren himself believes that his one-stage approach should be reserved to surgeons trained in this technique, and we agree that it should be employed in a limited fashion. Most sick infants with valves are most safely treated by high diversion with subsequent elective reconstruction.

Residual Urethral Dilatation

Valves may become elusive at endoscopy after the initial resection is begun. For this reason one should always make a postoperative cystogram to be certain that the obstruction has indeed been corrected. Williams found, in his large series, that 11 per cent needed repeat resections. The dilatation of the posterior urethra behind the valve is usually much reduced on voiding urethrograms made as soon as a few weeks after the initial surgery. However, in a minority of boys, perhaps 20 per cent, some posterior urethral dilatation persists for years. These patients need to be screened to be certain that there is no residual obstruction. Urinary flow rates are helpful in this regard, as is determination of residual urine. However, a second cystoscopy is necessary in many instances, particularly when hydronephrosis also remains unchanged after 3 to 6 months of follow-up.

Residual Hydroureteronephrosis

Some residual hydronephrosis is the rule in boys with relatively severe obstruction at the time of diagnosis. Though infants have a greater capacity for the kidney to return to normal in appearance on excretory urography than older children, calycectasis from congenital obstruction is usually fixed in degree after a year or two of age. This is not necessarily a bad prognostic sign, as the only result may be an unnoticed impairment of concentrating ability, but may cause the question of ureterovesical junction obstruction to arise. Residual hydroureteronephrosis usually turns out to be just that—residual hydronephrosis without obstruction. These ureters can be more accurately assessed and ureterovesical obstruction excluded by any of the maneuvers used to differentiate obstructed from nonobstructed megaureter. Pertinent tests include whether a ureteral catheter will pass, the volume of the hydronephrotic drip obtained, or a renogram or excretory urogram with furosemide given at the height of isotope or dye accumulation to estimate washout rates. If these are still equivocal, a Whitaker test may be necessary to definitely exclude obstruction. Happily, persistent obstruction of the dilated ureter by detrusor hypertrophy or obstruction cicatrix at the hiatus is an unusual occurrence, and ureteral reimplantation for ureterovesical junction obstruction is not often required in boys with valves.

Noncompliant bladder is a more common reason for increasing hydronephrosis and can often be shown by careful urodynamic studies to be the cause of elevated pressure in the upper tracts in such patients.

Posterior Urethral Strictures

Type III valves are sometimes described as congenital strictures. We believe that it is better to limit the term "stricture" to the acquired urethral narrowing seen after trauma or inflammatory disease.

The main causes of stricture of the posterior urethra in children are iatrogenic damage due to overdilatation; urethral rupture, which is usually associated with pelvic fracture or a fall astride; transurethral resection of valves; and inflammation secondary to catheter drainage. Strictures are usually diagnosed on a follow-up voiding cystourethrogram as a persistent narrowing of variable length and position, or by diminished urinary stream and flow rates. Although periodic dilatation of strictures is seldom a reasonable course in children with a whole lifetime ahead of them, a trial of one or two urethral dilatations is often desirable. A single dilatation will occasionally eradicate a stricture that is due only to mucosal adhesions. One hesitates to treat such strictures surgically until the scar has matured and the length of the stricture can be ascertained with accuracy. Simultaneous antegrade and retrograde uretherography is helpful in this regard. This examination should be performed several weeks or months after dilatation so that the stricture has a chance to recontract and the length of urethral involvement is not underestimated.

Short strictures may be treated endoscopically with the visual urethrotome. Intermittent catheterization once a day for several months then increases the chance that such strictures will not recur (Noe).

Short strictures, less than 0.5 cm in length and distal to the prostatic apex, may also be excised and the ends of the mobilized urethra reapproximated. The entire distal corpus spongiosum may be mobilized to prevent tension at the point of anastomosis. A stenting Silastic catheter is kept in place for 10 days to 2 weeks.

Longer strictures may be repaired in one stage with an island flap of skin rotated inward and sewn to the opened marsupialized strictured area with absorbable suture material. A free graft of defatted penile skin also gives generally good results. In any instance, the most important aspect of the operation is to ascertain that the augmenting skin patch is carried into healthy urethra above and distal to the stricture.

When the stricture is at the membranous urethra, as is often the case when it results from transurethral resection of valves, a two-stage repair is often desirable. A flap of perineal skin is elevated on a broad posterior perineal base. The tip of the flap is sutured to the opened prostatic urethra above the upper limit of the stricture. The edges of the skin flap are then sewn to the edges of the opened stricture. The urethra is intact dorsally. The external sphincter has been destroyed by the stricture, and continence depends on the intact bladder neck. Few problems with urinary control are encountered, however, after obstruction has been relieved.

After healing for 2 or 3 months, the urethral openings are calibrated. The distal defunctionalized urethral opening, especially, often becomes stenotic and requires minor revision to increase its caliber before the urethra is closed.

After 6 months, when healing is complete, the urethra is closed. Enough skin is tubularized, even in infants, to form a urethra 16 to 20 F in caliber. Absorbable subcuticular sutures are employed. As many layers as possible are closed over the newly tubularized urethra. A urethral catheter or cystostomy is left in place for 7 to 10 days.

Incontinence

As noted above, boys with valves may present because of overflow incontinence, and older boys with mild degrees of obstruction often have incontinence as their only symptom. However, persistence of incontinence or the onset of incontinence after valve resection is not uncommon. There are several possible causes. The incontinence may be a sign of inadequate valve resection, or of a stricture subsequent to the procedure which results in continued obstruction. Surgical correction will resolve these problems. The external sphincter may be damaged by the valve resection. More commonly, such incontinence is due to disruption of the sphincters by the dilatation of the posterior urethra caused by the valve. Neither sphincter may be able to coapt adequately to prevent stress incontinence. If a Y-V plasty or bladder neck resection has been performed, the internal sphincter has probably been ablated, and incontinence is more likely. This is one major reason why bladder neck enlargement should be reserved for very specific indications, the other being the risk of retrograde ejaculation that occasionally follows even an anterior Y-V plasty alone. If the bladder neck seems clearly the site of residual obstruction, intermittent catheterization on a temporary basis may be employed until the internal sphincter hypertrophy has subsided.

The incontinence due to sphincter weakness is usually self-limited and seems to resolve at or before puberty, probably because of prostatic growth. A formal incontinence operation is sometimes needed, but ephedrine, imipramine, or phenylpropanolamine (Orande) in appropriate doses is usually helpful if not temporarily curative.

Noncompliant Bladder

Another infrequent reason for persistent incontinence is a noncompliant bladder, which may also be the cause of functional but severe ureteral obstruction, as mentioned above. This too may be treated pharmacologically with anticholinergics, but with less chance of success. An augmentation cystoplasty, substituting a bowel segment for most of the bladder capacity to reduce tone, is apt to be required, usually by ileocecocystoplasty, sometimes moving the ureters away from the thickened bladder. Noncompliant bladders are occasionally also encountered when the urinary tract is reconstructed after temporary diversion, but are more commonly seen after one or more ureteral reimplantations, so scarring and denervation of the detrusor may often play some role in the pathogenesis. Diagnosis of the noncompliant bladder is discussed more fully in the articles in this chapter on the Ureter and Ureterovesical Junction and on the Bladder and Bladder Neck.

CONGENITAL HYPERTROPHY OF THE VERUMONTANUM

Early authors, Bugbee and Wollstein as well as Emmett among them, occasionally attributed outlet obstruction in male infants to hypertrophy of the vermontanum. The lesion was usually considered to be simple hypertrophy, perhaps in response to an endocrinologic imbalance. Presman has more recently suggested that such hypertrophy is a secondary change due to more distal obstruction, perhaps analogous to the secondary hypertrophy of the bladder neck that is usually seen proximal to a urethral valve. For whatever reason, this diagnosis is now seldom made. The normal verumontanum in the infant is much larger in proportion to the prostatic urethra than in older children or adults, and this may occasionally be a cause of confusion over the diagnosis. Also, some polyps of the verumontanum are sessile and may easily be mistaken for a very large verumontanum on endoscopic examination.

POLYPS OF THE VERUMONTANUM

More than 30 cases of polyps of the posterior urethra have been reported. Even so, this is misleading because such polyps are not

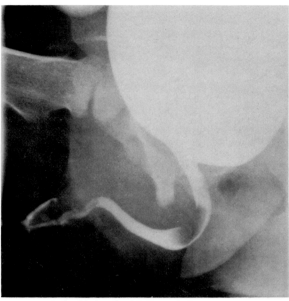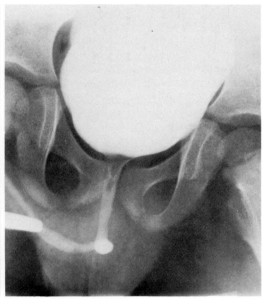

A   B

Figure 16–145. Congenital polyp of prostatic urethra as shown on voiding cystourethrograms. *A,* Lateral view. *B,* Anteroposterior view demonstrates pedunculated polyp as a filling defect in the posterior urethra. Note change of position. (From Stadaas JO: Pedunculated polyp of posterior urethra in children causing reflux and hydronephrosis. J Pediatr Surg 8:517–521, 1973. Reproduced by permission of the CV Mosby Company, St. Louis.)

rare. Many, however, are small, do not cause obstruction, and are incidental findings. Such polyps should probably be resected when encountered, as it is not known how likely it is that small lesions will enlarge enough to cause obstruction.

Obstructing polyps arise from the verumontanum or the floor of the prostatic urethra near the verumontanum (Fig. 16–145). They are usually pedunculated, and the stalk may be several cm in length. Such polyps are composed primarily of connective tissue covered by epithelium, but may contain smooth muscle, islands of glandular cells, and even nerve tissue (DeWolf and Fraley). The congenital nature of these polyps is suggested because they are often diagnosed in otherwise healthy infants and by histologic evidence that they are protrusions of the urethral wall and are not neoplasia (Downs).

At rest, the polyp usually lies in the bladder attached to the verumontanum by its stalk. During micturition, the polyp is pushed into the proximal urethra, where it acts like a plug and stops voiding abruptly, involuntarily, and prematurely. Polyps may pass down the urethra and through the external sphincter if the length of the stalk is great enough. Infants, of course, are not able to give the history of intermittent voiding and sometimes present with hematuria or signs of bladder outlet obstruction.

Boys are commonly not diagnosed until after an attempt at toilet training calls attention to the abnormal voiding pattern, and several cases have been described in adults.

Diagnosis is usually simple once bladder outlet obstruction is suspected. The voiding cystourethrogram will show the polyp as a filling defect in the bladder or in the urethra. Occasionally, if the polyp is large or if there is a good bit of edema of the posterior urethra, cystoscopy is necessary to differentiate a polyp from an obstructing rhabdomyosarcoma arising in the prostate.

Transurethral resection of the polyp is the best form of therapy. The base must be excised completely, usually necessitating partial resection of the verumontanum, as regrowth has been described after removal of the polyp and stalk alone.

When the polyp is too large for removal through the miniature resectoscope sheath, the base is simply resected. The filled bladder is then punctured with a 12 F Cystocath needle. An endoscopic forceps is passed into the bladder through the obturator and grasps the free polyp under vision through the cystoscope. When the polyp is firmly engaged, sheath, forceps, and polyp are withdrawn simultaneously, clearing the bladder of debris. An urethral catheter is then left for a day or two.

BIBLIOGRAPHY

Arey LB: Developmental Anatomy: A Textbook and Laboratory Manual of Embryology. Revised seventh ed. Philadelphia, WB Saunders Co., 1974.

Barry JM, Anderson JM, Hodges CV: The subcapsular C sign: a rare radiographic finding associated with neonatal urinary ascites. J Urol 112:836, 1974.

Bauer SB, Dieppa RA, Labib KK, et al: The bladder in boys with posterior urethral valves: a urodynamic assessment. J Urol 121:769, 1979.

Bazy P: Rétrècissement congenital de l'urètre chez l'homme. Presse Med 11:215, 1903.

Beck AD: The effect of intra-uterine urinary obstruction upon the development of the fetal kidney. J Urol 105:784, 1971.

Brandesky G: Conservatively treated urethral valves. J Pediatr Surg 8:945, 1973.

Budd G: Case of extraordinary dilatation of the kidneys, ureters and bladder. Lancet 1:767, 1839–1840.

Bueschen AJ, Garrett RA, Newman DM: Posterior urethral valves: management. J Urol 110:682, 1973.

Bugbee HG, Wollstein M: Retention of urine due to congenital hypertrophy of the verumontanum. J Urol 10:477, 1923.

Butt KM, Meyer A, Kountz SL, et al: Renal transplantation in patients with posterior urethral valves. J Urol 116:708, 1976.

Campbell MF: Obstruction of the posterior urethral valve in infancy and childhood: a study of eighteen cases. JAMA 96:592, 1931.

Campbell MF: Urology. Second ed. Philadelphia, WB Saunders Co., 1963.

Cass AS, Khan AU, Smith S, et al: Neonatal perirenal urinary extravasation with posterior urethral valves. Urology 18:258, 1981.

Cass AS, Stephens FD: Posterior urethral valves: diagnosis and management. J Urol 112:519, 1974.

Cendron J, DeBurge JP, Karlaftis C: Vulvules de l'urèthre postérieur. J Urol Nephrol (Paris) 75:13, 1969.

Churchill BM, Krueger RP, Fleisher MH, et al: Complications of posterior urethral valve surgery and their prevention. Urol Clin North Am 10:519, 1983.

Cornil C: Endoscopic diagnosis of posterior urethral valves. Birth Defects 13:51, 1977.

Counseller VS, Menville JG: Congenital valves of the posterior urethra. J Urol 34:268, 1935.

Cremin BJ: Urinary ascites and obstructive uropathy. Br J Radiol 48:113, 1975.

Crooks KK: The protean aspects of posterior urethral valves. J Urol 126:763, 1981.

Crooks KK: Urethral strictures following transurethral resection of posterior urethral valves. J Urol 127:1153, 1982.

Dahl DS: Reversible vesical hypertonicity, a consequence of the chronic empty state. Invest Urol 7:160, 1969.

Dean WM, Bourdeau EJ: Amniotic fluid alpha-fetoprotein in fetal obstructive uropathy. Pediatrics 66:537, 1980.

DeWolf WC, Fraley EE: Congenital urethral polyp in the infant: case report and review of the literature. J Urol 109:515, 1973.

Dockray KT: The perirenal P sign: a new roentgenogram index to the cause and treatment of urinary ascites in babies. Am J Dis Child 119:179, 1970.

Downs RA: Congenital polyps of the prostatic urethra: a review of the literature and report of two cases. Br J Urol 42:76, 1970.

Drouin G, Laperrière J, Grégoire A: Urethral valves as a cause of dilated Cowper's glands and perineal pain. J Urol 120:634, 1978.

Duckett JW Jr: Current management of posterior urethral valves. Urol Clin North Am 1:471, 1974.

Ellis DG, Fonkalsrud EW, Smith JP: Congenital posterior urethral valves. J Urol 95:549, 1966.

Emmett JL: Obstruction of the vesical neck of a male infant produced by hypertrophy of the verumontanum: report of case. Proc Staff Meet Mayo Clin 15:364, 1940.

Ericsson ND: Long-term results in surgical treatment of posterior urethral valves. Prog Pediatr Surg 10:197, 1977.

Esami K, Smith ED: A study of sequelae of posterior urethral valves. J Urol 127:84, 1982.

Everett HS, Brack CB: Unusual lesions of the female urethra. Obstet Gynecol 1:57, 1953.

Farkas A, Skinner DG: Posterior urethral valves in siblings. Br J Urol 48:76, 1976.

Field PL, Stephens FD: Congenital urethral membranes causing urethral obstruction. J Urol 111:250, 1974.

Fletcher JC: The fetus as patient: ethical issues. JAMA 246:772, 1981.

Forsythe WI, McFadden GDF: Congenital posterior urethral valves: a study of thirty-five cases. Br J Urol 31:63, 1959.

Friedland GW, Axman MM, Love T: Neonatal "urinothorax" associated with posterior urethral valves. Br J Radiol 44:471, 1971.

Gillenwater JY, Westervelt FB Jr, Vaughan ED Jr, et al: Renal function one week after release of chronic unilateral hydronephrosis in man. Kidney Int 7:179, 1974.

Glassberg KI, Schneider M, Haller JO, et al: Observations on persistently dilated ureter after posterior urethral valve ablation. Urology 20:20, 1982.

Golbus MS, Harrison MR, Filly RA, et al: In utero treatment of urinary tract obstruction. Am J Obstet Gynecol 142:383, 1982.

Gonzales ET Jr: Posterior urethral valves and bladder neck obstruction. Urol Clin North Am 5:57, 1978.

Gonzalez ET Jr: Valves in twins. Presented at Annual Meeting, American Academy of Pediatrics, 1983.

Gopal G: Treatment of congenital posterior urethral valves by "pressure necrosis." Indian Pediatr 13:359, 1976.

Graham SD Jr, Krueger RP, Glenn JF: Anterior urethral diverticulum associated with posterior urethral valves. J Urol 128:376, 1982.

Gray SW, Skandalakis JE: Embryology for Surgeons: The Embryologic Basis for the Treatment of Congenital Defects. Philadelphia, WB Saunders Co., 1972.

Griesbach WA, Waterhouse RK, Mellins HZ: Voiding cysto-urethrography in the diagnosis of congenital posterior urethral valves. Am J Roentgenol Radium Ther Nucl Med 82:521, 1959.

Harrison MR, Filly RA, Parer JT, et al: Management of the fetus with a urinary tract malformation. JAMA 246:635, 1981a.

Harrison MR, Golbus MS, Filly RA: Management of the fetus with a correctable congenital defect. JAMA 246:774, 1981b.

Harrison MR, Anderson J, Rosen MA, et al: Fetal surgery in the primate. I. Anesthetic, surgical and tocolytic management to maximize fetal-neonatal survival. J Pediatr Surg 17:115, 1982.

Harrison MR: Unborn: historical perspective of the fetus as a patient. Pharos 45:19, 1982.

Hasen HB, Song YS: Congenital valvular obstruction of the posterior urethra in two brothers. J Pediatr 47:207, 1955.

Hendren WH: A new approach to infants with severe obstructive uropathy: early complete reconstruction. J Pediatr Surg 5:184, 1970.

Hendren WH: Posterior urethral valves in boys: a broad clinical spectrum. J Urol 106:298, 1971.

Henneberry MO, Stephens FD: Renal hypoplasia in infants with posterior urethral valves. J Urol 123:912, 1980.

Johnston JH: Posterior urethral valves: an operative technic using an electric auriscope. J Pediatr Surg 1:583, 1966.

Johnston JH: Vesicoureteric reflux with urethral valves. Br J Urol 51:100, 1979.

Johnston JH, Kulatilake AE: The sequelae of posterior urethral valves. Br J Urol 43:743, 1971.

Kaplan GW: Posterior urethral valves. In Clinical Pediatric Urology. First ed. Edited by PP Kelalis, LR King, AB Belman. Philadelphia, WB Saunders Co., 1976.

Kimbrough HM Jr, Wyker AW Jr: Intraoperative compression cystourethrogram: a measure of adequate resection of posterior urethral valves. 117:239, 1977.

Kjellberg SR, Ericsson NO, Rudhe U: The Lower Urinary Tract in Childhood: Some Correlated Clinical and Roentgenologic Observations. Chicago, Year Book Medical Publishers, 1957.

Knox JHM, Sprunt TP: Congenital obstruction of the posterior urethra: report of a case in a boy aged five years. Am J Dis Child 4:137, 1912.

Knutrud O: Diversion vs. immediate reconstruction for megaureter. Presented at the meeting of the American Academy of Pediatrics, Surgical Section, Chicago, October 1973.

Kroovand RL, Weinberg N, Emami A: Posterior urethral valves in identical twins. Pediatrics 60:748, 1977.

Krueger RP: Posterior urethral valves masquerading as prune belly syndrome. Urology 18:182, 1981.

Krueger RP, Churchill BM: Megalourethra with posterior urethral valves. Urology 18:279, 1981.

Krueger RP, Hardy BE, Churchill BM: Growth in boys and posterior urethral valves. Primary valve resection vs upper tract diversion. Urol Clin North Am 7:265, 1980.

Kuppusami K, Moors DE: Fibrous polyp of the verumontanum. Can J Surg 11:388, 1968.

Kurth KH, Alleman ER, Schroder FH: Major and minor complications of posterior urethral valves. J Urol 126:517, 1981.

Landes HE, Rall R: Congenital valvular obstruction of the posterior urethra. J Urol 34:254, 1935.

Lattimer JK, Hubbard M: Relative incidence of pediatric urological conditions. J Urol 71:759, 1954.

Lome LG, Howat JM, Williams DI: The temporarily defunctionalized bladder in children. J Urol 107:469, 1972.

Lorenzo RL, Turner WR, Bradford BF, et al: Duplication of the male urethra with posterior urethral valves. Pediatr Radiol 11:39, 1981.

Lowsley OS: Congenital malformation of the posterior urethra. Ann Surg 60:733, 1914.

Lowsley OS, Kirwin TJ: A clinical and pathological study of congenital obstruction of the urethra: report of four cases. J Urol 31:497, 1934.

Mahony DT: Studies of enuresis. I. Incidence of obstructive lesions and pathophysiology of enuresis. J Urol 106:951, 1971.

Mahony DT, Laferte RD: Congenital posterior urethral valves in adult males. Urology 3:724, 1974.

Marsden RTH: Posterior urethral valves in adults. Br J Urol 41:586, 1969.

Martin J, Anderson J, Raz S: Posterior urethral valves in adults: a report of 2 cases. J Urol 118:978, 1977.

Matheson WJ, Ward EM: Hormonal sex reversal in a female. Arch Dis Child 29:22, 1954.

McCrea LE: Congenital valves of the posterior urethra. J Int Coll Surg 12:342, 1949.

Meadows JA Jr, Quattlebaum RB: Polyps of the posterior urethra in children. J Urol 100:317, 1968.

Moerman P, Fryns J-P, Goddeens P, et al: Pathogenesis of the prune belly syndrome: a functional obstruction caused by prostatic hypoplasia. Pediatrics 73:470, 1984.

Mogg RA: Congenital anomalies of the urethra. Br J Urol 40:638, 1968.

Morgagni GB: The Seats and Causes of Diseases Investigated by Anatomy. Translated by B Alexander. Book III. Article 40. New York, Hafner Publishing Company, 1960.

Morgan CL Jr, Grossman H: Posterior urethral valves as a cause of neonatal uriniferous perirenal pseudocyst (urinoma).

Myers DA, Walker RD III: Prevention of urethral strictures in the management of posterior urethral valves.

Nesbit RM, Labardini MM: Urethral valves in the male child. J Urol 96:218, 1966.

Nesbit RM, McDonald HP Jr, Busby S: Obstructing valves in the female urethra. J Urol 91:79, 1964.

Nieh PT, Hendren WH: Obstructing posterior urethral valves in octogenarian. Urology 13:412, 1979.

Noe HN: Complications and management of childhood urethral stricture disease. Urol Clin North Am 10:531, 1983.

North AF Jr, Eldredge DM, Talpey WB: Abdominal distention at birth due to ascites associated with obstructive uropathy. Am J Dis Child 111:613, 1966.

Osathanondh V, Potter EL: Pathogenesis of polycystic kidneys: type 4 due to urethral obstruction. Arch Pathol 77:502, 1964.

Presman D: Congenital valves of the posterior urethra. J Urol 86:602, 1961.

Rabinowitz R, Barkin M, Schillinger JF, et al: The influence of etiology on the surgical management and prognosis of the massively dilated ureter in children. J Urol 119:808, 1978.

Rabinowitz R, Barkin M, Schillinger JF, et al: Upper tract management when posterior urethral valve ablation is insufficient. J Urol 122:370, 1979.

Randall A: Congenital valves of the posterior urethra. Ann Surg 73:477, 1921.

Raper FP: The recognition and treatment of congenital urethral valves. Br J Urol 25:136, 1953.

Rattner WH, Meyer R, Bernstein J: Congenital abnormalities of the urinary system. IV. Valvular obstruction of the posterior urethra. J Pediatr 63:84, 1963.

Retief PJM: Urethral valve obstruction. S Afr Med J 44:181, 1970.

Rickham PP: Advanced lower urinary obstruction in childhood. Arch Dis Child 37:122, 1962.

Robertson WB, Hayes JA: Congenital diaphragmatic obstruction of the male posterior urethra. Br J Urol 41:592, 1969.

Saalfield JG, Lloyd LK, Evans BB: Management of severe hydroureteronephrosis in infants and young children. J Urol 115:587, 1976.

Savage JP: Urethral valves presenting as an encysted retroperitoneal urinary collection (pseudohydronephrosis). J Pediatr Surg 7:334, 1972.

Scott TW: Urinary ascites secondary to posterior urethral valves. J Urol 116:87, 1976.

Scott WF, Collins TA, Singer PL: Papilloma of urethra in infant. J Med Assoc State Ala 7:370, 1938.

Sober I: Pelvioureterostomy-en-Y. J Urol 107:473, 1972.

Stadaas JO: Pedunculated polyp of posterior urethra in children causing reflux and hydronephrosis. J Pediatr Surg 8:517, 1973.

Stephens FD: Urethral obstruction in childhood: the use of urethrography in diagnosis. Aust NZ J Surg 25:89, 1955.

Stephens FD: Congenital Malformations of the Rectum, Anus and Genitourinary Tracts. Edinburgh, E & S Livingstone, 1963.

Stephens FD: Congenital Malformations of the Urinary Tract. New York, Praeger, 1983.

Stoltz CR: Dystocia due to distention of the fetal bladder. Obstet Gynecol 20:268, 1962.

Stueber PJ, Persky L: Solid tumors of the urethra and bladder neck. J Urol 102:205, 1969.

Sullivan MJ, Lackner LH, Banowsky LHW: Intraperitoneal extravasation of urine: BUN/serum creatinine disproportion. JAMA 221:491, 1972.

Swain VAJ, Tucker S, Stimmler L, et al: Perinatal ascites due to extravasation of urine from ruptured kidneys: approaches to diagnosis and treatment. Clin Pediatr (Phila) 4:199, 1965.

Sweeney I, Kang BH, Lin P, et al: Posterior urethral obstruction caused by congenital posterior urethral valve: prenatal and postnatal ultrasound diagnosis. NY State J Med 81:87, 1981.

Tanagho EA: Surgically induced partial urinary obstruction in the fetal lamb. II. Urethral obstruction. Invest Urol 10:25, 1972.

Tanagho EA: Congenitally obstructed bladders: fate after prolonged defunctionalization. J Urol 11:102, 1974.

Tank ES, Carey TC, Seifert AL: Management of neonatal urinary ascites. Urology 16:270, 1980.

Tolmatschew N: Ein Fall von semilunaren Klappen der Harnröhre und von vergrösserter Vesicula Prostatica. Arch Pathol Anat 49:348, 1870.

Tsingoglou S, Dickson JAS: Lower urinary obstruction in infancy: a review of lesions and symptoms in 165 cases. Arch Dis Child 47:215, 1972.

Uehling, DT: Posterior urethral valves: functional classification. Urology 15:27, 1980.

Waldbaum RS, Marshall VF: Posterior urethral valves: evaluation and surgical management. J Urol 103:801, 1970.

Walker RD: Stricture formation after perineal urethrostomy. Presented at Annual Meeting, Section on Urology, American Academy of Pediatrics, 1982.

Waterhouse K, Hamm FC: The importance of urethral valves as a cause of vesical neck obstruction in children. J Urol 87:404, 1962.

Watson EM: The structural basis for congenital valve formation in the posterior urethra. J Urol 7:371, 1922.

Whitaker RH: The ureter in posterior urethral valves. Br J Urol 45:395, 1973.

Whitaker RH, Keeton JE, Williams DI: Posterior urethral valves: a study of urinary control after operation. J Urol 108:167, 1972.

Williams DI: Urology in Childhood. Encyclopedia of Urology. Vol 15 Suppl. New York, Springer-Verlag, 1974.

Williams DI, Abbassian A: Solitary pedunculated polyp of the posterior urethra in children. J Urol 96:483, 1966.

Williams DI, Eckstein HB: Obstructive valves in the posterior urethra. J Urol 93:236, 1965.

Williams DI, Rabinovitch HH: Cutaneous ureterostomy for the grossly dilated ureter of childhood. Br J Urol 39:696, 1967.

Williams DI, Whitaker RH, Barratt TM, et al: Urethral valves. Br J Urol 45:200, 1973.

Young BW: Lower Urinary Tract Obstruction in Childhood. Philadelphia, Lea & Febiger, 1972.

Young HH, Frontz WA, Baldwin JC: Congenital obstruction of the posterior urethra. J Urol 3:289, 1919.

Anterior Urethra

JAY D. BURSTEIN AND CASIMIR F. FIRLIT

ANTERIOR URETHRAL VALVES

Anterior urethral valves are a rare urethral congenital anomaly that must be excluded in the investigation of young males with evidence suggestive of outflow obstruction or recurrent infection. They can occur as single entities or in association with a proximal diverticulum (Colabawalla; Nesbit and Labardini; Texter and Enger). Some degree of urethral distention will always exist proximal to an anterior urethral valve. The point at which this distention becomes a saccular diverticulum continues to be debated (Kelalis et al). Several reports in the literature describe patients with anterior urethral valves, diverticula, and associated hydronephrosis (Firlit and King; Waterhouse and Scordamaglia; Small and Schoenfeld). In a series of 13 boys with anterior urethral valves, 6 valves were located at the bulbous urethra, 6 were found in the mid pendulous urethra, and 1 was located in the distal urethra. Among this group, 4 diverticula were associated with the valves. Frequently recognized as a filamentous cusp of mucosal tissue based on the ventral aspect of the urethra, anterior urethral valves may also assume an irislike or semilunar configuration (Golimbu et al). Frequently such valves produce only minimal obstruction. However, on occasion marked proximal obstructive changes associated with severe azotemia have required life-saving temporary proximal urinary diversion. The difficulty in distinction between valves alone and those associated with a urethral diverticulum may represent a spectrum of disease as opposed to each being a distinct and separate entity. However, when a sizable diverticulum is associated with local absence of surrounding corpus spongiosum, this appears as a different and perhaps distinct entity, a primary congenital diverticulum (Allen et al). The distal portions of such diverticula may undermine the urethra to produce cusplike flaps that are reminiscent of a valve and invite the diagnosis of a distal valve in many instances.

Embryology

The exact embryologic origin of anterior urethral valves is uncertain. They may arise from congenital cystic dilatation of normal or accessory periurethral glands that communicate with the urethra, resulting in a flaplike valve (Williams and Retik). Another explanation suggests that the valve is the result of an abortive attempt at urethral duplication.

Signs and Symptoms

The degree of obstruction produced by anterior valves is very variable. The neonate may present with a poor dribbling urethral stream, acidosis, azotemia, massive hydronephrosis, megacystis, bladder trabeculation, or severe urosepsis (Sawanishi; Texter and Engel). A small swelling resulting from an associated diverticulum may occasionally be appreciated at the penoscrotal junction during or after voiding. Obstructive changes accompanying these valves have been classified by Firlit as a continuity of pathology. This continuum is divided into four basic types. Type I demonstrates a urethral valve with minimal proximal urethral distention (Fig. 16–146). In type II the valve is associated with a well-defined urethral diverticulum, but the bladder and upper tracts are normal (Fig. 16–147). Type III demonstrates a distinct diverticulum associated with vesical distention, irregularity, mild trabeculation, and ureteral reflux (Fig. 16–148). Type IV are the most severely

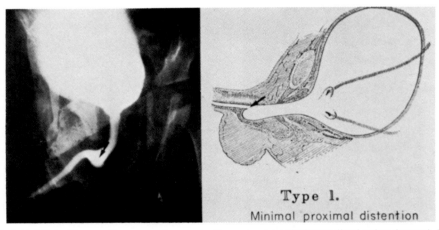

Type 1.
Minimal proximal distention

Figure 16–146. Micturition urethrogram demonstrating a type I anterior urethral valve *(arrow)*. Usually only minimal proximal urethral distention is noted. (From Firlit CF: Urethral abnormalities. Urol Clin North Am 5:1, 1978.)

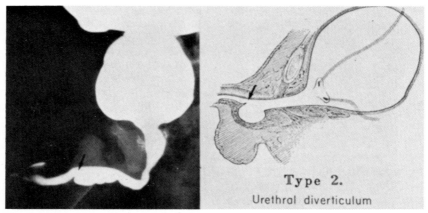

Type 2.
Urethral diverticulum

Figure 16–147. Voiding cystourethrogram illustrating a type II anterior urethral valve *(arrow)* associated with diverticulum formation. (From Firlit CF: Urethral abnormalities. Urol Clin North Am 5:1, 1978.)

obstructive, with Grade IV to V reflux, ureteral decompensation, and renal insufficiency (Fig. 16–149).

Diagnosis and Treatment

Presenting signs often include those of bladder outflow obstruction. In severely obstructed boys a weak stream may be associated with ventral urethral swelling during or after voiding. A large diverticulum can result in postvoiding incontinence. Minimally obstructive valves may fail to produce symptoms. However, such boys may present with enuresis, blood-stained shorts, or failure to thrive (Waterhouse and Scordamaglia). On occasion, patients may also present with progressive upper tract deterioration despite multiple prior endoscopic evaluations and surgical procedures (Chang; Firlit). Unless this lesion is considered in boys with outflow obstruction, it can be easily overlooked. A good voiding cystourethrogram (VCUG) is necessary to establish the diagnosis. Typically, some dilatation of the urethra proximal to a valve leaflet may be demonstrated (Fig. 16–150). Unless bladder expression is performed while searching the anterior urethra, recognition of the valve cusp may be difficult as retrograde flow flattens the valve against the urethral mucosa. The infant resectoscope can be used to elevate the leaflet with the ex-

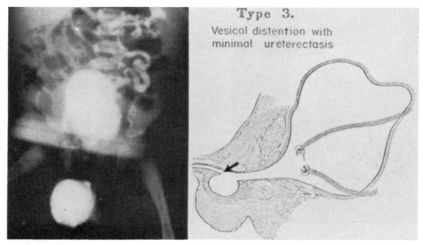

Type 3.
Vesical distention with minimal ureterectasis

Figure 16–148. Voiding cystourethrogram in a neonate demonstrating a large urethral diverticulum associated with a type III anterior urethral valve, bladder irregularity, and vesicoureteral reflux. (From Firlit CF: Urethral abnormalities. Urol Clin North Am 5:1, 1978.)

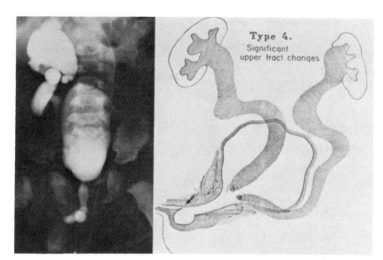

Figure 16–149. Type IV anterior urethral valve with significant hydroureteronephrosis and reflux. (From Firlit CF: Urethral abnormalities. Urol Clin North Am 5:1, 1978.)

tended loop. Electroresection can then effectively relieve the obstruction. When present, an associated diverticulum will require open excision and urethroplasty. Another suggestion is the use of a bougie or crochet hook in a gentle stroking fashion as it is withdrawn from the urethra. A snagging sensation will indicate the presence of a significant valve. Once the leaflet is engaged by the hook, aggressive traction can disrupt the leaflet and relieve the obstruction, although resection is usually preferred (Belman AB, personal communication, 1983).

COWPER'S GLAND DUCT CYSTS

Retention cysts of Cowper's gland have been rarely reported because they are rarely symptomatic and are often misdiagnosed. Englisch reported the first case of a Cowper's gland duct cyst. Elbogen presented detailed accounts of several cases of cysts arising in the bulbourethral glands, and found that 2.3 per cent of autopsied males, aged 7 to 60 years, had such cysts. He also noted that these lesions were incidental findings and of no apparent clinical significance. However, Cook and Shaw reported several pediatric patients in whom retention cysts resulted in urethral obstruction, urinary retention, and hydronephrosis.

Muschat classified Cowper's gland duct cysts into two categories. The first category describes those lesions which protrude into the urethral lumen, compressing the urethra and producing signs of obstruction. His second category includes cases in which cyst

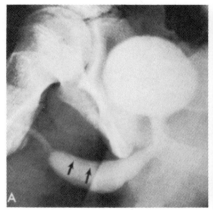
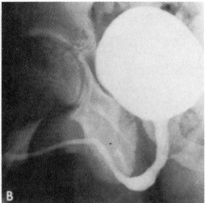

Figure 16–150. *A*, Anterior urethral valve *(arrows)* with diverticulum. *B*, Three months after open excision of valve. (From Firlit CF: Urethral abnormalities. Urol Clin North Am 5:1, 1978.)

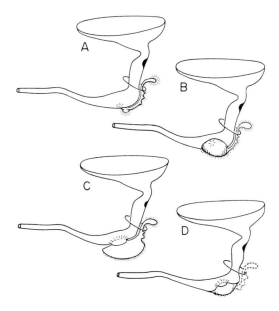

Figure 16–151. Schematic drawings of types of Cowper's syringoceles. Cowper's glands *(stippling)* are located above urogenital diaphragm *(black ring)*, along Cowper's duct, and at bulbar urethra. *A,* Simple syringocele. Cowper's duct is visualized by simple reflux into a minimally dilated duct. *B,* Imperforate syringocele. Orifice draining Cowper's duct is not apparent and is associated with dilatation of distal duct. Ectatic duct intrudes into bulbar urethra. *C,* Perforate syringocele. Orifice draining Cowper's duct is patulous and allows free reflux into duct. Ectatic duct appears as diverticulum of bulbar urethra. *D,* Ruptured syringocele. Bulbar portion of Cowper's duct is dilated and loses its communication with main duct. Rupture of this dilated duct leaves membranes as remnants of its wall. (From Maizels M, Stephens FD, King LR, et al: Cowper's syringocele: a classification of dilatations of Cowper's gland duct based upon clinical characteristics of 8 boys. J Urol *129*:114, 1983. ©1983, The Williams & Wilkins Co., Baltimore.)

enlargement occurred ouside the urethra filling the space of the triangular ligament between the urethral bulb and the ischiocavernosus muscle. This extraurethral enlargement becomes apparent on physical examination as a bulging perineal mass.

Maizels et al recently presented a classification of the various urethrographic appearances of dilated Cowper's gland ducts. He referred to them collectively as Cowper's syringoceles (Greek *syringo*, tube + *cele*, swelling). Four groups were defined: (1) simple syringocele—a minimally dilated duct; (2) perforate syringocele—a bulbous duct draining into the urethra by a patulous ostium

appearing as a diverticulum; (3) imperforate syringocele—a duct resembling a submucosal cyst appearing as a radiolucent mass protruding into the urethra on VCUG; and (4) ruptured syringocele—the membrane that remains after a dilated duct ruptures (Fig. 16–151). This system is useful in describing the lesions of Cowper's gland duct that occur in children.

Embryology

Cowper's glands arise as two solid ectodermal buds from the urogenital sinus at the site of the future bulbous urethra. The ducts course posteriorly, one on either side of the midline and parallel to the urethra. Numerous secondary ducts form as outgrowths from the main ducts. These remain in the area of the urethral bulb. Alveoli are formed at the ends of these ducts, and become functional at 4 months gestation. Final maturation into mucus-secreting cells simply involves growth changes in these areas. It is believed that cystic abnormalities of Cowper's gland occur because of obliteration of the ostia of the main duct, and therefore the cyst lies just beneath the mucosa of the bulbous urethra. Another theory suggests developmental arrest in ductal organization which then becomes a nonobstructed but dilated duct with an enlarged ostia. The female homologue of Cowper's glands is the Bartholin's (greater vestibular) glands.

Anatomy

The bulbourethral glands were first described by Mery in 1684. Cowper's account of their discovery published in 1699 earned him the eponym (Brock and Kaplan). These paired glands lie on either side of the membranous urethra within the urogenital diaphragm. They are approximately 0.5 cm in diameter. Comprised of tubuloalveolar glands, multiple lobules drain into individual ductules that unite to form a single duct for each gland, which drains into the urethra. The ducts pierce the inferior leaf of the triangular ligament and course obliquely through the corpus spongiosum to terminate in the bulbar urethra (Fig. 16–152). A second, smaller accessory gland lies within the spongiosum tissue. This second pair of glands appears to account for the difference between the intraurethral cyst-

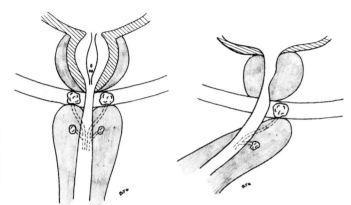

Figure 16–152. Anteroposterior and lateral diagrams show normal location of main and accessory Cowper's glands and ducts. (From Brock WA, Kaplan GW: Lesions of Cowper's glands in children. J Urol *122*:122, 1979. ©1979, The Williams & Wilkins Co., Baltimore.)

like obstructive variety and the extraurethral, nonobstructive lesions previously described as incidental findings.

Signs and Symptoms

A variety of initiating complaints can be elicited depending on the size and location of the Cowper's gland duct cyst. Several cases have been reported in stillborn babies with obstruction so severe that a probe could not be passed into the bladder (Firlit). In neonates who survive with these lesions, a diminished urinary stream, urinary retention, and occasionally hematuria may be noted. Less obstructive cysts in an older child may present as hematuria (Cook and Shaw), urinary infection, or an abnormal voiding pattern (Maizels et al). The low incidence of cystic anomalies of Cowper's gland ducts suggests that a majority of congenital Cowper's gland duct cysts do not become symptomatic. Moreover, when present, the associated signs and symptoms of these cysts are usually not severe in older children. Recurrent infection may be consequent to bacterial colonization of a stagnant collection of urine within the dilated duct. Hematuria can result from trauma to the delicate cyst membrane during micturition. In young adults a sudden decrease in the force and caliber of urinary stream, perineal pain, dysuria, hematuria, or bloody urethral discharge can be the presenting complaint. On occasion perineal pain may be associated with a bulging perineal mass.

Diagnosis

Bloody urethral discharge, postvoiding hematuria, a history of a narrow or interrupted urinary stream, or the inability to catheterize a patient who has no known urethral anomaly should alert the clinician to the possible presence of a Cowper's gland duct cyst. Voiding cystourethrography may demonstrate a filling defect in the bulbous urethra or a cystic submucosal lesion in the same area (Fig. 16–153).

Urethroscopy should be performed under direct vision while passing the panendoscope from the meatus proximally. It is suggested that the operator be in the standing position, maintaining traction on the penile urethra, while inserting the panendoscope (Cook and Shaw).

Treatment

Small, partially obstructive cysts are treated effectively by endoscopic unroofing with the resectoscope or Bugbee electrode. This form of treatment has proved ideal for the group of glands lying deep in the spongy tissue of the

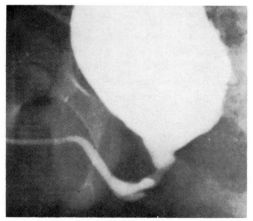

Figure 16–153. Cowper's gland duct cyst (dilated periurethral gland). (From Firlit CF: Urethral abnormalities. Urol Clin North Am 5:1, 1978.)

bulb. Treatment is simple and is associated with minimal morbidity. Small, asymptomatic lesions that are incidental urographic or endoscopic findings should probably be ignored. For the large obstructed gland that results in a perineal mass, open surgical excision and ligation of the cystic neck flush with the urethra is the treatment of choice.

ANTERIOR URETHRAL POLYPS

Urethral polyps occur exclusively in male patients, who most commonly present with symptoms of obstruction (Foster et al). The great majority of these lesions are located in the posterior urethra, attached to the verumontanum. Anterior urethral polyps are a very rare entity, as only 4 cases have been reported in the literature (Redman).

Signs and Symptoms

Presenting symptoms of anterior polyps include terminal hematuria, enuresis, and postvoid dribbling. One patient who also had a duplex urethra presented with recurrent infection (Falkowski and Cook).

Diagnosis and Treatment

Urethral polyps must be considered in the differential diagnosis of pediatric distal obstructive disease. Diagnosis is achieved by obtaining a retrograde urethrogram or voiding cystourethrogram. Treatment consists of excision by transurethral resection or through a urethrotomy.

Pathology

These lesions appear to arise from the ventral urethral wall (Fig. 16–154) and are believed to be congenital in nature. Salient features include a narrow stalk at the base with a transitional cell covering. The polyp itself contains a highly collagenous stroma. Chronic lesions may demonstrate squamous metaplasia.

URETHRAL DIVERTICULUM IN THE MALE

Congenital diverticula of the male anterior urethra are rare (Kelalis et al). The wide-mouthed (saccular) diverticulum and the small-mouthed pedunculated (globular) di-

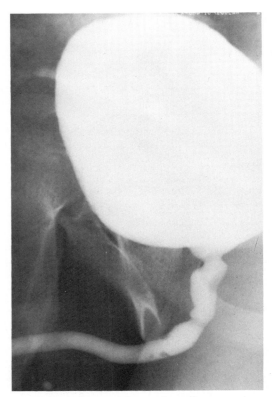

Figure 16–154. A voiding cystourethrogram shows anterior urethral polyps in bulbous urethra. (From Falkowski WS, Cook WA: Anterior urethral polyps: an unusual cause of hematuria in a child. J Urol 125:744, 1981. ©1981, The Williams & Wilkins Co., Baltimore.)

verticulum are two well-recognized varieties of the lesion. Located on the ventral aspect of the urethra from the bulbous to the mid pendulous urethra, the wide-mouthed diverticula lack a true neck. In contrast, the small-mouthed diverticula are usually located ventrally over the proximal urethra, and have a definite orifice and a narrow, communicating neck. These diverticula do not result from a distal obstructive lesion, but may cause urethral obstruction because of their propensity to poor drainage, bulging into the urethra and thereby contributing to urethral outflow resistance.

Large-mouthed diverticula undermine the urethra and are often associated with a mobile distal lip that functions like an anterior urethral valve. This pseudovalve formation is thought to be caused by progressive enlargement of the diverticulum. The question of whether an anterior valve was present initially and precipitated formation of the diverticulum is sometimes unresolvable. Moreover, when severe, the valvular obstruction associated with the diverticulum may result in upper tract decompensation (Boissonnat and Duhamel; Davis and Telinde; Mandler and Pool; Williams and Retik). Lesions causing less serious obstructions are often diagnosed incidentally when the boy is investigated for other disorders.

Embryology

There are many theories for the etiology of congenital urethral diverticula. Cystic dilatation of urethral glands that communicate eventually with the urethra has been suggested as a possible cause (Williams and Retik). Voillemier and DePaoli provide a somewhat more plausible explanation by suggesting that diverticula originate in an area in which there is defective or deficient corpus spongiosum. Another suggestion proposes formation of a distal congenital obstructing valve or membrane that results eventually in proximal diverticulum formation and then disappears (Boissonnat and Duhamel; Kaufman). In 1908, Suter postulated that the urethral gutter may leave behind an epithelial nest after closure of the urethral folds that may later give rise to dermoid cysts or urethral diverticula. This premise is consistent with the fact that congenital urethral diverticula are ventral midline structures (Mills).

The most obvious and convincing explanation is that such diverticula are formed as a result of a developmental defect in the corpus spongiosum. This may occur owing to focal arrest in the differentiation of periurethral mesenchyme into the spongy sheath. Subsequent lack of an effective tissue buttress may lead to urethral dilatation in this deficient area and result in the formation of a diverticulum. Histologically, diverticular walls are lined by epithelium and a delicate fibrous capsule. Supportive elements of the corpus spongiosum are lacking. The hypothesis of an arrest in mesenchymal differentiation is also analogous to explanations of deficiencies in other areas of the body such as absent abdominal musculature (Boissonnat and Duhamel) and posterior urethral valves (Graham et al).

Signs and Symptoms

In the neonatal period a large saccular obstructive urethral diverticulum may be seen and palpated on the ventral surface of the penis. Boys with this disorder void with a diminished, dribbling stream. Pressure on such diverticula after voiding results in further emptying of urine. The urinary tract is

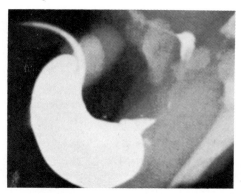

Figure 16–155. Saccular diverticulum of the anterior urethra resembling scaphoid megalourethra in a 2-day-old boy. (From Firlit CF: Urethral abnormalities. Urol Clin North Am 5:1, 1978.)

usually sterile, and hydronephrotic changes are not commonly seen on excretory urography. In other children urologic investigation is prompted by signs and symptoms of urinary tract obstruction or a penile mass. Some children complain of an enlarging penis during voiding and continuous dribbling incontinence due to subsequent emptying of the diverticulum. Frequency, dysuria, hematuria, and a firm penoscrotal mass may also be presenting complaints. The narrow-mouthed diverticulum may become a source of infection or result in stone formation as a consequence of poor emptying and urinary stasis (Virinder et al).

Diagnosis

Voiding cystourethrography or a retrograde urethrogram will confirm the diagnosis and define the location of the diverticulum (Fig. 16–155). Urethrography may demonstrate an accompanying obstructing anterior urethral leaflet (Fig. 16–156). The narrow neck of the globuolar variety can usually be delineated. Cystoscopy will further clarify the nature of the lesion, but is not always necessary as part of the diagnostic evaluation.

Treatment

Simple excision of the wide-mouthed diverticular sac with reapproximation of the urethral defect over a catheter will usually suffice. The closure should include a minimum of two layers, with urinary drainage by urethral catheter or suprapubic cystotomy. For the small wide-mouthed diverticulum with a distal valvelike leaflet, transurethral

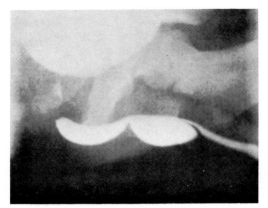

Figure 16–156. Bulbous urethral diverticulum with distal valvelike leaflet and dilatation of the. more proximal urethra. (From Firlit CF: Urethral abnormalities. Urol Clin North Am 5:1, 1978.)

and Stephens). The urethral plate tubularizes by midline fusion of the inner genital folds. This begins in the bulbous portion and proceeds through the penile portion to the base of the glans penis (Fig. 16–157B and C). This line of fusion is identified as the median raphe. The outer genital folds continue to fuse beyond the base of the glans penis to form the frenulum (Fig. 16–157D to F). An ectodermal core at the center of the glans canalizes downward to meet the glanular urethra to establish urethral continuity (Fig. 16–157C to F). This results in the formation of the urethral meatus and fossa navicularis (Fig. 16–157G). According to this theory, a diverticulum of the lacuna magna may result if the ectodermal ingrowth becomes abnormally long and its junction with the glanular urethra is not end-on.

incision, fulguration, or avulsion of the lip may be all that is necessary. When the distal leaflet is absent, open excision and two-layer closure provides satisfactory results. If the residual urethra appears too small for primary closure after diverticular excision, a two-staged procedure may be appropriate, as used for repair of urethral strictures.

DIVERTICULUM OF THE FOSSA NAVICULARIS (LACUNA MAGNA; VALVE OF GUÉRIN)

Dorsal urethral diverticula of the fossa navicularis has been described as a cause of hematuria and/or painful voiding in young boys (Sommer and Stephens). The largest depression in the fossa navicularis is termed the lacuna magna, and was first described by Morgagni. The septum between the lacuna magna and the urethral lumen is usually referred to as the valve of Guérin (Gray and Skandalakis). Symptoms appear to be related to overdistention of the lacuna magna. Of 21 boys undergoing routine endoscopic evaluation for various reasons, a discernible dorsal pit or lacuna magna was confirmed in 6 cases by probing the fossa navicularis and by urethroscopy.

Embryology

The studies of Sommer and Stephens support the concepts of Glenister in regard to formation of the glandular urethra (Sommer

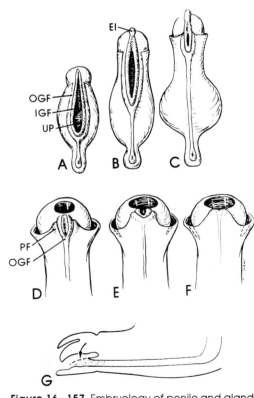

Figure 16–157. Embryology of penile and glandular urethra. OGF, outer genital folds; IGF, inner genital folds; PF, preputial folds; UP, urethral plate; EI, ectodermal ingrowth. *Arrow* indicates site of junction. When the junction is incomplete, a lacuna magna or dorsal diverticulum results (G). (From Sommer JT, Stephens FD: Dorsal urethral diverticulum of the fossa navicularis: symptoms, diagnosis and treatment. J Urol *124*:96, 1980. ©1980, The Williams & Wilkins Co., Baltimore.)

Signs and Symptoms

The clinical picture is usually one of sudden onset of dysuria or hematuria, which may be associated with intermittent spotting on the underpants. Hematuria and dysuria can also result from urethritis, cystitis, or urethral abnormalities such as a Cowper's gland duct cyst or urethral polyp. However, a diverticulum of the fossa navicularis should be suspected as a correctible lesion when the etiology of the patient's complaint remains obscure after physical examination and urinalysis.

Diagnosis

Voiding cystourethrography that visualizes the entire urethra may demonstrate a distended lacuna magna as a spherical diverticulum of the dorsal urethra at the junction of the glans and the penile shaft (Fig. 16–158). Caution must be used in the interpretation of this study, as droplets of opaque medium spilled on towels or over the area of the corona may lead to an erroneous diagnosis. Prior to endoscopy, a lacrimal duct probe guided along the dorsal aspect of the fossa navicularis may identify the diverticulum (Fig. 16–159A). Because of its proximity to the meatus, the orifice of the diverticulum may be difficult to visualize on urethroscopy.

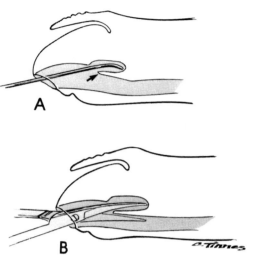

Figure 16–159. Dorsal diverticulum of glandular urethra. *A,* Identification and measurement of depth of diverticulum by lacrimal probe. *B,* Transmeatal marsupialization of lacuna by division of the valve of Guérin with scissors. (From Sommer JT, Stephens FD: Dorsal urethral diverticulum of the fossa navicularis: symptoms, diagnosis and treatment. J Urol *124*:96, 1980. ©1980, The Williams & Wilkins Co., Baltimore.)

Treatment

Marsupialization of the diverticulum by dorsal incision of the valve of Guérin is a simple and effective method of management. A pair of small blunt pointed scissors can be used to divide the common septum (Fig. 16–159B). Bleeding is seldom a serious problem after this maneuver, but if it occurs, a catheter may be inserted overnight.

URETHRAL DIVERTICULUM IN THE FEMALE

Congenital urethral diverticula in females are rare lesions. Those that are recognized are discovered because of a vaginal introital mass, urethral discharge, or recurrent urinary tract infections. The differential diagnosis of lesions of urinary tract origin also includes prolapsed urethra, prolapsed ureterocele, urethral polyp, and caruncle. In 1967, Andersen indicated that only one true documented congenital diverticulum had been described in the literature. Sumner recently described five cases of congenital urethral diverticulum in girls, however. None were associated with infection, unlike those in adult females, in

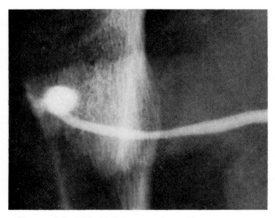

Figure 16–158. Voiding cystourethrogram shows rounded dorsal diverticulum of glandular urethra termed the lacuna magna and usually due to a valve of Guérin. The urethra is unobstructed. (From Sommer JT, Stephens FD: Dorsal urethral diverticulum of the fossa navicularis: symptoms, diagnosis and treatment. J Urol *124*:95, 1980. ©1980, The Williams & Wilkins Co., Baltimore.)

whom dysuria is usually the presenting complaint. Two cases were proved histologically to contain all layers of the urethra, and the three other lesions resolved spontaneously. Glassman et al described a urethral diverticulum in a newborn, and Newman reported a case of a Skene's duct abscess in a child. These lesions were considered to be similar to the diverticula seen in adult women resulting from infected paraurethral ducts. Davis and Telinde report a 6.5 per cent incidence of urethral diverticula in females under 20 years of age, so the lesion may not be as rare as it seems; it is diagnosed mainly in adolescents.

Embryology

The mechanism of urethral diverticulum formation in the female is unknown, but several theories have been proposed.

Various investigators consider such diverticula to be either remnants of ectopic ureteral orifices, portions of Gartner's duct, infected paraurethral glands, or an abortive attempt at urethral duplication (Silk and Lebowitz). The anterior urethra contains the prominent and persistent Skene's glands, which open on either side onto the floor of the urethra just within the meatus. If diverticula were to develop on a congenital basis from these paraurethral glands, they would be present at birth and be unassociated with infection (Sumner). If the ostia of their ducts become obstructed later in life, an acquired, infected diverticulum of the adult variety may result.

Symptoms and Diagnosis

The most prevalent presenting symptom is urinary frequency, reported in about 75 per cent of cases. Dysuria and burning occurred in 50 per cent, while hematuria or urethral discharge were present in 25 per cent. Awareness of a vaginal mass may also prompt the patient to seek medical attention.

The diagnosis of a urethral diverticulum is made upon suspicion and vaginal palpation. Palpation usually produces purulent discharge on urethral massage. Voiding cystourethrography or retrograde urethrography may further delineate the lesion (Fig. 16–160).

Treatment

Excision of the diverticulum is usually required. Marsupialization into the urethra may

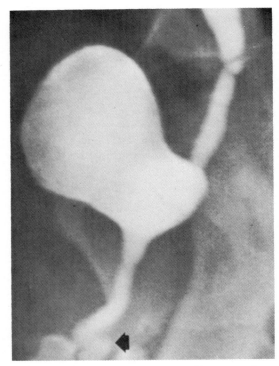

Figure 16-160. Voiding cystourethrogram demonstrating a congenital distal urethral diverticulum (arrow) in a 3-year-old girl with recurrent urinary tract infection. (From Firlit CF: Urethral abnormalities. Urol Clin North Am 5:1, 1978.)

be an attractive alternative. A urethral fistula is a recognized risk but has been reported only rarely. The neonatal female with an asymptomatic lesion is probably best treated expectantly, as the diverticulum may resorb, as it did in three of the five cases reported by Sumner.

ANTERIOR URETHRAL STRICTURES

Urethral strictures in boys are not rare lesions. There are many etiologies, of which the iatrogenic form is most common. Traumatic and inflammatory lesions occur with less frequency. Congenital strictures of the urethral bulb have become a controversial issue and may in fact represent what may be more accurately termed a perforate congenital urethral membrane or diaphragm.

Embryology

The male urethra is formed by the joining of the proximal endodermal urogenital sinus with the penile portion by fusion of the ectodermal genital folds along the genital ridge.

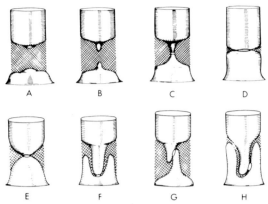

Figure 16-161. A to D, Concept of normal canalization of urogenital membrane. E, Congenital urethral membrane or stricture results from incomplete canalization, with formation of stenotic, mucosal aperture. F to H, Variations in formation of type III urethral valve. (From Gibbons MD, Koontz WW Jr, Smith JV: Urethral strictures in boys. J Urol *121*:220, 1979. ©1979, The Williams & Wilkins Co., Baltimore.)

These derivatives also give rise to the prostatic ducts and membranes. The phallic portion of the urogenital sinus contributes the cavernous urethra, which extends to the penis (Gray and Skandalakis). The ectodermal distal urethral anlage joins the prostatic endodermal anlage just distal to the bulbomembranous junction. This embryologic linkage suggests that incomplete rupture of the membrane could result in a soft, membranelike stricture (Fig. 16-161). This congenital membrane is not associated with ureteral fibrosis or deposition of abnormal tissue as is an acquired stricture. Several investigators consider this lesion to be embryologically identical to Young's type III urethral valve (Devereux and Williams; Sweetser; Duckett).

Other Etiologic Considerations

Iatrogenic injury accounted for stricture disease in nearly two thirds of the boys reported by Gibbons et al. In their series of 22 cases, strictures resulted from instrumentation (7), urethroplasty (5), fulguration of a posterior urethral valve (1), and an indwelling urethral catheter (1). Devereux and Williams reviewed 40 cases of anterior stricture, of which 17 were considered iatrogenic. These resulted from posterior valve fulguration (7), indwelling catheterization (3), anterior Y-V plasty of the bladder neck (5), and other causes (2). Less frequently, traumatic bulbar

urethral strictures can be attributed to straddle injury, a direct blow to the perineum, a penetrating injury, or pelvic fracture. Infectious urethritis may result in stricture formation. Gonococcal strictures are typically located in the bulbous urethra. This area contains a predominance of mucus-secreting glands. Gonorrhea in the prepubertal child is uncommon, but physicians treating the pediatric patient should be aware of the possibility (Meek et al). A form of "nonspecific" urethritis for which no causative agent could be identified was described by Williams and Mikhael in 17 boys between the ages of 5 and 15 years. A bulbar urethral stricture was diagnosed endoscopically in two of these patients, and Kaplan and Brock reported stricture formation in boys presenting with urethrorrhagia.

Cowper's gland duct abnormalities may have a role in stricture formation, as suggested by Currarino and Stephens. The location of the stricture often corresponds to the openings of these ducts. Opacification of Cowper's gland ducts is not unusual as an incidental finding on voiding cystourethrography in boys with stricture. Rupture of a Cowper's gland duct cyst may result in a fine, filmy membrane representing remnants of the ruptured duct wall (Maizels et al). However, the formation of a symptomatic bulbar stricture after rupture of a Cowper's gland duct cyst has never been reported.

The precise nature of congenital strictures in the proximal urethral bulb remains controversial. This is a rare lesion caused by a soft circumferential mucosal membrane. This congenital membrane or stricture differs from the acquired types of stricture in that there is a distinct lack of periureteral fibrosis or any abnormal tissue surrounding the urethra. In a report by Cobb et al, 26 cases of proximal urethral bulb strictures were identified and treated. These patients ranged in age from newborn to 16 years. None had a history of urethral or perineal trauma, urethroscopy, urethral surgery, or urethritis. Strictures were identified by retrograde urethrography, bougie calibration, or cystourethroscopy. Thirty-eight per cent of these boys had associated congenital anomalies including cerebral palsy, syndactyly, polydactyly, tetralogy of Fallot, cleft palate, myelomeningocele, and hypospadias. Stephens reported six patients who had recognizable congenital or idiopathic bulbous urethral strictures on postmortem examination. He also successfully treated four boys with similar strictures by urethral dilatation alone. All reported cases were associated with signs and symptoms of significant obstruction. The strictures were described as "soft," and all responded well to simple urethral dilatation which appears to permanently relieve such obstruction.

Congenital bulbar urethral stricture has been described in a family by Michon, occurring in a 42-year-old man and his 23- and 28-year-old sons. Additionally, Redman and Fraiser reported on two brothers aged 13 and 15 who both presented with hematuria and were found to have anterior urethral strictures of apparent congenital origin. In contrast, Currarino and Stephens were unable to determine whether short bulbous strictures found in six children were of an acquired or congenital origin. The lesions were not preceded by trauma, urethral instrumentation, or known urinary tract infection. Endoscopically they appeared to have thickened edges rather than the typical thin, delicate membrane.

Diagnosis and Treatment

Urethral strictures are best diagnosed with an excretory urogram and a voiding cystourethrogram (Fig. 16–162). A voiding or expression cystourethrogram can be made with an excretory urogram if there is adequate opacification of the bladder. Otherwise the bladder can be filled with contrast using a catheter or infant feeding tube. A voiding urethrogram can then document the location of the stricture. A retrograde urethrogram may be necessary if a feeding tube cannot be introduced. For a soft congenital urethral

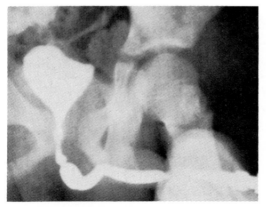

Figure 16–162. Congenital urethral stricture, proximal portion of bulbous urethra. (From Firlit CF: Urethral abnormalities. Urol Clin North Am 5:1, 1978.)

stricture, simple dilation may suffice, as noted above. Cobb et al suggest urethral dilation with infant sounds or pediatric Kollmann dilators. If this is ineffective, cold knife incision with the pediatric or infant resectoscope is then performed. In Devereux and Williams' series, 9 of the 37 children were treated by intermittent anterior urethral dilation, with success in 7 with mild strictures requiring only a single or infrequent dilation. Even though such an approach is unlikely to be effective in alleviating traumatic or iatrogenic strictures, spectacular results are occasionally obtained by single dilation (Fig. 16–163).

Repeated dilations are harmful, however, because they can accentuate the associated fibrous tissue reaction, making subsequent surgical repair more difficult. Furthermore, repetitive dilation entails frequent hospitalization because general anesthesia is necessary. Therefore, the treatment of the majority of urethral strictures in boys should be surgical correction.

Urethroplasty

It is imperative that no urethral dilation be performed immediately before a surgical procedure, because dilation makes it difficult to define, and sometimes to identify, the strictured area accurately. As a general rule, anterior urethral strictures are easier to repair than posterior ones, but, irrespective of the location, meticulous surgical technique and attention to details at all stages are mandatory. It is essential that the tissues be mobilized sufficiently to permit reconstruction without tension and that the tissues be accurately approximated after complete hemostasis.

For anterior urethral strictures, burying a longitudinal island flap of penile skin is ideal. For bulbar strictures, reconstruction from inlay tissue is preferable; scrotal tissue with its elasticity and rich blood supply is satisfactory. The main disadvantage of using scrotal tissue, at least in older children, is the need for epilation; however, this can be done easily by desiccating the hair follicles with electrocoagulation. In multistage urethroplasties, continuity should not be restored until one is certain that both distal and proximal urethrostomies are patent and that sufficient time has elapsed for the inlay (if used) to become solid. Finally, compression dressings should be used for several days postoperatively to decrease edema and prevent hematoma.

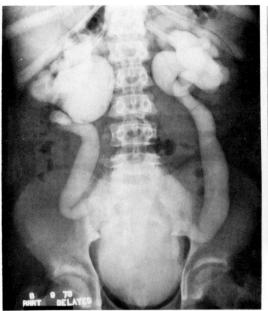

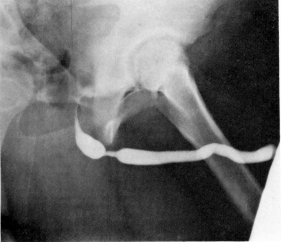

B

Figure 16–163. Urethral stricture in 15-year-old boy. *A*, Excretory urogram, showing bilateral hydroureteronephrosis. *B*, Retrograde urethrogram, showing bulbar stricture (iatrogenic): urethral dilatation. *C*, Postoperative (6 months) excretory urogram, showing regression of hydroureteronephrosis. Patient was doing well without further dilatation or significant recurrence of stricture 2 years later.

C

One-Stage Urethroplasty

The plethora of technical variations is proof that the ideal operation for the repair of urethral strictures remains elusive. The existence of a variety of techniques also emphasizes that strictures in various portions of the urethra pose different therapeutic problems for which no single type of urethroplasty suffices. Most, if not all, types of urethroplasty are purported to give satisfactory results, at least in adults, in whom the vast majority of strictures are encountered. From the limited number of urethroplasties reported in children, it would appear that, irrespective of the location of the strictures or the procedure used, the results are highly gratifying (Devereux and Williams).

For a single, localized urethral stricture, excision and end-to-end anastomosis of normal tissues without tension is ideal. Anastomosis of the dorsal wall with perineal diversion of urine for 10 to 14 days, to permit epithelialization of the lumen, is a procedure that has been used for many years. Recently, transfer of a full-thickness graft of hairless skin from

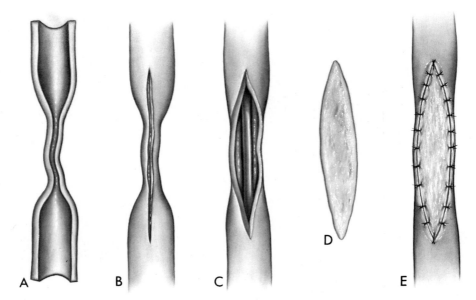

Figure 16-164. Urethroplasty with free full-thickness graft of penile skin.

the foreskin of the penile shaft to the incised strictured area has produced gratifying results (Fig. 16–164) (Devine et al). The defatted skin is sewn to the urethra with the subcutaneous surface superficial, and the urine is diverted by suprapubic cystostomy for 3 weeks. It is essential that voiding cystourethrography give evidence of complete healing before the catheter is removed. For longer strictures, a multistage approach is preferred.

Multistage Urethroplasty

ANTERIOR URETHRAL STRICTURES. In the first stage of multistage urethroplasty, the abnormal area may be excised completely

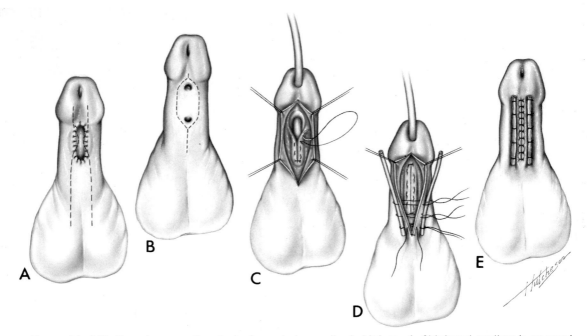

Figure 16-165. Two-stage urethroplasty for anterior urethral stricture. *A*, Strictured urethra is opened longitudinally and urethral mucosa is approximated to skin. *B*, Outlining of urethra several months later. *C*, Construction of new urethra. Normal urethra is exposed both proximally and distally. *D* and *E*, Skin closure with mattress sutures of fine nylon placed around strips of 8 F rubber tubing. Skin edges are approximated at midline with fine absorbable sutures.

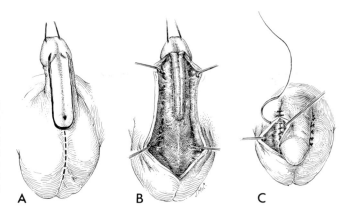

Figure 16–166. Cecil urethroplasty: When adequate skin is lacking, the neourethra may be "buried" in the scrotum during the second stage of this repair. At a third stage, about 4 months following the maneuver depicted in this diagram, the penis is released from the scrotum. Wide incisions are used to guarantee adequate scrotal skin for ventral skin coverage.

and the gap bridged with adjoining tissues. More often, the strictured area is opened longitudinally and the urethral mucosa is approximated to the skin with fine, interrupted, 5-0 temporary chromic catgut sutures (Fig. 16–165*A*). A urethral catheter is inserted via the proximal stoma.

Several months later, the second stage is completed. A new urethra is constructed, and the skin is closed with mattress sutures of fine nylon placed around strips of 8F rubber tubing (Fig. 16–165*B* to *E*). For longer strictures, the likelihood of fistula may be decreased

further by scrotal burial of the new urethra (Fig. 16–166). An alternative to this is simple burial of penile skin and subsequent closure of the skin flaps (Fig. 16–165*D* and *E*). With either method, temporary urinary diversion by suprapubic cystostomy or perineal urethrostomy is used.

In 19 boys treated by various techniques of urethroplasty for urethral strictures, Devereux and Williams encountered only two failures.

BULBAR STRICTURES. For bulbar strictures, the Leadbetter procedure using a poste-

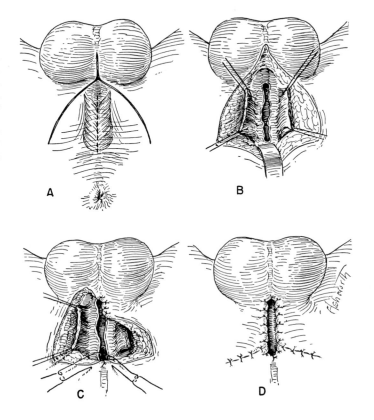

Figure 16–167. Leadbetter operation for stricture in the bulbous urethra: first stage. *A,* Incision. *B,* Bulbocavernosus muscle is retracted on either side and strictured area is incised. *C* and *D,* Completion of first stage. Subcutaneous tissue of skin flaps is approximated to periurethral tissue for relief of tension and skin closure. (From Hand JR: Surgery of the penis and urethra. *In* Campbell MF, Harrison JH: Urology. Vol 3, Third ed. Philadelphia, WB Saunders Co., 1970.)

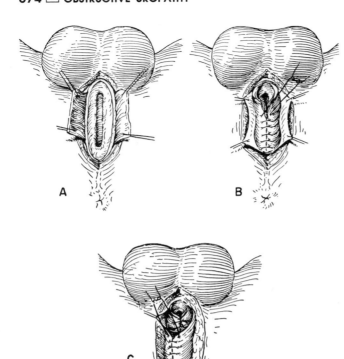

Figure 16–168. Leadbetter operation: second stage. *A,* Flap around marsupialized segment of urethra is mobilized. *B,* Bulbocavernosus muscle is approximated in midline over the closed urethra. *C,* Approximation of Colles' fascia lateral to midline to avoid superimposition of sutures (followed by approximation of subcutaneous tissue and skin—not shown). (From Hand JR: Surgery of the penis and urethra. *In* Campbell MF, Harrison JH: Urology. Vol. 3. Third ed. Philadelphia, WB Saunders Co., 1970.)

rior-based inlay of perineal skin is quite suitable. This is a modification of the Johansen technique. Lithotomy position is necessary. The first stage is illustrated in Figure 16–167. A urethral catheter is used. The second stage, performed 4 to 6 months later, is shown in Figure 16–168. A urethral catheter is again left indwelling for 7 to 10 days.

Conclusion

Congenital urethral stricture of the bulbous urethra is a distinct entity with an understandable embryologic basis. Persistence of the urogenital portion of the cloacal membrane accounts for the regular occurrence of these strictures in the proximal anterior urethra. However, the diagnosis of a congenital stricture must be made judiciously. Most case reports have included a majority of patients who are beyond the toddler years. Although a congenital origin is supported by reports of familial incidence, a lesion produced by a congenital anomaly should have its most common clinical presentation in the newborn and infancy periods. It is therefore also possible that previous straddle injury severe enough to result in bulbar urethral stricture may sometimes not be remembered by the patient or by parents. Therefore, to prevent inappropriate therapeutic measures, one must be cautious when ascribing stricture disease in the pediatric patient to congenital causes.

MEGALOURETHRA

Congenital megalourethra is an anomaly that is analogous to an extreme form of urethral diverticulum. The diverticulum is often associated with obstruction, however, whereas megalourethra is not associated with a recognizable obstructive lesion.

Megalourethra is a consequence of partial or complete agenesis of spongy and/or erectile tissue. Three distinct varieties of this disorder occur, ranging from a localized deficiency of corpus spongiosum to complete absence of both corpus spongiosum and corpora cavernosa (Stephens). The first type represents the mildest manifestation. A localized absence of corpus spongiosum predisposes to formation of a saccular diverticulum in the penile urethra. As the diverticulum enlarges, obstruction of the urethra may result from displacement of the tunica in a valvelike manner. The second form, or scaphoid megalourethra, is associated with greater deformity and also deficiency of erectile tissue (Fig. 16–169). If the corpora cavernosa are normal,

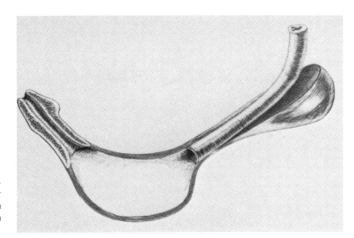

Figure 16–169. Scaphoid megalourethra. The corpus spongiosum is deficient at the site of urethral expansion. (From Firlit CF: Urethral abnormalities. Urol Clin North Am 5:1, 1978.)

micturition results in enlargement of the saccular ventral deformity, which deflects the penis superiorly and decreases the force of the urinary stream (Fig. 16–170). The fusiform type, representing the severest deficiency of erectile tissue, occurs as a result of nearly complete absence of the corpus spongiosum and corpora cavernosa. There have been eight reported cases of fusiform megalourethra, all of which were associated with severe congenital anomalies incompatible with life (Kelalis et al). Schwartz (cited by Firlit) reported a dramatic example in which an infant with congenital absence of the corpora cavernosa and corpus spongiosum also had an imperforate anus, bilateral cryptorchidism, left renal agenesis, and aberrant adrenal tissue (Fig.

16–171). A unique case of megalourethra representing features of both scaphoid and fusiform varieties was reported by Chehval and Mehan. The penis had a normal left corpus cavernosum, but the distal third of the corpus spongiosum and right corpus cavernosum was absent.

Embryology

Congenital megalourethra results from a failure of the mesodermal urethral folds and mesenchyme to differentiate adequately or completely into erectile tissue (Dorairajan; Stephens). The urethra consequently lacks adequate support on its dorsal and ventral aspects, and balloons during micturition.

Figure 16–170. Voiding cystourethrogram demonstrating scaphoid expansion of the penile urethra in a 3-year-old male with reflux. (From Firlit CF: Urethral abnormalities. Urol Clin North Am 5:1, 1978.)

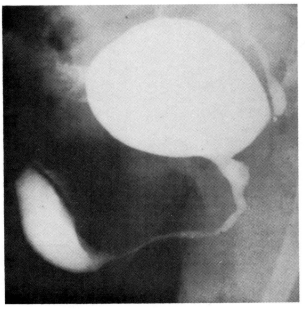

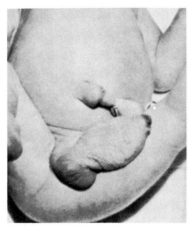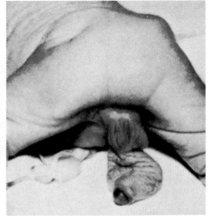

Figure 16–171. Fusiform megalourethra. Three-day-old infant with complete absence of corpora spongiosum and cavernosa and many other congenital anomalies, including imperforate anus. (From Firlit CF: Urethral abnormalities. Urol Clin North Am 5:1, 1978.)

Diagnosis

The diagnosis can often be made on simple inspection. Occasionally, urinary stasis can occur despite the lack of obstruction and may result in infection.

Hydroureteronephrosis, megacystis, and proximal urethral dilation may be demonstrable on urography. Dorairajan, and Johnston and Coimbra, describe upper tract abnormalities, deficiency in abdominal musculature, and rectourethral fistula as frequent associated findings. Clinically, when faced with the diagnosis of megalourethra, the physician should consider and investigate other mesodermal and nonmesodermal anomalies. In many instances these other anomalies are more serious and life-threatening than the nonobstructed megalourethra.

Treatment

Surgical reduction of the redundant dilated ventral urethra is required. Nesbit treated a scaphoid-type lesion by liberal excision of the redundant urethra. The narrowed urethra and skin were then reapproximated over a catheter used as a stent.

URETHRAL MEATAL STENOSIS IN THE MALE

Congenital stenosis of the distal urethral meatus that causes obstruction in boys is a rare phenomenon. Various reports in the older literature have emphasized the occurrence of meatal stenosis and have urged prompt recognition and treatment (Berry and Cross; Lattimer; Maynardt and Frederick). However, it now appears that congenital meatal stenosis has been tremendously overdiagnosed in the past as a cause of obstructive uropathy in childhood (Duckett).

To establish the incidence of neonatal meatal stenosis, Allen et al calibrated the urethral meatus of 100 consecutive newborn boys. The mean, median, and mode were each 8F. The authors concluded that there was a 10 per cent incidence of congenital stenosis (4 to 6F) as well as an additional 10 per cent incidence of equivocal meatal stenosis (6F). None of these asymptomatic neonates with stenosis were evaluated radiographically to rule out the presence of resultant obstructive uropathy.

Morton measured meatal size in 1000 circumcised boys aged 2 weeks to 16 years. Litvak et al later studied 200 boys with no urinary complaints using calibartion by bougies à boule. The results of these two studies were then combined and statistically analyzed (Table 16–15). These data revealed that the normal size of the urethral meatus could be differentiated into three age groups. These results also appear to define the lower limits of the normal urethral meatus size in boys. Meatal stenosis could be suspected in boys less than 4 years of age if the meatus measured less than 8F, and in boys over 10 if the meatus calibrated to less than 10F.

Embryology

The embryologic basis for neonatal urethral stenosis is considered to be a failure of the urethral membrane to canalize completely (Gray and Skandalakis). Partial canalization may result in stenosis. Complete failure to canalize would result in complete distal urethral obstruction, severe hydronephrosis, oligohydramnios, and quite possibly, a stillborn fetus.

Diagnosis and Treatment

Severe neonatal meatal stenosis with resultant obstructive uropathy has only rarely been documented. Visual inspection of the meatus is highly unreliable in determining caliber, which can be accurately ascertained only with the bougie à boule. Symptomatic meatal stenosis in infants and children usually results from inflammatory changes secondary to ammoniacal dermatitis, a complication of neonatal circumcision. Such patients may present with a pinpoint meatus, mucosal glandular fissuring, bleeding from fresh fissures with burning pain following micturition, or angulation of the urinary stream.

Stenosis has been well documented in the hypospadiac urethra. This tends to be a constrictive lesion and is occasionally associated with dysuria, frequency, meatal ulceration, and proximal urethral dilation (Stephens). Secondary bulbous urethritis caused by incomplete emptying of the obstructed urethra can result in stasis and infection. When significant neonatal or acquired meatal stenosis is present, a dorsal or ventral meatotomy be-

comes the treatment of choice. Close postoperative follow-up is necessary because of the high incidence of recurrence. Daily meatal dilatation by parents using a lubricant and a small eye dropper or an ophthalmic antibiotic applicator for 2 weeks sometimes helps to assure a satisfactory result (Firlit).

DISTAL URETHRAL RING

Therapy of recurrent urinary tract infection associated with voiding pattern abnormalities in females has evolved over many years. Such infection often presents with signs and symptoms compatible with bladder outlet obstruction. Various predisposing etiologies have been proposed. Historically, the "spinning top" deformity of the proximal urethra demonstrated frequently on voiding cystourethrography was explained as a poststenotic dilation. Y-V plasty of the bladder neck achieved cures in up to 50 per cent of cases. However, this aggressive approach has now been abandoned, and it has become apparent that the female urethra assumes various shapes in different stages of micturition (Fig. 16–172).

The distal urethral ring in females is a congenital structure first described by Lyon and Smith as an obstructive lesion detected in 70 of 100 girls who were evaluated for infection or dysuria. The "fibrotic" ring is recognized as a distinct, circumferential narrowing in the distal third of the urethra, readily detected by

Table 16–15. Normal Size of the Urethral Meatus in Male Children

Age	Size	No. (%)	Size	No. (%)
		Group 1		
6 wks. to 1 yr.	Below 8F	22/160 (14)	10F	138/160 (86)
1 yr.	Below 8F	10/63 (14)	10F	53/63 (86)
2 yrs.	Below 8F	17/109 (16)	10F	92/109 (84)
3 yrs.	Below 8F	13/93 (14)	10F	80/93 (86)
		Group 2		
4 yrs.	Tight 8F	7/83 (8)	12F	70/83 (84)
5 yrs.	Tight 8F	10/111 (9)	12F	92/111 (83)
6 yrs.	Tight 8F	8/87 (9)	12F	61/87 (82)
7 yrs.	Tight 8F	4/56 (7)	12F	43/56 (77)
8 yrs.	Tight 8F	5/61 (8)	12F	41/61 (67)
9 yrs.	Tight 8F	4/60 (7)	12F	40/60 (67)
10 yrs.	Tight 8F	3/50 (6)	12F	37/50 (74)
		Group 3		
11 yrs.	Below 10F	2/45 (4)	14F	36/45 (80)
12 yrs.	Below 10F	2/40 (5)	14F	28/40 (69)

From Litvak AA, Morris JD, McRoberts JW: Normal size of the urethral meatus in male children. J Urol 115:736, 1976. © 1976, The Williams & Wilkins Co., Baltimore.

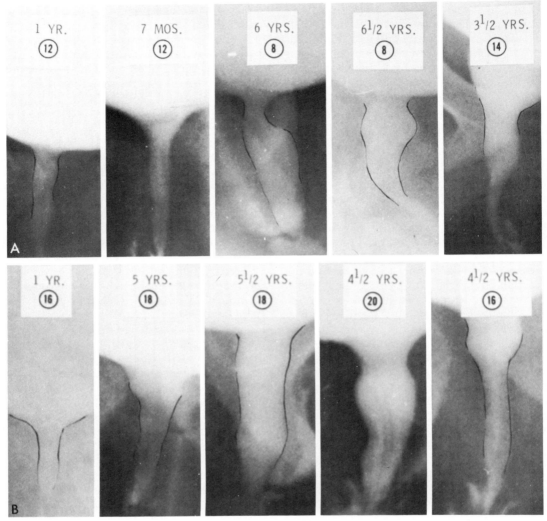

Figure 16–172. The appearance of the urethra on voiding cystogram in the female is seldom helpful in estimating the urethral caliber. In each instance, the age is given together with the size of the largest bougie à boule that could be withdrawn without detecting an obstruction at the distal urethral ring or the meatus. In the upper register *(A)*, calibers were relatively small, but the same urethral configurations were found during voiding in girls in whom the urethra was unequivocally normal in size. The distal urethral ring is a normal structure in girls and is analogous to meatal stenosis in boys. It is a narrow point in the urethra, but seldom the cause of obstruction. *B,* Lower register.

calibration with bougies. It can measure 6F or less in diameter and has a stiff, snug, and gritty feeling that can be appreciated as it snaps over the "shoulders" of the bougie during calibration. This condition is not meatal stenosis. The location of the narrowing in relation to the meatus is variable, depending on the length of the nonmuscular navicular fossa. However, it is distinctly separate from and above the meatus.

Immergut et al reported normal values for the caliber of the urethra in 136 females without urinary tract disease. The mean from ages 0 to 4 was 14.6F, from 5 to 9 years, 16.2F; and

from 10 to 14 years, 21.1F. The calibers of the distal urethral ring and the meatus were found to be essentially the same. This study and that of Graham et al, who found that urologically normal girls had slightly smaller urethral calibers than those with infection, suggest that Lyon's ring is a normal structure in prepubertal girls.

Embryology

The distal urethral ring is found at the junction between the urethral mucosa, which forms the proximal two thirds of the urethra, and the more squamous mucosa, which forms the distal third of the urethra. It is not apparent why this junctional area should become the site of a rigid ring or how it might produce irritative and obstructive symptoms in some girls. Lyon theorized that spontaneous reabsorption of the ring occurs at menarche, evidenced by the unexplained spontaneous recovery from a propensity to urinary infection in some girls at that age.

Arey considers the majority of the female urethra to be of endodermal origin. He states that the shortened neck connecting the bladder with the urogenital sinus elongates into the female urethra. The pelvic and phallic portions of the sinus merge to create the vestibule near the distal end of the urethra. It is in this region that the distal ring can be appreciated in some symptomatic girls and in normal girls as well.

Signs and Symptoms

Common complaints are those of dysuria, meatal burning, frequency, incontinence, and a history of recurrent urinary tract infection. Abnormal voiding patterns may include a low-velocity urinary stream, a staccato stream, or a hesitant stream. Although these signs and symptoms suggest a distal urethral ring, they are certainly not diagnostic as these symptoms are also those of detrusor-sphincter dyssynergy of childhood, and may also represent voluntary interruption of the stream due to dysuria or anxiety.

Diagnosis and Treatment

Patients with these symptoms require evaluation by voiding cystourethrography, excretory urography, and sometimes urodynamic evaluation and cystoscopy. A "spinning top" or "acorn" deformity of the proximal urethra will be demonstrated by the voiding cystourethrogram in about 67 per cent of girls with a history of urine infection. However, only 47 per cent demonstrate a distal urethral ring on bougie calibration. The remaining 20 per cent will be normal by calibration. Urodynamic evaluation of these children will often demonstrate a hyperactive external urethral sphincter or pelvic floor. The voluntary external sphincter and the urethral ring are in the same portion of the urethra. Consequently, voiding cystourethrography may produce similar urethral configurations when external sphincter dyssynergy is present (Fig. 16–173).

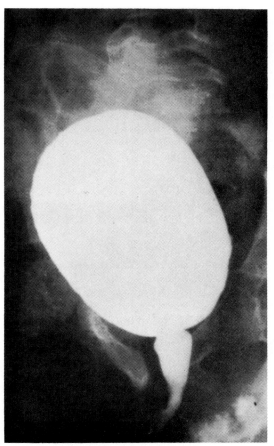

Figure 16–173. A voiding cystourethrogram in an 8-year-old girl with a history of recurrent cystitis, daytime wetting, and urge symptoms. This study demonstrates a urethra with the "spinning top" appearance. These urethral configurations with the above history are highly suggestive of the striated sphincter dyssynergy of childhood. These hyperdynamic sphincters contribute to outflow resistance and incomplete emptying, and ultimately may predispose to urinary infections. (From Firlit CF: Urethral abnormalities. Urol Clin North Am 5:1, 1978.)

Treatment of the distal urethral ring is by a single urethral overdilatation. Meatotomy by simple incision or by wedge resection may also be employed. Repeat dilatations are entirely contraindicated, as the ring does not reocclude after rupture. There are no hard data to support the notion that repeat urethral dilation prevents recurrent urinary infection (Kaplan et al). Treatment for external sphincter hyperactivity is by biofeedback or by pharmacologic therapy with diazepam, as much as 0.5 to 1.0 mg/kg/day in two divided doses, as discussed in Chapter 12.

The distal urethral ring is a congenital lesion, whereas the hyperactive external sphincter is acquired or learned. These distal obstructive lesions result in turbulent urethral flow, which may result in increased retrograde inoculation of urethral micro-organisms into the bladder. Since the majority of these patients fail to empty the bladder to completion at least at times, recurrent cystitis is common.

Conclusion

The meatus or distal urethral ring is only very rarely narrow enough to give rise to objective evidence of bladder outlet obstruction, manifested minimally by increased trabeculation. In the absence of such evidence, urethral dilatation, particularly repeated dilatation, is not a reasonable therapeutic approach in the management of girls with voiding problems or infection, and should be discouraged. On the other hand, if cystoscopy is being performed for other reasons, such as the evaluation of refluxing intravesical ureters or evaluation to rule out cystitis cystica, overdilatation of the urethra does not appear to increase the dysuria subsequent to the examination.

BIBLIOGRAPHY

Allen JS, Summers JD, Wilkerson JE: Meatal calibration in newborn males. J Urol 107:98, 1972.

Andersen MJF: Instrument for injection urethrography in women. Acta Radiol (Diagn) (Stockh) 2:523, 1964.

Andersen MJF: The incidence of diverticula in the female urethra. J Urol 98:96, 1967.

Arey LB: Developmental Anatomy. Revised seventh ed. Philadelphia, WB Saunders Co., 1974.

Berry CD, Cross RR: Urethral meatal caliber in circumcised and uncircumcised males. Am J Dis Child 92:152, 1956.

Boissonnat P, Duhamel B: Congenital diverticulum of the anterior urethra associated with aplasia of the abdominal muscles in a male infant. Br J Urol 34:59, 1962.

Brock WA, Kaplan GW: Lesions of Cowper's glands in children. J Urol 122:121, 1979.

Campbell MF: Urethral stricture in infants and children. J Pediat 35:169, 1949.

Campbell MF: Urology. Third ed. Philadelphia, WB Saunders Co. 1970, p 1589.

Chang C: Anterior urethral valves: a case report. J Urol 100:29, 1968.

Chehval MJ, Mehan DJ: Congenital megalourethra: report of a unique case. J Urol 123:433, 1980.

Cobb BG, Wolf JA, Ansell JS: Congenital stricture of the proximal urethral bulb. J Urol 99:629, 1968.

Colabawalla BN: Anterior urethral valve: a case report. J Urol 94:58, 1965.

Cook WA, Firlit CF, Stephens FD, et al: Techniques and results of urodynamic evaluation of children. J Urol 117:346, 1977.

Cook FE, Shaw JL: Cystic anomalies of the ducts of Cowper's glands. J Urol 85:659, 1961.

Currarino G, Stephens FD: An uncommon type of bulbar urethral stricture, sometimes familial, of unknown cause: congenital versus acquired. J Urol 126:658, 1981.

Davis HJ, Telinde RW: Urethral diverticula: an assay of 121 cases. J Urol 80:34, 1958.

DePaoli: Gaz Med Ital Torino, Obstr Zbl Chir 12:905, 1885.

Devereux MH, Williams DI: The treatment of urethral stricture in boys. J Urol 108:489, 1972.

Dorairajan T: Defects of spongy tissue and congenital diverticula of the penile urethra. Aust NZ J Surg 32:209, 1963.

Duckett JW Jr: Anomalies of the urethra. In Campbell's Urology. 4th ed. Edited by JH Harrison, RF Gittes, AD Perlmutter, et al. Philadelphia, WB Saunders Co. pp 1635–1658, 1979.

Elbogen A: Zur Kenntnis der Cystenbildung aus den Ausfuehrungsgaenge der Cowperschen Druesen. Heilkunde 7:221, 1886.

Englisch J: Veber Retentionscysten der Ausfuehrungsgaenge beider Cowperschen Druesen. Tageblatt d Deutsch Naturforscher u Aerzte, September 19, 1881, lib 18.

Falkowski WS, Cook WA: Anterior urethral polyps: an unusual cause of hematuria in a child. J Urol 125:744, 1981.

Firlit CF: Urethral abnormalities. Urol Clin North Am 5:1, 1978.

Firlit CF, King LR: Anterior urethral valves in children. J Urol 108:972, 1972.

Firlit RS, King LR, Firlit CF: Obstructive anterior urethral valves in boys. J Urol 119:879, 1978.

Foster RS, Weigerl JW, Mantz FA: Anterior urethral polyps. J Urol 124:145, 1980.

Gibbons MD, Koontz WW Jr, Smith JF: Urethral strictures in boys. J Urol 121:217, 1979.

Glassman TA, Weinerth TL, Glenn JF: Neonatal female urethral diverticulum. Urology 5:249, 1975.

Glenister TW: The origin and fate of the urethral plate in man. J Anat 88:143, 1954.

Golimbu M, Orca M, Al-Askari S, et al: Anterior urethral valves. Urology 12:343, 1978.

Graham SD Jr, Krueger RP, Glenn JF: Anterior urethral diverticulum associated with posterior urethral valves. J Urol 128:376, 1982.

Gray SW, Skandalakis JE: Embryology for Surgeons. Philadelphia, WB Saunders Co., 1972, p 624.

Guérin, A.: Elements de chirurgie operatoire. Third ed. Paris, F Chamerot, 1864, p 87.

Immergut M, Culp D, Flocks RH: The urethral 6 caliber in normal female children. J Urol 97:693, 1966.

Johnson CM: Diverticula and cyst of the female urethra. J Urol 39:506, 1937.

Johnson FP: The later development of the urethra in the male. J Urol 4:447, 1920.

Johnston JH, Coimbra JAM: Megalo-urethra. J Pediatr Surg 5:304, 1970.

Kaplan GW, Brock WA: Idiopathic urethrorrhagia in boys. J Urol 128:1001, 1982.

Kaplan GW, Sammons TA, King LR: A blind comparison of dilatation, urethrostomy and medication alone in the treatment of urinary tract infection in girls. J Urol 109:917, 1973.

Kaufman D: Dtsch Chir 8:123, 1886.

Kelalis PP, King LR, Belman AB (editors): Clinical Pediatric Urology. Philadelphia, WB Saunders Co., 1976.

Lattimer JK: Simlar urogenital anomalies in identical twins. Am J Dis Child 67:199, 1944.

Litvak AS, Morris JD, McRoberts JW: Normal size of the urethral meatus in male children. J Urol 115:736, 1976.

Lyon RP, Smith DR: Distal urethral stenosis. J Urol 89:414, 1963.

Maizels M, Stephens FD, King LR, et al: Cowper's syringocele: a classification of dilatations of Cowper's gland duct based upon clinical characteristics of 8 boys. J Urol 129:111, 1983.

Mandler JI, Pool TL: Primary diverticulum of the male urethra. J Urol 96:336, 1966.

Maynardt CR, Frederick AJ: Congenital imperforate urinary meatus. Urol Cutan Rev 47:78, 1943.

McGuire EJ, Weiss RN: Scrotal flap urethroplasty for strictures of the deep urethra in infants and children. J Urol 110:599, 1973.

Meek JM, Askari A, Belman AB: Prepubertal gonorrhea. J Urol 122:532, 1979.

Michon, J.: Rétrécissement "familial" de l'urètre. J Urol Nephrol 84:107, 1978.

Mills WGG: Chronic retention in boys caused by diverticula in the anterior urethra. Br J Urol 27:292, 1955.

Morgagni GB: Adversaria Anatomica Omnia. Padua, J Cominus. Part I, article 10, p 5, 1719.

Morton HG: Meatus size in 1000 circumcised children from two weeks to sixteen years of age. J Fla Med Assoc 50:137, 1963.

Muschat M: Occlusion of urethral meatus. Am J Dis Child 67:275, 1944.

Muschat M: Urethral and perineal cysts of the gland of Cowper. J Urol 22:239, 1929.

Nesbit RM, Labardini MM: Urethral valves in the male child. J Urol 96:218, 1966.

Nesbit TE: Congenital megalo-urethal. J Urol 73:839, 1955.

Newman DM: Skene's Abscess. Soc Ped Urol Newsletter May 23, 1978, p 36.

Redman JF: Anterior urethral polyp in a boy. J Urol 128:1316, 1982.

Redman JF, Fraiser LP: Apparent congenital anterior urethral strictures in brothers. J Urol 122:707, 1979.

Sawanishi K: Congenital valve of anterior urethra in an infant; a case report. Acta Urol Jpn 8:419, 1962.

Scott FB, Caffarena E: Diagnosis of anterior urethral valves. J Urol 110:261, 1973.

Silk MR, Lebowitz JM: Anterior urethral diverticulum. J Urol 101:66, 1969.

Small MP, Schoenfeld L: Anterior urethral valves. Urology 11:262, 1978.

Sommer JT, Stephens FD: Dorsal urethral diverticulum of the fossa navicularis: symptoms, diagnosis, and treatment. J Urol 124:94, 1980.

Smey P, Firlit CF: Micturition urodynamic flow studies in children. J Urol 119:250, 1978.

Stephens, F.D.: Congenital Malformation of the Rectum, Anus, and Genito-urinary Tracts. Edinburgh and London, E & S Livingstone, Ltd., 1963.

Sumner M: Urethral diverticula in young girls. Urology 17:243, 1981.

Suter F: Arch Klin Chir 87:225, 1908.

Sweetser TH: Congenital urethral diverticula in the male patient. J Urol 97:93, 1967.

Texter JH, Engel RME: Anterior urethral valve as a cause for urinary obstruction: a case report. J Urol 107:316, 1972.

Virinder MS, Gupta SK, Chernian J et al: Urethral diverticulum in male subjects: report of 5 cases. J Urol 123:592, 1980.

Voillemier LD: Traite des maladies des voies urinares. Paris, V Masson et Fils, 1868.

Waterhouse K, Scordamaglia LJ: Anterior urethral valve: a rare cause of bilateral hydronephrosis. J Urol 87:556, 1962.

Wharton LR, Kearns W: Diverticula of the female urethra. J Urol 63:1063, 1950.

Williams DI, Retik AB: Congenital valves and diverticula of the anterior urethra. Br J Urol 41:228, 1969.

Williams DI, Mikhael RB: Urethritis in male children. Proc Roy Soc Med 64:133, 1971.

17

URINARY DIVERSION

Temporary Diversion

A. Barry Belman

Urinary diversion can be divided into two major categories: temporary and permanent. Temporary diversion is subdivided further into intubated and nonintubated forms. Although at times useful as an independent procedure, the intubated type is employed most frequently in the short-term management of obstruction prior to definitive care or as an adjunct to other surgical procedures, for example, hypospadias repair or pyeloplasty. The major advantages of intubated urinary diversion are its simplicity of application and ease of reversibility; however, the drawbacks of constant infection (Rickham), risk of accidental removal, and stone formation make this form of diversion less than ideal for the long-term situation. Nonintubated forms of diversion, on the other hand, also allow the free flow of urine but can be kept intact for longer periods of time without the complications of infection and stone formation if residual urine is eliminated. Nonintubated temporary diversion may be considered useful when a definitive procedure must be postponed or when it is desirable to stabilize the function of a renal unit before engaging in definitive treatment, thus allowing time for complete evaluation. However, at times, temporary percutaneous methods are also applicable to these circumstances.

INTUBATED TEMPORARY DIVERSION

The clinical application of intubated diversion has changed drastically over the past years. Improved techniques and capabilities,

earlier and better treatment of urinary tract infection, and a more aggressive approach to primary reconstruction of conditions that had been managed in a staged fashion in the past have significantly altered the scope of this chapter since the publication of the first edition of this book in 1976. Realistically, in the modern pediatric health care center only a few of the techniques mentioned are employed with any degree of regularity. The pediatric urologist should be conversant with percutaneous nephrostomy and, it is hoped, will be part of the team when the procedures are employed. Percutaneous suprapubic cystotomy has simplified temporary lower tract diversion significantly; however, vesicostomy remains the pediatric urologist's salvation in infants with poor bladder emptying or severe reflux. Many of the other procedures may be useful in the occasional unusual situation.

Nephrostomy

The insertion of a tube directly into the kidney is a time-honored method of temporary high drainage. It remains the diversion of choice in the acute situation in the absence of significant pyelocalycectasis. One of its advantages, ease of reversibility, also becomes one of its major drawbacks. An inadvertently removed tube may have to be replaced by means of a formal operation. For this reason the more stable loop nephrostomy may be preferable when drainage is needed for a moderate period or when the patient is a small infant. One must be aware, however, that ureteropelvic junction obstruction has been reported as a complication of long-term nephrostomy drainage in infants (Parker and Perlmutter).

TECHNIQUE OF NEPHROSTOMY. The patient is placed in the standard flank position for a subcostal incision (Fig. 17–1A). The necessity for renal mobilization varies.

Radial Pyelotomy. *In the absence of caly-cectasis,* the renal pelvis is exposed and held

with silk sutures for a radial pyelotomy. A curved stone forceps is inserted into a lower calyx and, with a finger used for counterpressure, is bluntly worked through the overlying parenchyma (Fig. 17–1B). When the tip of the forceps is visible, the capsule is sharply incised and a length of moistened umbilical tape is grasped by or tied to the forceps (Fig. 17–1C). This tape is then withdrawn through the

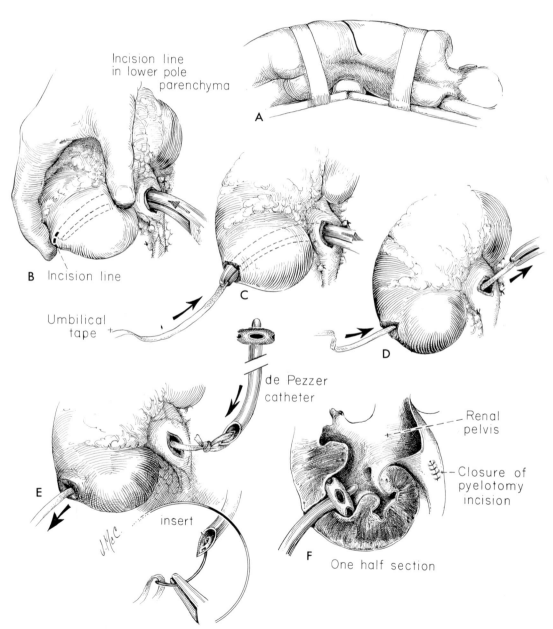

Figure 17–1. Technique for nephrostomy in the absence of significant calycectasis. (See text.) (From King LR, and Belman AB: A technique for nephrostomy in the absence of caliectasis. J Urol *108*:518, 1972. © 1972, The Williams and Wilkins Company, Baltimore.)

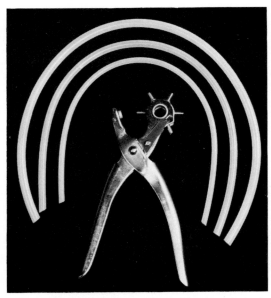

Figure 17–2. Leather punch used to place holes in Silastic tubing for loop nephrostomy.

capsular incision and through the pyelotomy (Fig. 17–1D). The end of the tape that has traversed the pyelotomy is sutured to a previously beveled nephrostomy tube (Fig. 17–1E). If the inferior calyces are narrow, trimming the flared end of the catheter may first be necessary to ensure adequate catheter fit and drainage. Using the umbilical tape as a guide, the surgeon then leads the tube into the collecting system while carefully avoiding sawing of the parenchyma.

Bleeding from the kidney is tamponaded by the catheter, which then may be fixed with absorbable sutures to the renal capsule. The renal capsule is usually fixed to the inner abdominal wall, ensuring a direct course for the tube from kidney to skin. The pyelotomy is approximated with a few interrupted 5-0 absorbable sutures, and the wound is closed in layers. The nephrostomy tube is brought through a separate stab wound and held with heavy silk sutures. A separate Penrose drain is advisable for a few days, since there may be drainage from the pyelotomy.

Loop Nephrostomy. The procedure of loop nephrostomy is carried out similarly. A variety of Silastic tubes and a leather punch are sterilized in advance (Fig. 17–2) or are used directly after removal from sterile commercial packaging. A site two thirds of the way down the length of the tube is selected and three or four paired holes are punched over a distance equal to the length of the renal pelvis. Since Silastic tears easily, these holes must be punched rather than cut to prevent disruption of the tube at that site (Binder et al).

Both pyelonephrostomy and ureteropyelonephrostomy have been described (Comarr), but it appears to be preferable to bring the limbs of the tubes through opposite renal poles, providing a more gentle curve to the tube and ensuring stability (Fig. 17–3). The ends of the tube are brought through separate stab wounds above and below the skin incision after it has been ascertained that the drainage holes lie within the renal collecting

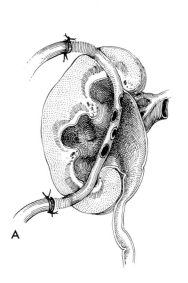

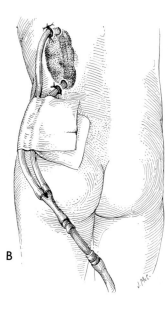

A   B

Figure 17–3. A, Loop nephrostomy using upper and lower calyces for exit of Silastic tubing. B, Tubing is stabilized to patient with sutures and tape.

system. Both limbs are then sutured to the skin and attached to a Y connector (Fig. 17–3B). A Penrose drain is inserted and the wound is closed in layers. The stability of this form of diversion makes it preferable to a standard nephrostomy when the need for proximal diversion becomes protracted.

When diversion is protracted, it may become necessary to change the tube. Weyrauch and Rous describe a means of assuring accurate placement of the drainage holes within the pelvis. A new length of tubing is intussuscepted or sutured to the upper limb of the old tube after it is cut at skin level. The old tube is withdrawn from below, with the new tube following. After the old tube is completely removed, it is used as a guide for proper hole placement in the new tube, which is then withdrawn back into the kidney and fixed in position with sutures.

Percutaneous Nephrostomy

The direct percutaneous insertion of a tube into the kidney is not a new idea; however, its application to children had been extremely limited until very recently. Improvement in localization techniques as well as instrumentation has made percutaneous nephrostomy applicable to patients of all ages. Sonographic visualization of the dilated collecting system followed by the direct insertion of a fine-gauge needle for infusion of contrast media allows the use of both sonographic and fluoroscopic monitoring techniques.

A variety of tubes have been inserted to drain the obstructed upper tract. These include pigtail angiographic catheters (Babcock et al), the Stamey suprapubic tube (Levy et al), and indwelling urethral catheters (Schilling et al). Prepackaged sets using a Malecot catheter are also available (Fig. 17–4).

The procedure can be performed under local anesthesia with sedation. After visualization of the collecting system by fluoroscopic or sonographic means, the collecting system may first be localized more accurately by insertion of a fine needle posteriorly and injection of contrast material or may be entered directly at the posterior axillary line with

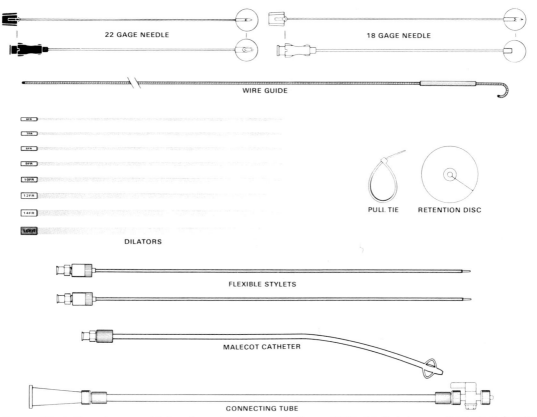

Figure 17–4. Percutaneous Malecot nephrostomy set. (From 1983–84 Catalogue: Urological Surgical Products. VPI, A Cook Group Company, P.O. Box 227, Spencer, Indiana 47460.)

an 18 gauge needle with a guide wire inserted. Fluoroscopic monitoring is used to ensure that the guide wire enters the collecting system, and the 18 gauge needle is removed. Dilators are passed over the guide wire to enlarge the tract and the appropriate tube is inserted following this maneuver. The tube is secured by whatever means are available in the kit employed.

Although complications of urine leak, hematoma, and abscess formation are potential risks (Perinetti et al), the success rate with percutaneous nephrostomy has been quite excellent. The significant prerequisite is a sufficiently dilated collecting system to allow insertion of the drainage device although with experience even relatively nondilated systems can be entered.

Application of this procedure is best suited to those children with obstruction and unresponsive infection in whom definitive surgery must be delayed while the infection is controlled (Fig. 17–5). Grossman et al reported control of acute hypertension in an infant with a solitary ureteropelvic junction obstruction. However, thickened intrapelvic material such as gross pus or fungus may not drain through the small percutaneous tubes, and a

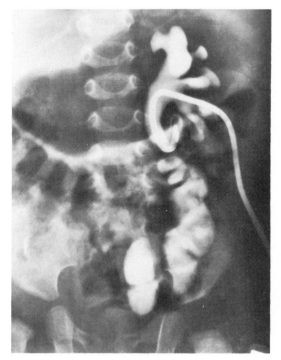

Figure 17–5. Percutaneous nephrostomy in septic infant with ureterovesical obstruction.

formal nephrostomy may be necessary under those circumstances (Eckstein et al).

Intubated Ureterostomy

Long-term use of an intubated cutaneous ureterostomy is not recommended. The chronic infection associated with a foreign body in the ureter provokes ureteral wall fibrosis, which may become irreversible. Additionally, the catheter may plug and obstruct drainage completely. Short-term intubation using Silastic or plastic feeding tubes is often employed, however, in conjunction with pyeloplasty, subsequent to closure of a loop ureterostomy and after a complicated or tapered ureteroneocystostomy. The tube may be brought out through its site of insertion (i.e., the flank wound) or, when used in conjunction with pyeloplasty, through an adjacent stab wound. Stents should be sutured to the skin for security.

Suprapubic Cystostomy

Suprapubic cystostomy is one of the oldest and most reliable methods of urinary diversion. Its current applicability in the pediatric population is mainly postoperative and short-term. Historically, cystostomy drainage had been used on a long-term or semipermanent basis in children with neuropathic disease or severe congenital outflow obstruction. As more definitive procedures have been perfected, this practice has been largely abandoned. The chronic infection and stone formation associated with this foreign body may progress to life-threatening and often fatal complications. This is particularly true in neonates, who tolerate cystostomy diversion poorly (Rickham). Nevertheless, the need for cystostomy drainage of several months' duration is still encountered in older children. Patients with severe traumatic urethral strictures or a complicated diagnostic or therapeutic problem in which temporization is judicious may be best served by cystostomy.

One must always keep in mind that no period of cystostomy drainage will alleviate obstruction at or above the ureterovesical junction. If upper tract improvement with this form of drainage is not apparent in a relatively short period of time, the situation requires re-evaluation. Edema at the ureterovesical junction, chronic ureteritis, or bladder thickening secondary to constant irritation due to

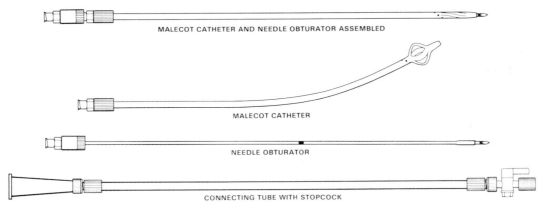

MALECOT CATHETER AND NEEDLE OBTURATOR ASSEMBLED

MALECOT CATHETER

NEEDLE OBTURATOR

CONNECTING TUBE WITH STOPCOCK

Figure 17–6. Stamey percutaneous suprapubic catheter set. (From 1983–84 Catalogue: Urological Surgical Products. VPI, A Cook Company, P.O. Box 227, Spencer, Indiana 47460.)

the presence of the suprapubic tube may exacerbate ureteral drainage problems, increasing the risk of renal parenchymal deterioration.

Percutaneous Cystostomy

Improved technology has made available a variety of simple kits for percutaneous cystostomy. Two that have become especially popular for use in children are the Stamey (Fig. 17–6) and the Cystocath (Fig. 17–7). Both employ the trochar technique, are relatively simple, and can be inserted in infants and children of all ages. The Stamey device employs a flanged catheter that can be retracted into the dome of the bladder. The Cystocath remains rolled up at the bladder base and, for that reason, may be responsible for a greater number of bladder spasms. Additionally, an occasional patient will void the tip of the Cystocath into the proximal urethra, thereby ending its ability to function properly until it is repositioned.

TECHNIQUE FOR INSERTION. Directions for application accompany these kits. The most important factor is the degree of bladder filling. The bladder must be distended to its maximum and, to ensure its staying that way as suprapubic pressure is applied with insertion of the trochar, simultaneous urethral compression may be neces-

Figure 17–7. Cystocath suprapubic drainage set. (From Medical Products, Bulletin 51–009b, Dow Corning Corporation, Midland, Michigan 48640.)

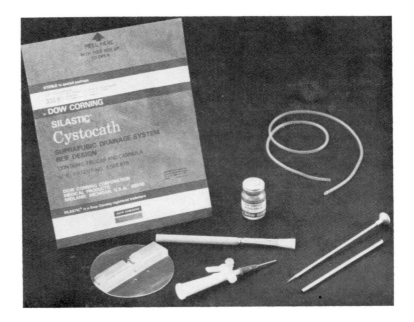

sary. Otherwise, voiding may occur with compression. Tiny skin and fascial incisions are made first, and then controlled pressure is applied to the trochar. Sometimes the amount of pressure required to perforate the fascia is significant and may provoke anxiety. However, steady pressure should obviate perforating the back wall of the bladder. The drainage tube is tied in at skin level and securely taped so that no loops can be available for grasping by the infant with subsequent inadvertent removal of the tube.

TECHNIQUE FOR OPEN CYSTOSTOMY. Although general anesthesia is ideal, under unusual circumstances suprapubic cystostomy can be performed with local anesthesia and sedation. Distention of the bladder greatly simplifies the procedure.

After appropriate skin preparation a short transverse skin incision is made a few centimeters above the symphysis (Fig. 17–8A). Since the skin is very elastic in children, a small incision will suffice. Subcutaneous tissue and superficial and deep fascia are incised in the direction of the skin incision, and the anterior rectus sheath cephalad to the incision is freed from the rectus muscles for a few centimeters.

The recti are bluntly separated, and the anterior bladder wall is visualized and grasped with Allis clamps or holding sutures (Fig. 17–8B). If there is doubt as to whether the viscus being held is truly the bladder, fluid can first be extracted with a small-bore needle and syringe. The bladder wall is then pulled into the wound and the peritoneum is bluntly pushed off its dome with a peanut dissector or a sponge. A small incision is then made in the dome between the Allis clamps or the sutures, the fluid previously inserted is aspirated, and a tube is inserted (Fig. 17–8C). In small children, a de Pezzer catheter with the button cut off to leave only a flange is the author's preference. It has staying power, yet it tends not to irritate the trigone and provoke bladder spasms.

The bladder incision is closed with interrupted absorbable sutures and the previously

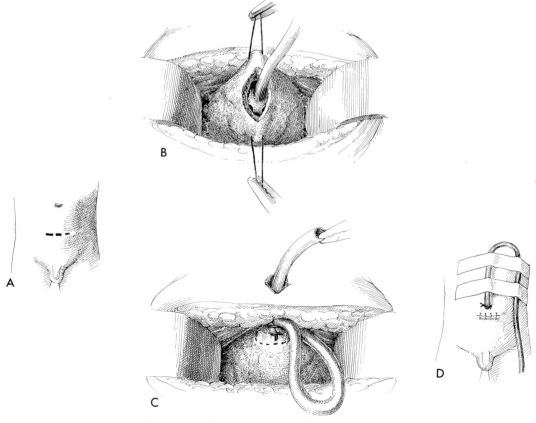

Figure 17–8. Suprapubic cystostomy. (See text.)

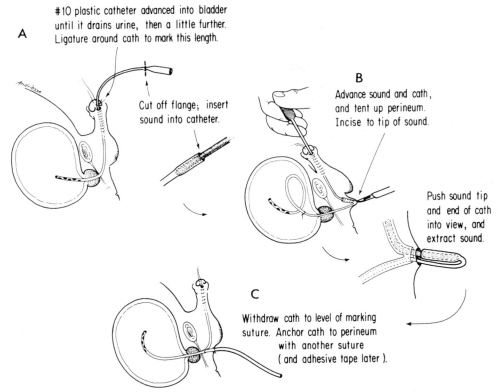

A

#10 plastic catheter advanced into bladder until it drains urine, then a little further. Ligature around cath to mark this length.

Cut off flange; insert sound into catheter.

B

Advance sound and cath, and tent up perineum. Incise to tip of sound.

Push sound tip and end of cath into view, and extract sound.

C

Withdraw cath to level of marking suture. Anchor cath to perineum with another suture (and adhesive tape later).

Figure 17–9. Technique for perineal urethrostomy. (From Kim SH, Hendren WH: Repair of mild hypospadias. J Ped Surg *16*:806–811, 1981. By permission of Grune & Stratton, Inc., New York.)

tapered end of the tube is brought out through a stab wound a few centimeters above the skin incision (Fig. 17–8C) Recall that the anterior rectus sheath had been dissected off the rectus earlier, simplifying this maneuver. Bringing the tube out of a separate wound and performing primary closure of the skin wound with subcuticular suture allows a more cosmetic closure. It is extremely important that the tube be snugged up and anchored to the skin so that its flange is against the bladder dome before the wound is closed. Careful taping of the tube in a child will prevent its inadvertent removal (Fig. 17–8D).

Perineal Urethrostomy

Perineal urethrostomy is a technique used by many as a means of temporary diversion following hypospadias repair (Coran; Kim and Hendren). A simple technique using a plastic catheter and urethral sound is demonstrated in Figure 17–9. Complications of perineal urethrostomy are rare, although stricture and persistent drainage can occur.

NONINTUBATED TEMPORARY DIVERSION

Ten years ago nonintubated temporary diversion was thought to be the treatment of choice by many for distal ureteral and bladder outlet obstruction in infants. With improved surgical and endoscopic techniques, primary treatment is pursued in the majority of cases, although it has been suggested that ultimate renal function can be improved by a period of temporary high diversion in some patients with posterior urethral valves (Krueger et al).

The major advantages of intubated diversion — ease of performance, simple nonoperative reversibility, and availability for urine collection — are lost with the nonintubated forms. A second major operation is necessary to reverse the diversion. Temporary diversion at the ureteral level has been said to delay definitive correction unnecessarily. Because a segment of ureter is devascularized, it may be more difficult to re-establish urinary tract continuity in the future (Hendren). It has also been suggested that, because of chronic irritation, vesicostomy may cause bladder changes that make definitive ureteral reimplantation more difficult. In addition, the stomal locations in both loop ureterostomy and vesicostomy make the fitting of a urine collecting device almost impossible.

In spite of these drawbacks, there are situations in which relatively long-term reversible diversion is desirable and may even be lifesaving. These include (1) nonresponsive sepsis in the child with obstructive uropathy, (2) the borderline situation in which the amount of renal reserve may not support life and extensive reconstruction not only is futile but may hasten the patient's demise, and (3) additional related or unrelated congenital abnormalities in infants, in whom a major definitive procedure is best postponed.

High, Reversible Nonintubated Diversion

Diversion at the renal level, if properly performed, assures free urinary drainage. Fears of missing partial obstruction in a sick infant at the level of the ureterovesical junction or the bladder outlet can be obviated with this procedure.

Another advantage afforded by all forms of high diversion is the availability for first-hand renal evaluation and biopsy. A renal unit capped by a tiny cystic parenchymal mass with little or no recognizably normal tissue may best be removed initially if the contralateral side has been shown to function by scan or excretory urogram or has already been observed at operation to appear fairly normal. When two severely abnormal units are encountered and it is apparent that overall long-term survival without renal augmentation (dialysis or transplantation) is unlikely, provisions for additional future care can be made at the outset.

Loop Cutaneous Ureterostomy

F. D. Stephens suggested a high, direct ureterocutaneous anastamosis as a method of ensuring excellent drainage when ureterectasis is severe (Johnston). In practice, this procedure has been performed most often in children with posterior urethral valves. Because of poor success with the tubed forms of diversion discussed previously, loop cutaneous ureterostomy became the preferred initial

form of management for patients with valves at many centers. More recently, primary valve resection has become more popular and is even being applied in septic infants following satisfactory medical stabilization.

Moderate to severe ureterectasis is an essential precondition for this procedure. If a ureter of normal or nearly normal size is brought directly to the skin, stenosis is very common. Innovation may be required if one finds an unsuspected duplication of the collecting system at the time of operation. A form of ipsilateral ureteroureterostomy, pyelopyelostomy or ureteropyelostomy, would then seem appropriate.

In loop ureterostomy as described by Johnston, it is inadvisable to bring the ureter to the skin at any level other than immediately below the ureteropelvic junction. Straightening of all kinks between the renal pelvis and the stoma has been said to be essential for the success of this procedure.

TECHNIQUE OF LOOP URETEROSTOMY. Theoretically, the patient may be placed in a variety of positions for the procedure. These include the prone position with a roll under the abdomen, allowing the surgeon to approach the ureters posteriorly; the supine position, with the infant's skin surgically prepared circumferentially, in which two subcostal incisions are made while the patient is rolled slightly from one side to the other; and the supine position, with the approach made through a midline incision. However, the standard flank position is simplest, has the lowest incidence of obstruction, and affords the best opportunity to approach the ureter at its highest level. The obvious disadvantage of this approach is the necessity for turning and redraping the patient when a bilateral procedure is required. Nevertheless, the overall operative success will be improved by using the flank approach as described below.

The child is taped in place with a roll under the flank. A subcostal incision through the skin and muscles is made down to and through the lumbodorsal fascia (Fig. 17–10A). In young infants the peritoneal reflection swings markedly posterior. To avoid inadvertently opening the peritoneum, the retroperitoneal space must be well dissected before the surgeon incises what he believes to be Gerota's fascia. The iliopsoas muscle may be used as a landmark. One is generally safe in assuming that the fascia adjacent to it is Gerota's fascia and not peritoneum.

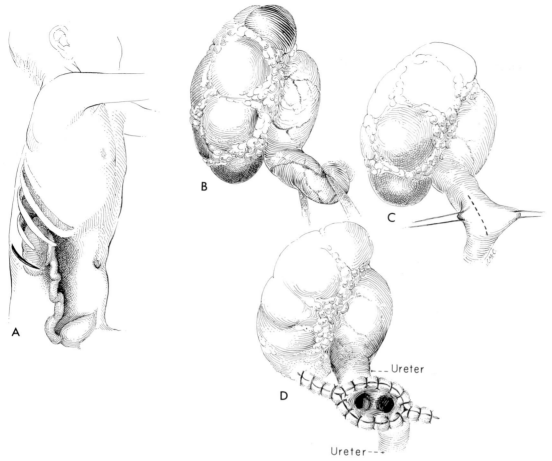

Figure 17–10. Loop ureterostomy. (See text).

The ureter in this situation is often as large in diameter as the infant's bowel. Even the most experienced urologist has, at times, wondered if he is not about to grasp the intestine during the initial dissection. The sight of urine aspirated from the viscus with a small-gauge needle may greatly allay this anxiety.

The ureter is then held with umbilical tape and dissected proximally to the ureteropelvic junction, all kinks being straightened along the way (Fig. 17–10B). Additional distal dissection may also be necessary to gain length sufficient to prevent tension on the completed suture line. With stay sutures used as guides, a longitudinal incision is made to open the ureter for a few centimeters (Fig. 17–10C). The most proximal apex of this ureterotomy is sutured to the most posterior aspect of the skin wound. A catheter is passed into the renal pelvis through the orifice created to ensure unencumbered drainage. Muscle layers are closed under the ureter to prevent retraction, and the ureteral edges are sutured to the skin (Fig. 17–10D). Either absorbable or nonabsorbable sutures may be employed.

REVERSING THE LOOP URETEROSTOMY. A major operative procedure is required to reverse the loop ureterostomy. Although the cutaneous segment may be detached, closed, and dropped into the retroperitoneal space, most who use loop ureterostomy prefer to remove the externalized segment with its metaplastic mucosa and to perform end-to-end ureteroureterostomy. The disadvantage of excising the cutaneous segment is that if a procedure at the ureterovesical junction is required, simultaneous operation on the lower ureter risks devascularization. Nevertheless, successful reimplantation at the time of loop closure has been reported by Dwoskin and by Novak and Gonzales. A ureteral stent brought out below the anastomosis, or a short-term nephrostomy, is advisable at the time of closure of the ureterostomy, particularly if distal obstruction is known to persist and definitive distal repair is being postponed. Antegrade flow studies may then be carried out to assess the distal ureter by this route if indicated (Rabinowitz et al). The technique of ureteroureterostomy is discussed in Chapter 16.

Y-Ureterostomy

In 1972, Sober offered a modification of loop ureterostomy with two advantages: closure without risk of distal devascularization, and the opportunity for some urine to enter the bladder. Irreversible bladder contracture after loop ureterostomy has been reported (Lome et al). This is thought to be in part secondary to total bladder defunctionalization in association with chronic infection, and may be preventable if some urine continues to flow down the distal ureter into the bladder.

TECHNIQUE OF Y-URETEROSTOMY. The approach for Y-ureterostomy is similar to that for loop ureterostomy; however, diversion is achieved with a high end-on ureterostomy (Fig. 17–11A). Again, it is stressed that this portion of the ureter must pursue a straight course to the skin. The remaining distal upper ureter is mobilized to obtain length sufficient to reach the renal pelvis, to which it is attached in an end-to-side fashion. Most of the urine drains primarily directly out to the skin through the high, end-on cutaneous ureterostomy, but part of it may go to the bladder through this new ureteropelvic anastomosis (Fig. 17–11B).

The takedown of this procedure is simpler than that for loop ureterostomy and does not risk ureteral devascularization. The cutaneous limb is simply excised to its origin at the pelvis and closed with running absorbable sutures. Narrowing or kinking of the previously constructed ureteropelvic anastomosis must be cautiously avoided.

Cutaneous Pyelostomy

Cutaneous pyelostomy is similar to the two methods of diversion just discussed. It has similar indications and some of the same drawbacks (Immergut et al; Schmidt et al). Its primary advantage is that the ureter need not be disturbed at the time of either formation or takedown, thereby making it preferable to loop ureterostomy. A large extrarenal pelvis is

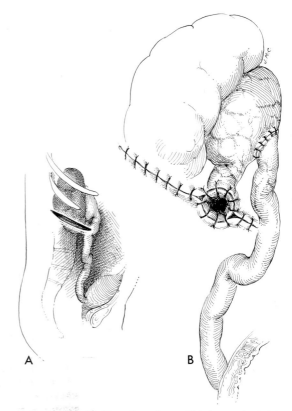

Figure 17–11. Y-ureterostomy. This form of urinary diversion allows some urine to drain into bladder, thus avoiding total defunctionalization.

a prerequisite, however. Closure of a cutaneous pyelostomy is simpler than closure of a ureteroureterostomy. Cutaneous pyelostomy also allows simultaneous closure and uteroneocystostomy, if indicated, without concern about ureteral devascularization.

TECHNIQUE OF CUTANEOUS PYELOSTOMY. The approach is the same as those previously described, except that the proximal ureter is not mobilized (Fig. 17–12A). The ureter is traced cephalad to the renal pelvis. The pelvis is held with silk sutures and incised in its midportion in the direction of the skin incision. Care must be taken neither to extend the pyelotomy into the ureteropelvic junction nor to make it excessively large. An overly large cutaneous pyelostomy has resulted in prolapse of the kidney through its stoma (Francis and Bucy; Glassberg et al).

Reversal of the cutaneous pyelostomy involves dissection of the redundant pelvis and its closure. Care must be taken to avoid distortion and obstruction of the ureteropelvic junction.

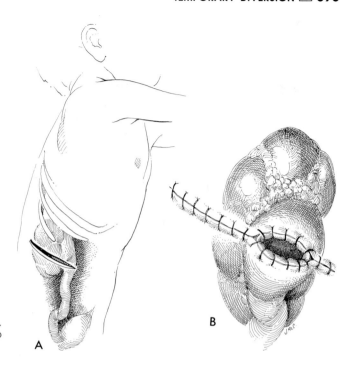

Figure 17–12. Cutaneous pyelostomy. The renal pelvis itself is sutured directly to the skin.

A

B

End Ureterostomy

The concept of constructing an end ureterostomy with the stoma in the lower abdomen would appear to violate the dogma espoused in the section on high temporary diversion; that is, the creation of a short straight segment from the kidney to the skin. Experience in those children with primary valve resection has demonstrated that these dilated ureters are capable of conveying urine into the bladder, provided that distal ureteral obstruction does not exist. Therefore, a distal end ureterostomy should be considered as a viable option when dealing with the child with obstructive megaureter in whom a primary procedure is not a reasonable alternative. This avoids the potential risk to the ureter of a double procedure (proximal and distal) when definitive reconstruction is carried out and simplifies future surgical repair (Rabinowitz et al). Distal ureterostomy has also been applied to the obstructed ureter in a duplicated system in cases in which it has been impossible to ascertain the degree of function at the time of initial evaluation or in which percutaneous nephrostomy or high ureteral diversion might jeopardize the normal renal segment. Options for future reconstruction after this approach is used include ipsilateral ureteropyelostomy or proximal or distal ureteroureterostomy.

TECHNIQUE OF END URETEROSTOMY. A lower midline incision gives excellent ureteral exposure yet preserves a scarfree area for the stoma (Fig. 17–13A). By dividing the fascia in the midline and bluntly separating the recti, the surgeon can keep the operation entirely extraperitoneal. A significant length of ureter can be freed, although excessive straightening and adventitial dissection are to be discouraged. A core of anterior abdominal wall is removed for the stoma, and the ureter is sutured directly to the skin (Fig. 17–13B). Stomal formation is described in more detail in the section on permanent urinary diversion.

Vesicostomy

One of the simplest forms of temporary diversion, one that has gained a great acceptance over the past 10 years in pediatric urologic circles, is vesicostomy (Bruce and Gonzales; Allen). None of the operations described is applicable to all situations — these procedures are highly individualized and their usefulness extends only to limited situations. This may be most true of vesicostomy, since any degree of supravesical obstruction immediately precludes its applicability. The task, then, is to rule out high obstruction when considering this method.

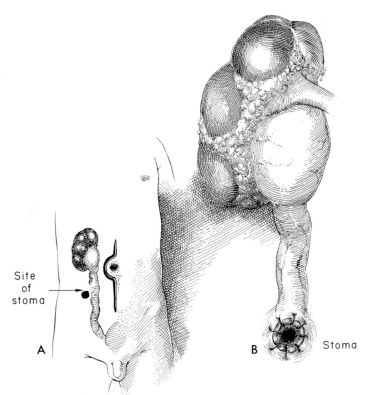

Site
of
stoma

A

B

Stoma

Figure 17–13. End ureterostomy. The anterior approach is preferred for accurate stomal location.

Cystography may be used to evaluate ureteral function. If reflux is present a post-drainage film with a catheter indwelling will help to determine the degree of impairment of upper tract drainage and possibly will suggest the presence of coexisting ureterovesical obstruction (Belman and King). If there is no reflux, an excretory urogram or a renal scan with a urethral catheter indwelling will often give the same information.

Vesicostomy is most appropriate for newborn infants with infravesical obstruction in whom definitive correction cannot be performed. An example is the premature boy with a posterior urethral valve in whom valve resection may not be technically possible because of the small urethral size (Duckett, 1974). Additionally, vesicostomy may be the most conservative means of managing the small baby with severe (grade IV to V) vesicoureteral reflux in whom both recurrent infection and complications of reimplantation constitute a great risk to future renal function. Finally, its application in the child with neuropathology (Cohen et al) or a prune belly (Duckett, 1976) as a means of controlling infections cannot be sufficiently extolled.

Vesicostomy should not be considered as a form of permanent diversion. The location of the stoma makes fitting a urinary collection device exasperating and often impossible (Carlson). Additionally, pubic hair growth compounds this problem by contributing to stomal incrustation and stone formation. When vesicostomy is used as a temporary diversion in infants, the lower abdominal position of the stoma allows the inconspicuous wearing of routine diapers until reversal is elected.

TECHNIQUE OF VESICOSTOMY. Filling the bladder to capacity simplifies the operation. The transverse skin incision should be made as near to the level of the bladder dome as possible but no higher than 2 cm below the umbilicus (Fig. 17–14A). The fascia is opened in the same direction and the rectus muscles are bluntly separated in the midline. Wedges of rectus and fascia may be removed laterally if these impinge upon the wound (Fig. 17–14B). The bladder is grasped with an Allis clamp and delivered into the wound while the peritoneum is simultaneously bluntly rolled off the dome to the level of the urachal remnant (Fig. 17–14C).

A transverse cystotomy on the dorsal aspect of the dome is followed by anastomosis of the bladder to the fascia and the skin with 3-0 or 4-0 absorbable suture (Fig. 17–14E and F).

The stoma should be large enough to admit at least one finger.

A complication of vesicostomy is bladder prolapse, which may obstruct outflow of urine. Prolapse can generally be prevented by avoiding redundancy between the base of the bladder and its point of fixation at the stoma. This requires sweeping peritoneum off the dome prior to incising the bladder. If it is discovered at that time that excessive bladder

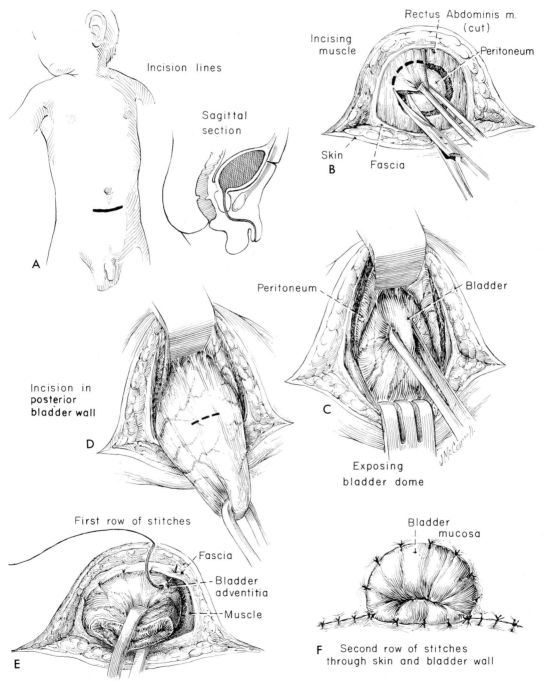

Figure 17–14. Vesicostomy in infants. The abdominal location of the bladder allows direct anastomosis of the dome to the skin. (See text.) (From Belman AB, King LR: Vesicostomy: useful means of reversible urinary diversion in selected infants. Urology *1*:208, 1973.)

redundancy persists, a more posterior cystotomy may be made and the original bladder incision closed. If prolapse produces obstruction, revision may require relocation of the stoma at a slightly higher level.

Stomal revision occasionally becomes necessary as the child grows, since the circumferential scar sometimes contracts or becomes relatively stenotic. In this instance, revision is a simple matter accomplished by excising the scar and resuturing the bladder wall to the skin.

Closure. Closing the vesicostomy is also simple and is usually done at the time of definitive operation such as reimplantation or valve ablation. Excision of the metaplastic mucosa and closure in layers, reapproximating the fascia with absorbable suture, is recommended. Successful closure with or without a temporary cystostomy can be achieved; however, a drain should be left in the prevesical space until urinary drainage has ceased.

BIBLIOGRAPHY

INTUBATED TEMPORARY DIVERSION

Babcock JR, Schkolnik A, Cook WA: Ultrasound-guided percutaneous nephrostomy in the pediatric patient. J Urol 121:327, 1979.

Binder C, Gonick P, Ciavarra V: Experience with Silastic U-tube nephrostomy. J Urol 106:499, 1971.

Comarr AE: Experience with the U-tube for renal drainage among patients with spinal cord injury. J Urol 95:741, 1966.

Coran AG: A simplified technique for performing perineal urethrostomy. Surg Gynecol Obstet 150:735, 1980.

Crawford ED, Borden TA: New instrument for placement of circle tube nephrostomy. J Urol 124:324, 1980.

Eckstein C, Kass EJ, Koff SA: Anuria in a newborn secondary to bilateral ureteropelvic fungus balls. J Urol 127:109, 1982.

Grossman IC, Cromie WJ, Wein AT, et al: Renal hypertension secondary to ureteropelvic junction obstruction. Urology 17:69, 1981.

Kim SH, Hendren WH: Repair of mild hypospadias. J Ped Surg 16:806, 1981.

King LR, Belman AB: A technique for nephrostomy in the absence of caliectasis. J Urol 108:518, 1972.

Levy JM, Potter WM, Stegman CJ: A new catheter system for permanent percutaneous nephrostomy. J Urol 122:442, 1979.

Parker RM, Perlmutter AD: Upper urinary tract obstruction in infants. J Urol 102:355, 1969.

Perinetti E, Catalona WJ, Manley CB, et al: Percutaneous nephrostomy: indications, complications and clinical usefulness. J Urol 120:156, 1978.

Rickham PP: Advanced lower urinary obstruction in childhood. Arch Dis Child 37:122, 1962.

Schilling A, Goettinger H, Mark FJ, et al: A new technique for percutaneous nephrostomy. J Urol 125:475, 1981.

Weyrauch HM, Rous SN: U-tube nephrostomy. J Urol 97:225, 1967.

NONINTUBATED TEMPORARY DIVERSION

Allen TD: Vesicostomy for the temporary diversion of the urine in small children. J Urol 123:929, 1980.

Belman AB, King LR: Vesicostomy: useful means of reversible urinary diversion in selected infants. Urology 1:208, 1973.

Blocksom BH Jr: Bladder pouch for prolonged tubeless cystostomy. J Urol 78:398, 1957.

Bruce RR, Gonzales ET Jr: Cutaneous vesicostomy: a useful form of temporary diversion in children. J Urol 123:927, 1980.

Carlson HE: Tubeless cystostomy in childhood. J Urol 83:669, 1960.

Cohen JS, Harbach LB, Kaplan GW: Cutaneous vesicostomy for temporary diversion in infants with neurogenic bladder dysfunction. J Urol 119:120, 1978.

Duckett JW Jr: Cutaneous vesicostomy in childhood: the Blocksom technique. Urol Clin North Am 1:485, 1974.

Duckett JW Jr: The prune-belly syndrome. In Clinical Pediatric Urology. First ed. Edited by PP Kelalis, LR King, AB Belman. Philadelphia, WB Saunders Co., 1976.

Dwoskin JY: Management of the massively dilated urinary tract in infants by temporary diversion and single-stage reconstruction. Urol Clin North Am 1:515, 1974.

Francis DR, Bucy JG: Inside-out kidney: an unusual complication of cutaneous pyelostomy. J Urol 112:514, 1974.

Glassberg KI, Laungani G, Macchia RJ, et al: Bilateral kidney herniation: complications of cutaneous pyelostomy. Urology 16:504, 1980.

Hendren WH: Urinary tract refunctionalization after prior diversion in children. Ann Surg 180:494, 1974.

Immergut MA, Jacobson JJ, Culp DA, et al: Cutaneous pyelostomy. J Urol 101:276, 1969.

Ireland GW, Geist RW: Difficulties with vesicostomies in 15 children with myelomeningocele. J Urol 103:341, 1971.

Johnston JH: Temporary cutaneous ureterostomy in the management of advanced congenital urinary obstruction. Arch Dis Child 38:161, 1963.

Karafin L, Kendall AR: Vesicostomy in the management of neurogenic bladder disease secondary to meningomyelocele in children. J Urol 96:723, 1966.

Krueger RP, Hardy BE, Churchill BM: Growth in boys with posterior urethral valves. Urol Clin North Am 7:265, 1980.

Lapides J, Ajemian EP, Lichtwald TR: Cutaneous vesicostomy. J Urol 84:609, 1960.

Leadbetter GW Jr: Skin ureterostomy with subsequent ureteral reconstruction. J Urol 107:462, 1972.

Leape LL, Holder TM: Temporary tubeless urinary diversion in children. J Pediatr Surg 5:288, 1970.

Lome LG, Howat JM, Williams DI: The temporarily defunctionalized bladder in children. J Urol 107:469, 1972.

Lome LG, Williams DI: Urinary reconstruction following temporary cutaneous ureterostomy diversion in children. J Urol 108:162, 1972.

Novak ME, Gonzales ET: Single stage reconstruction of urinary tract after loop cutaneous ureterostomy. Urology 11:134, 1978.

Perlmutter AD: Temporary urinary diversion in the management of the chronically dilated urinary tract in childhood. In Reviews in Paediatric Urology. Edited by JH Johnston, WE Goodwin. Amsterdam, Excerpta Medica, 1974.

Perlmutter AD, Patil J: Loop cutaneous ureterostomy in infants and young children: late results in 32 cases. J Urol 107:655, 1972.

Perlmutter AD, Tank ES: Loop cutaneous ureterostomy in infancy. J Urol 99:559, 1968.

Rabinowitz R, Barkin M, Schillinger JF, et al: Surgical treatment of the massively dilated ureter in children. Part I. Management by cutaneous ureterostomy. J Urol 117:658, 1977.

Schmidt JD, Hawtrey CE, Culp DA, et al: Experience with cutaneous pyelostomy diversion. J Urol 109:990, 1973.

Sober I: Pelviureterostomy-en-Y. J Urol 107:473, 1972.

Williams DI, Rabinovitch HH: Cutaneous ureterostomy for the grossly dilated ureter of childhood. Br J Urol 39:696, 1967.

Permanent Urinary Diversion

Alan B. Retik

Despite increasing experience and facility with extensive reconstruction of the urinary tract, the use of pharmacologic agents, intermittent catheterization, and artificial, mechanical devices for urinary continence and decompression, and increasing emphasis on urinary undiversion, there are still several conditions that require the urine to be diverted permanently. The most common conditions requiring permanent diversion in children are neuropathic bladder dysfunction, unreconstructable exstrophy of the bladder, and tumors of the lower urinary tract. In addition, a few children with markedly diminished renal reserve and very severe dilatation of the urinary tract who have been unresponsive to reconstructive surgical procedures may also require diversion. Many children who underwent "permanent" diversion in the past for conditions now amenable to rehabilitative efforts have subsequently been "undiverted." Very careful selection is mandatory before deciding upon permanent diversion in a child. Permanent urinary diversion should be used only after all other methods of therapy have been considered and exhausted.

Most of the types of permanent diversion that have been performed in our institution during the past decade have utilized one of the nonrefluxing colon conduits. Ureterosigmoidostomy has been infrequently performed because of reports of malignancy at the site of the ureterointestinal anastomoses. This will be discussed below. I have performed a few continent urinary diversions as well.

For the sake of completeness, however, procedures that were formerly performed frequently but that would appear to have little current application in the surgery of infants and children will also be discussed.

INTERNAL DIVERSION

Ureterosigmoidostomy

Ureterosigmoidostomy is a method of internal diversion that has been primarily used in children with exstrophy of the bladder (with an intact anal sphincter) or lower urinary tract malignancies. Prior to the popularization of the submucosal tunnel technique of Leadbetter with accurate mucosa-to-mucosa anastomosis, ureterosigmoidostomy frequently led to pyelonephritis, stone formation, and eventual renal deterioration. However, long-term results (Bennett, Spence et al, 1975) with the antireflux technique have been reasonably good, and this method of urinary diversion has received prime consideration (Allen), especially in the child with exstrophy who is not a candidate for primary closure.

This operation is contraindicated in children with impaired renal function, significant bilateral ureterectasis, or a lax anal sphincter. This obviously precludes its use in children with neuropathic vesical dysfunction. Spence recommended that ureterosigmoidostomy be done in the patient with exstrophy between the ages of 3 and 6 months. Hendren advocates a two-stage ureterosigmoidostomy. The first stage is the formation of a nonrefluxing sigmoid conduit; subsequent anastomosis of the conduit to the intact sigmoid colon is done at a later date if there is no evidence of reflux or obstruction and anal sphincter tone is satisfactory. One can usually adequately evaluate anal sphincter tone between the ages of 6 and 12 months. Sphincter control can be tested preoperatively by the child's ability to retain an oatmeal enema.

TECHNIQUE. Following adequate mechanical and antibacterial bowel preparation, the abdomen is opened through a left paramedian incision (Fig. 17–15). Both ureters are identified as they cross the iliac vessels. They are isolated, traced inferiorly, and divided close to the bladder. The sigmoid colon is grasped between Babcock clamps or stay sutures, and the site for the right anastomosis is prepared first. A 5-cm area along the tenia is infiltrated submucosally with a dilute epi-

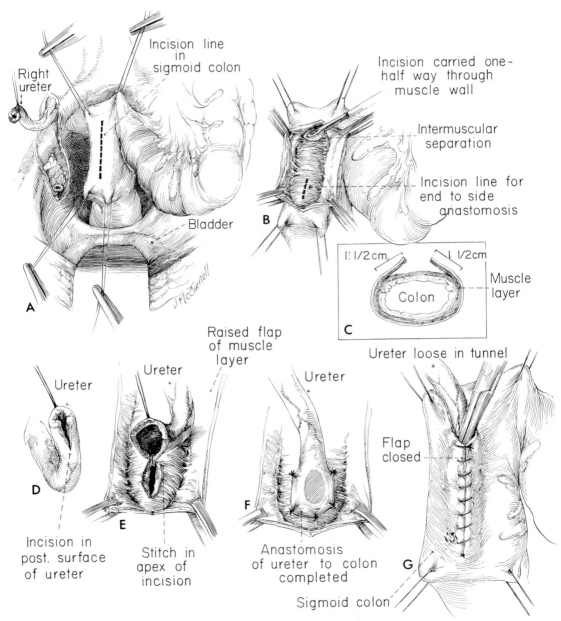

Figure 17–15. Ureterosigmoidostomy. (See text.) (From Current Controversies in Urologic Management. Edited by R Scott. Philadelphia, WB Saunders Co., 1972.)

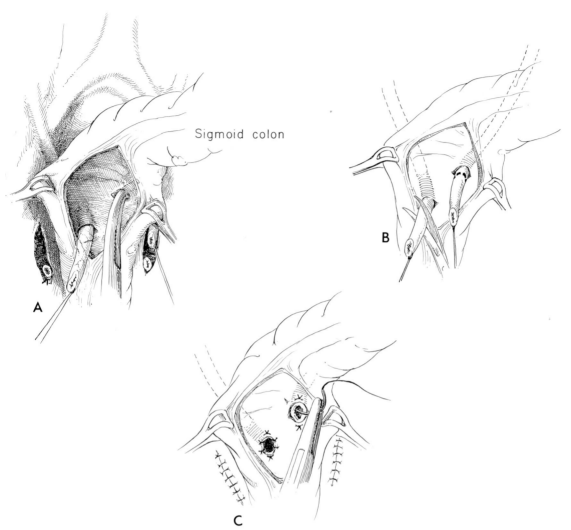

Figure 17–16. Intracolonic ureteral anastomosis and creation of submucosal tunnel for sigmoid conduit.

nephrine solution introduced through a fine-gauge needle. This aids both hemostasis and the development of the proper plane. An incision is then made along the tenia until the submucosa pouts up. The muscle is separated from the submucosa with scissors. It is important to reflect the muscle widely to ensure that the tunnel is wide. An incision is made at the distalmost portion of the exposed submucosa, and the spatulated ureter is anastomosed to the mucosa with interrupted 5-0 chromic catgut. The seromuscular layer is then reapproximated over the ureter with interrupted 4-0 silk. The most proximal portion of the tunnel should allow passage of a right-angle clamp, to avoid constricting the ureter. The ureteral adventitia is then sutured to the serosa of the

sigmoid with one or two 5-0 silk sutures just proximal to the tunnel to take tension off the anastomosis. The left ureteral anastomosis is performed at a slightly higher level on the sigmoid. It is important that both ureters have a smooth course without angulation. The anastomoses are retroperitonealized if at all possible. A Penrose drain is placed in the pelvis for 48 hours. Stents are not employed. A large-caliber rectal tube is taped in place and left indwelling for several days following the procedure.

Others have recommended different types of ureterosigmoid anastomoses. Goodwin uses a transcolonic anastomosis (Fig. 17–16). Mathisen devised a nipple-valve technique that is useful when ureteral length is lacking.

COMPLICATIONS AND RESULTS. One major complication, with an incidence of approximately 15 per cent, has been ureterosigmoid anastomotic obstruction; this sometimes has occurred rather late. Because the lower colon is highly absorptive, electrolyte imbalance is a common postoperative complication of ureterosigmoidostomy. Hyperchloremic acidosis with potassium depletion has been consistently observed. These findings are accentuated in children with marginal renal function. It is often desirable to use bicarbonate and potassium supplementation on a regular basis after surgery to correct acidosis and maximize growth potential.

Probably the major long-term complication of ureterosigmoidostomy is the increased risk for the development of adenocarcinoma at the site of the ureterocolic anastomosis. There is a several hundred–fold increased risk of carcinoma in these patients; these malignancies generally appear at a much earlier age in these patients than among the general population (Bennett; Eraklis and Folkman; Leadbetter; Parsons et al; Rabinovitch; Warren et al). For this reason, some have rejected ureterosigmoidostomy as a form of urinary diversion for benign disease (usually bladder exstrophy) in children (Rabinovitch). Excretory urograms must therefore be obtained annually for the life of the individual who has ureterosigmoidostomies. The finding of hydronephrosis in a child with a previously undilated upper urinary tract should suggest a tumor at the anastomosis. I have also been performing colonoscopy on a routine basis starting at the seventh postoperative year.

The exact etiology of the adenocarcinoma is unknown. It is fascinating that a number of tumors have occurred at the ureterosigmoid junction left in situ many years even after diversion of the urine to an ileal conduit (Eraklis and Folkman; Parsons et al; Shapiro et al; Spence et al, 1979) or nephrectomy (Oetjen). It has been shown in a rat model that adenocarcinoma does not develop at the bladder-bowel junction if the fecal stream is diverted (Crissey et al). The staged ureterosigmoidostomy using a nonrefluxing colon conduit initially, with later reanastomosis to the intact colon, may reduce the incidence of tumor growth by excluding the ureterocolic anastomoses from the fecal stream. This may be particularly successful when a nonrefluxing ileocecal conduit, with the plicated ileocecal valve protecting the ureteroileal anastomoses from contact with the fecal stream, is employed.

EXTERNAL (CUTANEOUS) DIVERSIONS

The Stoma

Perhaps the most important consideration in the construction of the various types of cutaneous diversions to be discussed is the site and construction of the stoma. Certainly, it is the most important to the patient and to a great extent determines the patient's acceptance of the procedure. Stomas that are poorly located or constructed predispose to leakage around the appliance, local inflammation and encrustation, bleeding, and resultant stomal stenosis.

In general, the site of the stoma should not be near the umbilicus or abdominal scars and should not impinge on any adjacent bony structure. The stomal site should be flat and should ideally be chosen preoperatively after the child is examined in both erect and supine positions. It is advisable to have the child wear an appliance on the proposed stomal location for a few days prior to operation to ascertain that the placement is correct. Although the conventional location for a urinary stoma is usually described as just below the center of the line connecting the anterior superior iliac spine to the umbilicus, in practice stomal locations are usually higher, especially in children with myelodysplasia. The most suitable locations in many of these children are in the upper quadrant or even in the epigastrium.

TECHNIQUE. It is advisable to mark the stomal location with a needle in the operating room prior to preparing the abdomen. In most instances, it is possible and desirable to prepare the stomal site prior to making the abdominal incision. This avoids the baffle effect of the abdominal wall, which can cause relative obstruction. When it is not feasible to create the stoma prior to making the abdominal incision, all layers of the abdomen should be grasped in alignment during the creation of the stoma.

A segment of skin that is somewhat larger than a quarter is excised. A core of fascia and muscle is also removed. The subcutaneous tissue is left intact to help avoid inversion of the stoma. The posterior fascia and peritoneum are incised in cruciate fashion and spread to allow passage of two fingers. In this manner, the opening from the skin into the abdominal cavity should be straight. The peritoneum and posterior fascia are marked with 4-0 silk sutures, which are eventually used to reapproximate these tissues to the serosa of the bowel. In addition, the fascia is sutured to the serosa with interrupted 3-0 chromic catgut. It is desirable to have a stomal bud of approximately 2 cm to allow proper application of the permanent appliance. The bud is created by first placing quadrant sutures of 4-0 Dexon in subcuticular fashion through the skin, the seromusculature layer of the bowel just above the fixation of the bowel to the fascia, and the full thickness of the bowel edge. Tying the sutures will allow a very adequate bud, and the anastomosis can be completed by suturing skin to edge of bowel (Fig. 17–17).

Some authors have reported a reduced incidence of postoperative stomal stenosis with incorporation of one or more skin flaps into the wall of the stoma (Fig. 17–18).

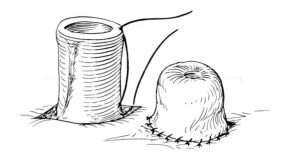

Figure 17–17. Creation of the stoma. The sutures include the subcuticular portion of the skin and the serosa of the bowel at the level of the skin with the muscularis and mucosa of the distal end of the segment. This creates a mature nipple stoma. (From Skinner DG, Richie JP: Ureterointestinal diversion. *In* Campbell's Urology. Fourth ed. Vol. 3. Edited by JH Harrison, RF Gittes, AD Perlmutter. Philadelphia, WB Saunders, Co., 1979.)

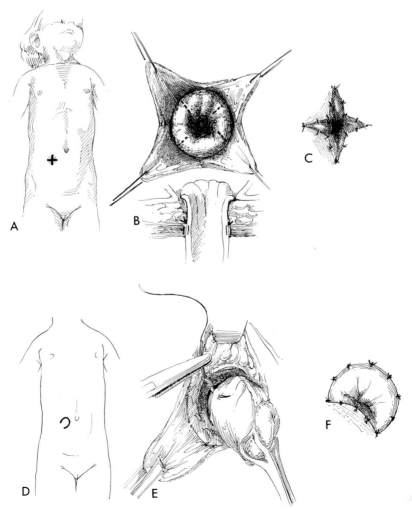

Figure 17–18. Two methods of formation of the stoma incorporating one or more skin flaps into the bowel itself to lessen the incidence of stomal stenosis.

A particular problem has been encountered with stomas created from large intestine. This has been the undesirable increase in the diameter and bulkiness of the stoma, especially when compared with the small delicate ileal stomas that many of these children have had previously. This can be circumvented by tapering the stoma. A V-shaped wedge is excised from the antimesenteric wall of the large bowel with the base positioned distally and closed with two layers of chromic catgut. This decreases the diameter of the stoma without significantly reducing the capacity of the conduit.

End Cutaneous Ureterostomy

End cutaneous ureterostomy is currently infrequently used as a method of either tem-

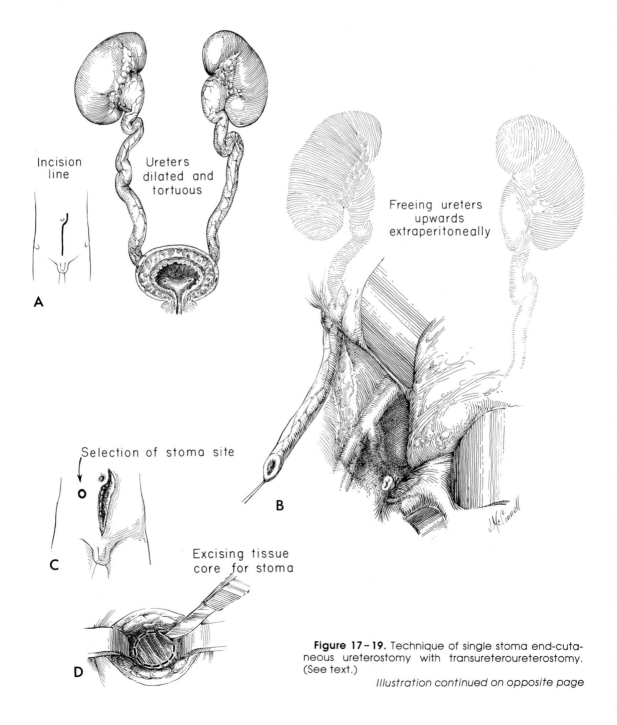

Figure 17–19. Technique of single stoma end-cutaneous ureterostomy with transureteroureterostomy. (See text.)

Illustration continued on opposite page

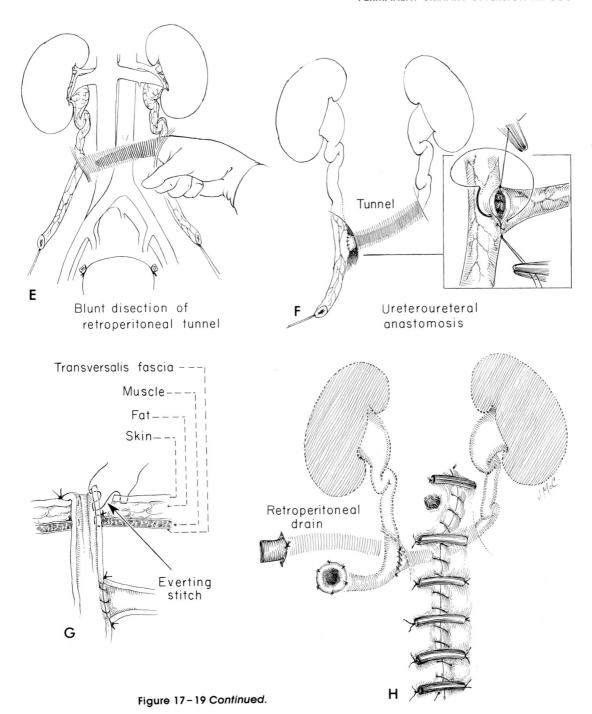

E   Blunt disection of
     retroperitoneal tunnel

F   Ureteroureteral
     anastomosis

Transversalis fascia ---
Muscle---
Fat---
Skin---

Everting
stitch

G

Retroperitoneal
drain

H

Figure 17–19 Continued.

porary or permanent urinary diversion. As a temporary diversionary procedure it can be applied:

1. In the child with severe uremia who requires supravesical diversion and who may be a candidate for renal transplantation.

2. To divert the upper pole ureter associated with an ectopic ureterocele at the time

of excision of the ureterocele and reconstruction of the trigone. This allows a delay before deciding upon anastomosis of the upper pole ureter to the lower pole pelvis or removal as the definitive procedure for the upper pole.

3. As a temporary diversion, with the option of ureteroneocystostomy at a later date if justified by the return of renal function.

As a permanent method of diversion, cutaneous ureterostomy offers a simple method of supravesical urinary diversion. It is probably most applicable in the child with markedly dilated ureters who is perhaps azotemic and who does not have a reconstructable urinary tract. As mentioned previously, this occurs very rarely. In the reasonably healthy child with severe bilateral hydroureter, most surgeons would prefer one of the nonrefluxing colon conduits as a method of permanent diversion with perhaps tapering one or both ureters if necessary. It is mandatory that cutaneous ureterostomy be employed only with ureters that are dilated (greater than 1 cm) and *thick-walled*. The basic advantages of cutaneous ureterostomy over nonrefluxing colon conduits are that it is simpler to perform, it may be done through a retroperitoneal approach, electrolyte reabsorption does not occur (Williams and Rabinovitch), and the incidence of stomal stenosis has been reported to be lower than in ileal conduits (Filmer and Honesty).

TECHNIQUE. Several techniques have been described for cutaneous ureterostomy. My preference is a bud stoma with an inlay skin flap similar to that described in the discussion of stomas. The procedure is accomplished, when possible, via an extraperitoneal approach, but is also frequently done transperitoneally. The stomal site is marked out in advance, although this cannot always be done if there is some doubt as to which ureter will be exteriorized. The more dilated ureter is exteriorized and the contralateral ureter is anastomosed to it as a transureteroureterostomy (Fig. 17–19).

The ureter can be approached by a low transverse, paramedian, or Gibson incision. Mobilization is done carefully to preserve ureteral blood supply. A retroperitoneal tunnel is made bluntly just above the aortic bifurcation through which the contralateral ureter will be anastomosed to the exteriorized one. Between holding sutures of fine silk, the recipient ureter is incised on its anteromedial surface. The anastomosis is then done with interrupted 5-0 chromic catgut. Both ureters should have smooth courses without angulation. The anastomosis is drained in retroperitoneal fashion. The stoma is made as described above with an inlay U-shaped skin flap. The ureter should be brought out 2 to 3 cm beyond the skin without tension.

Bilateral cutaneous ureterostomy through a single stoma has been described (Straffon) for bilateral dilated ureters (Fig. 17–20).

Ileal Conduit

Although no form of urinary diversion is ideal, for many years the ileal conduit was considered to offer the best possibility of stable renal function, absence of electrolyte problems, and a decent stoma. During the past decade, however, a number of authors (Schwarz and Jeffs; Shapiro et al; Richie) have reported major long-term complications of this form of diversion. Stomal stenosis has always been recognized as a problem, and revisions may be necessary in at least 40 per cent of children. Some children have required two or even more revisions.

Of greater concern are the observations of ureteroileal or intrinsic loop strictures occurring as late as 10 to 15 years postoperatively. It is also felt that a combination of reflux, refluxed mucus, and infection has caused chronic pyelonephritis and stone formation in many of these children. Increasing concern with these problems has led to the increased utilization of nonrefluxing colon conduits. In our institution, construction of an ileal conduit has not been performed as a method of permanent urinary diversion since 1974. It remains to be seen whether the nonrefluxing types of diversion will ultimately prove to be better. The technique for the ileal conduit is mentioned briefly.

TECHNIQUE. After the stomal site has been prepared, the abdomen is opened though a left paramedian incision (Fig. 17–21). Both ureters are isolated as they cross the iliac vessels, traced distally for several centimeters, ligated, and divided. The proximal ends of the ureters are mobilized superiorly, the left ureter being mobilized more than the right, and then brought under the sigmoid mesentery to lie in a smooth, gentle curve. A segment of ileum is chosen approximately 15 to 20 cm from the ileocecal valve: the segment should be 12 to 15 cm in length and supplied by two radial arteries. The distal mesentery is incised 5 to 6 cm to ensure adequate mobility of the isolated segment. The proximal mesentery need be incised only 2 to 3 cm. The pedicle should be a broad one. The bowel is divided, with the ileal segment allowed to fall inferiorly, and continuity of the intestine is restored.

The proximal end of the ileal segment is inverted with a Parker-Kerr continuous catgut stitch reinforced by fine silk Lembert sutures. This end of the ileum is tacked down to the sacral promontory or small bowel mesentery with fine catgut. Both ureteroileal anasto-

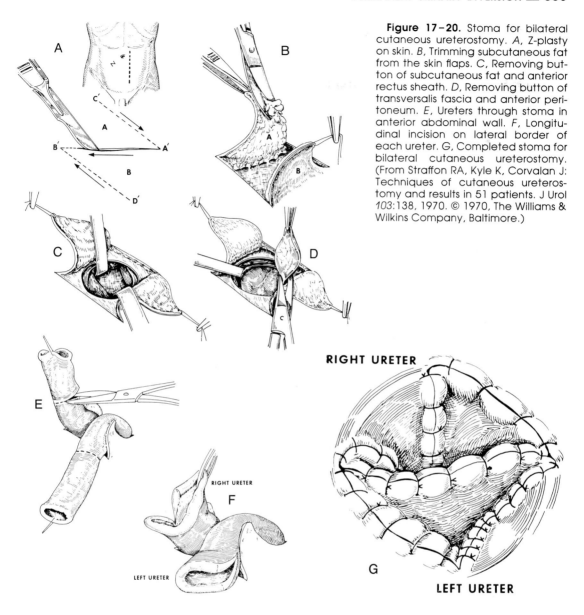

Figure 17–20. Stoma for bilateral cutaneous ureterostomy. *A*, Z-plasty on skin. *B*, Trimming subcutaneous fat from the skin flaps. *C*, Removing button of subcutaneous fat and anterior rectus sheath. *D*, Removing button of transversalis fascia and anterior peritoneum. *E*, Ureters through stoma in anterior abdominal wall. *F*, Longitudinal incision on lateral border of each ureter. *G*, Completed stoma for bilateral cutaneous ureterostomy. (From Straffon RA, Kyle K, Corvalan J: Techniques of cutaneous ureterostomy and results in 51 patients. J Urol *103*:138, 1970. © 1970, The Williams & Wilkins Company, Baltimore.)

moses are made on the antimesenteric surface of the ileum, the left one no more than 2.5 cm from the turned-in proximal end of the conduit. Fine chromic catgut is used to suture the ureter to the bowel serosa to eliminate tension on the anastomosis. An incision is made in the bowel and a small portion of mucosa is excised. The right ureter is anastomosed to the ileum approximately 2 cm from the left using 5-0 chromic catgut.

Wallace has advocated joining both ureters together in gun-barrel fashion and anastomosing them to the end of the conduit. This prevents pooling of urine in the blind end and may allow formation of a shorter conduit. The isolated ileal segment is then brought through the opening previously made in the abdominal wall and any excess of the conduit may be resected. Any bowstring effect of the mesentery or the conduit can be corrected by incising the mesentery further. The formation of the stoma has been described above. It is usually not necessary to stent the ureteroileal anastomoses.

Pyeloileal Conduit

Pyeloileocutaneous diversion was advocated by Holland et al (1967) as a method of stabilizing kidney function in children with large, adynamic ureters. With increasing emphasis on reconstructive surgery of the large ureter, the initial enthusiasm for this procedure has waned. Perhaps it might be considered in the child who continues to form stones to permit easier passage of these calculi to the exterior. Otherwise, for practical purposes it is of historical interest only.

TECHNIQUE. A rather long segment (20 to 25 cm) of high ileum or jejunum is isolated and is placed above the intestinal anastomosis (Fig. 17–22), rather than below it as in the ileal conduit. The proximal and distal incisions in the mesentery should be at least 5 to 6 cm long to ensure adequate mobility of the segment. This is more easily accomplished with the proximal ileum or jejunum than with the distal ileum. The hepatic and splenic flexures are mobilized medially to expose both renal pelves. The segment of intestine is passed through a retroperitoneal tunnel behind the duodenum and pancreas and anterior to the aorta and vena cava. An end-to-end pyeloileal anastomosis is carried out on the left and an end-to-side union on the right.

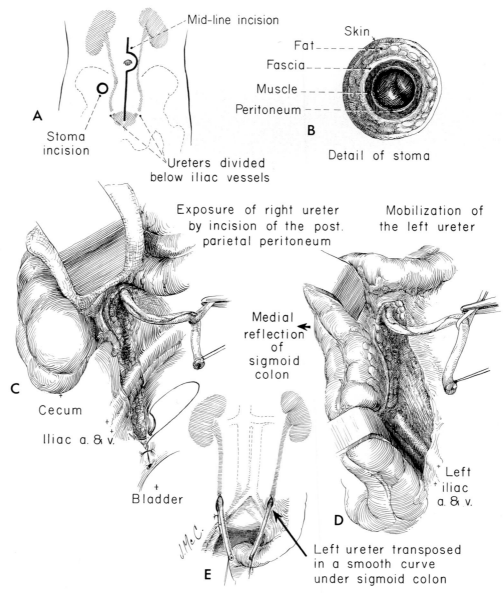

Figure 17–21. Technique for creation of an ileal conduit. (See text.) (From King LR, Urological Research: Papers presented in honor of Scott WW, Plenum Publishing Co., 1972.)

Illustration continued on opposite page

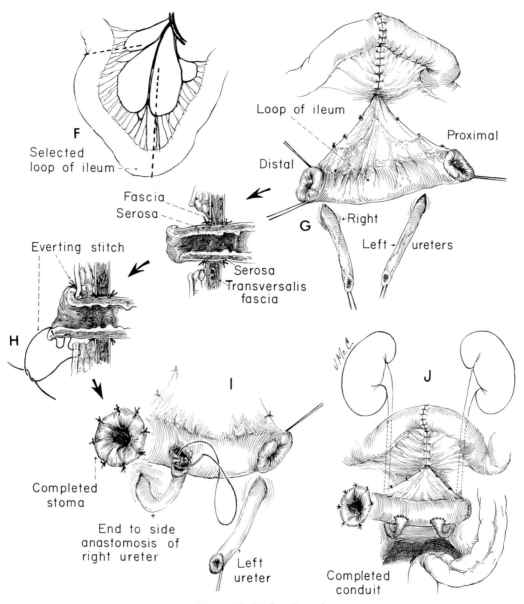

F Selected loop of ileum

Loop of ileum

Distal

Proximal

G Right

Left ureters

Fascia
Serosa

Serosa
Transversalis fascia

Everting stitch

H

I

Completed stoma

End to side anastomosis of right ureter

Left ureter

J

Completed conduit

Figure 17–21 *Continued.*

This procedure has also been modified by employing two smaller segments of bowel, anastomosing each to a renal pelvis and then anastomosing one segment to the other in a Roux-en-Y fashion. This procedure may allow a straighter course of the intestine from kidneys to skin.

Nonrefluxing Colon Conduits

The increasing number of late complications with ileal conduit diversion has prompted the use of the colon as a urinary conduit. The occurrence of pyelonephritis following ileal conduit diversion has been attributed to reflux with infection. Richie et al have also shown in animal experiments the increased incidence of histologic pyelonephritis in freely refluxing ileal conduits when compared with nonrefluxing colon conduits. In addition, the incidence of stomal stenosis appears lower with the colon than with the small intestine. The following methods of diversion are being employed in children with increasing frequency as methods of permanent or, in some instances, temporary urinary diversion. The initial results with these proce-

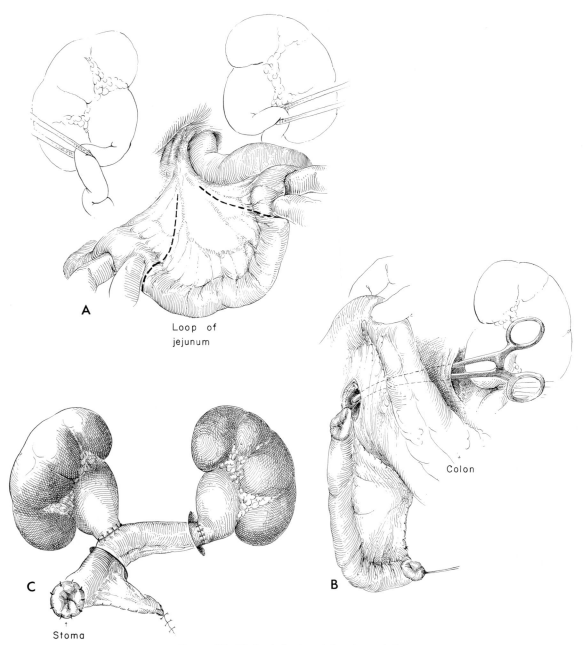

A

Loop of
jejunum

C

Stoma

B

Colon

Figure 17–22. Pyeloileal or -jejunal conduit.

dures have been excellent. The incidence of reflux, ureteral obstruction and stomal stenosis has been low. However, follow-up in this group has been relatively short-term to date.

Sigmoid Conduit

The indications for sigmoid conduit diversion are similar to those for the ileal conduit; it is indicated in children with neuropathic bladder dysfunction with repeated attacks of

pyelonephritis or severe incontinence unresponsive to conventional therapy and some tumors of the lower urinary tract. The transverse colon conduit might be preferable in the latter situation, as discussed in detail later in this article. We have employed the sigmoid conduit primarily to convert failing ileal conduits to a nonrefluxing type of diversion. Hendren has recommended the use of the sigmoid conduit as a temporary method of urinary diversion in infants with exstrophy of the bladder, to be later reconnected to the sigmoid colon after it is ascertained that the conduit is functioning well without reflux and that the child has acceptable rectal control.

TECHNIQUE. Stomal considerations are analogous to those described previously, with the exception that the stoma is usually located on the left side of the abdomen. In children with ileal conduits being converted to sigmoid conduits, I usually prefer to use the previously located stomal site. The mobility of the sigmoid colon in children readily allows this.

The abdomen is opened through a paramedian incision, and the ureters are isolated and divided over the pelvic brim. The lateral attachments of the sigmoid colon are incised and a 15-cm segment is chosen, with due care to insure a broad-based blood supply (Fig. 17-23). The isolated segment may be placed lateral or medial to the bowel anastomosis. The conduit is rotated 180 degrees to make it isoperistaltic, and the proximal end is closed with a Parker-Kerr stitch of chromic catgut and interrupted fine silk Lembert sutures. The ureteral anastomoses, done by a submucosal tunnel technique, should provide a tunnel length of 4 to 5 cm. The tunnels are staggered along the teniae, which are infiltrated with dilute epinephrine solution to minimize bleeding and help establish the correct plane. Each tenia is incised and the seromuscular wall is reflected from the submucosa. Most of the undermining is done laterally to avoid devitalizing the medial portion between the two ureteral tunnels. It is important to provide a tunnel adequate in width as well as length. The mucosa is incised at the distal portion of the tunnel, and the ureters are spatulated slightly and anastomosed to the mucosa with interrupted 5-0 chromic catgut. The seromuscular layer is then closed over the ureter with interrupted 4-0 silk. It is important to be able to insert a right-angled clamp alongside the ureter easily into the entrance of the tunnel to ensure that the ureter is not constricted. The stoma is constructed in a manner similar to that for the ileal conduit.

Large ureters may be implanted in the sigmoid conduit after being tapered. In this situation, 5 F infant feeding tubes are left indwelling to protect the suture lines. With two very dilated ureters, it is often advisable to obtain one very long (greater than 5 cm) tunnel for a tapered ureter, performing a transureteroureterostomy above the tapered area.

An alternative technique for sigmoid conduit diversion has been advocated by Kelalis.

The antireflux effect is achieved by burying the anastomosis and 3 cm of ureter in a seromuscular tunnel created with Lembert sutures of 4-0 chromic catgut (Fig. 17-24).

RESULTS. A number of authors have reported encouraging results with sigmoid conduit diversion (Altwein et al; Morales and Golimbu). Althausen et al found no cases of stomal stenosis, a 10 per cent incidence of ureterocolic stenosis, and a 14 per cent incidence of low pressure reflux in 40 children with sigmoid conduits followed from 1 to 8 years. However, a recent long-term follow-up report on 41 children with the sigmoid conduit (Elder et al) contrasted with the initial encouraging findings. In this series from Wales, with an average follow-up of 13.2 years, there was a 61 per cent incidence of stomal stenosis, a 22 per cent incidence of ureterocolic obstruction, a 58 per cent incidence of colouretal reflux, and a 48 per cent incidence of upper urinary tract deterioration. Therefore, it is imperative to reserve final judgment on any of the nonrefluxing colon conduits until further long-term results become available.

Ileocecal Conduit

The ileocecal segment has been used for many years primarily for bladder augmentation. The use of this segment of bowel as a urinary conduit has not received much attention. In 1975 Zinman and Libertino reported its use in this regard and emphasized the effectiveness of the ileocecal valve as an antirefluxing mechanism. Subsequently, the use of the ileocecal segment has been described in children as a means of permanent urinary diversion (Retik et al). The ileocecal segment has certain anatomic advantages as a conduit over other colonic segments. The ileocolic vessels supplying it are constant and are easily mobilized with a long mesentery providing an excellent blood supply to the bowel. These vessels can be isolated accurately even in obese children with thick mesenteric attachments by palpation of the ileocolic and right colic arteries. Other advantages of ileocecal segments are:

1. Subsequent undiversion can be done relatively easily by cecocystoplasty.
2. There are minimal stomal problems.
3. The ileocecal segment can be added on to a pre-existing ileal segment if the ureteroileal anastomoses are functioning well.

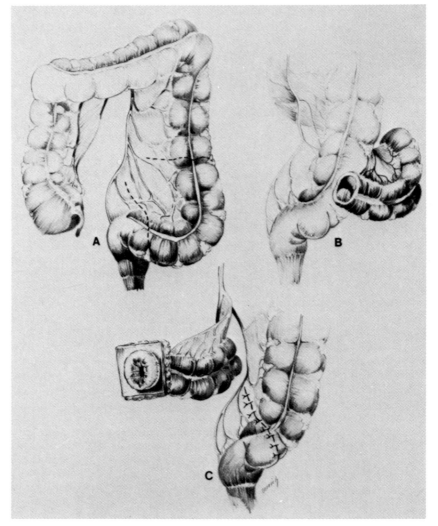

Figure 17-23. Technique for creation of a sigmoid conduit. *A*, A segment of sigmoid colon approximately 15 cm long is chosen. Incisions are made in the mesentery to ensure a broad-based blood supply. *B* and *C*, The isolated segment may be placed lateral or medial to the bowel anastomosis. The conduit is rotated 180° to make it isoperistaltic and the proximal end is closed.

Illustration continued on opposite page

4. It is the diversion of choice for absent, short, or dilated ureters.

5. It may lower the incidence of tumor development following later internal diversion (ureterosigmoidostomy).

In our series of more than 50 children who have had ileocecal urinary diversion performed, approximately 80 per cent had failed ileal conduits. The majority of these were patients with myelodysplasia. We have also employed this method of diversion in the few children with neuropathic bladder dysfunction who cannot be successfully managed by intermittent catheterization, pharmacologic means, bladder neck surgery, or implantation of an artificial sphincter. Ileocecal urinary diversion has also been used in children with malignant bladder or prostatic tumors and as a temporary method of urinary diversion as part of a series of operations to reconstruct complex anomalies such as exstrophy of the bladder or cloaca, severe female epispadias with maldevelopment of the bladder, and bilateral single ectopic ureters.

The ileocecal segment should also be strongly considered if internal diversion via a two-stage ureterosigmoidostomy is to be performed. An increasing number of malignant tumors have been reported in patients who have had ureterosigmoidostomies for 7 years

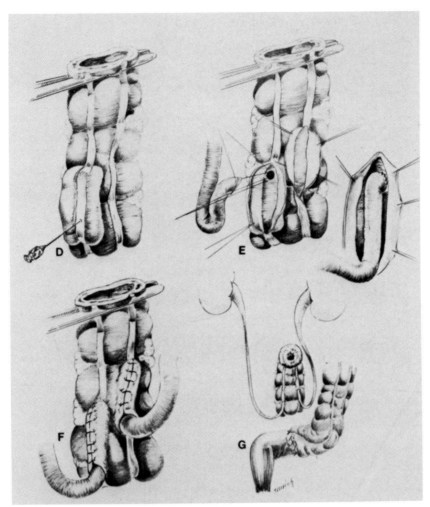

Figure 17–23 *Continued.* *D*, A dilute epinephrine solution is injected along the tenia. This minimizes bleeding and defines the correct plane. *E*, The tenia is incised and the seromuscular wall is reflected from the submucosa. Most of the undermining is done laterally to avoid devitalizing the area between the two tunnels. The mucosa is incised at the distal portion of the tunnel, and the ureters are spatulated slightly and anastomosed to the mucosa with interrupted 5-0 chromic catgut. *F*, The seromuscular layer is closed over the ureter with interrupted fine silk. The proximal portion of the tunnel should allow the insertion of a right-angled clamp to ensure that the ureter is not constricted. *G*, The completed sigmoid conduit, after the stoma is constructed in a manner similar to that for the ileal conduit stoma. (From Retik AB: Urinary diversion. *In* Pediatric Surgery. Third ed. Edited by MM Ravitch. Copyright © 1979 by Year Book Medical Publishers, Inc., Chicago.)

or longer. Experimental evidence (Crissey et al) has indicated that uroepithelium in contact with fecal material and a carcinogen is necessary for tumor induction. If an ileocecal conduit that has a well-functioning antireflux mechanism is anastomosed to the colon, contact between the uroepithelium and fecal stream will be minimized.

TECHNIQUE. Through a midline incision, the cecum, right colon, and hepatic flexure are mobilized. The right ureter is isolated below the pelvic brim. The constant ileocolic vessels are identified and the ileum is divided approx-

imately 10 cm proximal to the ileocecal valve (Fig. 17–25). The ascending colon is divided proximal to the right colic artery and the mesentery is incised appropriately. A 28 F catheter is introduced into the ileum, through the ileocecal valve, to emerge through the colonic end; the antireflux mechanism is obtained by intussuscepting the cecum into the terminal ileum in a collarlike fashion (Fig. 17–25C). The use of a catheter avoids too much narrowing of the distal ileum during this process. The anterior and posterior walls of the cecum are then wrapped like a collar around the

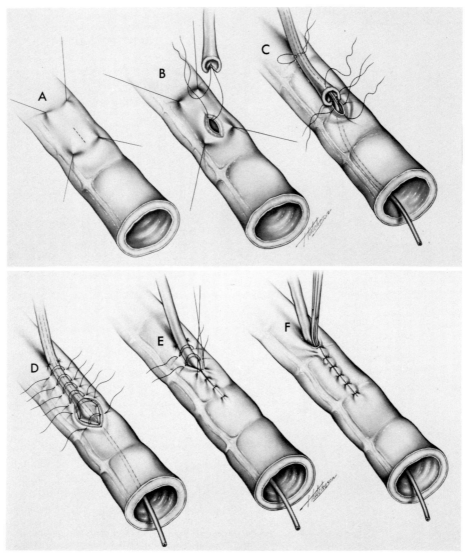

Figure 17–24. Seromuscular tunnel technique for ureterocolic anastomosis. (From Kelalis PP: Urinary diversion in children by the sigmoid conduit: its advantages and limitations. J Urol 112:666, 1974. © 1974, The Williams & Wilkins Company, Baltimore.)

terminal 4 cm of ileum in a 270-degree encircling fashion with interrupted seromuscular Tevdek incorporating ileum into the cecal wall on either side of the mesentery. (Fig. 17–25D). An alternate technique for reflux prevention has been outlined by Hendren in which 6 to 8 cm of terminal ileum which has been scarified is intussuscepted into the cecum (Fig. 17–26).

After this is completed, the large red rubber catheter is removed and the antireflux mechanism is tested by inflating the ascending colon and measuring pressures. The valve mechanism should be continent to at least 50 cm of water. It is also advisable to make absolutely

certain that the plication has not caused obstruction by ascertaining that fluid can pass in antegrade fashion from the ileum to the colon at low pressure (<20 cm H_2O). The left ureter is then isolated lateral to the simoid colon and brought under the sigmoid mesentery through the peritoneal opening on the right side. The ureteroileal anastomoses are performed in a manner similar to that described for the ileal conduit after the proximal ileum has been closed. Alternatively, I often prefer a conjoint ureteroureterostomy (Wallace technique), which is constructed by incising the ureters medially for 3 cm, suturing their walls with interrupted 5-0 chromic catgut, and anastomosing the resultant single opening to the open proximal ileum (Fig. 17–25F). The stoma is then created in the fashion described in the discussion of stoma formation earlier in this article.

RESULTS. In adults, the results of ileocecal conduit diversion have been excellent. Zinman and Libertino have reported almost uniform success with antireflux plication of the ileocecal valve. The incidence of obstruction has been minimal. Long-term results of the ileocecal conduit in children are lacking, although the short-term results are very encouraging. The incidence of obstruction is negligible and the incidence of low-pressure reflux is minimal. Reflux at higher pressures is seen more often, and this in general is not a problem when the ileocecal segment is used

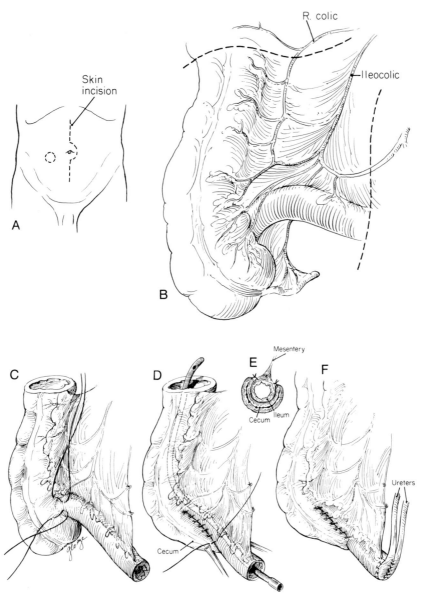

Figure 17–25. A, and B, Technique for creation of an ileocecal conduit. A, The stomal site is in the right lower quadrant. B, The ileocecal segment is isolated from its blood supply based on the reliable ileocolic vessels. C to F, Reinforcement of the ileocecal valve. C, The ileum is intussuscepted into the cecum with seromuscular sutures. D and E, the redundant cecum is then wrapped around the terminal ileum in a 200 to 270° encircling fashion over a large catheter inserted into the segment. The seromuscular sutures are placed on either side of the mesentery. F, An antirefluxing ileocecal conduit is completed with a Wallace conjoint ureteral anastomosis to the proximal end of the ileum. (From Zinman SL, Libertino JA: Antirefluxing ileocecal conduit. Urol Clin North Am 7:503, 1980.)

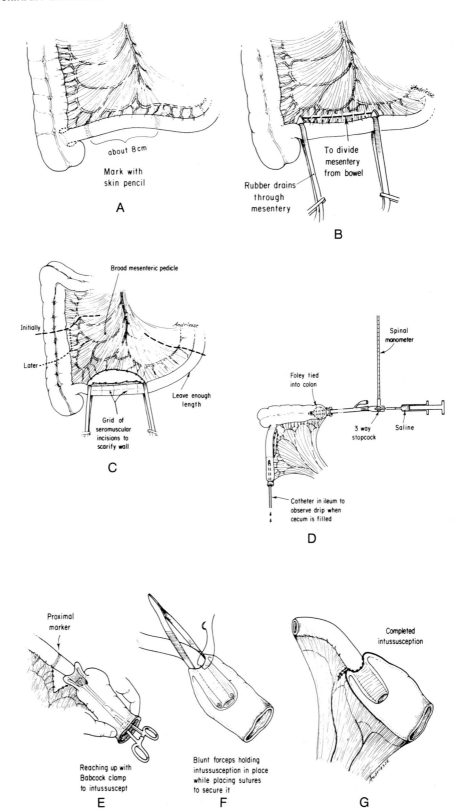

Figure 17–26. Technique of intussuscepting terminal ileum to prevent reflux. (From Hendren WH: Reoperative ureteral reimplantation: management of the difficult case. J Ped Surg *15*:770–786, 1980. By permission of Grune & Stratton, Inc.)

as a conduit. However, if the conduit is subsequently anastomosed to the bladder and subjected to higher intravesical pressures, the nipple often is completely reduced and free reflux sometimes occurs.

The other major complication that has frequently been observed with the ileocecal conduit has been prolapse of the stoma. The etiology of this is not completely clear. This is best prevented and treated by tapering the stoma, as mentioned above, and making the opening in the abdominal wall smaller.

Transverse Colon Conduit

The transverse colon conduit is infrequently used as a method of diversion in chil-

dren. It is almost exclusively employed in those children with pelvic rhabdomyosarcoma undergoing cystectomy and extensive pelvic radiation requiring high cutaneous diversion. It is an excellent method of diversion permitting the use of nonirradiated bowel. Construction of long tunnels to prevent reflux is easily accomplished, as with the sigmoid conduit. Some of the long-term survivors of malignancy merit consideration for internal diversion by anastomosis of the transverse colon conduit to the sigmoid colon.

CONTINENT URINARY DIVERSIONS

There has been some emphasis in recent years on continent urinary diversions. These

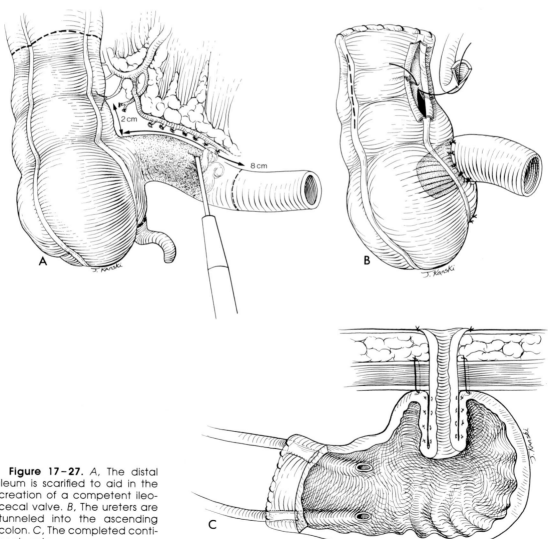

Figure 17-27. *A,* The distal ileum is scarified to aid in the creation of a competent ileocecal valve. *B,* The ureters are tunneled into the ascending colon. *C,* The completed continent ureter.

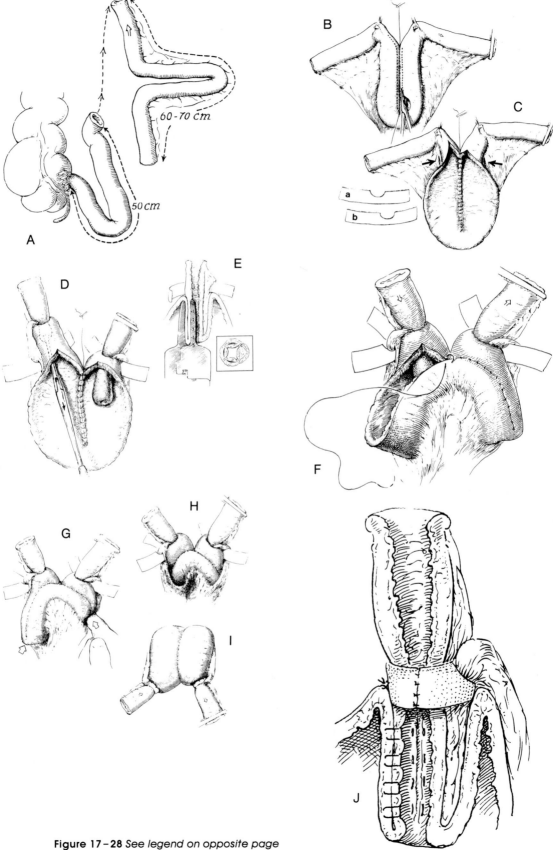

Figure 17–28 *See legend on opposite page*

have been of most appeal to adolescents and young adults who simply cannot tolerate wearing an appliance. Certainly the concept of a continent urinary diversion is quite attractive, especially to someone in a young age group who has a benign condition and a normal life expectancy.

Schneider et al have reported their technique for a continent vesicostomy. The continence mechanism relies upon an intussuscepted bladder flap. This procedure has had some success in adults, but in general has been disappointing in children. Bauer (personal communication, 1983) has bridged the gap between the bladder and the abdominal wall in a teenager with an isolated segment of ileum; the proximal end of the segment was intussuscepted into the bladder, and this procedure has provided total continence. The bladder neck in such patients must be surgically closed, which may be difficult to achieve at times.

A more popular form of continent urinary diversion involves the use of the ileum or ileocecal segment. In 1973, Sullivan et al reported the results of the continent ureterocecocutaneous ileostomy developed by Gilchrist et al in 1950. The success rate was 94 per cent in 40 patients followed at least 10 years. This technique was never widely used. It involves the isolation of an ileocecal segment in which the ureters are tunneled in antireflux fashion along the tenia in the cecum, the ileum is intussuscepted into the cecum to provide continence, and the proximal portion of the ileum is brought out as a stoma (Fig. 17–27). We have done this recently on one older child who is completely continent between catheterizations.

Kock et al (1981, 1982) have described their experiences with urinary diversion via a continent ileal reservoir in 12 patients. An isolated ileal reservoir was constructed using the techniques described for patients with a continent ileostomy. The ureters were implanted into an afferent segment provided with a reflux-preventing nipple valve (Fig. 17–28). Reoperation was necessary in 7 of the 12 patients

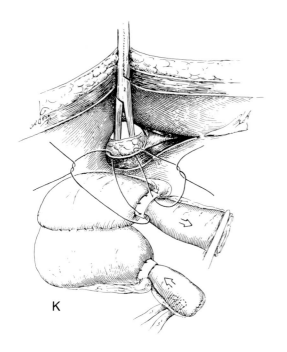

K

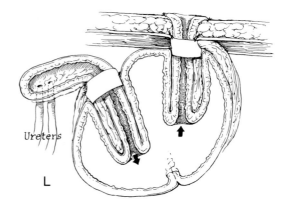

Ureters

L

Figure 17–28. *A*, Continent ileal reservoir. Bowel segment measuring 60 to 70 cm is isolated approximately 50 cm from the ileocecal valve and positioned as the letter U with the terminal end directed toward the head of the patient and the bottom of the U toward the left side of the patient. *B*, Legs of U are united at antimesenteric border with continuous 3-0 polyglycolic acid. Intestine is divided along suture line and incision is continued for 3 cm on afferent limb. *C*, Mucous membrane is sutured with continuous 3-0 polyglycolic acid. Openings are made in mesentery supplying the future base of the nipple valves. *D*, Intussusception at parts of afferent and efferent segments into future reservoir. *E*, Nipple valves are secured with staples. *F*, Closure of reservoir with two continuous inverting 3-0 polyglycolic acid sutures. *G to I*, Reservoir is brought into final position by pushing corners of reservoir downward between mesenteric leaves. *J*, Fascia or Marlex mesh encircles the base of the nipple valve and ends are approximated with three to four nonabsorbable sutures. Reservoir wall is sutured to the cylinder with 3-0 polyglycolic acid sutures. *K*, Cylinder at efferent segment is attached to the opening and anterior rectus sheath with nonabsorbable sutures. *L*, The completed continent ileal reservoir. (From Kock et al: Urinary diversion by a continued ileal reservoir: clinical results in 12 patients. J Urol *128*:469, 1982. © 1982, The Williams & Wilkins Company, Baltimore.)

because of malfunction of the continence-producing valve. Follow-up in this group of patients ranged between 9 months and 6½ years. All patients were continent without reflux. The reservoir generally was emptied by intermittent catheterization 3 to 6 times per day. The volume capacity of the reservoir was more than 50 ml.

These continent methods of diversion certainly seem both reasonable and encouraging. It is to be hoped that the long-term results will continue to be encouraging and allow broader usage of these methods of diversion.

BIBLIOGRAPHY

URETEROSIGMOIDOSTOMY

Allen TD: Ureterosigmoidostomy in urinary diversion. Dial Pediatr Urol 3:11, 1980.

Bennett AH: Exstrophy of the bladder treated by ureterosigmoidostomies: long-term evaluation. Urology 2:165, 1973.

Coffey RC: Transplantation of the ureters into the large intestine in the absence of the functioning urinary bladder. Surg Gynecol Obstet 32:383, 1921.

Cordonnier JJ: Ureterosigmoid anastomosis. Surg Gynecol Obstet 88:441, 1949.

Crissey MM, Steele GD, Gittes RF: Rat model for carcinogenesis in ureterosigmoidostomy. Science 207:1079, 1980.

Eraklis AJ, Folkman J: Adenocarcinoma at the site of ureterosigmoidostomies for exstrophy of the bladder. J Ped Surg 13:730, 1978.

Goodwin WE, Harris AP, Kaufman JJ, et al: Open, transcolonic ureterointestinal anastomosis: a new approach. Surg Gynecol Obstet 97:295, 1953.

Goodwin WE, Scardino PT: Ureterosigmoidostomy. J Urol 118:169, 1977.

Hendren WH: Exstrophy of the bladder—an alternative method of management. J Urol 115:195, 1976.

Leadbetter GW Jr, Zickermin P, Pierce E: Ureterosigmoidostomy and carcinoma of the colon. J Urol 121:732, 1979.

Leadbetter WF: Consideration of problems incident to performance of uretero-enterostomy: report of a technique. J Urol 65:818, 1951.

Mathisen W: A new method for ureterointestinal anastomosis: a preliminary report. Surg Gynecol Obstet 96:255, 1953.

Mogg RA: Neoplasms at the site of ureterocolic anastomosis. Br J Surg 64:758, 1977.

Oetjen LH Jr, Campbell JL, Tomley MW, et al: Carcinoma of the colon following ureterosigmoidostomy: report of a case. J Urol 104:536, 1970.

Parsons CD, Thomas MH, Garrett RA: Colonic adenocarcinoma: a delayed complication of uretero-sigmoidostomy. J Urol 118:31, 1977.

Rabinovitch HH: Ureterosigmoidostomy in children: revival or demise? J Urol 124:552, 1980.

Shapiro SR, Baez A, Colodny AH, et al: Adenocarcinoma of colon at ureterosigmoidostomy site 14 years after conversion to ileal loop. Urology 3:229, 1974.

Spence HM: Ureterosigmoidostomy for exstrophy of the bladder: results in a personal series of 31 cases. Br J Urol 38:36, 1966.

Spence HM, Hoffman WW, Fosmire GP: Tumor of the colon as a late complication of ureterosigmoidostomy for exstrophy of the bladder. Br J Urol 51:466, 1979.

Spence HM, Hoffman WW, Pate VA: Exstrophy of the bladder. I. Long-term results in a series of 37 cases treated by ureterosigmoidostomy. J Urol 114:133, 1975.

Stamey TA: The pathogenesis and implications of the electrolyte imbalance in ureterosigmoidostomy. Surg Gynecol Obstet 103:736, 1956.

Warren RB, Warner TF, Hafez GR: Late development of colonic adenocarcinoma 49 years after ureterosigmoidostomy for exstrophy of the bladder. J Urol 124:550, 1980.

Zincke H, Segura JW: Ureterosigmoidostomy: critical review of 173 cases. J Urol 113:324, 1975.

THE STOMA

Cordonnier JJ, Nicolai CH: An evaluation of the use of an isolated segment of ileum as a means of urinary diversion. J Urol 83:834, 1960.

Dicus DR: New perspectives in the construction of the ileal stoma. J Urol 112:591, 1974.

Filmer RB, Honesty H: Problems with urinary conduit stomas in children. Urol Clin North Am 1:531, 1974.

Habib HN, McDonald DF: A technique for prevention of intramural obstruction of Bricker's ileal loop. J Urol 88:211, 1962.

Jeter K, Bloom S: Management of stomal complications following ileal or colonic conduit operations in children. J Urol 106:425, 1971.

Kelalis PP: Urinary diversion in children by the sigmoid conduit: its advantages and limitations. J Urol 112:666, 1974.

Richardson JR Jr, Linton PC, Leadbetter GW Jr: A new concept in the treatment of stomal stenosis. J Urol 108:159, 1972.

Smith ED: Ileo-cutaneous ureterostomy in children: operative technique and complications. Aust NZ J Surg 34:89, 1964.

END CUTANEOUS URETEROSTOMY

Beland G, Laberge I: Cutaneous transureterostomy in children. J Urol 114:588, 1975.

Claman M, Shapiro AE, Orecklin JR: Cutaneous ureterostomy, the preferred diversion of the solitary functioning kidney. Br J Urol 51:352, 1979.

Eckstein HB: Cutaneous ureterostomy. Proc R Soc Med 56:749, 1963.

Feminella JG Jr, Lattimer JK: A retrospective analysis of 70 cases of cutaneous ureterostomy. J Urol 106:538, 1971.

Filmer RB, Honesty H: Problems with urinary conduit stomas in children. Urol Clin North Am 1:531, 1974.

Flinn RA, King LR, McDonald JH, et al: Cutaneous ureterostomy: an alternative urinary diversion. J Urol 105:358, 1971.

Halpern GN, King LR, Belman AB: Transureteroureterostomy in children. J Urol 109:504, 1973.

Hendren WH, Hensle TW: Transureteroureterostomy: experience with 75 cases. J Urol 123:826, 1980.

Sadlowski RW, Belman AB, Filmer RB, et al: Follow-up of cutaneous ureterostomy in children. J Urol 119:116, 1978.

Straffon RA: Urinary diversion by cutaneous ureterostomy. In Current Controversies in Urologic Management. Edited by R Scott, HL Gordon, FB Scott, et al. Philadelphia, WB Saunders Co., 1972, p 299.

Swenson O, Smyth BT: Aperistaltic megaloureter: treatment by bilateral cutaneous ureterostomy using a new technique; preliminary communication. J Urol 82:62, 1959.

Udall DA, Hodges CV, Pearse HM, et al: Transureteroureterostomy: a neglected procedure. J Urol 109:817, 1973.

Williams DI, Rabinovitch HH: Cutaneous ureterostomy for the grossly dilated ureter of childhood. Br J Urol 39:696, 1967.

ILEAL CONDUIT

Cordonnier JJ, Nicolai CH: An evaluation of the use of an isolated segment of ileum as a means of urinary diversion. J Urol 83:834, 1960.

Delgado GE, Muecke EC: Evaluation of 80 cases of ileal conduit in children. Indications, complications and results. J Urol 109:311, 1973.

Derrick WA Jr, Hodges CV: Ileal conduit stasis: recognition, treatment and prevention. J Urol 107:747, 1972.

Dretler SP: The pathogenesis of urinary tract calculi occurring after ileal conduit diversion. J Urol, 109:204, 1973.

Malek RS, Burke EC, DeWeerd JH: Ileal conduit urinary diversion in children. J Urol 105:892, 1971.

Perlmutter AD, Tank ES: Ileal conduit stasis in children: recognition and treatment. J Urol 101:688, 1969.

Retik AB, Perlmutter AD, Gross RE: Cutaneous ureteroileostomy in children. N Engl J Med 277:217, 1967.

Richie JP: Intestinal loop urinary diversion in children. J Urol 111:687, 1974.

Schwarz GR, Jeffs RD: Ileal conduit urinary diversion in children: computer analysis of follow-up from 2 to 16 years. J Urol 114:285, 1975.

Shapiro SR, Lebowitz R, Colodny AH: Fate of ninety children with ileal conduit urinary diversion a decade later: analysis of complications, pyelography, renal function and bacteriology. J Urol 114:289, 1975.

Smith ED: Follow-up studies on 150 ileal conduits in children. J Pediatr Surg 7:1, 1972.

Wallace DM: Ureteric diversion using a conduit: a simplified technique. Br J Urol 38:522, 1966.

Wallace DM: uretero-ileostomy. Br J Urol 42:529, 1970.

PYELOILEAL CONDUIT

Holland JM, King LR, Schirmer HKA, et al: High urinary diversion with an ileal conduit in children. Pediatrics, 40:816, 1967.

Holland JM, Schirmer HKA, King LR, et al: Pyeloileal urinary conduit: an 8-year experience in 37 patients. J Urol 99:427, 1969.

King LR: Technique of ileal conduit. Evolution of the Brady method. Papers presented in honor of WW Scott. New York, Plenum Publications, 1972.■

King LR, Scott WW: Ileal urinary diversion: success of pyeloileocutaneous anastomosis in correction of hydroureteronephrosis persisting after ureteroileocutaneous anastomosis. JAMA, 181:831, 1962.

King LR, Scott WW: Pyeloileocutaneous anastomosis. Surg Gynecol Obstet 119:281, 1964.

NONREFLUXING COLON CONDUITS

Richie JP, Skinner DG: Urinary diversion: the physiological rationale for non-refluxing colonic conduits. Br J Urol 47:269, 1975.

SIGMOID CONDUIT

Althausen AF, Hagen-Cook K, Hendren WH: Non-refluxing colon conduit: experience with seventy cases. J Urol 120:35, 1978.

Altwein JE, Jonas U, Hohenfellner R: Long-term follow-up of children with colon conduit urinary diversion and ureterosigmoidostomy. J Urol 118:832, 1977.

Dagen JE, Sanford EJ, Rohner TJ Jr: Complications of the non-refluxing colon conduit. J Urol 123:585, 1980.

Elder DD, Moisey CU, Rees RWM: A long-term follow-up of the colonic conduit operation in children. Br J Urol 51:462, 1979.

Hendren WH: Non-refluxing colon conduit for temporary or permanent urinary diversion in children. J Pediatr Surg 10:381, 1975.

Kelalis PP: Urinary diversion in children by the sigmoid conduit: its advantages and limitations. J Urol 112:666, 1974.

Mogg RA: Urinary diversion using the colonic conduit. Br J Urol 39:687, 1967.

Mogg RA, Syme RRA: The results of urinary diversion using the colonic conduit. Br J Urol 41:434, 1969.

Morales P, Golimbu M: Colonic urinary diversion: ten years of experience. J Urol 113:302, 1975.

Richie JP, Skinner DG, Waisman J: The effect of reflux in the development of pyelonephritis in urinary diversion: an experimental study. J Surg Res 16:256, 1974.

ILEOCECAL CONDUIT

Hendren WH: Re-operative ureteral reimplantation: management of the difficult case. J Ped Surg 15:770, 1980.

Retik AB, Colodny AH, Bauer SB: The ileocecal segment in children. Presented at the American Urological Association meeting, Boston, May, 1981.

Skinner DG: Further experience with the ileo-cecal segment in urinary reconstruction. J Urol 128:252, 1982.

Zinman L, Libertino JA: The ileo-cecal conduit for temporary and permanent urinary diversion. J Urol 113:317, 1975.

CONTINENT URINARY DIVERSIONS

Gilchrist RK, Merricks JW, Hamlin HH, et al: Construction of a substitute bladder and urethra. Surg Gynecol Obstet 90:752, 1950.

Kock NG, Nilson AE, Nilsson LO, et al: Urinary diversion via continent ileal reservoir: clinical results in 12 patients. J Urol 128:469, 1982.

Kock NG, Myrvold HE, Nilsson LO, et al: Continent ileostomy. An account of 314 patients. Acta Chir Scand 147:67, 1981.

Schneider KM, Reid RE, Fruchtman B, et al: Continent vesicostomy: surgical technique. Urology 6:741, 1975.

Sullivan H, Gilchrist RK, Merricks JW: Ileo-cecal substitution bladder; long-term follow-up. J Urol 109:43, 1973.

Urinary Undiversion and Augmentation Cystoplasty

W. Hardy Hendren

There are many patients with various types of urinary diversions whose urinary tracts can be "undiverted." From 1969 to February 1983, the author refunctionalized the previously diverted urinary tract in 130 patients. This chapter will describe some of the important considerations in doing such reconstructive surgery. Selected cases will demonstrate some of the necessary technical maneuvers.

The types of urinary diversions in these patients are shown in Table 17–1. Nearly half (58 of 130 patients) had ileal loops. In the majority of cases (100 of 130) the diversion had been considered to be a permanent one when originally performed. Eight of the diversions had been done by the author; 122 had originally been done elsewhere.

Figure 17–29 shows the age of these patients, a broad spectrum from infancy to age 28 years.

Figure 17–30 shows the duration of the urinary diversions in these patients. In 41 of the patients the diversion had been present for 10 years or longer. One patient had worn an appliance for 21 years. Clearly, experience has shown that long-term disuse of the bladder does not preclude its refunctionalization.

ASSESSMENT OF BLADDER FUNCTION

The majority of patients in this series did not have neurogenic bladders; their diver-

sions had been done for severe obstructive uropathy, such as urethral valves, or after failed surgery for the prune-belly syndrome, megaureter, or massive vesicoureteral reflux. More recently this type of reconstructive surgery has been applied in patients with neurogenic bladder, that is, previous myelomeningocele or sacral agenesis. This latter group of patients with neurologically impaired bladders presents a special challenge to the reconstructive surgeon. Artificial sphincters have been placed by some surgeons in this type of case. I believe, however, that the failure rate of these devices is still too high and prefer to avoid their use.

Urodynamic evaluation is often not very helpful in predicting how well a defunctionalized bladder will function when urine flow to it is re-established. It is important to know why the diversion was done in the first place. A cystogram will show bladder size and sensation and can demonstrate the presence of diverticula, urethral valves, and refluxing ureteral stumps. Cystoscopy will supplement that information. The long-diverted bladder usually (but not always) is of small capacity and has a smooth lining. It generally bleeds readily when filled with irrigating fluid under pressure. It is important not to overfill the bladder with too much pressure, which can cause it to rupture. We had this complication occur in four patients in whom excessive pressure was applied in an attempt to stretch the bladder.

During cystoscopy a small Silastic catheter is introduced by the percutaneous trocar technique (Kogan et al). This allows subsequent irrigation with saline to test continence and ability to void and to see whether the bladder will increase its capacity by being used once again. Urethral valves in boys can be destroyed with a cutting electrode at the time the suprapubic catheter is placed, since pseudofunction will be instituted immediately by using the irrigation regimen. On the other hand, valves should never be fulgurated in a completely defunctionalized urethra; they can scar shut into impermeable strictures. We

Table 17–1. 130 Cases of Urinary Undiversion

58 Ileal loop (12 pyeloileal)
30 Loop ureterostomy
17 End ureterostomy
19 Cystostomy
7 Nephrostomy
100 Permanent diversions
30 Temporary diversions
40 Females
90 Males
33 Patients had one kidney

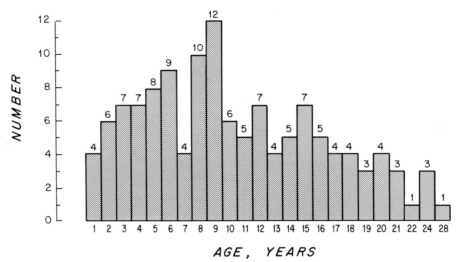

Figure 17-29. Age of 130 patients at time of undiversion.

have treated several patients in whom this has occurred.

The type of catheter used deserves mention. I prefer to thread several inches of an 8 F Cystocath (Dow Corning) into the bladder. This catheter has the disadvantage that it can be voided out the urethra, as I have seen several times. This requires pulling it back enough so that its end is in the bladder. An alternative is the Stamey Malecot-type percutaneous catheter. In two cases, however, the contracting bladder pulled away from the Malecot catheter placed in its dome, allowing the irrigating fluid to enter the prevesical space.

There is a wide range of results with placement of an irrigating catheter into a diverted bladder. An occasional patient will void in an almost normal manner the first time the bladder is filled. Other patients will not void at all initially. Some small bladders will stretch remarkably in just a few days; others will not, making it likely that augmentation will be needed. The patient is instructed to fill the bladder by rapid drip from a reservoir bottle 3 to 4 feet above the level of the bladder. To the

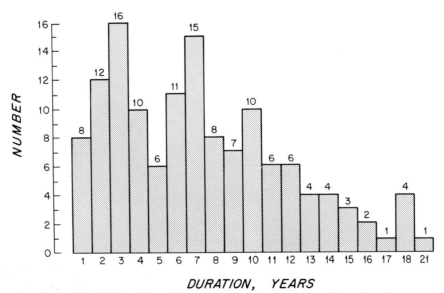

Figure 17-30. Duration of diversions in 130 patients prior to undiversion.

saline is added 0.5 per cent neomycin solution to avert infection. Usually within a week one can obtain a fairly reliable estimate of the patient's bladder size, continence, sensation, and ability to void. If some of this is not clear, the patient can continue this regimen at home for several weeks more to gain this information. Irrigating fluid is tap water to which 2 teaspoons of salt are added per quart, boiled to obtain sterility.

TECHNICAL PRINCIPLES IN UNDIVERSION SURGERY

These are long, technically difficult procedures which must be done with technical precision to avoid complications such as leak, stricture, massive reflux, or loss of a kidney. Each case will differ from every other. It is essential to delay deciding exactly how reconstruction will be done in a given case until all of the anatomy is laid out at the operating table. Only then can various options be determined and the best chosen.

Operations often last many hours. Skillful anesthesia and careful monitoring are mandatory. Intraoperative fluid losses are usually large during these major cases. Thus, maintaining normal blood volume and adequate urinary output is essential. These patients can

ill afford inadequate replacement, which can cause shock and renal tubular necrosis. I have found that the fluid replacement needed is usually in the range of 20 to 25 ml/kg per hour in young patients. This is four to five times greater than the volume replacement generally given during ordinary intra-abdominal operations. For older patients the volume requirements are 10 to 20 ml/kg per hour. I routinely monitor central venous pressure, arterial pressure, urinary output (estimate), blood gases, hematocrit, and serum electrolytes.

Wide transabdominal exposure is used, through a vertical midline incision, usually from the symphysis pubis to the xiphisternum. The right and left colon are mobilized and reflected medially to expose kidneys and ureters. Mobilization of a ureter is performed as shown in Figure 17–31. The ureter is mobilized with all of its periureteral tissue, skeletonizing the surrounding anatomic structures, not the ureter. The gonadal vessels are divided above the ovarian hilum in the female or at the internal ring in the male, maintaining the vessels with the ureter for collateral blood supply. This will not damage the gonad. A ureter can be mobilized all the way to the kidney, without loss of its blood supply, if it is done in this fashion. A little additional length can be obtained by mobilizing the kidney just

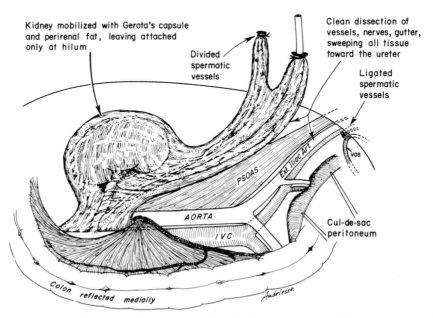

Figure 17–31. Technique for mobilizing kidney and ureter to gain additional length by wide dissection of structures, preserving periureteral tissue for ureteral blood supply, including gonadal vessels. (From Hendren WH: Some alternatives to urinary diversion in children. J Urol *119*:652, 1978. © 1978, The Williams and Wilkins Co., Baltimore.)

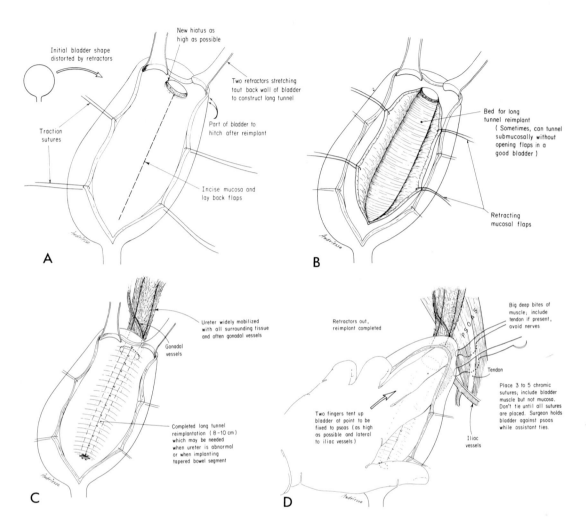

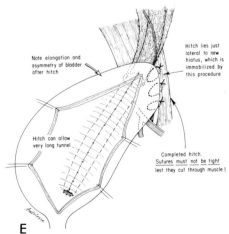

Figure 17–32. Technique of psoas hitch fixation of bladder. This allows creation of a superlong ureteral reimplantation tunnel. It also fixes the point of entry of the ureter into the bladder so that it does not become angulated when the bladder fills. *A,* Bladder is stretched upward using two retractors, selecting a point for the new ureteral hiatus as high as possible on the back wall of the bladder. *B,* Dissecting back flaps to expose the bed in which the ureter will be placed. This technique is necessary in most bladders, which are scarred and pock-marked with cellules. *C,* Placement of ureter in tunnel. *D,* Placement of fixation sutures. This can be done with chromic catgut, although monofilament nonabsorbable suture material may be more effective in holding the bladder in position. If nonabsorbable suture material is used it must not enter the bladder lumen, lest it cause stone formation. *E,* Completed hitch. (From Hendren WH: Reoperative ureteral reimplantation: management of the difficult case. J Ped Surg *15:*770–786, 1980. By permission of Grune & Stratton, Inc.)

as would be done for a radical nephrectomy, sliding it down and pexing it at a lower level.

Transureteroureterostomy or transureteropyelostomy is often used in these cases (Hendren and Hensle; Hodges et al; Sharpe). Only occasionally is it feasible to join two ureters to the bladder. It is generally better to reimplant the better ureter, usually with the adjunct of a psoas hitch, draining the other ureter across into it. In transureteroureterostomy the ureter to be drained is brought across to the contralateral ureter, with absolutely no tension. It must be anastomosed accurately to the medial aspect of the recipient ureter; an anastomosis placed in the anterior wall can angulate and obstruct. The ureter to be drained must not be wedged beneath the inferior mesenteric or other artery, which can obstruct it. Two soft, small-caliber plastic catheters (usually 5 F feeding tubes) are passed through the bladder wall, up the reimplanted ureter, and one to each kidney. Contrast medium is injected into these (a "stent study") about 8 to 10 days postoperatively to be certain there is no leak. I have not encountered a leak in more than 150 transureteroureterostomies. Subsequent reoperation was necessary in 4, however; in 3 it was for vascular compression of the ureter, and in 1 there was angulation at the anastomosis.

Psoas hitch, shown in Figure 17–32, is used in most cases, whether implanting a ureter or a tapered bowel segment. The latter requires an especially long tunnel to prevent reflux. The ratio of tunnel length to ureteral diameter should be about 5 to 1.

Augmentation is needed when the bladder is small and inelastic and fails to respond to preoperative hydrostatic stretching. In many such bladders a reimplantation procedure is not technically feasible. Further, the patient must not be left with a small-capacity, noncompliant, high-pressure bladder, which can cause secondary hydronephrosis. Augmentation can be done with a segment of small intestine or colon, or an ileocecal segment.

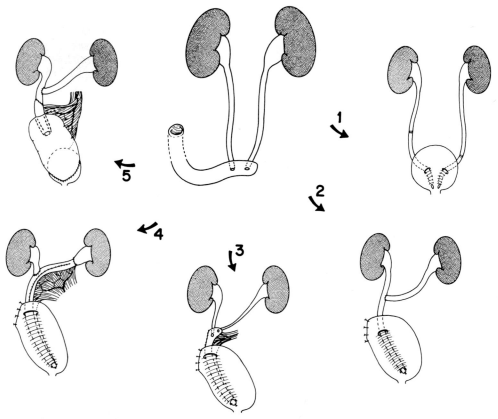

Figure 17–33. Most common options for ileal loop undiversion. When ureters can be used, that is best. Tapered bowel can work well if a very long tunnel is constructed. Bladder augmentation should be used when the bladder is small and scarred. Another option, autotransplantation of the kidney, is not shown. (From Hendren, WH, Radopoulos D: Complications of ileal loop and colon conduit urinary diversion. Urol Clin North Am *30*:451, 1983.)

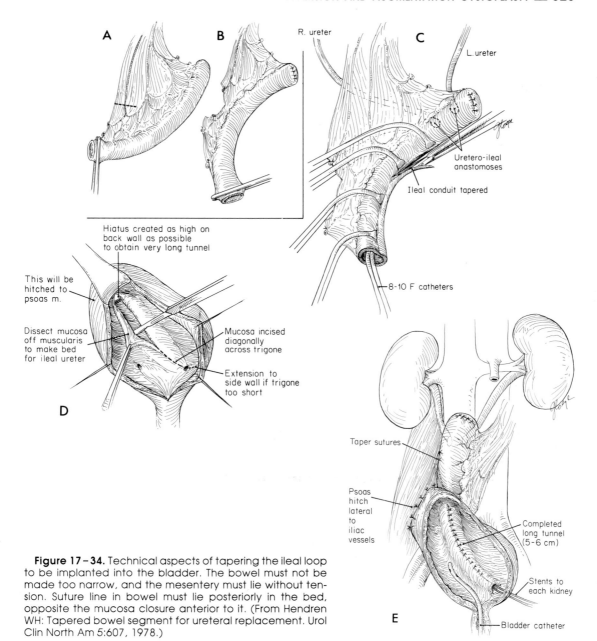

Figure 17–34. Technical aspects of tapering the ileal loop to be implanted into the bladder. The bowel must not be made too narrow, and the mesentery must lie without tension. Suture line in bowel must lie posteriorly in the bed, opposite the mucosa closure anterior to it. (From Hendren WH: Tapered bowel segment for ureteral replacement. Urol Clin North Am 5:607, 1978.)

SELECTED UNDIVERSION CASES

Previous publications have described technical details in reconstructing many of the patients in this series of cases (Hendren, 1973, 1974, 1976b, 1979b, 1983). The following additional cases will show the spectrum of the types of patients who may benefit from undiversion as well as the use of the various technical adjuncts mentioned above, which should be in the armamentarium of the surgeon who undertakes operating for undiversion.

Ileal Loop

The principal options to consider in taking down an ileal loop urinary diversion and reconnecting the upper tract to the bladder are shown in Figure 17–33. Not shown is the option of autotransplantation, which we have used on one occasion. Whenever it is possible to discard the loop, that is preferred. It may be necessary to use the ileal loop, however, to bridge the gap between the upper tract and the bladder.

Figure 17–34 shows the technical details of

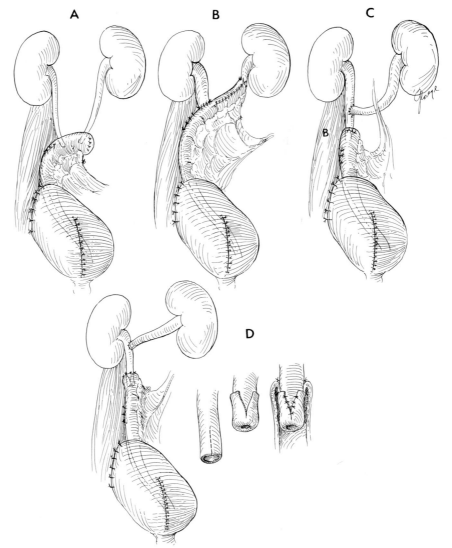

Figure 17–35. Some variations in the use of bowel as a substitute ureter. *A,* A usual ileal loop. *B,* A pyeloileal conduit with no remaining ureter. *C,* One ureter reimplanted into bowel with transureteroureterostomy. *D,* Optional use of a nipple at the upper end of the conduit as a second line of defense against reflux. If a nipple is subjected to considerable back pressure, it becomes effaced and ineffective. (From Hendren WH: Tapered bowel segment for ureteral replacement. Urol Clin North Am 5:607, 1978.)

tapering and implanting an ileal loop to serve as a ureter.

Figure 17–35 shows variations in the anatomic scheme of using tapered small bowel as ureter. Although some surgeons (Goodwin; Goodwin et al; Skinner and Goodwin) believe that a simple end-to-side anastomosis of untapered bowel to the bladder is adequate, that has not been my experience. I believe that it is far better to prevent reflux which in combination with infection or voiding dysfunction has the potential to damage the upper tracts through the years.

Case 1 (Figs. 17–36 and 17–37)

This 16-year-old boy was evaluated in April 1981 for possible undiversion. In 1967, when he was 3 years of age, hydronephrosis had been discovered. Right nephrectomy and left cutaneous ureterostomy were performed. The ureterostomy never drained well. In 1974, when he was 10 years of age, diversion of the left kidney was changed to a jejunal conduit diversion. Because there was continuing infection and progressive hydronephrosis, he was referred for further reconstructive surgery.

A loopogram showed extensive stricture of the bowel segment. Contrast instilled by antegrade pressure perfusion technique showed no passage of contrast from the kidney to the stoma at pressures of 40 cm of water. A cystogram showed a bladder consistent with what would be expected in a patient with urethral valves.

Cystoscopy showed typical urethral valves. They were resected. A Silastic suprapubic cystostomy tube was inserted by trocar technique to begin stretching and testing the bladder. In just 5 days this long-defunctionalized bladder increased in capacity from 60 to 250 ml. The patient demonstrated good control. He could empty instilled saline with a good stream. Undiversion was performed. This included removing the previous bowel loop, which appeared ischemic from too narrow a vascular pedicle. A new bowel conduit was made from ileum, with its distal end tapered and placed in the bladder with a long tunnel to prevent reflux. A psoas hitch was performed. This reconstruction was well tolerated. Convalescence was uneventful. Follow-up in March 1982 was satisfactory. Bladder volume, control, and urinary stream were normal. There was no reflux up the reimplanted bowel segment. Excretory urography showed satisfactory function and drainage. Antegrade pressure perfusion pyelography showed an opening pressure of only 7 cm of water. This rose to only 9 cm after perfusing 10 ml per minute, even with a full bladder. The segment emptied rapidly upon ceasing perfusion. Serum BUN was 29 mg/dl, creatinine was 1.6 mg/dl, and creatinine clearance was 82 L absolute.

COMMENT. This patient is one of many we have treated with severe obstruction from urethral valves that had not been diagnosed previously. That should occur less often today with availability of improved fiberoptic endoscopes and the realization that valves are more common than previously suspected (Hendren, 1971, 1976a). There was an immediate increase in capacity of this bladder after only 5 days of suprapubic instillation of saline. This hydrostatic stretching is done as often as the patient can do it, with instillation of as much fluid as can be tolerated short of provoking pain. If an existing bowel segment is inadequate (this was strictured) a new one should be constructed. Note that the tunnel in this case was 9 cm long. This proved adequate to prevent reflux. No attempt should be made to implant a tapered bowel segment into a small, scarred bladder in which a long tunnel cannot be constructed. Of the 58 ileal loop cases I have undiverted, in 28 the bowel was tapered and reimplanted into the bladder. Nine of these patients required reoperation because of reflux. In 6 it was possible to make a longer tunnel, which stopped the reflux. These were patients with basically good bladders. In 3 of the patients the tapered bowel segment had been placed in a small, fibrotic,

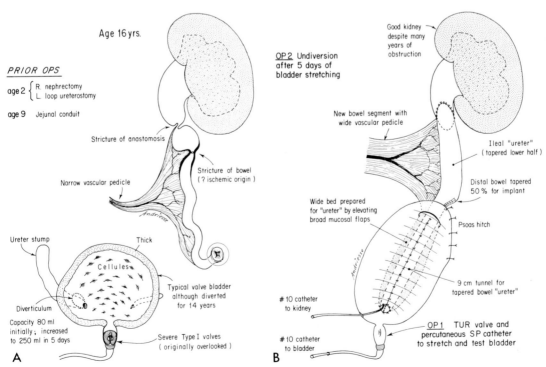

Figure 17–36. Case 1 before (A) and after (B) reconstruction. (See text.)

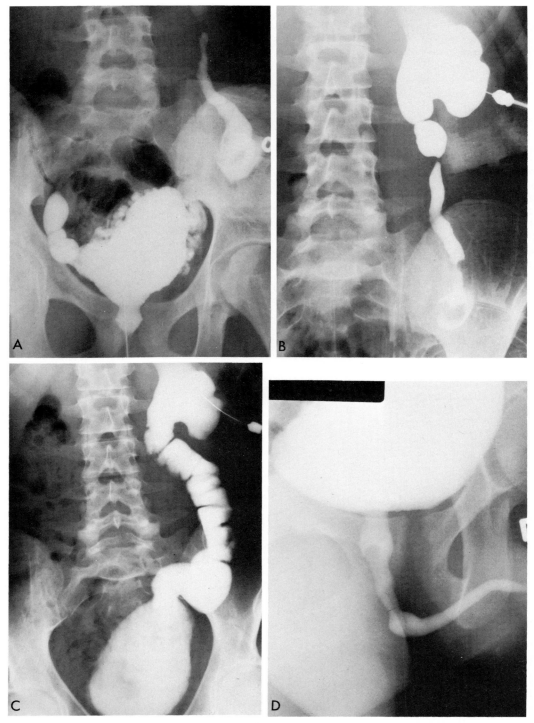

Figure 17–37. Selected roentgenograms from Case 1. *A,* Simultaneous preoperative loopogram and cystogram. Note bladder with many cellules, typical of that seen in boys with severe urethral valve obstruction of urethra. Note reasonable size of bladder despite many years of diversion. *B,* Simultaneous preoperative antegrade study (note needle in kidney) and loopogram, showing multiple strictures of bowel conduit and its anastomosis of kidney. *C,* Antegrade study 7 months postoperatively showing free flow from kidney to bladder. *D,* Cystogram 7 months postoperatively, with satisfactory bladder size and function. No urethral obstruction, and no reflux up tapered bowel conduit.

noncompliant bladder in which only a short tunnel could be attained. At reoperation, reconstruction was altered to cecal cystoplasty, using the ileal cecal segment to prevent reflux. From this experience it can be emphasized that a tapered bowel segment should be placed only in a favorable bladder in which a very long tunnel can be attained. Otherwise it will reflux.

When bowel is used as a substitute ureter, indefinite long-term follow-up is required. It is well known that spontaneous stricture is a complication of ileal loop urinary diversion. As reported recently, three of our undiversion cases with a small bowel ureter later developed such a spontaneous stricture requiring reoperation (Hendren and McLorie).

The ureteral stumps in this patient were not suitable for use, and so they were discarded. Some ureteral stumps can be utilized. If they show reflux on preoperative cystogram in the defunctionalized state, that does not necessarily mean that reimplantation is necessary. In some patients reflux will stop spontaneously

when the bladder is put back to work, stretching the trigone and elongating the ureterovesical tunnels. On the other hand, if reflux was known to be present before the patient's diversion was done, or if the lower ureteral segment is obviously dilated, is ectopically placed in the side wall of the bladder, is associated with a diverticulum, or demonstrates no tunnel at all, reimplantation should be done during undiversion. This is generally better than reoperation later to correct reflux.

Case 2 (Figs. 17–38 and 17–39)

This 24-year-old college student was referred for possible undiversion. She was born with myelomeningocele. After various orthopedic operations, ileal loop urinary diversion was performed for the problems of urinary incontinence and infection when she was age 14 years.

In October 1982, a Silastic suprapubic tube was passed percutaneously to test bladder function. During the next 3 months, which the patient spent at home, it was clear that her maximum bladder volume was less than 100 ml. Saline instilled

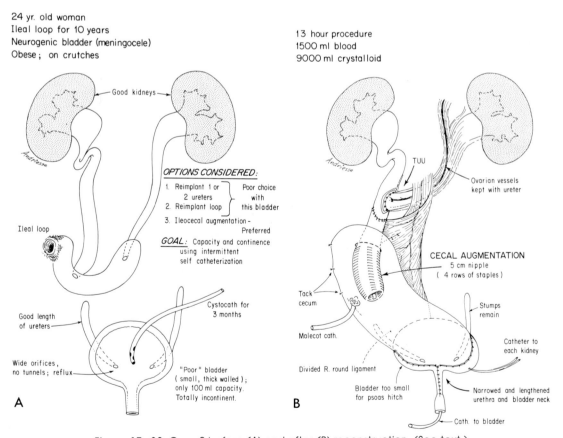

Figure 17–38. Case 2 before (A) and after (B) reconstruction. (See text.)

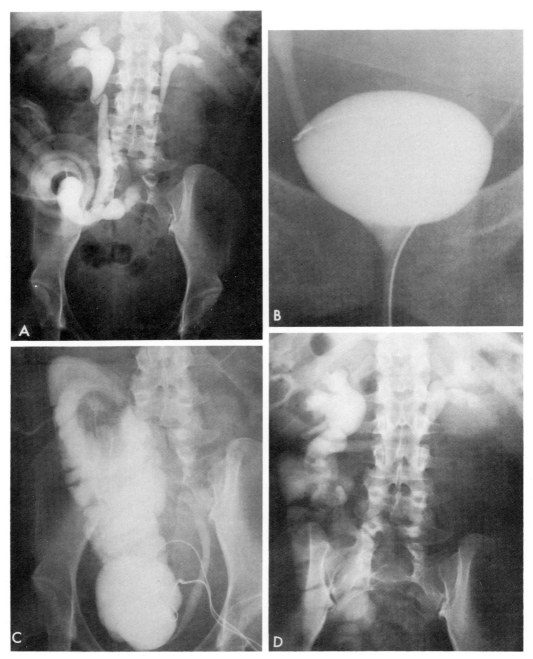

Figure 17–39. Selected roentgenograms from Case 2. *A,* Preoperative loopogram with moderate upper tract dilatation. Note strictures of ileal loop. *B,* Preoperative cystogram showing small capacity, completely incontinent bladder, with refluxing ureteral stumps. *C,* Cystogram 10 days following reconstructive procedure. Various postoperative catheters still in place. Note cecum and ascending colon added to small bladder. The intussuscepted ileum is evident as a filling defect in cecum. Staples are visible. *D,* Excretory urogram 9 months postoperatively. Stable upper tracts. Cystogram shows no reflux. Patient is dry.

through the tube ran freely from the urethra. An extensive reconstruction was performed in January 1983. The urethra and bladder neck were narrowed as much as possible to create more outlet resistance. The bladder was small and thick-walled. It was felt unwise to attempt reimplantation of even one ureter into this particular bladder.

It was augmented using the cecum, creating a nonrefluxing mechanism with the ileocecal junction. The dilated right ureter was joined to the terminal ileum of the ileocecal cystoplasty. The left ureter was drained via transureteroureterostomy.

Convalescence following this extensive reconstruction was uneventful. Postoperative radiographic study showed satisfactory drainage of the upper tract into her augmented bladder, and no reflux on cystographic examination. The patient returned to college, emptying her bladder by intermittent self-catheterization. Although socially continent, she was not absolutely dry for the first 4 postoperative months. It was contemplated that she would probably require a urethral extension procedure to gain more resistance. However, by 8 months postoperatively she was completely dry on the program of intermittent self-catheterization.

COMMENT. There are many young adults like this who had ileal loop urinary diversion for neuropathic bladder during the heyday of the ileal loop, from about 1955 to 1975. Although some patients with long-standing ileal loops are free from infection and have stable, normal upper tracts, there is overall an unacceptable rate of upper tract deterioration in these patients (Hendren and Radopoulos; Middleton and Hendren; Pitts and Muecke; Retik et al; Schwarz and Jeffs; Shapiro et al; Smith). Therefore, I have not performed ileal loops on young patients since 1969. If bowel conduit diversion is needed, we use a nonrefluxing colon conduit or nonrefluxing ileocecal conduit (Althausen et al; Hendren, 1975b; Richie and Skinner; Richie et al; Skinner et al). Recently the suggestion was made that the nonrefluxing colon conduit does not protect against upper tract deterioration, based on a large series done by the late Richard Mogg (Dagen et al; Elder et al). This comparison is not valid, in my opinion, however, because those colon conduits were not made with long ureterocolic tunnels to prevent reflux. We are firmly convinced by both clinical follow-up and laboratory studies that an effective tunneling ureterocolic implantation will usually prevent reflux and upper tract deterioration.

It is fruitless to rejoin the upper tract to a bladder that was once incontinent unless some measure is taken to create outlet resistance. To be effective, the Young-Dees narrowing of the proximal urethra and bladder neck must be made very small in caliber. It should be snug to passage of a 10 F catheter when the mucosa adjacent to that segment is resected and the muscle is closed over it. After return of function, the remaining bladder will expand. In a small-capacity bladder like this, augmentation must be used also, to avoid having the upper tract empty into a small-volume, high-pressure bladder. The ureters in this case were actually long enough to justify consideration of ureteral reimplantation. It was decided against, however, because the bladder was small and thick-walled, reducing

the likelihood of successful reimplantation. It was felt that it would be safer to rely on a nipple of terminal ileum intussuscepted into the cecum.

Special mention should be made of altering the ileocecal valve to prevent reflux. In testing the ileocecal segment for reflux at the operating table, we learned that most will resist reflux until the pressure exceeds 15 cm of water. The ileocecal junction can be reinforced by the technique described by Zinman and Libertino, plicating cecal wall in several layers over the terminal ileum, except on its mesenteric side. At the operating table this will be competent to withstand pressures of 60 cm of water or greater. If the segment is used as an isolated conduit to the surface, this nonrefluxing mechanism continues to be competent. However, in our experience, when the ileocecal segment is joined to the bladder, thereby intermittently filling and emptying, this antireflux mechanism breaks down. For this reason we began creating a 4- to 5-cm nipple by intussuscepting 8 to 10 cm of terminal ileum. Some of these nipples held up, and continued to protect against reflux when joined to the bladder. However, others broke down. Therefore, subsequently, the bowel was scarified and its mesentery was removed before it was intussuscepted, in an effort to maintain the nipple. Some of these also broke down. Still later we placed many tacking sutures into the nipple; this also proved unreliable. Finally, three to four rows of staples were placed, because it was thought that this would surely maintain the nipple. Even this measure proved unreliable. Nipples that early postoperatively could be seen hanging down into the cecum, and that did not show reflux on early follow-up cystograms, later popped out of the cecum and refluxed. The currently employed technique consists of creating the nipple as before, using staples, but then incising its back wall the full length of nipple through the ileocecal valves, and down a corresponding distance along the adjacent wall of the cecum. The nipple is then sewn to the adjacent cecal wall to hold it in place. Early follow-up of this method during the past year has shown it to be effective. It maintains the nipple within the cecum. It also appears effective when revising nipples that have broken down and allowed reflux. Most staples become covered by mucosa. In three cases, small stones were seen on exposed staples at follow-up cystoscopy. These were easily plucked out using alligator forceps. Long-term follow-up will be needed. We have employed cecal augmentation of the bladder in 41 young patients. In 28, the ileocecal junction was used to prevent reflux. I believe it is better to implant a ureter into the bladder or into the cecal wall as the means for preventing reflux, if the length and quality of ureter will permit. Only if this is not feasible do we use the ileocecal junction to prevent reflux.

I have undiverted 11 patients with neuropathic bladders. All but one were similar to this case, needing bladder augmentation and more outlet resistance. Most of these patients prefer intermittent self-catheterization as a way of life compared with drainage of the urinary tract through an abdominal stoma. If and when mechanical artificial sphincters become perfected in the future, it might be possible to resect the narrowed bladder neck endoscopically, reducing the resistance created and allowing the bladder to empty without catheterization. Continence could then be attained by placing a sphincter. In my opinion, however, mechanical sphincters are not yet sufficiently reliable to warrant this approach.

End Ureterostomy

End ureterostomy has been used widely for urinary diversion. End ureterostomies are prone to stenosis if the ureters are small in caliber, but may be a satisfactory means for long-term permanent drainage when the ureters are dilated. Seventeen patients who had undergone end ureterostomy were referred for reconstruction.

Case 3 (Figs. 17-40 and 17-41)

This 27-month-old girl was referred for undiversion in January 1983. A lumbar meningomyelocele had been closed shortly after birth. When she was 7 months old, bilateral cutaneous ureterostomy was performed because there was severe hydronephrosis with multiple urinary infections.

At the time of evaluation the kidneys were improved compared with their condition as shown by films taken prior to ureterostomy. Cystography showed a small bladder with complete incontinence of instilled contrast medium. Cystoscopy performed with the patient under anesthesia showed a maximum bladder capacity of 30 ml. A small Silastic catheter was introduced through a trocar. Two weeks of attempted hydrostatic stretching of the bladder showed no improvement in bladder size or continence.

At undiversion both ureters had good length. Although the bladder was small, it was not thick-walled. It was suitable for reimplantation of one ureter; the second ureter was drained via transureteroureterostomy. The bladder neck was narrowed as much as possible to provide greater outlet resistance. The bladder was augmented with cecum. This procedure was lengthy but well tolerated.

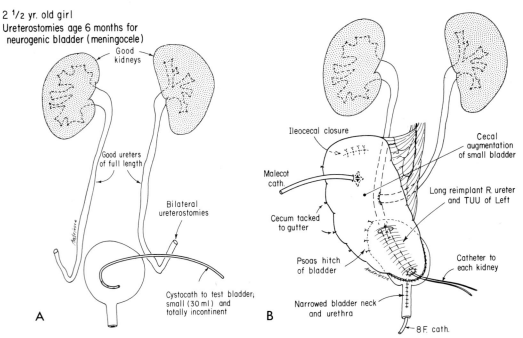

Figure 17-40. Case 3 before *(A)* and after *(B)* reconstruction. (See text.)

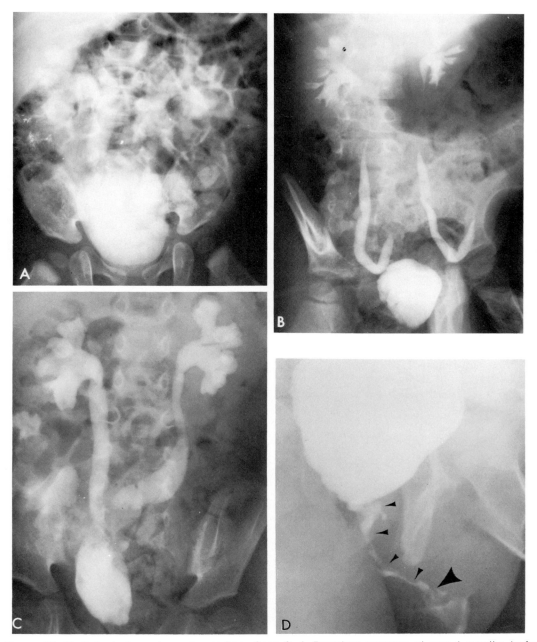

Figure 17–41. Selected roentgenograms from Case 3. *A*, Excretory urogram at age 6 months, before ureterostomy, showing severe hydronephrosis secondary to neurogenic bladder. *B*, Simultaneous cystogram and ureterograms before undiversion. The small bladder did not increase in size with attempted hydrostatic stretching. Freely incontinent. *C*, Excretory urogram 2 weeks after undiversion. Note cecum added to bladder, transureteroureterostomy, and long tunnel implantation of right ureter. The dilatation of upper tracts is due to postoperative edema, which was shown to be resolved on excretroy urogram 3 months postoperatively. *D*, Cystogram to show long, narrow urethra *(small arrows)* that resulted from narrowing of bladder neck and proximal urethra during indiversion, and later lengthening of urethra from below, out to the level of the clitoris *(large arrow)*.

Cystoscopy 2 weeks later showed a bladder volume of 110 ml. Initially the patient was absolutely dry, on a program of intermittent catheterization. This happy state did not continue, however, and she began to be wet despite catheterization every 4 hours.

Urodynamic evaluation 2 months after undiversion showed contractions of the cecum producing pressures of 35 cm of water. There was no significant resistance in the urethra despite the previous narrowing procedure. The bladder could be emptied easily with a good stream by moderate suprapubic pressure. Obviously, greater resistance was needed. Various drugs to inhibit contraction of the bladder and cecal muscle were used, together with therapy to contract urethral muscle, all to no avail. Therefore, 5 months after undiversion, urethral lengthening was done from below (Hendren, 1980a, 1980b). This involved tubularizing the introitus from her urethral opening distal to the clitoris; the neourethra was covered with a buttock flap. Six weeks later the base of the flap was divided, restoring the vaginal introitus to a normal anatomic appearance. Subsequently the patient returned home dry, on intermittent catheterization every 4 hours by her parents.

COMMENT. Review of this child's original films, before diversion, shows why children with myelodysplasia must have close continuing follow-up of their urinary tracts, which can deteriorate rapidly. There was severe hydronephrosis at age 7 months when her ureterostomies were performed. The upper tracts improved dramatically on drainage. Intermittent catherization instituted then might well have produced the same benefit without the need for diversion.

It is a very large responsibility to take down a urinary diversion that is working well in a patient with myelodysplasia in whom a dry state is provided, albeit with a stoma, while also protecting the upper tracts. This is a much more difficult decision than in cases in which function should be normal when restored. It requires having a highly motivated patient who strongly wants undiversion and whose physical state will allow intermittent self-catheterization. This approach is therefore precluded in a retarded patient or one physically unable to perform self-catheterization. This youngster was deemed a suitable candidate despite her age because she is exceptionally intelligent and her parents are highly motivated professionals.

Undiversion from Loop Ureterostomy

Loop ureterostomy has been used widely as a means of temporary diversion of the urinary tract of infants and children with severe obstructive uropathy (Johnston; Leape and Holder; Perlmutter and Patil; Perlmutter and Tank; Sober; Williams and Cromie). It is easily performed and will usually provide immediate improvement in high-grade obstruction with renal failure. It is not intended as a permanent means of diversion. The procedure

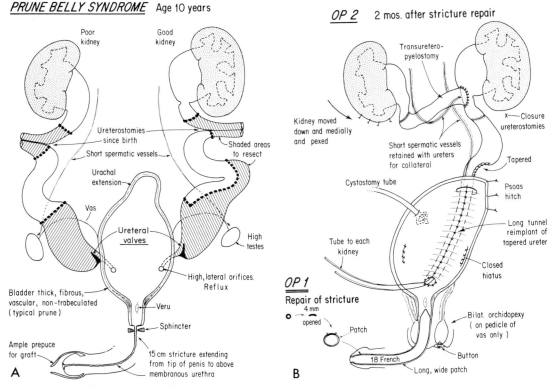

Figure 17–42. Case 4 before (A) and after (B) reconstruction. (See text.)

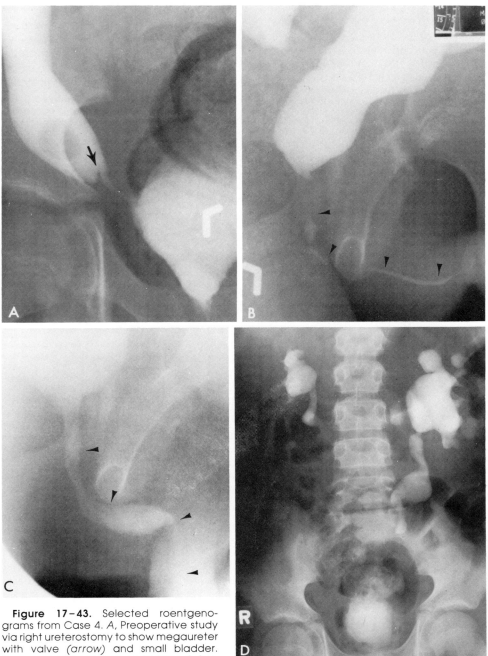

Figure 17–43. Selected roentgenograms from Case 4. *A*, Preoperative study via right ureterostomy to show megaureter with valve *(arrow)* and small bladder. There was also reflux on cystogram. *B*, Preoperative cystogram showing hypoplasia of entire urethra through which the patient could squeeze only a few drops of fluid instilled into the bladder *(arrows)*. *C*, Cystogram after long patch graft to urethra, showing satisfactory caliber of new urethral passage *(arrows)*. *D*, Excretory urogram 2 weeks after reconstructive surgery.

comes at a high price, however, for it greatly complicates the ultimate reconstruction that must be done (Hendren, 1978). All but one of the 30 loop ureterostomy cases in this series were diverted elsewhere. The following two representative cases will illustrate the problem.

Case 4 (Figs. 17–42 and 17–43)

This 10-year-old boy was referred for reconstruction of the urinary tract, which had been diverted at birth via bilateral cutaneous loop ureterostomies. Subsequent evaluation of the urinary tract elsewhere led to the conclusion that reconstruction was probably not feasible because there were such extensive anatomic abnormalities. There was, paradoxically, both obstruction and reflux at both ureterovesical junctions. The ureteral orifices were placed high in this typical prune-belly bladder, and they refluxed. Antegrade filling of the ureters showed a flap valve above each ureterovesical junction, a rare finding. There was an extensive stricture of the urethra extending from just distal to the verumontanum all the way to the meatus.

At the preliminary procedure, a 15-cm patch graft for the urethral stricture was fashioned by cutting the prepuce in a spiral fashion. Later hydrostatic testing of the bladder through a suprapubic cystocath showed satisfactory relief of urethral obstruction. The patient was able to empty the bladder surprisingly well considering that it had been defunctionalized since birth. Therefore, 2 months after stricture repair, reconstruction was performed in August 1982. Both ureterostomies were resected. The left ureter was tapered and reimplanted with a long tunnel. The right ureter was drained via transureteropyelostomy. Both kidneys were moved downward and pexed inferiorly. Both testes were placed in the scrotum by the Fowler-Stephens orchiopexy technique. Fluid replacement during this 13-hour procedure included 9 L of lactated Ringers' solution, 750 ml of normal saline, 500 ml of packed red cells, and 500 ml of albumin solution. Postoperative radiographic evaluation showed satisfactory drainage of the upper tracts; there was no reflux on cystographic examination. Postoperatively the patient was able to void, although the stream was not forceful. Continence was good, but is not yet perfect.

COMMENT. There are several interesting aspects of this case. First was the presence of a long urethral stricture. Obviously, reconstruction would have been of no avail if there had been continuing urethral obstruction. If prepuce had not been available as a long graft, a long strip of bladder mucosa could have been used. Alternatively, a thick (0.020 inch) skin graft from a non–hair-bearing area can be employed. It is uncommon to see reflux and obstruction in the same ureter unless the orifice is ectopic in the bladder neck or the urethra, where it is compressed most of the time but refluxes during micturition.

Some patients with loop ureterostomy have been reconstructed in stages, with the lower ureteral surgery at one operation, closing the ureterostomies in another. I believe, however, that it is better to expose the entire urinary tract simultaneously through a long transabdominal approach in order to repair all pathology in one sitting. There are several reasons for this. First, it often proves best to reimplant one ureter and drain the other by transureteroureterostomy. This would be difficult except with generous operative exposure. Second, when ureters have been tethered upward by ureterostomies, gaining enough length for reimplantation may be impossible without taking down the ureterostomies. Third, reimplanting ureters that are diverted runs a high risk of stricture during "dry reimplant" healing. If a ureter is reimplanted while diverted, a Silastic stent should remain in the lower ureter until the ureterostomy is closed to avert that complication. Simultaneous operation on both ends of a ureter, as done in this case, can be performed safely if all of the periureteral tissue is maintained with the ureter during its mobilization.

It has been stated that ureterostomy will allow a dilated ureter to decompress, so that when reconstruction is done later it will not require tapering. Sometimes that is true, but sometimes it is not. We believe that the additional difficulty of reconstructing a patient with prior loop ureterostomies more than outweighs that possible advantage. Tapering a ureter is not difficult if done with care (Hendren, 1969, 1975a, 1979a).

Case 5 (Figs. 17–44 and 17–45)

This 5-year-old girl was referred in September 1980. She had been born with a cloacal anomaly with high confluence of the bladder, two vaginas, and the colon. More than half of her life had been spent in hospitals. There was a right nephrostomy and left loop ureterostomy. The bladder was badly scarred. Both previously reimplanted ureters were obstructed. A perineal flap had been advanced into the urogenital sinus, which was unfortunate because the urogenital sinus should have been preserved as a urethra.

The initial reconstructive approach in this patient was to make a urethra and widen the introitus to provide entry to the vagina(s). Six months later undiversion was performed. The better ureter was reimplanted into the small, contracted bladder, simultaneously closing the ureterostomy. The right ureter was drained via transureteroureterostomy. The bladder was augmented using a patch of ileum. There was a subsequent complication regarding the newly created urethra when an oversized sound was passed during cystoscopy, creating a urethrovaginal fistula. Another buttocks flap procedure was required to close that fistula. A dressing that was too snug then caused necrosis of the second flap. A third flap procedure succeeded. Since August, 1983, the patient has been without a tube for the first time in her life. She empties her bladder easily every 4 hours by passing a 16 F Walther catheterizing sound. Her mother gives a soapsuds enema every 2 days to evacuate the colon, which keeps her continent of feces.

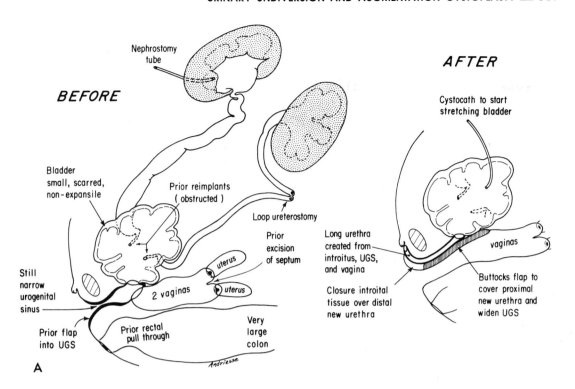

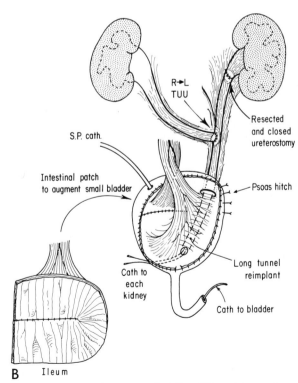

Figure 17–44. Case 5 before and after reconstruction (A) and 6 months postoperatively (B).

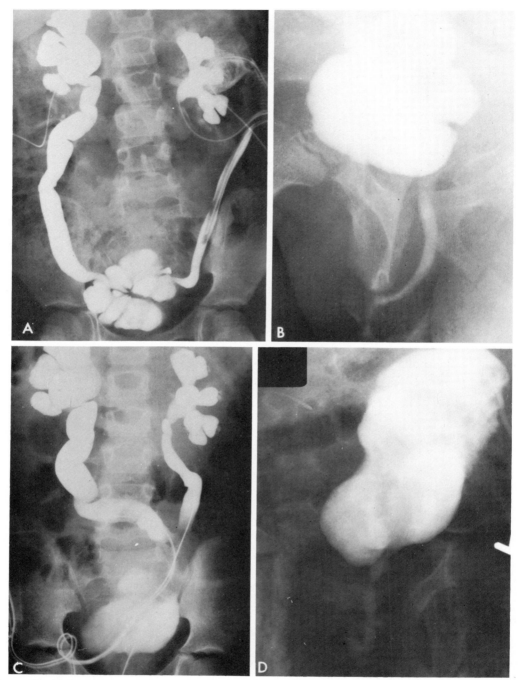

Figure 17–45. Selected roentgenograms from Case 5. *A,* Preoperative study of urinary tract made by filling through the right nephrostomy, and right loop ureterostomy. Both ureters are partially obstructed as they enter the badly scarred, deformed bladder. The bladder had looked normal on original cystograms several years previously. *B,* Cystogram after construction of urethra, before undiversion. *C,* Postoperative "stent study" 12 days after the undiversion, showing closed ureterostomy on the left, and right-to-left transuretero-ureterostomy. Note the long tunnel implant of left ureter into bladder, which has been augmented. *D,* Cystogram 2 weeks following undiversion. Note Malecot catheter *(arrow)* in dome of the bladder, through small bowel patch augmentation.

COMMENT. This case illustrates many important points. First is the need to study the anatomy in patients with cloacal malformations in order to plan an appropriate reconstruction. A perineal flap exteriorization had been attempted initially. This will suffice with low malformations. In a high confluence case, however, the vagina(s) should be separated from the urogenital sinus, and joined to the perineum by one of several possible means. The urogenital sinus should be saved as the urethra. This would have avoided a great deal of subsequent surgery in this child. Additionally, the rectal pull-through had been performed too anteriorly and was partially obstructed. There was an enormous fecal impaction. All of this needed to be revised. In our experience reconstruction in these patients is best done at a single extensive procedure, not doing the colon pull-through on one occasion and the urinary tract reconstruction on another. Details of these operative approaches have been described previously (Hendren, 1977, 1980c, 1982). Some girls with extensive cloacal reconstructions will require intermittent self-catheterization for an extended time after reconstructive surgery; most will eventually learn to empty the bladder spontaneously.

This child's original cystogram showed a normal bladder. Somehow surgery caused remarkable scarring as well as ureteral obstruction. That had been relieved on one side by nephrostomy and on the other by loop ureterostomy. Reconstruction would not have been possible without augmenting what had once been a normal bladder. Small bowel was chosen for patch augmentation in this case because the blood supply of the adjacent sigmoid colon was not normal, since there had been an abdominal perineal pull-through. This patient's undiversion, along with two other cases, is the subject of a motion picture on undiversion (Hendren and Skinner).

Case 6 (Figs. 17-46 and 17-47)

This 16-year-old boy was seen in April 1980 for undiversion. Six previous operations included: (1) transperineal resection of urethral valves at age 5½ years; (2) transurethral resection of urethral valves again at age 6 years; (3) Y-V plasty to the bladder

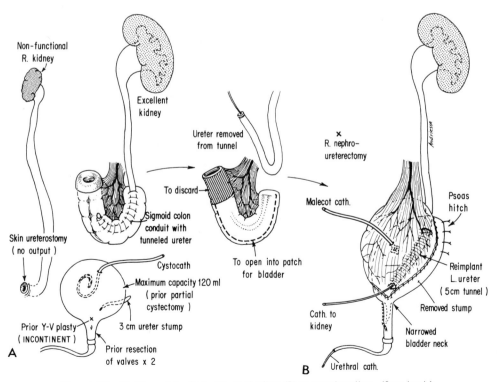

Figure 17–46. Case 6 before *(A)* and after *(B)* reconstruction. (See text.)

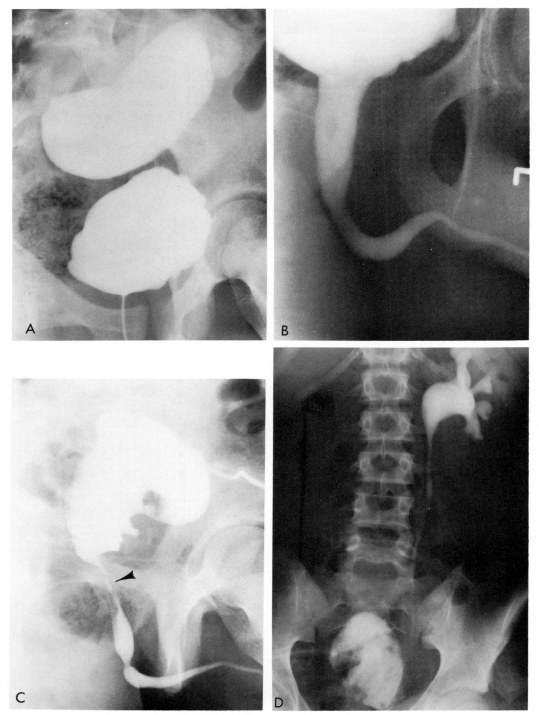

Figure 17–47. Selected roentgenograms from Case 6. *A*, Simultaneous preoperative cystogram and loopogram. Loop and bowel conduit are about the same size. *B*, Preoperative voiding study, showing wide open bladder neck, as a result of previous Y-V plasty. *C*, Cystogram 2 weeks after undiversion, via Malecot catheter in bladder. Note narrowing of bladder neck and proximal urethra to gain continence *(arrow)*. *D*, Excretory urogram 2 weeks after undiversion.

neck at age 7½ years; (4) partial cystectomy at age 9½ years; (5) right end ureterostomy at age 14 years; (6) sigmoid loop diversion of the left kidney at age 14½ years.

A small Silastic catheter was introduced into the bladder using the percutaneous technique to test bladder sensation, continence, and size. The bladder held as much as 150 ml. The patient could empty it voluntarily, but there was some degree of incontinence.

At undiversion the nonfunctioning right kidney was removed. The bladder neck was narrowed to provide greater outlet resistence. Although consideration was given to simply adding the nonrefluxing colon conduit to the small bladder, maintaining the ureterocolic tunnel, ureter length was ample, and so we opted to reimplant the ureter into the bladder, together with a psoas hitch, utilizing the isolated sigmoid loop for augmentation of the bladder. In more than 3 years postoperatively, there have been stable upper tracts, no reflux, good continence, and normal bladder volume.

Although he was instructed to avoid contact sports, the patient enrolled in competitive karate classes. A kick to the bladder ruptured it through the sigmoid patch. This was closed successfully and no further complications have occurred.

COMMENT. Ureterostomy had been performed on the right side in this patient to test renal function. There was none. Today improved radiographic techniques, particularly renal scans, make it possible to predict which renal segments are nonfunctional and best removed. If there is reflux, a radionuclide scan to measure function should be done while the bladder is drained by catheter, so that contrast excreted by one kidney will not reflux from the bladder to a nonfunctional renal segment giving a spurious indication of "function."

This patient had previously undergone a Y-V plasty to the bladder neck. Although that was done widely 10 to 20 years ago, experience has shown that it is seldom indicated. It can create stress incontinence and also retrograde ejaculation in the male. This patient had previously undergone partial cystectomy, but the reason for that was unclear. The sigmoid colon with its blood supply so near to the bladder makes an ideal bowel patch for bladder augmentation. Because there was ample ureteral length, the ureter was reimplanted into the bladder. If it had been too short, or if the bladder had been unsuited for accepting a ureter reimplant, the conduit could have been simply added on to the bladder with its ureterocolic anastomosis intact.

SOME CONCLUSIONS ABOUT UNDIVERSION AND BLADDER AUGMENTATION

Urinary undiversion should be considered for many patients who have undergone diversion in the past. The surgeon must have a broad spectrum of experience, because each case will differ from all others in some respects. This makes considerable judgment necessary in deciding how best to deal with a particular anatomic problem. Reconstructions of this magnitude require meticulous attention to all technical details. It would be catastrophic for a patient to have a serious complication such as a leaking anastomosis or a sloughed ureter. There has been no major immediate postoperative complication of that sort in the 130 cases I have undiverted, although some patients have required later reoperation to stop reflux. One patient died at age 28 years, 11 years after undiversion, from sepsis during hemodialysis. His original creatinine clearance at the time of undiversion had been only 20 per cent of normal.

Many of these patients had poor renal function when they presented for reconstruction. Eight have subsequently undergone transplantation. About 20 more will likely require transplantation when they become older. We have not felt that poor renal function is a contraindication for undiversion, because often several years of normal life has been made possible before transplantation was needed. When transplantation becomes necessary, it is better that the kidney drain into a functional urinary tract than into a urinary diversion. If reconstruction requires incorporation of a bowel segment into the urinary tract, such as cecal augmentation of the bladder, close metabolic surveillance must be maintained, because serum electrolyte exchange occurs across the bowel surface. Hyperchloremic acidosis and hypokalemia can be managed by administration of supplemental sodium bicarbonate and potassium. All of the patients with marginal renal function are followed in collaboration with the nephrology service to best direct dietary and metabolic management.

BIBLIOGRAPHY

Althausen AF, Hagen-Cook K, Hendren WH: Non-refluxing colon conduit: experience with 70 cases. J Urol *120*:35, 1978

Dagen JE, Sanford EJ, Rohner TJ Jr: Complications of the non-refluxing colon conduit. J Urol 123:585, 1980.

Elder DD, Moisey CU, Rees RWM: A long term follow up of the colonic conduit operation in children. Br J Urol 51:462, 1979.

Goodwin WE, Winter CC, Turner RD: Replacement of the ureter by small intestine: Clinical application and results of the "ileal ureter." J Urol 81:406, 1959.

Goodwin WE: Editorial comment. J Urol 129:589, 1983.

Hendren WH: Operative repair of megaureter in children. J Urol 101:491, 1969.

Hendren WH: Posterior urethral valves in boys: a broad clinical spectrum. J Urol 106:298, 1971.

Hendren WH: Reconstruction of previously diverted urinary tracts in children. J Pediatr Surg 8:135, 1973.

Hendren WH: Urinary tract refunctionalization after prior diversion in children. Ann Surg 180:494, 1974.

Hendren WH: Complications of megaureter repair in children. J Urol 113:238, 1975a.

Hendren WH: Non-refluxing colon conduit for temporary or permanent urinary diversion in children. J Pediatr Surg 10:381, 1975b.

Hendren WH: Urethral Valves: Diagnosis and Endoscopic Resection. Catalogue no. 850. Norwich, Conn., Eaton Film Library, 1976a.

Hendren WH: Urinary diversion and undiversion in children. Surg Clin North Am 56:425, 1976b.

Hendren WH: Surgical management of urogenital sinus abnormalities. J Pediatr Surg 12:339, 1977.

Hendren WH: Complications of ureterostomy. J Urol 120:269, 1978.

Hendren WH: Megaureter. In Campbell's Urology. Fourth ed. Edited by JH Harrison, RF Gittes, AD Perlmutter, et al. Philadelphia, WB Saunders Co., 1979a, p 1697.

Hendren, WH: Urinary tract undiversion. In Pediatric Surgery. Third ed. Edited by MM Ravitch, KJ Welch, CD Benson, et al. Chicago, Year Book Medical Publishers, 1979b, p 1275.

Hendren WH: Construction of female urethra from vaginal wall and a perineal flap. J Urol 123:657, 1980a.

Hendren WH: Reconstructive problems of the vagina and the female urethra. Clin Plastic Surg 7:207, 1980b.

Hendren WH: Urogenital sinus and anorectal malformation: experience with 22 cases. J Pediatr Surg 15:628, 1980c.

Hendren WH: Further experience in reconstructive surgery for cloacal anomalies. J Pediatr Surg 17:695, 1982.

Hendren WH: Urinary undiversion. In Urologic Surgery. Edited by JF Glenn. Philadelphia, JB Lippincott Co., 1983.

Hendren WH, Hensle TW: Transureteroureterostomy: experience with 75 cases. J Urol 123:826, 1980.

Hendren WH, McLorie GA: Late stricture of intestinal ureter. J Urol 129:584, 1983.

Hendren WH, Radopoulos D: Complications of ileal loop and colon conduit urinary diversion. Urol Clin North Am 10:451, 1983.

Hendren WH, Skinner DG: Undiversion. A Visit in Urology. Norwich, Conn., Eaton Film Library, 1980.

Hodges CV, Moore RJ, Lehman TH, et al: Clinical experiences with transuretero-ureterostomy. J Urol 90:552, 1963.

Johnston JH: Temporary cutaneous ureterostomy in the management of advanced congenital urinary obstruction. Arch Dis Child 38:161, 1963.

Kogan SJ, Kim K, Levitt SB: Preoperative evaluation of bladder function prior to renal transplantation or urinary tract reconstruction in children: description of a method. J Pediatr Surg 11:1007, 1976.

Leape LL, Holder TM: Temporary tubeless urinary diversion in children. J Pediatr Surg 5:288, 1970.

Middleton AW Jr, Hendren WH: Ileal conduits in children at the Massachusetts General Hospital from 1955 to 1970. J Urol 115:591, 1976.

Perlmutter AD, Patil J: Loop cutaneous ureterostomy in infants and young children: late results in 32 cases. J Urol 107:655, 1972.

Perlmutter AD, Tank ES: Loop cutaneous ureterostomy in infancy. J Urol 99:559, 1968.

Pitts WR Jr, Muecke EC: A 20-year experience with ileal conduits: the fate of the kidneys. J Urol 122:154, 1979.

Retik AB, Perlmutter AD, Gross RE: Cutaneous uretero-ileostomy in children. N Engl J Med 177:217, 1967.

Richie JP, Skinner DG: Urinary diversion: the physiological rationale for non-refluxing colonic conduits. Br J Urol 47:269, 1975.

Richie JP, Skinner DG, Waisman J: The effect of reflux on the development of pyelonephritis in urinary diversion: an experimental study. J Surg Res 16:256, 1974.

Schwarz GR, Jeffs RD: Ileal conduit urinary diversion in children: computer analysis of follow-up from 2 to 16 years. J Urol 114:285, 1975.

Shapiro SR, Lebowitz R, Colodny AH: Fate of 90 children with ileal conduit urinary diversion a decade later: analysis of complications, pyelography, renal function and bacteriology. J Urol 114:289, 1975.

Sharpe NW: Trans-uretero-ureteral anastomosis. Ann Surg 44:687, 1906.

Skinner DG, Goodwin WE: Indications for the use of intestinal segments in management of nephrocalcinosis. J Urol 113:436, 1975.

Skinner DG, Gottesman JE, Richie JP: The isolated sigmoid segment: its value in temporary urinary diversion and reconstruction. J Urol 113:614, 1975.

Smith ED: Follow up studies on 150 ileal conduits in children. J Pediatr Surg 7:1, 1972.

Sober I: Pelviureterostomy-en-Y. J Urol 107:473, 1972.

Williams DI, Cromie WJ: Ring ureterostomy. Br J Urol 47:789, 1975.

Zinman L, Libertino JA: Ileocecal conduit for temporary and permanent diversion. J Urol 113:317, 1975.

Index

Page numbers in *italics* indicate illustrations.
Page numbers followed by (t) indicate tables.

i